Sleep Medicine

Sleep Medicine: Essentials and Review

Teofilo Lee-Chiong Jr

Medical Director, Sleep Center
National Jewish Medical and Research Center
Associate Professor of Medicine
University of Colorado Health Sciences Center
Denver, Colorado

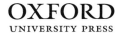

OXFORD
UNIVERSITY PRESS

2008

OXFORD
UNIVERSITY PRESS

Oxford University Press, Inc., publishes works that further
Oxford University's objective of excellence
in research, scholarship, and education.

Oxford New York
Auckland   Cape Town   Dar es Salaam   Hong Kong   Karachi
Kuala Lumpur   Madrid   Melbourne   Mexico City   Nairobi
New Delhi   Shanghai   Taipei   Toronto

With offices in
Argentina   Austria   Brazil   Chile   Czech Republic   France   Greece
Guatemala   Hungary   Italy   Japan   Poland   Portugal   Singapore
South Korea   Switzerland   Thailand   Turkey   Ukraine   Vietnam

Published by Oxford University Press, Inc.
198 Madison Avenue, New York, New York 10016
www.oup.com

Library of Congress Cataloging-in-Publication Data
Lee-Chiong, Teofilo L., 1960-
Sleep medicine : essentials and review / by Teofilo Lee-Chiong Jr.
p. ; cm.
Includes bibliographical references.
ISBN 978-0-19-530659-0
1.   Sleep disorders. 2.   Sleep--Physiological aspects. I. Title.
[DNLM: 1.   Sleep Disorders. 2.   Sleep--physiology. WM 188 L477s 2007]
RC547.L44 2007
616.8'498--dc22
2007019539

9 8 7 6 5 4 3 2 1

Printed in the United States of America

on acid-free paper

Preface

This book does not contain *everything* about Sleep Medicine—you do not need *all* that information to practice excellent clinical sleep medicine (or to pass the Sleep Medicine Examination). What it does include is enough know-how about Sleep Medicine to care for your patients with sleep disorders (and pass its Board).

Painstaking research had been undertaken to ensure the accuracy and timeliness of the data in this book. Nonetheless, the disciplines of sleep and dreaming are constantly evolving. Each day, new discoveries prompt us to redefine old concepts and formulate new ones—these will be incorporated in future editions of this book.

Remember, the Board is not the culmination of your Sleep Medicine career; rather, it is its beginning. Strive to learn something new each day.

I wish to dedicate this book to my wife, *Dolores Grace Zamudio*, and my daughter, *Zoë Lee-Chiong*, whose unwavering spirit, good humor and *joie de vivre* have found their way into many pages of this book.

T. Lee-Chiong, MD

Contents

Sleep Medicine: Essentials and Review

Basic Science of Sleep　1

Sleep is a complex rapidly reversible neurologic state that is actively generated by different neuronal systems using several neurotransmitters; it is regulated by homeostatic, circadian, and ultradian influences.

History of Sleep Medicine

Table 1–1 presents the chronology of sleep medicine.

Table 1-1. **Chronology of sleep medicine**	Date	Events
	1818	John Cheyne and John Stokes described Cheyne-Stokes respiration
	1880	Gelineau described the clinical features constituting narcolepsy
	1907	Legendre and Pieron induced sleep in dogs by administering serum obtained from sleepy dogs
	1920	Kleitman reported that sleep deprivation resulted in increased sleepiness
	1928	Discovery of electroencephalography by Berger
	1930	Berger first described beta waves
	1936	Harvey and Loomis proposed classifying sleep electroencephalography as stages A,B,C,D and E
	1939	Publication of Nathaniel Kleitman's book *Sleep and Wakefulness*
	1944	First description of delta and theta waves by Walter and Dovey
	1945	Karl Ekbom described restless legs syndrome
	1949	Discovery of reticular formation by Moruzzi and Magoun
	1953	Discovery of REM sleep by Aserinski and Kleitman
	1960	Sleep onset REM periods (SOREMPs) in narcolepsy described by Vogel
	1965	Clinical description of obstructive sleep apnea by Gastault, Tasinari, Duron, Jung, and Kuhlo
	1968	Publication of Rechtschaffen and Kales' *Manual of Standardized Terminology, Techniques and Scoring System for Sleep Stages of Human Subjects*
	1970	Dement established first clinical sleep laboratory at Stanford
	1975	Creation of American Sleep Disorders Association
	1977	Publication of Carskadon's Multiple Sleep Latency Test
	1978	First actigraphy device described by Krupke
	1981	First report on uvulopalatopharyngoplasty by Fujita
	1981	Sullivan described continuous positive airway pressure therapy of obstructive sleep apnea

Table 1-1.	Date	Events
Chronology of sleep medicine—cont'd	1982	Mittler introduced the Maintenance of Wakefulness Test
	1982	First oral device described by Samuelson
	1986	Schenck reported on features of REM sleep behavior disorder
	1991	Publication of Epworth Sleepiness Scale by Johns
	1992	Guilleminault described upper airway resistance syndrome
	1999	Description of link of hypocretin (orexin) and narcolepsy

REM = Rapid eye movement.

Behavioral Definition of Sleep

Human existence could be divided, based on behavioral and physiologic criteria, into three distinct states: namely wakefulness, non–rapid eye movement (NREM) sleep, and rapid eye movement (REM) sleep.

Wakefulness is a state in which the person is aware of and responds to sensory input from the environment. Sleep can be defined as a state of behavioral quiescence accompanied by an elevated arousal threshold and a species-specific sleep posture. Behavior characteristic of human sleep includes a typical recumbent sleep posture, closed eyes, and decrease in or absence of movements (Box 1–1).

Box 1-1.	
Behavioral characteristics of sleep	• Absence or marked reduction of movement
	• Diminished responsiveness to external stimuli (easy reversibility)
	• Recumbent body position
	• Closed eyes
	• Slow and regular respiratory pattern

Function of Sleep

A comprehensive theory explaining the function of sleep remains elusive. Sleep is believed to be important for facilitation of anabolic processes (restorative theory), regulation of body temperature, immune defense, energy conservation, survival adaptation (protective behavior), removal of "toxins" generated during wakefulness, and promotion of neuronal synaptic plasticity and integrity (eg, brain development, restoration, learning, and memory), and facilitation of overall neuronal function.

However, current theories fail to incorporate the various aspects of sleep, including the function of sleep across the lifespan of the individual (ontogeny of sleep), in the course of development of the species (evolution of sleep), and in the diversity of the animal kingdom (phylogeny of sleep), as well as its unique characteristics compared to the state of rest (eg, loss of consciousness, homeostatic drive, and differing sleep stages of NREM and REM sleep). The functions of sleep are summarized in Box 1–2.

Box 1-2. **Proposed functions of sleep**	• Regulation of somatic growth (growth hormone release during NREM stages 3 and 4 sleep) • Neural growth and processing • Memory consolidation (REM sleep) • Thermoregulation • Energy conservation

NREM=non-rapid eye movement; REM = rapid eye movement.

Normal Sleep Requirements

There is great individual variability as well as age-related differences in the total duration of sleep required each day. Most adults sleep between 6 to 9 hours (average of 8 hours) nightly. Sleep duration less than 5 to 6 hours per day is commonly associated with symptoms of sleep deprivation.

Regulation of Sleep and Wakefulness

Two basic intrinsic components, namely circadian rhythm (process C) and sleep homeostasis (process S), interact to regulate the timing and consolidation of sleep and waking (Borbely's model). Sleep homeostasis is dependent on the sleep-wake cycle, whereas circadian rhythms are independent of it.

Sleep homeostasis is characterized by an increase in sleep pressure following sleep deprivation that is related to the duration of prior wakefulness (ie, a person is sleepier the longer one is awake), followed by a decline in sleep need as sleep accumulates. The increase in sleep that occurs after sleep deprivation or sleep fragmentation is referred to as "sleep rebound." Electroencephalographic (EEG) slow-wave activity is often used as a marker for process S.

Circadian process promotes wakefulness during the day. There are two circadian peaks in wakefulness (wake-maintenance zones): one occurring near the maximum core temperature about 8 hours before the minimum core body temperature [CTmin] (early evening) and a second peak about 4 to 8 hours after CTmin (late morning). Sleep propensity is least during these peaks of circadian rhythms of arousal (early evening, about 2 to 3 hours before bedtime, and late morning). Optimal sleep occurs when the desired sleep time coincides with the circadian timing of greatest sleep propensity during periods of circadian troughs in arousal (overnight between 3:00 and 5:00 AM; early-mid afternoon between 3:00 and 5:00 PM). Thus, there are two peaks in sleep propensity: a primary peak occurring near CTmin (early morning), and a secondary peak about 9 hours after CTmin (early-mid afternoon).

Sleep latency and subsequent sleep duration and quality are influenced by both sleep deprivation and circadian factors.

A third component, sleep inertia (process W), refers to the short-lived reduction of alertness that occurs immediately following awakening from sleep and disappears within 2 to 4 hours. This postsleep effect is stronger following awakenings from NREM stages 3 and 4 sleep or after sleep of more prolonged duration.

Finally, the timing of sleep is determined by behavioral influences, such as volitional attempts to stay up later at night due to social activities, as well as autonomic nervous system tone (ie, decrease in sympathetic activation and increase in parasympathetic discharge is required for sleep).

Sleep in Animals

Mammals have cycling of NREM (quiet) and REM (paradoxical) sleep. Sleep spindles and delta waves can be seen during NREM sleep. Mammalian REM sleep is defined by low-amplitude, mixed-frequency EEG; muscle atonia; and rapid eye movements. Among mammals, unihemispheric sleep (EEG showing wakefulness in one hemisphere and sleep on the opposite hemisphere) can be seen in dolphins, eared seals, and manatees.

Although sleep spindles are present in primates, they are absent in birds. Avian sleep is characterized by the absence of spindles during NREM sleep, and brief REM sleep periods. Unihemispheric sleep has also been described among birds.

Among the many early animal brain transection studies of sleep, the experiments conducted by Frederick Bremmer are particularly noteworthy. He described two different brain sections, namely *encephale isole* and *cerveau isole*, that produced EEGs demonstrating alternating waking and sleeping states, or only sleeping state, respectively. For characteristics of sections of the cat brain, See Table 1–2.

Table 1–2. Two different cat brain sections (Frederick Bremmer)

Brain section	Electrical rhythms
Encephale isole	Transection at C1 vertebral level in the lower part of the medulla between the brain and spinal cord EEG demonstrates alternating wake and sleep states
Cerveau isole	Transection at the midcollicular level caudal to the origin of the oculomotor nerves in the midbrain, that disrupts the projections of the brainstem ascending reticular activating system EEG demonstrates sleep state

EEG = electroencephalography.

Human Sleep

Sleep architecture is a term used to describe the division of sleep among the different sleep stages using specific EEG, electro-oculographic (EOG), and chin electromyographic (EMG) criteria. It also involves the relationship of the individual sleep stages to each other.

Sleep can be differentiated into NREM sleep and REM sleep. NREM sleep can be further subdivided into stages 1, 2, 3, and 4 sleep (Box 1–3). NREM stages 3 and 4 sleep are often collectively referred to as *slow wave* or *delta wave* sleep.

Table 1–3. Percentages of sleep stages in healthy adults

Sleep stage	Percentage of total sleep time
Stage 1	2–5%
Stage 2	45–55%
Stage 3/4	5–20%
Stage REM	20–25%

A sleep cycle refers to the period from NREM stages 1 to 4 to REM sleep. There are commonly three to five NREM-REM sleep cycles, each occurring every 90 to 120 minutes in adults (every 60 minutes in infants and young children) during the night. Each sleep stage is not necessarily present in every sleep cycle. The percentage of NREM stages 3 and 4 sleep is greater during the initial part of sleep, whereas REM sleep is relatively more common during the latter part of sleep. REM density (frequency of rapid eye movements during REM sleep) also increases during the latter portion of the night. Whereas NREM stages 3 and 4 sleep is related to the length of prior wakefulness and to sleep onset, REM sleep is related to circadian rhythms of body temperature. The percentages spent by adults in the different sleep stages is presented in Table 1–3.

Arousal threshold is lowest during NREM stage 1 sleep (easiest to awaken) and highest during NREM stages 3 and 4 sleep (most difficult to awaken).

Box 1–3.

Sleep stages

STAGE WAKE

Electroencephalography

Low-voltage, high-frequency activity when a person is alert and eyes are open
Lower frequency activity when a person is relaxed
Prominent alpha (8–13 Hz) activity, > 50% of the epoch, when a person is drowsy and eyes are closed

Electro-oculography

Blinking or rapid eye movements when a person is awake and alert
Slow rolling eye movements when a person is drowsy and eyes are closed

Electromyography

High chin muscle activity (ie, high chin EMG amplitude)

Associated features

EEG and EOG tracings may demonstrate muscle artifacts when the person is tense
Alpha activity is generally more prominent in the occipital leads compared to central leads
Recording occipital leads can facilitate the recognition of alpha waves as well as the timing of sleep onset
Eye opening suppresses alpha activity

STAGE 1 SLEEP

Electroencephalography

Low-voltage, mixed-frequency activity
Prominent theta activity; beta rhythms may be present
Alpha activity occupies < 50% of the epoch
Vertex sharp waves (high-amplitude, brief, negative deflections) may be present (more prominent in central leads)
Absence of sleep spindles or K-complexes

Electro-oculography

Occasional slow rolling eye movements
No rapid eye movements

(continued from page 6)
Box 1–3.

Sleep stages

Electromyography

High chin muscle activity (ie, high chin EMG amplitude) that is less than or equal to that during wakefulness

Associated features

Person is unresponsive but easily aroused
Occurs at sleep onset or following arousals from sleep
Accounts for about 2% to 5% of total sleep time in an adult
Transitions into stage 2 sleep within a few minutes

STAGE 2 SLEEP

Electroencephalography

Low-voltage, mixed-frequency activity
Presence of sleep spindles and K complexes (generally maximal over the vertex)
Delta activity occupies < 20% of the epoch

Electro-oculography

No movements

Electromyography

Low chin muscle activity

Associated features

Accounts for the greatest proportion (45% to 55%) of total sleep time in adults

Three-minute stage 2 sleep scoring rule: Sleep spindles and K complexes are episodic and may not be present in every epoch. An epoch is scored as stage 2 sleep if the intervening period between sleep spindles or K complexes is less than 3 minutes, would otherwise meet criteria for stage 1 sleep (low-amplitude, mixed-frequency EEG), and is not associated with an arousal. An epoch is scored as stage 1 sleep if the intervening period is equal to or greater than 3 minutes.

STAGE 3 SLEEP

Electroencephalography

Delta activity occupies between 20% and 50% of the epoch
Sleep spindles may be present

Electro-oculography

No movements

Electromyography

Low chin muscle activity (generally less than that in stages 1 and 2 sleep)

Associated features

Accounts for about 10% of total sleep time in an adult
Along with NREM stage 4 sleep, has the highest arousal threshold by external stimuli among the different sleep stages

(continued from page 7)
Box 1–3.

Sleep stages

Certain parasomnias (disorders of arousal such as sleep terrors or sleepwalking) occur during NREM stages 3 and 4 sleep

Amount of NREM stages 3 and 4, and EEG amplitude of delta waves are increased among adolescents and reduced in older adults

More prominent during the first half of sleep

STAGE 4 SLEEP

Electroencephalography

Delta activity occupies > 50% of the epoch
Sleep spindles may be present

Electro-oculography

No movements

Electromyography

Low chin muscle activity (generally less than that in stages 1 and 2 sleep)

Associated features

Accounts for about 10% of total sleep time in an adult
Along with NREM stage 3 sleep, has the highest arousal threshold by external stimuli among the different sleep stages
Certain parasomnias (disorders of arousal such as sleep terrors or sleepwalking) occur during stages 3 and 4 sleep
Amount of NREM stages 3 and 4, and EEG amplitude of delta waves are increased among adolescents and reduced in older adults
More prominent during the first half of sleep

REM SLEEP

REM sleep is composed of two components, namely, tonic (without rapid eye movements) and phasic (with rapid eye movements) sleep.

Electroencephalography

Low-voltage, mixed-frequency activity (theta and beta rhythms)
Saw-tooth waves may be present (more prominent over the vertex and frontal leads)
Alpha waves are 1 to 2 Hz slower than those occurring during wakefulness and NREM stage 1 sleep
Vertex sharp waves are not prominent

Electro-oculography

No movements (tonic REM sleep)
Bursts of conjugate (out-of-phase) rapid eye movements (phasic REM sleep)

Electromyography

Amplitude of chin EMG is reduced or absent (ie, at least equal to or, more commonly, lower than the lowest amplitude during NREM sleep)
Loss of postural muscle tone due to postsynaptic hyperpolarization of the spinal motoneurons
May have "bursts" of chin EMG activity during phasic REM sleep

(continued from page 8)

Box 1–3.

Sleep stages

Associated features

Accounts for about 25% of total sleep time in an adult

Often three to five periods of REM sleep occur during the night, with progressively greater REM sleep during the latter part of sleep

REM and NREM stages cycle every 90 to 120 minutes throughout the night in an adult

High arousal threshold by external stimuli

Generalized skeletal muscle atonia or hypotonia (with sparing of the diaphragm, extraocular muscles, and sphincter muscles)

Increase in middle ear muscle activity (phasic REM sleep)

Presence of periorbital integrated potentials

Occurrence of penile tumescence among men and vaginal vascular engorgement and clitoral erection in women

Dreaming is more frequent and more complex compared to NREM sleep

Increase in sympathetic activation (phasic REM sleep)

Irregular respiratory pattern with decrease in tidal volume accompanying rapid eye movements

Decrease in hypoxic and hypercapnic ventilatory responses

Decrease in activity of the upper airway dilator muscles

Variable heart rate and blood pressure

Increase in brain metabolism and temperature

Certain parasomnias (REM sleep behavior disorder and nightmares) occur during stage REM sleep

REM sleep rebound refers to an increase in duration of REM sleep above baseline, often accompanied by greater REM density, during recovery following selective REM sleep deprivation

Ponto-geniculo-occipital waves during REM sleep in the cat

Note: REM sleep rule. EEG, EOG, and EMG do not necessarily change simultaneously at the start or end of REM periods. Any epoch contiguous with stage REM sleep with an EEG showing a relatively low-amplitude, mixed-frequency activity is scored as REM sleep if the EMG shows atonia or hypotonia and if no intervening arousals occur, whether or not rapid eye movements are observed.

If an arousal occurs at the transition between NREM and REM sleep, the epochs prior to the arousal with REM-like EEG and EMG are considered stage REM sleep unless the arousal occurred less than three minutes after a sleep spindle or K complex in which case the epoch is scored as NREM stage 2 sleep.

EEG = electroencephalography; EOG = electro-oculography; EMG = electromyography.

Normal Adult Sleep

Normal sleep in an adult is characterized by short sleep latency (95%), and few and relatively brief awakenings. Sleep is typically entered into through NREM sleep. NREM sleep predominates in the first half of the night, whereas REM sleep percentage is greatest during the second half of the night. REM sleep occurs in three to five episodes during the night that alternates with NREM sleep every 90 to 120 minutes.

Changes in sleep architecture in the older adult include a decrease in total sleep time, increase in frequency of arousals, reduced sleep efficiency, and decrease in percentage of both NREM stages 3 and 4 sleep and REM sleep.

Chemical Neuroanatomy of Sleep and Wakefulness

Specific neural systems located in specific areas of the brain that contain specific neurotransmitters generate and maintain the states of wakefulness, NREM sleep, and REM sleep (Table 1–4). These systems are generally redundant, and destruction of any particular system is unlikely to completely abolish sleep or wakefulness.

Table 1–4. Neuroanatomy of sleep and wakefulness

State	Neural systems	Neurotransmitters
Wakefulness	Brainstem reticular formation (RF) (medullary, oral pontine, and midbrain) Caudal diencephalon (posterior hypothalamus, subthalamus, and ventral thalamus) Intralaminar thalamic nuclei Dorsolateral tegmental and pedunculopontine nuclei Locus ceruleus Dorsal raphe Ventral tegmental area Basal forebrain Rostral basal forebrain Note: RF has two major ascending projections into the forebrain: 1. Dorsal pathway → thalamus → cerebral cortex (thalamocortical system) 2. Ventral pathway → subthalamus and posterior hypothalamus → basal forebrain and septum → cerebral cortex Neurons of the locus ceruleus, midbrain reticular formation, thalamus and lateral hypothalamus, and basal forebrain have a tonic high rate of discharge during wakefulness. The ascending reticular activating system also receives input from visceral, somatic, and special sensory systems. Specific neural systems: 1. Locus ceruleus in the dorsal pontine tegmentum *Neurotransmitter*: noradrenaline *Neural projections*: cerebral cortex, subcortical areas, brainstem, and spinal cord *Discharge rates*: increase during waking; decrease during NREM sleep stages 3 and 4 and absent during REM sleep *Effect of stimulation*: cortical activation *Effect of lesions*: no reduction in waking or cortical activation 2. Substantia nigra and ventral tegmental area *Neurotransmitter*: dopamine *Neural projections*: frontal cortex and basal ganglia	Acetylcholine Dopamine Glutamate Histamine Hypocretin (orexin) Norepinephrine Serotonin Peptides that are important in enhancing the effect of these neurotransmitters include adrenocorticotropic hormone, corticotropin-releasing factor, neurotensin, substance P, thyroid-stimulating hormone, thyrotropin-releasing factor, and vasoactive intestinal peptide.

Table 1–4. Neuroanatomy of sleep and wakefulness—cont'd

State	Neural systems	Neurotransmitters
	3. Tuberomammillary nucleus in the posterior hypothalamus *Neurotransmitter:* histamine *Neural projections:* forebrain *Discharge rates:* increase during waking and absent during REM sleep *Effect of lesions:* decrease in arousal without a decrease in waking amount 4. Perifornical neurons in Lateral hypothalamus *Neurotransmitter:* orexin or hypocretin *Neural projections:* cerebral cortex *Effect of lesions:* narcolepsy in animals with orexin gene deletion no change in total amount of waking with destruction of neurons 5. Brainstem tegmentum (laterodorsal and pedunculopontine tegmental nuclei) *Neurotransmitter:* acetylcholine *Neural projections:* thalamus, posterior hypothalamus and basal forebrain *Discharge rates:* increase during both waking and REM sleep 6. Basal forebrain (substantia innominata and diagonal band of Broca and septum) *Neurotransmitter:* acetylcholine *Neural projections:* cerebral cortex and hippocampus *Discharge rates:* increase during both waking and REM sleep 7. Dorsal raphe *Neurotransmitter:* serotonin Note: Lesions of the central midbrain tegmentum produce cortical inactivation without affecting behavioral responsiveness to sensory stimulation, whereas lesions of the ventral tegmentum produce behavioral somnolence and unresponsiveness without loss of cortical activation.	
NREM sleep	Forebrain (anterior hypothalamus-preoptic region, including ventrolateral preoptic area [VLPO] and basal forebrain) Solitary tract nuclei Midbrain raphe Orbitofrontal cortex Amygdala Anterior and dorsomedial thalamic nuclei Reticular nucleus of the thalamus (generates spindles) Note: Activity of acetylcholine- and hypocretin-containing cells is lowest or absent during NREM sleep.	The main NREM neurotransmitters are serotonin and gamma-aminobutyric acid (GABA). Other neurotransmitters include adenosine, norepinephrine, and peptides (alpha melanocyte-stimulating hormone, cholecystokinin, cortistatin, growth hormone–releasing hormone, interleukins, muramyl peptides, opiates, and somatostatin).

Continued

Table 1-4.   Neuroanatomy of sleep and wakefulness—cont'd

State	Neural systems	Neurotransmitters
REM sleep	Pons (pedunculopontine tegmental nuclei and the laterodorsal tegmental nuclei) Brainstem reticular formation, especially oral pontine reticular formation Other brainstem (lower medullary) and spinal cord neurons Note: REM sleep is associated with activation of "REM-on" cholinergic neurons and inhibition of "REM-off" noradrenergic neurons (locus ceruleus), serotonergic neurons (dorsal raphe) and histaminergic neurons (posterior hypothalamus). In animal models, ponto-geniculo-occipital (PGO) waves are generated by the mesopontine neurons, accompanied by activation of the lateral geniculate and occipital cortex (P = pons, G = geniculate, O = occipital). Muscle atonia or hypotonia is a result of inhibitory postsynaptic potentials originating from the pons, projecting to the alpha and gamma motor neurons of the anterior horn cells of the spinal cord via the medullary magnocellular nucleus and lateral reticulospinal tract.	The main REM sleep neurotransmitter is acetylcholine. Other neurotransmitters include GABA and glycine. Note: Muscle atonia results from inhibition of motor neurons *Note:* Cholinergic agonists (physostigmine) decrease REM sleep latency. Serotonin inhibits PGO wave generation.

a Main transmitters.
NREM = non-rapid eye movement; REM = rapid eye movement.

Neurotransmitters Associated With Sleep-Wake Regulation

Wakefulness, NREM sleep, and REM sleep are each generated and maintained by specific neural networks utilizing different neurotransmitters, neuropeptides, immunomodulators and hormones (Table 1–5). Other chemicals, including enkephalins, growth hormone (GH), prolactin, and vasoactive intestinal peptide, also regulate sleep and wakefulness.

Table 1-5.   Neurotransmitters involved in sleep-wake regulation

Neurotransmitter	Role
Acetylcholine	*Location of neurons*: Basal forebrain and laterodorsal tegmentum/pedunculopontine tegmentum (LDT/PPT) *Neurotransmitter release*: Increase during wake and REM sleep; decrease during NREM sleep

Table 1–5.   Neurotransmitters involved in sleep-wake regulation—cont'd

Neurotransmitter	Role
	Characteristics: Acetylcholine causes cortical EEG desynchronization during wakefulness and REM sleep (role in REM sleep regulation via muscarinic (M2/M3) cholinergic receptors in the pontine reticular formation). REM abnormalities in narcolepsy may be related to hypersensitivity of cholinergic systems.
Adenosine	*Location of neurons:* Basal forebrain *Neurotransmitter release:* Occurs during sleep deprivation *Characteristics:* Levels of adenosine increase during prolonged wakefulness and decrease during sleep recovery. The methylxanthines, including caffeine and theophylline, are psychostimulants that block the action of adenosine.
Dopamine	*Location of neurons:* Ventral mesencephalic tegmentum and substantia nigra *Neurotransmitter release:* Occurs during both wake and REM sleep; increased by amphetamines and related compounds *Characteristics:* D2/D3 dopamine receptor agonists cause sedation. A decrease in arousal follows lesions of dopamine neurons.
Gamma-amino-butyric acid (GABA)	*Location of neurons:* Ventrolateral preoptic area, thalamus, hypothalamus, basal forebrain, cerebral cortex *Neurotransmitter release:* Sleep *Characteristics:* GABA is the main CNS inhibitory neurotransmitter. Alcohol, barbiturates, benzodiazepines, and nonbenzodiazepine benzodiazepine receptor agonists (eg, zolpidem) act on the GABA-A receptor, whereas sodium oxybate acts on the GABA-B receptor.
Glutamate	*Characteristics:* Glutamic acid is the main excitatory CNS neurotransmitter.
Glycine	*Neurotransmitter release:* Occurs during REM sleep *Characteristics:* Glycine is the main inhibitory neurotransmitter in the spinal cord and causes REM sleep-related paralysis via hyperpolarization of spinal motoneurons.
Histamine	*Location of neurons:* Tuberomammillary nucleus of the posterior hypothalamus *Neurotransmitter release:* Occurs during wakefulness *Characteristics:* Histamine H-1 receptor blockers increase sleepiness.
Hypocretin 1 and 2 (orexin)	*Location of neurons:* Perifornical region of lateral hypothalamus *Neurotransmitter release:* Occurs during wakefulness

Continued

Table 1–5. Neurotransmitters involved in sleep-wake regulation—cont'd

Neurotransmitter	Role
	Characteristics: Hypocretin acts on other CNS centers related to sleep-wake regulation, including the dorsal raphe, locus ceruleus, tuberomammillary nuclei, and spinal cord. Hypocretin system dysfunction is associated with narcolepsy-cataplexy.
Immunomodulators	*Neurotransmitter release:* NREM sleep *Characteristics:* A variety of immunomodulators promote NREM sleep, including interleukin-1 and -6, tumor necrosis factor alpha (TNFα), prostaglandin D2, arginine vasotocin, cholecystokinins, cortistatin, C-reactive protein, delta sleep-inducing peptides, growth hormone-releasing factors, muramyl peptides, somatostatin, and vasoactive intestinal peptide.
Melatonin	*Location of neurons:* Pineal gland *Neurotransmitter release:* Occurs during the night *Characteristics:* Melatonin receptors are present in the suprachiasmatic nuclei and hypothalamus.
Norepinephrine	*Location of neurons:* Locus ceruleus *Neurotransmitter release:* Occurs during wake, decreases during NREM sleep, and is absent during REM sleep *Characteristics:* Norepinephrine is involved with maintenance of wakefulness.
Serotonin	*Location of neurons:* Raphe nuclei, thalamus *Neurotransmitter release:* Highest during wake, decreased during NREM sleep, and lowest during REM sleep *Characteristics:* Agents that inhibit serotonin reduce REM sleep.

CNS = central nervous system, EEG = electroencephalography; GABA = gamma-aminobutyric acid; NREM = non-rapid eye movement; REM = rapid eye movement.

Autonomic Nervous System

The autonomic nervous system consists of two components: sympathetic nervous system and parasympathetic nervous system (Table 1–6). Homeostasis is maintained by precise interactions between these two components.

Table 1–6. Anatomic features of the automatic nervous system

Component	Anatomic features
Sympathetic nervous system	Originates in the thoracolumbar portion of the spinal cord
Parasympathetic nervous system	Originates in the brainstem and sacral portion of the spinal cord

There is an overall reduction in sympathetic activity and increase in parasympathetic activity during the transition from wakefulness to NREM sleep. There is a further increase in parasympathetic activity and reduction in sympathetic activity during REM sleep (except for the transient increases in sympathetic tone during phasic REM).

Respiratory Physiology During Sleep

The principal function of the respiratory system is the maintenance of adequate ventilation and gas exchange in order to achieve optimal levels of acid-base levels (pH), arterial carbon dioxide ($PaCO_2$), and arterial oxygen (PaO_2). Breathing is an automatic behavior generated by a network of respiratory neurons, which are active during the inspiratory, postinspiratory or late-expiratory phases, or which spans different phases of respiration (Table 1–7). Receptors involved with the metabolic control of respiration include peripheral carotid body chemoreceptors (pH, PaO_2, and $PaCO_2$), central nervous system (CNS) chemoreceptors (acidity and CO_2), lung mechanoreceptors (lung volume), and hypothalamus (thermal receptors). Respiratory neurons are described in Table 1–8.

Table 1–7. Three phases of the respiratory cycle

Respiratory neurons	Respiratory cycle
Inspiratory	Active inhalation
Post-inspiratory	Passive exhalation
Late-expiratory	Active exhalation

Respiration During the Different Sleep Stages

Wakefulness, NREM sleep, and REM sleep are associated with characteristic patterns of respiration, with state-dependent changes in respiratory rate, tidal volume, and minute ventilation. Respiration is controlled by two systems: metabolic (ie, pH, PaO_2, and $PaCO_2$) and behavioral. Both systems are operational during wakefulness, whereas only the metabolic system operates during NREM sleep, as described in Table 1–9.

Hypoxic and hypercapnic ventilatory responses decrease during sleep compared with wakefulness, with a greater reduction seen during REM sleep than during NREM sleep. PaO_2 may decrease by 2 to 12 mm Hg, and $PaCO_2$ may increase by 2 to 8 mm Hg during sleep compared with levels during wakefulness. SaO_2 may fall by about 2% during sleep.

Upper airway muscle tone is diminished during sleep secondary to decreased respiratory neuron excitatory activity to pharyngeal motor neurons. This decreases airway diameter and

Table 1–8. Respiratory neurons

Neuron group	Definiton
Ventrolateral reticular formation	Location: Dorsal brainstem and upper spinal cord Actions: Pre-Botzinger neurons (maintenance of respiratory rhythm) Botzinger complex (late expiratory and phase-spanning neurons) Ventral respiratory group (rostral inspiratory and caudal expiratory neurons) Upper cervical group (inspiratory neurons)

Continued

Table 1-8. Respiratory neurons—cont'd

Neuron group	Definiton
Dorsal respiratory group	Location: Dorsal medulla (ventrolateral section of solitary tract nucleus) Action: Primarily inspiratory neurons
Pontine respiratory group	Location: Parabrachial region of the dorsolateral pons Action: Not essential for generation of basic respiratory rhythm Note: Lesions cause apneustic breathing
Nucleus ambiguus	Location: Parallel to the ventrolateral respiratory group Action: Modulates respiration by its action on laryngeal and pharyngeal muscles

Table 1-9. Respiration during wakefulness and sleep

Wakefulness	NREM sleep	REM sleep
Pattern of breathing is controlled by metabolic processes (involuntary respiration) and influenced by nonrespiratory processes such as phonation and deglutition (voluntary respiration).	Due to the loss of the wake-related stimulus for breathing and the absence of nonrespiratory factors affecting respiration, breathing becomes regular in amplitude and frequency. Respiration is under the sole control of centrally driven processes. Periodic breathing, with hypopnea and hyperpnea, can occur at sleep onset and may persist until NREM stage 2 sleep. NREM stages 3 and 4 sleep is associated with: 1. Stable and regular pattern of respiration 2. Decrease or no change in respiratory rate 3. Decrease in tidal volume and functional residual capacity 4. Reduction in minute ventilation (relative hypoventilation) 5. Increase in $PaCO_2$ 6. Decrease in PaO_2 7. Decrease in inspiratory airflow and increase in upper airway resistance 8. Diminished activity of the accessory muscles of respiration (intercostals muscles) and dilator muscles of the nose, pharynx, and larynx	REM sleep is associated with: 1. Variable and irregular pattern of respiration 2. Variability in respiratory rate 3. Variability in tidal volumes 4. Central apneas or periodic breathing (especially during phasic REM sleep) 5. Diminished activity of the motor neurons (eg, hypoglossal nerve innervating the pharyngeal dilator muscle genioglossus) leading to muscle atonia during REM sleep 6. Atonia or hypotonia of the intercostal muscles 7. Intact activity of the phrenic motor neurons innervating the diaphragm 8. Increase in $PaCO_2$ 9. Decrease in PaO_2 10. Decrease in functional residual capacity

NREM = non-rapid eye movement; REM = rapid eye movement.

increases its vulnerability to collapse. Sleep also blunts the ventilatory response to added inspiratory resistance.

In addition, there are gender differences in respiratory control. The hypoxic ventilatory response may be similar during both wakefulness and NREM sleep among women (ie, there is a greater fall in hypoxic drive in men than in women from wakefulness to sleep).

Excitatory (serotonin and catecholamine) respiratory neurons have greater activity during wakefulness compared to NREM sleep and REM sleep, with least activity during REM sleep.

The Upper Airway as a Collapsible Cylinder

The upper airway can be conceptualized as a collapsible cylinder, with air flow within its lumen being driven by changes between upstream (nasal) pressure and downstream pressure, as well as by airway resistance. Airflow is greater with higher upstream nasal pressure and lower airway resistance, and vice versa. Upper airway patency is influenced by several factors, including its collapsibility, length, and caliber, and pressure gradient against its wall.

Intraluminal extrathoracic airway pressure decreases during inspiration, leading to a narrowing of the airway. Narrowing of the airway initially accelerates airflow, which further promotes airway narrowing (Bernoulli effect). The critical closing pressure (P_{crit}) is the intraluminal pressure at which the upper airway collapses and airflow ceases. P_{crit} is progressively less negative as one goes from nonsnorers, to snorers, to persons with predominantly hypopnea, and, finally, to those with apnea whose P_{crit} is generally near atmospheric pressure.

Activation of upper airway dilator muscles decreases P_{crit} (reduces airway collapsibility) and increases airflow. The activity of the upper airway dilator muscles is diminished by sleep, alcohol ingestion, and the use of muscle relaxants. In addition, during wakefulness, reflex upper airway dilator muscle activation is triggered by negative subatmospheric intraluminal pressure. This reflex is diminished as sleep progresses from NREM to REM sleep. Furthermore, upper airway dilator response to hypoxia and hypercapnia is suppressed during NREM sleep and may be completely abolished during REM sleep. Finally, activity of the genioglossus muscle is inhibited by increases in blood pressure that accompanies obstructive respiratory events and the subsequent arousals that follow them.

In summary, upper airway patency depends on activation of upper airway dilator muscles that is sufficient to counteract the forces promoting airway closure and properly synchronized to specific segments of the respiratory cycle (ie, activation of upper airway muscles preceding activation of the diaphragm). The muscles of the upper airway are named in Table 1–10.

Table 1–10. Upper airway dilator muscles

Anatomic region	Muscle(s)
Nose	Alai nasi
Palate	Levator veli palatini, palatoglossus, tensor veli palatini
Oropharynx	Genioglossus, geniohyoid, sternohyoid, sternothyroid
Larynx	Cricothyroid, posterior cricoarytenoid

Upper Airway Function in Obstructive Sleep Apnea and Snoring

Compared to control subjects, individuals with obstructive sleep apnea (OSA) often have anatomically narrower retropalatal (behind the palate) and retroglossal (behind the tongue) airspaces that narrows further during sleep. The causes of upper airway narrowing in OSA are listed in Box 1–4. Increase in activity of upper airway dilators (eg, genioglossus) is often present during wakefulness to compensate for the narrower airways. This compensatory dilator muscle activity is abolished during sleep.

Autonomic Nervous System and Sleep Apnea

Sympathetic neural activity, during both sleep and wakefulness, is increased in persons with OSA. This may be responsible, in part, to the greater risk of cardiovascular events observed in this patient group. A number of mechanisms may account for this elevated sympathetic activity, including repetitive arousals, hypoxemia, and hypercapnia occurring during sleep. Effective positive airway pressure therapy of OSA reduces this elevation in sympathetic neural tone. The increase in blood pressure associated with OSA may also result from sodium retention due to activation of the renin-angiotensin system.

Box 1–4. **Causes of upper airway narrowing in obstructive sleep apnea**	• Adenoidal and tonsillar hypertrophy • Macroglossia • Micrognathia or retrognathia • Pharyngeal fat deposits • Reduction in lung volume • Supine position-related effect of gravity on the tongue and mandible

Nocturnal Asthma

Stimulation of the sympathetic nervous system (adrenergic beta-2 receptors) produces bronchodilation, whereas greater parasympathetic neural activity leads to bronchoconstriction and increased mucus production. The nocturnal decrease in sympathetic activity and enhanced parasympathetic tone can give rise to worsening of lung function and asthma symptoms in the early morning hours.

Cardiovascular Physiology During Sleep

Activation of the parasympathetic nervous system leads to decreased cardiac contractility and heart rate. In contrast, sympathetic nervous stimulation generally produces vasoconstriction (alpha-1 receptors), vasodilatation (beta-2 receptors), tachycardia, and increased cardiac contractility.

Both heart rate and systolic blood pressure decrease at night. Nighttime systolic blood pressure is often about 10% less than that during the daytime ("dipping" phenomenon). This is believed to be secondary to circadian rhythm–related nocturnal reductions in catecholamine levels. In addition, there are sleep stage–dependent changes in autonomic neural tone, with a decrease in sympathetic output during NREM sleep. Autonomic activity during REM sleep is more complicated, with fluctuating parasympathetic and sympathetic tone during tonic and phasic REM sleep.

Enhanced sympathetic activity accompanies awakenings and results in increases in heart rate, peripheral vascular resistance and blood pressure. Autonomic nervous system changes related to the cardiovascular system are described in Table 1–11.

Table 1-11.   The autonomic nervous system and the cardiovascular system

Sleep state	Features
NREM sleep	Compared to wakefulness: ↓ Sympathetic tone ↑ Parasympathetic tone Decrease in heart rate and blood pressure
REM sleep	Compared to NREM sleep: ↑ Sympathetic tone (phasic REM sleep) Higher mean heart rate and blood pressure Note: During tonic REM sleep, increase in parasympathetic tone can give rise to relative bradycardia and periods of asystole
Arousals and awakenings	Compared to NREM and REM sleep: ↑ Sympathetic tone Increase in heart rate and blood pressure

NREM = non-rapid eye movement; REM = rapid eye movement.

The prevalence of ischemic cardiac events, including angina, myocardial infarction, and cardiac arrest, peak in the morning hours between 6:00 and 11:00 AM and are lowest during sleep. Nonetheless, the risk of cardiovascular events in persons with ischemic cardiac disease may increase during both REM sleep (due to coronary vasospasm) and NREM sleep (due to relative hypotension and bradycardia). Cardiovascular features of sleep are summarized in Table 1–12.

Gastrointestinal Physiology During Sleep

Swallowing, salivary production, and esophageal motility decrease during sleep. All of these changes delay esophageal acid clearance and prolong mucosal acid contact in patients with gastroesophageal reflux.

Basal gastric acid secretion displays a circadian rhythmicity, with a peak secretion between 10:00 PM and 2:00 AM (as a result of increased parasympathetic activity) and a nadir in the morning between 5:00 and 11:00 AM. Gastric acid secretion increases during sleep in patients with peptic ulcer disease, with no difference in secretion between NREM sleep and REM sleep.

Intestinal motility (ie, migrating motor complex) has the lowest velocity during sleep.

Table 1-12.   Cardiovascular features of sleep

Feature	NREM sleep (compared to wakefulness)	Tonic REM sleep (compared to NREM sleep)	Phasic REM sleep (compared to NREM and tonic REM sleep)
Heart rate	Decrease	Decrease	Increase
Stroke volume	Minimal change	Minimal change	Minimal change
Peripheral vascular resistance	Minimal change or slight decrease	Decrease	Increase

Continued

Table 1–12. Cardiovascular features of sleep—cont'd

Feature	NREM sleep (compared to wakefulness)	Tonic REM sleep (compared to NREM sleep)	Phasic REM sleep (compared to NREM and tonic REM sleep)
Cardiac output	Decrease	Decrease	Increase
Systemic blood pressure	Decrease	Decrease	Increase
Coronary circulation	Decrease	Increase	Increase
Cerebral circulation	Decrease Intact autoregulation; under metabolic control	Increased to certain brain areas (eg, hypothalamus and brainstem[1]) Intact autoregulation; under metabolic control	Increased to certain brain areas (eg, hypothalamus and brainstem[1]) Intact autoregulation; under metabolic control
Renal circulation	Unchanged	Unchanged or slight increase	Unchanged or slight increase
Splanchnic circulation	Unchanged	Unchanged or slight increase	Unchanged or slight increase
Cutaneous circulation	Increase (due to vasodilatation)	Variable (dependent on ambient temperature)	Variable (dependent on ambient temperature)
Skeletal circulation	Unchanged	Unchanged or slight decrease	Unchanged or slight decrease

[1] *Increased cerebral blood flow during REM sleep is seen in the amygdala, anterior cingulate, dorsal mesencephalon, pontine tegmentum, and thalamus. NREM = non-rapid eye movement; REM = rapid eye movement.*

Renal Physiology During Sleep

Urine volume decreases during sleep due to an increase in water reabsorption, decrease in glomerular filtration, and increase in release of renin. Vasodilation of the renal vessels occurs during REM sleep as a result of a decrease in sympathetic activity.

Genitourinary Physiology During Sleep

Due to increased parasympathetic activity, REM sleep is associated with penile tumescence in men and clitoral tumescence and vaginal engorgement in women.

Endocrine Physiology During Sleep

Oscillations in hormone levels occur throughout the 24-hour day related to circadian rhythm-related and sleep-related changes in secretions of hormones.

Growth Hormone

Biosynthesis and secretion of GH by the anterior pituitary gland is stimulated by growth hormone–releasing hormone (GHRH) and inhibited by somatostatin. GH is involved with protein anabolism and tissue growth. Release of GH is linked to sleep, occurring among adults during NREM stages 3 and 4 sleep. However, GH secretion can also occur without NREM stages 3 and 4 sleep. Sleep disturbance leading to decreases in NREM stages 3 and 4 sleep can diminish GH release.

In young healthy adults, the daily peak in GH secretion occurs near the onset of sleep, often associated with the first period of NREM stages 3 and 4 sleep. GH secretion is lower during the second half of the sleep period. In some patients, sleep deprivation may suppress GH secretion. Unlike men in whom there is one peak in secretion of GH at sleep onset, there may be several peaks in GH secretion in women throughout the day and night. With aging, GH secretion declines, paralleling the decrease in NREM stages 3 and 4 sleep.

GHRH promotes sleep in men (in women GHRH may inhibit sleep), and increases NREM stages 3 and 4 sleep. Somatostatin, by antagonizing GHRH, inhibits sleep. Administration of octreotide, a somatostatin analogue, reduces NREM stages 3 and 4 sleep. On the other hand, gamma hydroxybutyrate and ritanserin increase NREM stages 3 and 4 sleep, and may increase GH secretion.

Prolactin

Levels of prolactin, an anterior pituitary hormone, increase shortly following the onset of sleep, with peak levels occurring during the second half of the evening prior to awakening. Prolactin secretion increases during NREM stages 3 and 4 sleep and decreases during REM sleep. Prolactin secretion is suppressed by sleep fragmentation. Prolactin secretion is also influenced by circadian rhythms, with lower hormone levels at noon and higher levels in the evening in awake individuals. Like GH, prolactin secretion declines with aging, paralleling the decrease in NREM stages 3 and 4 sleep. Administration of benzodiazepines can increase prolactin secretion during sleep.

Corticotropin-Releasing Hormone, Adrenocorticotropic Hormone, and Cortisol

Release of corticotropin-releasing hormone (CRH) from the hypothalamus stimulates the secretion of adrenocorticotropic hormone (ACTH) by the anterior pituitary, which, in turn increases cortisol release from the adrenal cortex in a pulsatile fashion. Secretion of cortisol appears to be linked to circadian rhythm rather than to sleep. Levels increase in the early morning, peak at midmorning (ie, 8:00 AM), and decline to the nadir in the evening. Sleep is associated with a modest decline in cortisol secretion. The nadir of cortisol levels occurs following the onset of sleep. Cortisol is then released in pulses starting in the early morning (ie, between 2:00 and 4:00 AM) until final awakening. Sleep fragmentation and awakenings give rise to increased secretion of cortisol.

CRH increases vigilance and inhibits sleep. Administration of CRH, ACTH, or cortisol decreases REM sleep. CRH decreases NREM stages 3 and 4 sleep, whereas cortisol enhances NREM stages 3 and 4 sleep.

Thyroid-Stimulating Hormone and Thyroid Hormone

Thyroid stimulating hormone (TSH) levels are lowest during the daytime, increase progressively during the night, reaching their peak prior to sleep onset, and they decline thereafter.

Sleep, particularly NREM stages 3 and 4 sleep, inhibits the secretion of TSH. Levels of TSH increase with awakenings and during sleep deprivation. Thus, TSH secretion appears to be linked to both circadian rhythms and sleep.

Thyroid hormone levels are high during the daytime and low at night.

Parathyroid Hormone

Levels of parathyroid hormone increase during sleep.

Luteinizing Hormone

Among pubescent children, there is a sleep-related increase in levels of luteinizing hormone (LH). LH secretion occurs mainly during NREM sleep. In adult men, increase in secretion of LH continues to be related to sleep. In contrast, sleep does not appear to have a prominent effect on LH secretion in adult women, in whom LH secretion may even decline during sleep, particularly during the follicular phase of the menstrual cycle.

Testosterone

Levels of testosterone in adult men increase at night during sleep.

Renin

Plasma levels of renin increase during NREM sleep and decrease during REM sleep.

Antidiuretic Hormone

Although antidiuretic hormone secretion increases during the night, secretion is not related to sleep.

Aldosterone

Levels of aldosterone increase in the early morning prior to awakening.

Melatonin

Synthesis and secretion of melatonin is suppressed by light exposure. Minimal melatonin is secreted in infants younger than 3 months of age; levels increase gradually and peak at 1 to 3 years of age, and they decline thereafter. Levels of melatonin rise in the evening, peak in the early morning (between 3:00 and 5:00 AM), and then decline. This pattern persists even if no sleep occurs during the night. Evening melatonin secretion is decreased among older adults with insomnia.

Insulin

Blood levels of glucose and insulin may decline during sleep. Insulin resistance may develop, and levels of insulin may decrease during sleep deprivation.

Leptin

Leptin, a product of the obese (*ob*) gene, is involved with the regulation of energy balance by reducing the intake of food. It is released from peripheral adipocytes, with highest serum levels between 12:00 PM to 4:00 AM.

Ghrelin

Ghrelin, like leptin, also regulates energy balance. Serum levels increase at night. Ghrelin promotes NREM sleep.

Neuropeptide γ

Neuropeptide γ (NPγ) antagonizes CRH. NPγ promotes sleep (ie, decrease in sleep latency and increase in NREM stage 2 sleep).

Sleep and Endocrinology

Some changes in hormone secretion during the night are presented in Table 1–13. Other sleep-related endocrine activity associated with diseases is described in Table 1–14.

Table 1–13.   Hormone secretion during the night

During the first half of the night	During the second half of the night
↑ Growth hormone	↓ Growth hormone
↓ Cortisol	↑ Cortisol
↓ Adrenocorticotropic hormone (ACTH)	↑ Adrenocorticotropic hormone (ACTH)

Aging and the Endocrine System

Except for prolactin, most hormones have reduced amplitudes with aging. GHRH activity and GH secretion decrease in parallel with the reduction of NREM stages 3 and 4 sleep. Other hormones that are reduced during aging include testosterone (among males) and melatonin.

Table 1–14.   Changes of sleep-endocrine activity related to diseases

Disorder	Sleep features	Endocrine features
Cushing disease	↑ Sleep latency ↑ Wake time after sleep onset ↓ NREM stages 3 and 4 sleep	↑ Levels of cortisol
Growth hormone deficiency	↓ NREM stages 3 and 4 sleep	↓ Levels of growth hormone (GH)
Acromegaly	↓ NREM stages 3 and 4 sleep ↓ REM sleep	↑ Levels of GH

Continued

Table 1–14.   Changes of sleep-endocrine activity related to diseases—cont'd

Disorder	Sleep features	Endocrine features
Hyperprolactinoma	↑ NREM stages 3 and 4 sleep	↑ Levels of prolactin
Brain injury	↓ NREM stage 2 sleep	↓ Levels of GH
Blindness (with no light perception)	Free-running sleep-wake rhythms	Free-running cortisol and melatonin rhythms
Depression	↑ Wake time after sleep onset ↓ NREM stages 3 and 4 sleep ↓ REM sleep latency ↑ REM density	↑ Cortisol ↑ ACTH ↓ GH ↑ Leptin (nocturnal) ↓ Testosterone (males)
Insomnia (primary)	↑ Sleep latency ↓ Total sleep time ↑ Wake time after sleep onset	↑ Cortisol ↑ ACTH
Jet lag	↑ Sleep latency ↓ Total sleep time ↑ Wake time after sleep onset	Initial sleep-wake and cortisol rhythm dissociation GH adapts more rapidly than cortisol to new environmental time
Shift work	↑ Sleep latency ↓ Total sleep time ↑ Wake time after sleep onset	↓ Cortisol during nighttime work ↑ Cortisol during daytime sleep ↓ Thyroid-stimulating hormone during daytime sleep

ACTH = adrenocorticotropic hormone. NREM = non-rapid eye movement; REM = rapid eye movement.

Immune Function and Sleep

Acute infectious and inflammatory processes can give rise to sleepiness, mediated, in part, via CNS cytokines, particularly interleukin-1 and tumor necrosis factor-alpha (Table 1–15). Sleep deprivation can impair antibody response to vaccination, and alter specific immune parameters (Box 1–5).

Temperature Regulation

Sleep is affected by changes in body and environmental temperatures. Sleep, in turn, affects body temperature.

Table 1–15.   Cytokines and their effects on sleep

Sleep enhancement	Sleep inhibition
Fibroblast growth factor Interleukins IL-1, IL-2, IL-6, IL-8, IL-15, and IL-18 Nerve growth factor Tumor necrosis factor (TNF) α	Insulin-like growth factor Interleukins IL-4, IL-10, and IL-13

Box 1–5.	• Increase in interleukin-1, interferon, and tumor necrosis factor
Effect of sleep deprivation on immune parameters	• Changes in numbers of T lymphocytes and natural killer cells
	• Changes in lymphocyte mitogenesis and phagocytosis
	• Changes in circulating immunoglobulins and immune complexes

Sleep propensity and quality are influenced by both environmental and body temperatures. There is a tight coupling of body temperature and sleep-wake circadian rhythms, both of which are regulated by the suprachiasmatic nucleus of the hypothalamus.

Neurons involved with thermoregulation and sleep regulation are related anatomically. Thermoregulation is controlled by the preoptic and anterior hypothalamus. Receiving afferents from thermal receptors located in the skin, these cold- or warmth-sensing neurons reduce or increase heat production or loss to maintain thermal homeostasis. Activity of cold-sensing neurons is decreased during sleep and increased during wakefulness. In contrast, warmth-sensing neurons are more active during sleep onset, when they inhibit ascending activating pathways.

Core body temperature peaks in the late afternoon and early evening from 6:00 to 8:00 PM and falls at the onset of sleep. This is due to a number of factors, including:

• Greater heat loss mediated by sweating and peripheral vasodilatation

• Less heat generation secondary to a decrease in both metabolism and wake-related muscle activity

• Decrease in thermoregulation with a readjustment of the thermal set point to a lower level. The responsiveness to thermal challenges declines during NREM sleep, and diminishes further during REM sleep. Sweating and shivering are still present during NREM sleep. Heat production with shivering is absent during REM sleep because of the associated muscle atonia.

Among healthy adults, minimum core body temperature occurs at about 4:00 to 5:00 AM, or nearly 2 hours prior to usual wake time. Exposure to bright lights before the nadir of body temperature gives rise to a phase delay of the circadian rhythm. Conversely, a phase advance of the circadian rhythm is produced by exposure to light after the minimum body temperature.

The onset of the major sleep period typically occurs during the declining phase of the temperature rhythm, with acceleration in the rate of fall in body temperature, following a temperature peak. The degree of heat loss at sleep onset also influences the quantity of sleep that follows.

Table 1–16 presents the sleep changes that occur based on temperature at sleep onset. Sleep onset and NREM stages 3 and 4 sleep are enhanced by mild increases in body temperature

Table 1–16. Changes in sleep architecture based on temperature at sleep onset

Body temperature	Sleep characteristics
Initiating sleep during the falling phase of the temperature rhythm (increase heat loss and decrease heat production)	↓ Sleep latency ↑ Total sleep time ↑ NREM stages 3 and 4 sleep
Initiating sleep during the rising phase of the temperature rhythm (decrease heat loss and increase heat production)	↑ Sleep latency ↓ Total sleep time ↓ NREM stages 3 and 4 sleep ↑ REM sleep

NREM = non-rapid eye movement; REM = rapid eye movement.

(eg, exposure to warm environment) 1 to 2 hours prior to bedtime, whereas moderate to severe alterations in ambient temperature (either excessively warm or cold) suppress sleep. Furthermore, sleep is disrupted by extremes of environmental temperature. Awakening occurs during the rising phase of the temperature rhythm following the temperature nadir.

Changes in thermoregulation are present in certain sleep disorders such as insomnia and sleep disturbance related to mood disorders (Table 1–17).

Table 1-17. Sleep disorders and thermoregulation

Sleep disorder	Changes in thermoregulation
Insomnia	Phase delay in temperature rhythm leads to sleep initiation occurring closer to the body temperature peak
Mood disorders	Reduced amplitude of the temperature rhythm

Metabolism and Sleep

Among humans, metabolic rate is decreased during NREM sleep compared to wakefulness. Metabolic rates during REM sleep are either similar or higher than that during NREM sleep.

Musculoskeletal Physiology and Sleep

Sleep is associated with skeletal muscle relaxation (hypotonia or atonia) and inhibition of deep tendon reflexes. There is a reduction in sympathetic activity during NREM sleep that increases during REM sleep. Vasoconstriction of the skeletal muscle vasculature develops during REM sleep due to this increase in sympathetic activity.

Pupillary Changes during Sleep

Constriction of the pupils secondary to parasympathetic stimulation occurs during NREM and tonic REM sleep. Dilation of the pupils due to parasympathetic inhibition is present during phasic REM sleep.

Cognitive Function

For many individuals, short-term memory is greatest in the morning.

Dreaming

Dreams can occur during both REM (accounting for 80% of dreams) and NREM (20% of dreams) sleep. Compared to REM sleep-related dreams that tend to be more complex and irrational, NREM dreams are generally simpler and more realistic. Dreams are thought to be associated with processing and consolidation of memory, and activation and stimulation of CNS neural networks. Theories of dreaming include the *cognitive hypothesis* (dreaming is an extension of awake thought that is governed by different processes) and the *activation synthesis hypothesis* (dreaming is produced by cortical interpretation of randomly generated intrinsic subcortical activity).

Sleep Deprivation

Sleep Deprivation in Animals

In animal models of sleep deprivation, one or more of the following have been described:

1. *Increase in homeostatic sleep drive* with sleep rebound (eg, increase in behavioral quiescence, slow wave sleep and paradoxical sleep) following periods of sleep deprivation

2. *Changes in metabolism* with decrease in anabolic hormones, weight loss despite high amounts of food intake, and an increase in metabolic rate

3. *Neuroendocrine abnormalities* (increase in plasma norepinephrine levels)

4. *Impaired response to infectious agents*

5. *Skin lesions*, including hyperkeratosis and ulcerations

6. *Increase in heart rate*

7. *Decrease in body temperature* and failure of thermoregulation

8. *Death* with prolonged sleep deprivation.

Table 1–18. Classification of sleep deprivation

Type	Description
Acute and total	One or several nights of complete lack of sleep
Acute and partial	One or several nights of inadequate sleep
Chronic and partial (sleep restriction)	At least a week of inadequate sleep
Sleep fragmentation	Reduced total sleep time secondary to repeated awakenings

Table 1–19. Etiology of sleep deprivation among humans

Etiologic category	Specific causes
Primary sleep disorders	Insomnia Restless legs syndrome, periodic limb movement disorder Sleep-related breathing disorders
Medical disorders	Asthma, chronic obstructive pulmonary disease Coronary syndromes Endocrine disorders Fibromyalgia and chronic pain syndromes Gastroesophageal reflux disease, peptic ulcer disease Infectious disorders (HIV infection, Lyme disease) Renal disorders
Neurologic disorders	Dementia Parkinson disease

Continued

Table 1-19.   Etiology of sleep deprivation among humans—cont'd

Etiologic category	Specific causes
Psychiatric disorders	Anxiety disorder
	Mood disorder
	Schizophrenia
	Substance use disorder
Medication and substance use	Caffeine
	Cardiac medications
	Corticosteroids
	Nasal decongestants
	Nicotine
	Opiates
	Theophylline

Sleep Deprivation in Humans

Sleep deprivation may be voluntary or involuntary, and can be related to absent or decreased sleep, or abnormal sleep consolidation (ie, sleep disruption). The classification and etiology of sleep deprivation are presented in Tables 1–18 and 1–19, respectively.

Consequences of Sleep Deprivation

The most important consequence of sleep deprivation is *excessive sleepiness*. Sleep deprivation can also affect general health, and alter mood, cognition, performance, cerebral function, cardiovascular disorders, endocrine function, metabolism, immunity, inflammation, and safety (Table 1–20).

There is significant inter-individual vulnerability to sleep deprivation, with some individuals demonstrating more adverse neurocognitive effects to sleep loss than others. For instance, compared with the elderly, younger individuals appear to be more susceptible to the effects of total sleep deprivation with greater negative impact on alertness and cognitive performance. However, this variability among individuals becomes less prominent as the duration of sleep deprivation increases. The adverse physiologic, neurocognitive, and behavioral consequences of acute total sleep deprivation differ from that generally observed with chronic partial sleep deprivation (sleep restriction).

Table 1-20.   Consequences of sleep deprivation

Consequence	Specific result
Sleepiness	Sleep deprivation is associated with increases in homeostatic sleep drive and propensity to fall asleep (eg, napping and sleep attacks). Microsleeps, or brief lapses into sleep, can occur during wakefulness due to heightened sleep pressure. Decrease in sleep latency may be observed during polysomnography, Multiple Sleep Latency Test and Maintenance of Wakefulness Test. Greater sleep deprivation produces shorter sleep latencies. Polysomnography also demonstrates an increase in slow wave activity and NREM stages 3 and 4 sleep, and decrease in NREM stages 1 and 2 sleep. REM sleep may also increase (usually during the second recovery night after NREM stages 3 and 4 have normalized). Wake time after sleep onset is reduced. There is a decrease in alpha activity, and increase in delta and theta activity.

Table 1–20. Consequences of sleep deprivation—cont'd

Consequence	Specific result
	Hyperactivity may paradoxically develop in children. In selective sleep deprivation, rebound of the specific sleep stage that is reduced occurs during recovery sleep. EEG during wakefulness may show an increase in the slower theta and delta rhythms. Greater frequency of slow eye movements while awake has been described.
General health	Sleep deprivation is associated with an increase in morbidity and mortality. Excess mortality has been observed in persons sleeping either less than 6.5 hours or more than 8 hours each day. The mechanisms responsible for the association between duration of sleep and elevated mortality are unknown.
Mood	Sleep deprivation has a negative impact on mood. Among adolescents, it can give rise to irritability, nervousness, and impulsiveness. Interestingly remission of major depressive episodes has been described following sleep deprivation.
Cognition and performance	Sleep deprivation results in diminished attention, alertness, vigilance, vigor, cognition, concentration, learning, memory, psychomotor performance, executive function, reaction time, and motivation. There is an increase in fatigue, confusion and errors of both omission and commission.
Neurologic function	Total sleep deprivation is associated with a fall in cerebral glucose metabolism. Ptosis, nystagmus, slurring of speech, hyperactive gag reflexes, and tremors may develop. Corneal reflexes are sluggish. Deep tendon reflexes may become hyperactive. Pain sensitivity increases.
Cardiovascular disorders	An increase in cardiovascular morbidity has been described in sleep-deprived individuals.
Endocrine function and metabolism	Sleep deprivation can produce an increase in sympathetic activation, evening levels of cortisol, and levels of ghrelin. Sleep deprivation blunts the sleep-dependent secretion of growth hormone and prolactin. Decreases in glucose tolerance (insulin resistance) may develop. Levels of thyroxine and leptin may decrease. Low leptin and increased ghrelin stimulate appetite and may lead to weight gain and obesity. Metabolic rate increases. Hypothermia may occur.
Immunity and inflammation	Sleep deprivation has been reported to decrease febrile response to endotoxin, and antibody titers to influenza vaccination. It can also alter levels of cytokines, interleukin-6 and tumor necrosis factor-alpha, and leukocytes, and affect activity of natural killer cells. Finally, there is a decrease in granulocytes and lymphocytes in response to antigens.
Safety issues	Sleep deprivation is associated with an increase in risk of motor vehicle accidents.

EEG = electroencephalography; NREM = non-rapid eye movement. REM = rapid eye movement.

References

General References

American Academy of Sleep Medicine. *The International Classification of Sleep Disorders: Diagnostic and Coding Manual.* 2nd ed. Westchester, IL: American Academy of Sleep Medicine, 2005.

Bowman TJ. *Review of Sleep Medicine.* Burlington, MA: Butterworth-Heinemann, 2002.

Berry RB. *Sleep Medicine Pearls.* 2nd ed. Philadelphia, PA: Hanley & Belfus, 2002.

Chokroverty S. *Clinical Companion to Sleep Disorders Medicine.* 2nd ed. Butterworth-Heinemann, 2000.

Hirshkowitz M. Normal human sleep: an overview. In: *Sleep Disorders.* Medical Clinics of North America. Philadelphia, PA: Elsevier Saunders, 2004.

Lavie P, Pillar G, Malhotra A. *Sleep Disorders Handbook.* New York, NY: Taylor & Francis, 2002.

Lee-Chiong TL, (ed. *Sleep: A Comprehensive Handbook.* Hoboken, NJ: John Wiley & Sons, 2006.

Lee-Chiong TL, Sateia M, Carskadon M, eds. *Sleep Medicine.* Philadelphia, PA: Hanley & Belfus (Elsevier), 2002.

Perlis ML, Lichstein KL, eds. *Treating Sleep Disorders: Principles and Practice of Behavioral Sleep Medicine.* Hoboken, NJ: John Wiley & Sons, 2003.

Rechtschaffen A, Kales A. *A Manual of Standardized Terminology, Techniques and Scoring System for Sleep Stages of Human Subjects.* Los Angeles, CA: University of California, Brain Information Service/Brain Research Institute, 1968.

Reite M, Ruddy J, Nagel K. *Concise Guide to Evaluation and Management of Sleep Disorders.* 3rd ed. Arlington, VA: American Psychiatric Publishing, April 2002.

Sleep Disorders. Medical Clinics of North America. Elsevier Saunders. 2004.

Sleep Medicine. Primary Care: Clinics in Office Practice. Philadelphia, PA: Elsevier Saunders, 2005.

Sleep Research Society. *SRS Basics of Sleep Guide.* Westchester, IL: Sleep Research Society, 2005.

History of Sleep Medicine

Bowman TJ. *Review of Sleep Medicine.* Burlington, MA: Butterworth-Heinemann, 2002.

Behavioral Definition of Sleep

Perlis ML, Lichstein KL, eds. *Treating Sleep Disorders: Principles and Practice of Behavioral Sleep Medicine.* Hoboken, NJ: John Wiley & Sons, 2003.

Sleep Research Society. *SRS Basics of Sleep Guide.* Westchester, IL: Sleep Research Society, 2005.

Function of Sleep

Benington J. Sleep homeostasis and the function of sleep. *Sleep.* 2001;23:959–966.

Benington JH, Frank MG. Cellular and molecular connections between sleep and synaptic plasticity. *Progress in Neurobiology.* 2003;69:77–101.

Frank MG. The function of sleep. In: Lee-Chiong TL, ed. *Sleep: A Comprehensive Handbook.* Hoboken, NJ: John Wiley & Sons, 2006.

Inoue S, Honda K, Komoda Y. Sleep as neuronal detoxification and restitution. *Behav Brain Res.* 1995;69:91–96.

Rechtschaffen A. Current perspectives on the function of sleep. *Perspect Biol.* Med 1998;41:359–90.

Shaw PJ, Tononi G, Greenspan RJ, Robinson DF. Stress response genes protect against lethal effects of sleep deprivation in Drosophila. *Nature.* 2002;417:287–91.

Normal Sleep Requirements

Lee-Chiong TL, ed. Sleep: A Comprehensive Handbook. Hoboken, NJ: John Wiley & Sons, 2006.

Lee-Chiong TL, Sateia M, Carskadon M, eds. *Sleep Medicine.* Philadelphia, PA: Hanley & Belfus (Elsevier), 2002.

Sleep Research Society. *SRS Basics of Sleep Guide.* Westchester, IL: Sleep Research Society.

Regulation of Sleep and Wakefulness

Lee-Chiong TL, ed. *Sleep: A Comprehensive Handbook.* Hoboken, NJ: John Wiley & Sons, 2006.

Lee-Chiong TL, Sateia M, Carskadon M, eds. *Sleep Medicine.* Philadelphia, PA: Hanley & Belfus (Elsevier), 2002.

Sleep Research Society. *SRS Basics of Sleep Guide.* Westchester, IL: Sleep Research Society.

Sleep in Animals

Lee-Chiong TL, ed. *Sleep: A Comprehensive Handbook.* Hoboken, NJ: John Wiley & Sons, 2006.

Lee-Chiong TL, Sateia M, Carskadon M, eds. *Sleep Medicine.* Philadelphia, PA: Hanley & Belfus (Elsevier), 2002.

Human Sleep

Lee-Chiong TL, ed. *Sleep: A Comprehensive Handbook.* Hoboken, NJ: John Wiley & Sons, 2006.

Lee-Chiong TL, Sateia M, Carskadon M, eds. *Sleep Medicine.* Philadelphia, PA: Hanley & Belfus (Elsevier), 2002.

Sleep Research Society. *SRS Basics of Sleep Guide.* Westchester, IL: Sleep Research Society.

Normal Adult Sleep

Lee-Chiong TL, ed. *Sleep: A Comprehensive Handbook.* Hoboken, NJ: John Wiley & Sons, 2006.

Lee-Chiong TL, Sateia M, Carskadon M, eds. *Sleep Medicine.* Philadelphia, PA: Hanley & Belfus (Elsevier), 2002.

Sleep Research Society. *SRS Basics of Sleep Guide.* Westchester, IL: Sleep Research Society.

Chemical Neuroanatomy of Sleep and Wakefulness

Jones BE. Basic mechanisms of sleep-wake states. In: Kryger MH, Roth T, Dement WC, eds. Principles and Practice of Sleep Medicine. 3rd ed. Philadelphia, PA: WB Saunders, 2000;134–154.

Morruzi G, Magoun HW. Brainstem reticular formation and activation of the EEG. *Electroencephalogr Clin Neurophysiol*. 1949;1:455.

Norgren R. Projections from the nucleus of the solitary tract in the rat. *Neuroscience*. 1978;3:207.

Shneerson JM. Physiological basis of Sleep and wakefulness. In: Schneerson JM. *Handbook of Sleep Medicine*. Malden, MA: Blackwell Science Ltd, 2000;16–32.

Siegel JM. Brainstem mechanisms generating REM sleep. In: Kryger MH, Roth T, Dement WC, eds. *Principles and Practice of Sleep Medicine*. 3rd ed. Philadelphia, PA: WB Saunders, 2000;112–133.

Steriade M, Pare D, Parent A, Smith Y. Projections of cholinergic and non-cholinergic neurons of the brainstem core to relay and associational thalamic nuclei in the cat and macaque monkey. *Neuroscience*. 1988;25:47.

Neurotransmitters Associated With Sleep-Wake Regulation

Jouvet M. The role of monoamines and acetylcholine containing neurons in the regulation of the sleep-waking cycle. *Ergeb Physiol*. 1972;64:165.

Monnier M, Sauer R, Hatt AM. The activating effect of histamine on the central nervous system. *Int Rev Neurobiol*. 1970;12:265.

Mugnaini E, Oertel WH. An atlas of the distribution of GABAergic neurons and terminals. In: Bjorklund A, Hokfelt T, eds. *Handbook of Chemical Neuroanatomy*. Vol 4, GABA and neuropeptides in the CNS, Part 1. Amsterdam, The Netherlands: Elsevier; 1985:436.

Radulovacki M, Virus RM, Djuricic-Nedelson M et al. Adenosine and adenosine analogs: effects on sleep in rats. In: McGinty DJ, Morrison A, Drucker-Colin R, et al., eds. *Brain Mechanisms of Sleep*. New York, NY: Raven Press; 1985:235.

Steriade M, Pare D, Parent A, Smith Y. Projections of cholinergic and non-cholinergic neurons of the brainstem core to relay and associational thalamic nuclei in the cat and macaque monkey. *Neuroscience*. 1988;25:47.

Autonomic Nervous System

Lee-Chiong TL, ed. *Sleep: A Comprehensive Handbook*. Hoboken, NJ: John Wiley & Sons, 2006.

Lee-Chiong TL, Sateia M, Carskadon M, eds. *Sleep Medicine*. Philadelphia, PA: Hanley & Belfus (Elsevier), 2002.

Sleep Research Society. *SRS Basics of Sleep Guide*. Westchester, IL: Sleep Research Society.

Respiratory Physiology During Sleep

Simon PM, Landry SH, Leiter JC. Respiratory control during sleep. In: Lee-Chiong TL, Sateia M, Carskadon M, eds. *Sleep Medicine*. Philadelphia, PA: Hanley & Belfus (Elsevier), 2002.

Cardiovascular Physiology During Sleep

Verrier RL. Cardiac physiology during sleep. In: Lee-Chiong TL, Sateia M, Carskadon M, eds. *Sleep Medicine*. Philadelphia, PA: Hanley & Belfus (Elsevier), 2002.

Gastrointestinal Physiology During Sleep

Orr WC. Sleep and the gastrointestinal tract. In: Lee-Chiong TL, ed. *Sleep: A Comprehensive Handbook*. Hoboken, NJ: John Wiley & Sons, 2006.

Renal Physiology During Sleep

Parker K. Renal disease. In: Lee-Chiong TL, ed. *Sleep: A Comprehensive Handbook*. Hoboken, NJ: John Wiley & Sons, 2006.

Genitourinary Physiology During Sleep

Lee-Chiong TL, ed. Sleep: A Comprehensive Handbook. Hoboken, NJ: John Wiley & Sons, 2006.
Endocrine Physiology During Sleep

Vgontzas AN, Vela-Bueno A, Chrousos GP. Endocrine disorders and sleep. In: Lee-Chiong TL, ed. *Sleep: A Comprehensive Handbook*. Hoboken, NJ: John Wiley & Sons, 2006.

Immune Function and Sleep

Krueger JM, Majde JA. Sleep and the immune response. In: Lee-Chiong TL, ed. *Sleep: A Comprehensive Handbook*. Hoboken, NJ: John Wiley & Sons, 2006.

Lange T, Perras B, Fehm HL, Born J. Sleep enhances the human antibody response to hepatitis A vaccination. *Psychosom Med*. 2003;65:831–835.

Larson SJ, Dunn AJ. Behavioral effects of cytokines. *Brain Behav Immun*. 2001;15:371–387.

Majde JA. Viral double-stranded RNA, cytokines and the flu. *J Interferon Cytok Res*. 2000;20:259–272.

Majde JA, Krueger JM. Neuroimmunology of sleep. In: *Biological Psychiatry*. London, England: John Wiley & Sons, 2002;1247–1257.

Obal Jr F, Krueger JM. Biochemical regulation of sleep. *Front Biosci*. 2003;8:511–519.

Spiegel K, Sheridan JF, Van Cauter E. Effect of sleep deprivation on responses to immunization. *JAMA*. 2002;288:1471–1472.

Temperature Regulation

Skinner RD. Temperature regulation during sleep. In: Lee-Chiong TL, Sateia M, Carskadon M, eds. *Sleep Medicine*. Philadelphia, PA: Hanley & Belfus (Elsevier), 2002.

Metabolism and Sleep

Lee-Chiong TL, ed. *Sleep: A Comprehensive Handbook*. Hoboken, NJ: John Wiley & Sons, 2006.

Lee-Chiong TL, Sateia M, Carskadon M, eds. *Sleep Medicine*. Philadelphia, PA: Hanley & Belfus (Elsevier), 2002.

Sleep Research Society. *SRS Basics of Sleep Guide*. Westchester, IL: Sleep Research Society.

Musculoskeletal Physiology and Sleep

Lee-Chiong TL, ed. *Sleep: A Comprehensive Handbook*. Hoboken, NJ: John Wiley & Sons, 2006.

Lee-Chiong TL, Sateia M, Carskadon M, eds. *Sleep Medicine*. Philadelphia, PA: Hanley & Belfus (Elsevier), 2002.

Pupillary Changes During Sleep

Lee-Chiong TL, ed. *Sleep: A Comprehensive Handbook*. Hoboken, NJ: John Wiley & Sons, 2006.

Lee-Chiong TL, Sateia M, Carskadon M, eds. *Sleep Medicine*. Philadelphia, PA: Hanley & Belfus (Elsevier), 2002.

Cognitive Function

Lee-Chiong TL, ed. *Sleep: A Comprehensive Handbook*. Hoboken, NJ: John Wiley & Sons, 2006.

Lee-Chiong TL, Sateia M, Carskadon M, eds. *Sleep Medicine*. Philadelphia, PA: Hanley & Belfus (Elsevier), 2002.

Dreaming

Kramer M. Biology of dreaming. In: Lee-Chiong TL, ed. *Sleep: A Comprehensive Handbook*. Hoboken, NJ: John Wiley & Sons, 2006.

Hartmann E. Dreaming. In: Lee-Chiong TL, Sateia M, Carskadon M, eds. *Sleep Medicine*. Philadelphia, PA: Hanley & Belfus (Elsevier), 2002.

Sleep Deprivation

Carskadon MA. Sleep deprivation: health consequences and societal impact. *Sleep Disorders*. Medical Clinics of North America. Philadelphia, PA: Elsevier Saunders. 2004.

Malik SW, Kaplan J. Sleep deprivation. *Sleep Medicine*. Primary Care: Clinics in Office Practice. Philadelphia, PA: Elsevier Saunders. 2005.

Rosenthal L, Meixner R. Sleep deprivation. In: Lee-Chiong TL, Sateia M, Carskadon M, eds. *Sleep Medicine*. Philadelphia, PA: Hanley & Belfus (Elsevier), 2002.

Evaluation of Sleep, and Sleep Disorders 2

- **Sleep History**
  - Family History
  - Medication Use
  - Nighttime Events
- **Manifestations of Sleep Disorders**
- **Sleep Diaries**
- **Sleep Questionnaires**
  - Epworth Sleepiness Scale
  - Stanford Sleepiness Scale
  - Visual Analog Scale
- **Physical Examination**
- **Polysomnography**
  - Electroencephalography
  - Electro-oculography
  - Electromyography (Chin)
  - Electrocardiography
  - **Measurement of Airflow**
  - Pneumotachography
  - Nasal Pressure
  - Thermal Sensors
  - Expired Carbon Dioxide
  - **Measurement of Respiratory Effort**
  - Esophageal Pressure
  - Surface Diaphragmatic Electromyography
  - Strain Gauges
  - Respiratory Inductance Plethysmography
  - Thoracic Impedance
  - **Measurement of Oxygenation and Ventilation**

- Pulse Oximetry
- Transcutaneous Oxygen ($PtcO_2$) Monitoring
- Transcutaneous Carbon Dioxide ($PtcCO_2$)
- Expired End Tidal Carbon Dioxide ($PetCO_2$)
- Pulse Transit Time
- Snoring
- Electromyography (Anterior Tibialis)
- **Sleep-Related Breathing Disorders**
- **Sleep Staging**
- **Scoring Sleep in Newborns**
- **Factors Affecting Sleep Architecture**
- **Definitions of Common Polysomnographic Parameters**
- **Performing a Polysomnography: An Overview**
  - Understanding the Polygraph Equipment
  - Patient Preparation
  - Electrode Application
  - Physiologic Calibrations
  - Starting and Monitoring the Study
  - Artifact Recognition and Troubleshooting
  - Ending the Study
- **Indications for Polysomnography**
- **Portable Polysomnography**
- **Multiple Sleep Latency Test**
- **Maintenance of Wakefulness Test**
- **Actigraphy**
- **References**

Sleep History

Inquiry should be made into the patient's history of medical, surgical, or psychiatric disorders; family history of sleep conditions; medication and substance use; and nighttime activities.

Family History

The interview should include a thorough family history. Many disorders tend to be more prevalent among children, siblings, and other close relatives of patients. These include snoring, restless legs syndrome, narcolepsy, obstructive sleep apnea, enuresis, sleepwalking, sleep terrors, familial fatal insomnia, mood disorders, and schizophrenia. A positive family history is present in up to 30% of patients with narcolepsy or restless legs syndrome.

Medication Use

A complete medication list must be obtained. Many medications can cause insomnia or excessive sleepiness, or they can precipitate or aggravate parasomnias or restless legs syndrome.

Nighttime Events

Patients should be asked about their usual nighttime activities and bedroom environment, including:

1.   Time of arrival home from work

2.   If the patient is a shift worker, the various work schedules and the interval between shift changes

3.   Responsibilities at home including house chores and child care

4.   Exercise or any recreational pursuits prior to and after supper

5.   Time of supper and other evening snacks

6.   Bedtime

7.   Activities performed in bed (eg, reading or watching television)

8.   Factors that may interfere with sleep onset such as bright lights, excessive noise, extremes of bedroom temperature, concerns regarding safety in the house, responsibility of caring for children, elderly parents or sick family members, an uncomfortable bed, or a restless or snoring bed partner

9.   Effect of a new sleep environment (eg, living room or hotel room) on sleep

10.   Changes in sleep patterns during weekends

11.   Time in bed before sleep occurs

12.   Number of awakenings during the night and reasons for these nighttime awakenings

13.   Duration of awakenings as well as the ease or difficulty of returning to sleep following these events

14.   Time of awakening in the morning

15.   Whether sleep is adequate or unrefreshing

16.   Presence of any daytime fatigue or sleepiness

17.   Daytime performance at work and in school

18.   General mood during the day (eg, irritability, anger, impatience, or apathy)

19.   Occurrence of profound, uncontrollable sleepiness (eg, while driving or as a passenger in the car; when reading; while watching television or in a movie theater; when working, especially if operating heavy and dangerous machinery; during conversations or at meals)

20.   Frequency, timing, and duration of napping (patients with narcolepsy may describe occurrence of dreaming during brief naps)

21.   Presence of persistent, low-level sleepiness throughout the day or if unexpected and unpredictable sleep attacks occur in a background of otherwise full daytime alertness

Many events that occur during the night may increase the likelihood of developing insomnia or excessive sleepiness. Individuals may not be aware of their occurrence during their sleep; thus input from bed partners may be invaluable. Patients and their bed partners should be asked about the occurrence of snoring, sleep apnea, parasomnias, nocturnal seizure activity, restless legs, periodic limb movements, painful leg cramps, recurrent sleep starts, night terrors, nightmares, nocturnal chest pain, severe choking sensation, dyspnea, wheezing, bruxism, and urinary or fecal incontinence.

Manifestations of Sleep Disorders

Sleep-related disorders can present in a variety of ways, including insomnia, excessive sleepiness, snoring, sleep apnea, cataplexy, sleep paralysis, sleep hallucinations, nocturnal dyspnea, nocturnal pain, and nocturnal physical phenomena. Proper evaluation of sleep disorders requires an understanding of the differential diagnosis for each of these complaints.

1.   *Insomnia*—Persons who complain of insomnia report an inability to fall asleep or to remain asleep. They may feel that their sleep is short and inadequate, light and easily disrupted, or non-restorative.

2.   *Excessive sleepiness*—Persons complain of being unable to consistently achieve and sustain wakefulness and alertness to accomplish the tasks of daily living, with sleep occurring unintentionally or at inappropriate times.

3.   *Sleep apnea*—Apnea is defined as the absence of airflow for ten or more seconds. When airflow is diminished but not absent, the event is termed hypopnea. Both obstructive sleep apnea (OSA) and central sleep apnea can result in either insomnia or excessive somnolence. In contrast to obese persons with severe OSA who typically present with excessive sleepiness, those with complaints of insomnia generally have less severe sleep-disordered breathing and are less likely to be obese. Apnea frequency and duration tend to be lower, and oxygen desaturation milder, in persons with insomnia compared with hypersomnolent individuals who have OSA.

4.   *Cataplexy*—Patients report an abrupt, transient, and bilateral loss or reduction of postural muscle tone occurring during wakefulness and precipitated by intense emotion such as laughter.

5.   *Sleep paralysis*—Patients describe an inability to move while awake at the transition between sleep and wakefulness.

6.   *Sleep hallucinations*—Hallucinatory phenomena that can be visual, auditory, tactile, or kinetic occur while awake either at sleep onset or upon awakening.

7.   *Nocturnal dyspnea*—Respiratory disorders including sleep-related asthma and chronic obstructive pulmonary disease might cause nighttime awakenings due to dyspnea. Other causes of nocturnal dyspnea include OSA, nocturnal cardiac ischemia, congestive heart failure with paroxysmal nocturnal dyspnea, central alveolar hypoventilation syndrome, sleep-related gastroesophageal reflux, sleep-related laryngospasm, sleep choking syndrome, and sleep-related abnormal swallowing syndrome.

8. *Nocturnal pain*—Chronic pain is the chief cause of sleep disturbance in many medical disorders. Pain may arise from sleep-related headaches, cancer and rheumatologic conditions, including fibromyalgia. Persons with fibromyalgia often complain of chronic fatigue, nonrestorative sleep, and generalized muscle discomfort. Nocturnal cardiac ischemia, left ventricular failure (paroxysmal nocturnal dyspnea), sleep-related gastroesophageal reflux, peptic ulcer disease, or a primary respiratory disorder such as chronic obstructive pulmonary disease may also produce nocturnal chest pain.

9. *Nocturnal physical phenomena*—The list of etiologies responsible for nocturnal movements is lengthy and includes OSA with forceful arousals, periodic limb movement disorder, disorders of arousal (confusional arousals, sleepwalking, and sleep terrors), rhythmic movement disorder, sleep starts, sleep talking, nocturnal leg cramps, nightmares, rapid eye movement (REM) sleep behavior disorder, sleep bruxism, benign neonatal sleep myoclonus, sleep-related epilepsy, fragmentary myoclonus, terrifying hypnagogic hallucinations, sleep-related laryngospasm, and sleep choking syndrome. Some are evident predominantly during certain sleep stages, whereas others emerge sporadically throughout the sleep cycle.

10. *Aggressive behavior during sleep*—REM sleep behavior disorder and somnambulism can present as aggressive, potentially injurious, behavior during sleep.

Sleep Diaries

Patients are often requested to complete a sleep log daily for 1 to 2 weeks prior to their office visit. Although the exact questions may vary, sleep logs typically contain information regarding both the quality and quantity of nighttime sleep as well as any daytime consequences of sleep disruption. Patients are asked to monitor the following in their sleep logs:

1. *Bedtime*—Time they went to bed and when they actually tried to sleep

2. *Sleep latency*—Estimated length of time it took them to fall asleep

3. *Awakenings*—Number of awakenings during the evening and the duration of each awakening

4. *Time in bed*—Total amount of time spent in bed during the night

5. *Total sleep time*—Estimated total amount of actual sleep during the night

6. *Arising time*—Time they woke up in the morning and when they got out of bed

7. *Sleep quality*—Subjective assessment of the quality of their sleep

8. *Medications, caffeine, tobacco and alcohol use*—Use of hypnotic agents, other medications, coffee, tobacco products, and alcohol

9. *Daytime napping*—Whether any naps were taken during the day

10. *Unusual events*—Any special or unusual events that they had in the preceding weeks that may have influenced the entries in the sleep log.

The data in the sleep diary are discussed with the patient during the office interview. Data from actigraphy may be used to support the subjective reports from sleep diaries.

Sleep Questionnaires

Epworth Sleepiness Scale

The Epworth Sleepiness Scale (ESS) measures general sleep propensity (likelihood of dozing off or falling asleep) using an eight-item questionnaire. Patients are asked to rate their chance of dozing in eight situations (Box 2–1). The aggregate score (0 to 24) determines the degree of sleepiness. The correlation between ESS and multiple sleep latency test (MSLT) is low but significant; however, changes in one may not correlate with changes in the other.

Box 2–1.
 	
Epworth sleepiness scale
	Situations in Recent Times
	
	  1. Sitting, and reading
	
	  2. Watching television
	
	  3. Sitting, inactive in a public place (eg, a theater or a meeting)
	
	  4. As a passenger in a car for an hour without a break
	
	  5. Lying down to rest in the afternoon
	
	  6. Sitting, talking to someone
	
	  7. Sitting quietly after lunch without alcohol
	
	  8. In a car, while stopped for a few minutes in traffic
	
	Chances of dozing: 0 (Never); 1 (Slight chance); 2 (Moderate chance); 3 (High chance)
	
	Score: 0–9: normal; 10–12: mild sleepiness; 13–17: moderate sleepiness; 18, and above: severe sleepiness
	
	Source: Adapted from Johns MW. A new method for measuring daytime sleepiness: the Epworth Sleepiness Scale. Sleep. 1991;14: 540-545.

Stanford Sleepiness Scale

The Stanford Sleepiness Scale is a seven-point subjective measure of the perception of sleepiness (Box 2–2).

Box 2–2. **Stanford sleepiness scale**	1. Active, wide awake, vital, and alert 2. Able to concentrate, and functioning at high level, but not at peak 3. Relaxed, awake, responsive but not fully alert 4. Feeling a little foggy, and not at peak 5. Feeling foggy, losing interest in staying awake 6. Sleepy, woozy, preferring to lie down 7. Unable to remain awake, sleep onset is imminent *Source: Adapted from Hoddes E, Zarcone V, Smythe H, et al. Quantification of sleepiness: a new approach. Psychophysiology. 1973;10:431-436.*

Visual Analog Scale

Subjective sleepiness is indicated by an arbitrary point on a straight line.

Physical Examination

Physical examination may help confirm the presence of medical or neurologic conditions identified from clinical history. Alternatively, it may uncover unsuspected disorders that might contribute to sleep disturbance.

Polysomnography

Polysomnography refers to the simultaneous and continuous recording of several physiologic variables (eg, electroencephalography [EEG], electro-oculography [EOG], electromyography [EMG], electrocardiography [EKG], airflow, respiratory effort, and oxygen saturation) during sleep. These various components are listed in Box 2–3.

Box 2-3.
 	
Typical polysomnography montage
	Electroencephalography (EEG)
	
	    Central EEG
	
	    Occipital EEG
	
	Electro-oculography (EOG)
	
	    Right EOG
	
	    Left EOG
	
	Electromyography
	
	    Chin
	
	    Right leg
	
	    Left leg
	
	Electrocardiography (EKG)
	
	Snoring
	
	Airflow
	
	Thoracic movement
	
	Abdominal movement
	
	Oxygen saturation (SaO$_2$)
	
	Body position
	
	Additional channels
	
	    Esophageal pressure

(continued from page 40)
Box 2–3.

Typical polysomnography montage

End-tidal carbon dioxide ($PetCO_2$)

Transcutaneous carbon dioxide ($PtcCO_2$)

Positive airway pressure level

Additional EEG channels (for evaluation of suspected nocturnal seizures)

Video-monitoring (for evaluation of suspected parasomnias or seizures)

Esophageal pH sensors (for evaluation of suspected gastroesophageal reflux)

Electroencephalography

The voltage recorded from scalp electrodes originates from the summed potential activity of neuronal somas and dendrites within the cortex. EEG waveforms have voltages between 5 and 200 microvolts (mV) and frequencies between 0.5 and 45 Hz. Wakefulness is associated with EEG frequencies from 14 to 45 Hz, whereas sleep EEG frequencies are generally restricted to 0.5 to 14 Hz. Table 2–1 lists the frequencies of the different types of EEG waves.

Table 2–1.		
Frequency of electroencephalography waves	**Wave**	**Frequency**
	Delta	< 4
	Theta	4-7
	Alpha	8-13
	Beta	> 13

Electrode placement is based on the International 10–20 system. In this system, electrodes are placed at 10% or 20% of the distance between specific landmarks (eg, bridge of nose [nasion], occipital prominence [inion], vertex, and preauricular location).

Each electrode is provided with a letter that represents the corresponding region of the brain (F = frontal; Fp = frontopolar; O = occipital; P = parietal; and T = temporal) and a numerical subscript (left-sided electrodes = odd numbers; right-sided electrodes = even numbers). Reference electrodes are placed over the mastoid process (A).

A derivation is the difference in voltage between two electrodes. Standard electrode derivations for monitoring EEG are C3/A2 or C4/A1 (based on Rechtschaffen and Kales criteria), or 01/A2 or 02/A1. Additional EEG electrodes are necessary to evaluate nocturnal seizure activity. A montage or set of derivations can either be bipolar (two standard electrodes are matched to each other), or referential (a standard electrode is compared to a reference electrode, such as a mastoid electrode).

EEG is commonly recorded using either gold cup or silver silver-chloride electrodes. Electrode impedance should ideally be less than 5000 Ω. Standard gain for EEG electrodes is a deflection of 1 cm for every 50 μV. Excessively high low-frequency filter settings can decrease wave amplitude. Table 2–2 describes the EEG waveforms.

Table 2–2. **Electroencephalographic (EEG) waveforms**

Wave type	Waveform
Alpha waves	EEG oscillations with a frequency of 8–13 Hz (slower among children, and elderly adults compared to younger adults) Variable amplitude (generally < 50 μV among adults) Present when a person is relaxed, and drowsy, and eyes are closed Also present during arousals from sleep Originate in the occipital cortex; more prominent in the occipital leads compared with central leads Eye opening suppresses alpha activity
Alpha-delta	Alpha waves occurring during NREM stages 3, and 4 (slow wave or delta) sleep
Beta waves	EEG oscillations with a frequency of 13–35 Hz, and an amplitude that is usually < 30 μV Present during alert wakefulness
Delta waves	High-amplitude (peak to peak of > 75 μV), slow (< 2–4 Hz) EEG activity Seen in NREM stages 3, and 4 sleep Originate in the cortex
Sleep spindles	Brief oscillations with a frequency of 12–14 Hz lasting 0.5–1.5 seconds, and an amplitude generally < 50 μV More prominent, and with highest voltage over the central leads May occur during NREM stages 2, 3, and 4 sleep; not seen in NREM stage 1 sleep, and REM sleep Generated in midline thalamic nuclei Compared to sleep spindles, alpha waves are slower (8–13 Hz) "Pseudo–spindles" or "drug spindles" secondary to benzodiazepines have a higher frequency (about 15 Hz)
K complex	High-amplitude, biphasic wave (an initial sharp negative deflection followed by a positive high-voltage slow wave) with a duration of at least 0.5 seconds Seen maximally over the vertex (central, and central-parietal leads) Believed to represent evoked responses to internal, and external stimuli
Saw-tooth waves	Theta waves with a notched waveform More prominent over the vertex, and frontal leads Occur during REM sleep
Theta waves	EEG oscillations with a frequency of 4 to 7 Hz Originate in the hippocampus Maximal over the central, and temporal leads
Vertex sharp deflections	Sharp negative deflections with amplitudes < 250 μV that are maximal over the vertex

NREM = non-rapid eye movement; REM = rapid eye movement.

Electro-oculography

EOG records the difference in potentials (dipole) between the cornea (positively charged) and the retina (negatively charged). This dipole changes with eye movements. A positive voltage (downward deflection) is recorded when the eye moves *toward* an electrode, and a negative voltage (upward deflection) accompanies an eye movement *away* from an electrode.

Electrodes are placed (using adhesive and *not collodion*) 1 cm lateral and superior to the outer canthus of one eye (right outer canthus) and 1 cm lateral and inferior to the outer canthus of the other eye (left outer canthus). Electrodes are connected either to the opposite or same mastoid process (A) of the temporal bone.

Conjugate eye movements create out-of-phase deflections in the two EOG channels, whereas high-voltage EEG artifacts produce in-phase deflections. Patterns of eye movements may be:

1. Slow rolling movements consist of slow undulating deflections that are present during drowsiness with closed eyes, non–rapid eye movement (NREM) stage 1 sleep, or brief awakenings. They disappear during stage NREM stage 2 sleep.

2. Rapid movements are composed of sharper deflections that can occur during wakefulness with open eyes (eye blinks), or rapid eye movement (REM) sleep. Rapid eye movement density (frequency of rapid eye movements per minute of REM sleep) is less during early REM sleep episodes and progressively increases during later REM sleep periods.

Patients taking selective serotonin reuptake inhibitors (SSRIs) (eg, fluoxetine) and tricyclic antidepressants (TCAs) may have eye movements during NREM stages 2, 3, and 4 sleep (so-called "Prozac eyes").

Electromyography (Chin)

Leads are placed in the mental and submental areas to identify REM sleep. An additional electrode can be placed over the masseter muscle to detect bruxism

Electrocardiography

A single channel, with one electrode placed near the sternum at the area of the right clavicle and another over the left lateral chest wall near the seventh rib, is used to monitor cardiac rate and rhythm.

Measurement of Airflow

Techniques to measure airflow include nasal pressure, pneumotachography, thermistors, thermocouples, and end-tidal carbon dioxide ($PetCO_2$) monitoring. Only pneumotachography measures airflow directly. Thermal sensors and $PetCO_2$ monitoring provide indirect estimates of airflow based on the changing thermal and chemical characteristics of inspired ambient air and expired air originating from the lungs and airways.

Apneas are reliably detected by most indirect methods of measuring respiratory airflow. However, it is uncertain whether indirect methods can consistently identify hypopneas.

Pneumotachography

A pneumotachometer, placed in a well-fitted face mask, can measure total oronasal airflow by detecting changes in pressure between inspiration and expiration. A pneumotachometer is the reference standard for detecting obstructive apnea-hypopnea.

Nasal Pressure

The presence of airflow can be inferred by changes in nasal pressure during respiration. Nasal airflow can be measured quantitatively and directly with a pneumotachograph consisting of a standard oxygen nasal cannula connected to a pressure transducer and placed in the nares. Respiration produces fluctuations on the nasal pressure transducer signals (decreases during inspiration and increases during expiration) that are proportional to flow. Nasal pressure is recorded either as a direct current (DC) signal or as an alternating current (AC) signal if used with appropriate filters.

The shape and amplitude of the nasal cannula signal are comparable to those obtained from face mask pneumotachographs. The presence of a *plateau* (flattening) on the inspiratory flow signal is associated with increased upper airway resistance and airflow limitation (obstructive event). In contrast, the signal is reduced but rounded in central events.

Nasal pressure monitoring is better able to detect hypopneas compared to thermal sensors. However, it is not recommended for patients who are predominantly mouth breathers or have nasal obstruction in whom airflow may be underestimated. Simultaneous use of an oral thermal sensor can be used for such patients.

Thermal Sensors

Thermal sensing devices provide an indirect and semiquantitative measurement of airflow. Thermal sensors, placed over the nose and mouth, sense airflow by differences in the temperature between warmer expired air and cooler inhaled ambient air. The flow signal generated is related directly to the sensor temperature (measured as electrical resistance by a thermistor and as change in voltage by a thermocouple) and indirectly to airflow. It is also dependent on the pattern of airflow and the placement of the sensor in relation to the nostril.

Signals obtained from thermal sensors provide only qualitative data regarding airflow. As a rule, they are unable to reliably identify the presence of hypopneas, or distinguish central from obstructive apnea-hypopneas.

Expired Carbon Dioxide

Expired carbon dioxide monitoring using infrared analyzers placed in front of the nose and mouth can provide a qualitative measure of airflow because ambient air contains negligible amounts of carbon dioxide (CO_2) compared with expired air from the lungs, which have a higher concentration of CO_2. One can also infer the occurrence of hypoventilation by a rising $PetCO_2$ level.

With central apnea, cardiac oscillations in the CO_2 tracing may be noted. These are produced by small fluctuations in lung volume accompanying each heartbeat that is transmitted to the sensor via a patent upper airway.

Measurement of Respiratory Effort

Respiratory effort can be identified using esophageal pressure monitoring, surface diaphragmatic EMG, strain gauges, respiratory inductance plethysmography, or thoracic impedance. Measurement of respiratory effort is important in distinguishing central from obstructive apneas.

Esophageal Pressure

Measurement of esophageal pressures during polysomnography is the reference standard for detecting respiratory effort. Respiratory effort is accompanied by changes in pleural pressure, which can be accurately measured by esophageal pressure monitoring using either traditional esophageal balloons or newer catheter transducers. This method is particularly useful in distinguishing between obstructive and central apneas.

During episodes of respiratory event–related arousals (RERAs) in patients with upper airway resistance syndrome (UARS), esophageal pressures become increasingly more negative immediately preceding an arousal, after which the esophageal pressure rapidly returns to baseline levels.

Surface Diaphragmatic Electromyography

Signal tracings derived from electrodes placed on the chest wall may infer respiratory effort indirectly.

Strain Gauges

Strain gauges, which are length-sensitive, can be positioned below the axilla and at the level of the umbilicus to measure rib cage and abdominal excursions, respectively. A single uncalibrated abdominal or chest gauge can be used to detect respiratory movements. Quantitative measurements of volume change require calibration of the rib cage and abdominal gauges against another volume-measuring device.

Signal quality from strain gauges is affected by sleep position, movements during sleep, and displacement, overstretching or understretching of the strain gauges during the monitoring period. The summed rib cage–abdominal volume signals cannot distinguish central (no net volume change due to absence of respiratory effort) from obstructive (no net volume change due to rib cage–abdominal paradox) sleep apnea. It is, therefore, advisable to verify the absence of respiratory effort by esophageal pressure monitoring whenever most apneas detected by strain gauges appear central in origin.

Respiratory Inductance Plethysmography

Changes in chest and abdominal volume during respiration can be measured semi-quantitatively using respiratory inductance plethysmography (RIP). Transducers placed around the chest (at the level of the nipples) and abdomen (at the level of the umbilicus) monitor changes in the cross-sectional area of the respective body compartments as reflected in changes in inductance (resistance to change in flow of current) of the transducers. The sum of the signals from calibrated chest and abdominal sensors can afford an estimate of tidal volume and respiratory patterns during sleep. Although RIP provides data on movements of the rib cage and abdomen, it does not offer information regarding airflow.

Paradoxical motion of the chest and abdomen suggests an obstructive event rather than a central process. This is most pronounced during REM sleep due to chest wall muscle hypotonia.

The accuracy of RIP in monitoring the presence and volume of respiration depends on its initial calibration as well as the constancy of calibration during body movements and changes in lung volumes. Inaccuracies in measurements may arise due to displacements of the transducer bands or alterations in posture during sleep. Sleep-related thoracoabdominal distortion or movement asynchrony and changes in body position also affect the accuracy of quantitative measurements using RIP during sleep.

Thoracic Impedance

With impedance pneumography, a current is applied across the thorax, which serves as an electrical conductor. Impedance varies with the relative amounts of conductive materials (body fluids and tissue) and nonconductive air between a pair of electrodes placed at opposite sides of the thoracic cage. Total impedance decreases as the volume of conductive material increases in proportion to air and vice versa, affording a qualitative measure of respiratory effort.

Measurement of Oxygenation and Ventilation

Direct measurements of arterial oxygen tension (PaO_2), arterial carbon dioxide tension ($PaCO_2$), and SaO_2 via arterial blood sampling are more accurate than estimates derived from noninvasive methods. However, they afford only a static measure of oxygenation and ventilation at discrete points of time rather than continuous monitoring. Oxygenation and ventilation change rapidly during sleep in patients with sleep-related breathing disorders (SRBDs). Thus, to be accurate and reliable, methods to assess blood gases must be capable of rapid and repetitive measurements. However, repetitive sampling of arterial blood during sleep is painful, time-consuming, inconvenient, expensive and intrusive of the patient's sleep. Noninvasive assessments include pulse oximetry, transcutaneous oxygen tension ($PtcO_2$) measurement, transcutaneous carbon dioxide tension ($PtcCO_2$) measurement, or airway CO_2 ($PetCO_2$) monitoring.

Pulse Oximetry

Pulse oximeters respond rapidly to changes in SaO_2 and permit continuous monitoring of SaO_2. Using either spectrophotometric technique or photoelectric plethysmography, pulse oximeters are routinely utilized during overnight polysomnography to monitor SaO_2. A pulsating vascular bed (eg, earlobe or fingertip) is placed between a two-wavelength light source and a sensor.

Altering the pulse oximeter response time influences the accuracy of pulse oximeters in measuring changes in SaO_2. For instance, SaO_2 recordings may be inaccurate if the oximeter response time approximates the duration of oxygen desaturation events. Sensitivity is greater with shorter sampling intervals, and the least filtering to achieve the most rapid response is recommended. Signal amplitude is affected by reduced skin perfusion due to hypothermia, hypotension or vasoconstriction and by poor sensor attachment. In addition, oximetry readings may overestimate low oxygen saturation values. Lastly, due to its reliance on only two light wavelengths, the presence of dyshemoglobin species such as carboxyhemoglobin or methemoglobin produces errors in measurement.

Transcutaneous Oxygen ($PtcO_2$) Monitoring

A modified Clark electrode can be used to measure oxygen tension at the skin surface ($PtcO_2$). Cutaneous perfusion, temperature, and metabolism influence the surface oxygen tension. Blood flow to the skin can be increased by local application of heat (43°C), with periodic site changes every 4 to 6 hours to prevent cutaneous thermal injury.

Several factors limit the application of $PtcO_2$ monitoring during adult sleep studies including the variable relationship between PaO_2 and $PtcO_2$, slow response time that fails to mirror rapid changes in PaO_2, and the need for periodic site changes.

Transcutaneous Carbon Dioxide ($PtcCO_2$)

Transcutaneous carbon dioxide ($PtcCO_2$), the CO_2 tension at the epidermal surface, can be monitored noninvasively using a silver chloride electrode or an infrared capnometer. Although $PtcCO_2$ affords continuous monitoring during sleep, $PtcCO_2$ often differs significantly from a simultaneously obtained $PaCO_2$.

PtcCO$_2$ monitoring is most commonly used during neonatal or pediatric polysomnography. It has less clinical utility among adults because its slow response time makes it unsuitable for monitoring blood gas tensions during sleep when rapid and short-lasting changes can occur. PtcCO$_2$ monitoring may be of some use in patients with waking hypercapnia and in those with suspected sleep-related alveolar hypoventilation.

Expired End Tidal Carbon Dioxide (PetCO$_2$)

Infrared spectrophotometers or respiratory mass spectrometers can be utilized to continuously monitor airway carbon dioxide (CO$_2$). The measured level of CO$_2$ at the end of a complete expiration (PetCO$_2$) is related to PaCO$_2$. PetCO$_2$ may underestimate PaCO$_2$ when the dead space to tidal volume ratio is increased during sleep due to a reduction in tidal volume, and may be less accurate during supplemental oxygen or positive airway pressure therapy.

Pulse Transit Time

In persons with OSA, blood pressure (BP) fluctuates during sleep with transient increases in BP accompanying arousals from sleep, and falls in BP seen during inspiration. Pulse transit time (PTT), which is inversely related to BP, is the transmission time taken by the arterial pulse pressure wave as it travels from the aortic valve to the periphery (interval between the EKG R-wave and the subsequent pulse shock wave at the finger); the PSS is typically about 250 ms. The speed of the shock wave is affected by the stiffness of the arterial walls and BP. PTT increases during inspiratory falls in BP and decreases during arousal-induced increases in BP.

Reportedly, PTT is useful in distinguishing between central and obstructive apnea-hypopneas. In addition, it may help differentiate patients requiring nasal continuous positive airway pressure (CPAP) from those who do not.

Snoring

Sound or vibration originating from the upper airways can be detected using a microphone.

Electromyography (Anterior Tibialis)

Electrodes placed over the anterior tibialis of both legs are used to detect periodic leg movements during sleep. Additional electrodes can be placed over the upper limbs (extensor digitorum communis) to identify REM sleep behavior disorder.

Sleep-Related Breathing Disorders

The American Academy of Sleep Medicine (AASM) Task Force report on SRBDs in adults, published in 1999, defined four separate syndromes associated with abnormal respiratory events during sleep: obstructive sleep apnea-hypopnea, central sleep apnea-hypopnea, Cheyne-Stokes breathing, and sleep hypoventilation syndrome. UARS was not regarded as a distinct syndrome; instead, RERAs were considered to be part of obstructive sleep apnea-hypopnea. These four SRBDs are outlined in Table 2–3.

Sleep Staging

Polysomnographic data are divided into 30-second time periods, or *epochs*. The standard sleep study paper speed is 10 millimeters per second (ie, 30 centimeters per epoch page). In contrast,

Table 2–3. Sleep-related breathing disorders

Syndrome	Features
Obstructive sleep apnea-hypopnea syndrome	Repetitive reduction or cessation of airflow despite the presence of respiratory efforts due to partial or complete upper airway occlusion during sleep. Episodes are accompanied by oxygen desaturation, arousals, and sleep disruption. This syndrome includes mixed apneas, in which an initial period of apnea secondary to an absence of respiratory efforts precedes the upper airway obstruction. In routine clinical care, it is not necessary to distinguish apneas from hypopneas, and often the two respiratory events are scored, and reported together. Measurement techniques that identify hypopneas are able to detect apneas as well; in contrast, methods that measure apneas may not necessarily be adequate in identifying hypopneic events. A reduction in total oronasal airflow detected by a pneumotachometer placed in a well-fitted face mask is the reference standard for measuring obstructive apnea-hypopneas. Other methods that can be utilized to identify obstructive apnea-hypopneas include measurement of nasal pressure, respiratory inductance plethysmography (RIP), piezo sensors, strain gauges, thoracic impedance, thermal sensors, and expired carbon dioxide ($PetCO_2$.) Respiratory effort–related arousals (RERAs) consist of increasing respiratory efforts (progressively more negative esophageal pressures), lasting 10 seconds or longer, culminating in arousals (or a change in esophageal pressure to a less negative level). These events do not fulfill the criteria for either apnea or hypopnea. The reference standard for identifying a RERA is the measurement of esophageal pressure. RERAs can also be detected using measurements of nasal pressure, and surface diaphragmatic EMG. The sum of apneas, and hypopneas divided by the total sleep time is commonly referred to as the apnea-hypopnea Index. Respiratory disturbance index is the sum of apneas, hypopneas, and RERAs divided by the total sleep time.
Central sleep apnea-hypopnea syndrome	Presence of repetitive episodes of apneas or hypopneas during sleep that are not accompanied by upper airway obstruction. A central apnea-hypopnea event consists of a reduction of airflow lasting 10 seconds or longer along with a reduction in esophageal pressure excursions compared to baseline. Respiratory events are often associated with oxygen desaturation, and arousals. Esophageal pressure monitoring is the reference standard measurement of central apnea-hypopneas. RIP, surface diaphragmatic EMG, thermal sensors, expired carbon dioxide ($PetCO_2$), piezo sensors, and strain gauges are relatively insensitive in identifying central apnea-hypopneas.
Cheyne-Stokes breathing syndrome	Cyclical waxing, and waning of respiration with central apnea or hypopnea alternating with hyperpnea. Transient arousals often occur at the crest of hyperpnea, leading to sleep fragmentation, and excessive somnolence. Measurements of airflow using a pneumotachometer, and esophageal pressure monitoring are the reference standards for measuring airflow, and respiratory effort, respectively. Other techniques for detecting Cheyne-Stokes breathing include RIP, surface diaphragmatic EMG, oronasal airflow monitoring, and oximetry.
Sleep hypoventilation syndrome	Both oxygen desaturation, and hypercapnia (increase in $PaCO_2$ during sleep by greater than 10 mm Hg compared to levels during wakefulness), unrelated to distinct periods of apnea-hypopnea, are present during sleep. Periods of central hypoventilation are more frequent and more severe during REM sleep than in NREM sleep. Diurnal hypercapnia is frequently present. $PaCO_2$ is the reference standard measurement. Other techniques that have been utilized to monitor sleep hypoventilation include continuous oximetry (decline in SaO_2 without accompanying respiratory events), transcutaneous carbon dioxide ($PtcCO_2$) monitoring, calibrated RIP (reduced tidal volume, and minute ventilation), and $PetCO_2$ measurements.

EMG = electromyography; NREM = non-rapid eye movement; REM = rapid eye movement.

EEG evaluation of seizure activity usually utilizes 10-second time periods (30 millimeters per second). Each epoch is assigned a sleep stage according to the stage that occupies the majority of the epoch.

Scoring Sleep in Newborns

Sleep scoring in newborns also follows an "epoch" approach using behavior, respiration, EEG, EOG, and EMG data to classify sleep into active REM sleep or quiet sleep. The term "*intermediate sleep*" is used when epochs do not fully meet criteria for active or quiet sleep.

Scoring in newborns is described in Table 2–4. Scoring in children older than 2 years of age follow the criteria established by Rechtschaffen and Kales.

Table 2–4. Scoring sleep and wakefulness in newborn infants

Feature	Awake	Active REM sleep	Quiet sleep
Behavior	Eyes open Visible movements Vocalizations	Eyes closed Visible movements (facial grimaces, smiles, movements of body, and limbs) Vocalizations	Eyes closed No body movements
Respiration	Variable	Irregular	Regular
EEG	Mixed slow-wave (theta) pattern with occasional beta, and delta waveforms	Low-voltage irregular pattern Mixed pattern	High-voltage slow pattern Trace alternant pattern Mixed pattern
EOG	Waking eye movements	Positive	Negative
EMG	Sustained tone with burst of phasic activity	Low	High

Note:
1. Respiration is classified as either regular (rate varies < 20 breaths per minute), or irregular (rate varies > 20 breaths per minute).
2. Electroencephalography (EEG) is classified as:
   a. High-voltage slow pattern—Continuous, medium- to high-amplitude (between 50, and 150 μV) waveforms; frequencies between 0.5, and 4.0 Hz; present in both quiet, and active REM sleep
   b. Low-voltage irregular pattern—Low-amplitude (between 14, and 35 μV) waveforms; frequencies between 5.0, and 8.0 Hz; present in active REM sleep
   c. Trace alternant pattern—Bursts of slow (0.5-3 Hz), high-amplitude waves (0.5-3 Hz), fast low-amplitude waves, and sharp waves (2-4 Hz) lasting several seconds interspersed with periods of relative quiescence (mixed frequency waveforms) lasting 4-8 seconds; present in quiet sleep
   d. Mixed pattern—High-, and low-voltage waveforms; present in both quiet, and active REM sleep
3. Electro-oculography (EOG) is classified as either positive (rapid eye movements are present) or negative (no rapid eye movements).
4. Electromyography (EMG is classified as either high (tonic activity occupies > half of epoch) or low (tonic activity occupies < half of epoch).

Factors Affecting Sleep Architecture

Many factors can change the relative percentages of sleep stages throughout the night. These include age, medication use, and medical, neurologic, and psychiatric disorders. Aging is associated with an increase in NREM stage 1 and 2 sleep, decrease in NREM stages 3 and 4 sleep, diminished amplitude of delta waves, and no significant change in REM sleep after young adulthood.

Recovery from sleep deprivation can give rise to an increase in NREM stages 3 and 4 sleep, as well as REM sleep. Antidepressants generally decrease REM sleep and increase REM sleep latency; conversely, discontinuation of antidepressants can cause an increase in REM sleep and decrease in REM sleep latency. Finally, patients unaccustomed to sleeping in the sleep laboratory may demonstrate a "first-night effect" characterized by a decrease in NREM stages 3 and 4 sleep as well as REM sleep.

Definitions of Common Polysomnographic Parameters

Several terms are routinely used to characterize sleep architecture and its many subdivisions (Table 2–5). REM sleep latency is defined as the period from the first epoch of sleep (sleep onset)

Table 2–5.   Definitions of polysomnographic parameters

Term	Definition
Apnea	Absence of airflow at the nose, and mouth for at least 10 seconds Classification of apneas: 1. Obstructive–absence of airflow despite the presence of respiratory efforts 2. Central–absence of airflow accompanying an absence of respiratory effort 3. Mixed–period of apnea consisting of an initial central component, and a terminal obstructive component
Apnea index	Number of apneas per hour of sleep
Apnea-hypopnea index	Number of apnea *plus* hypopneas per hour of sleep
Arousal	Sudden, and brief (3–14 seconds) change in EEG from sleep to wakefulness, or from a "deeper" (stages 3, and 4) to a "lighter " (stages 1, and 2) NREM sleep stage. It may be accompanied by an increase in EMG activity, body movements, or heart rate. Usually identified during NREM sleep by an abrupt change in EEG frequency of at least 3 seconds in duration, including alpha, theta, or beta activity (but not spindles or delta waves), following at least 10 seconds of continuous sleep NREM sleep arousals do not need to be accompanied by changes in chin EMG. During REM sleep arousals, EEG changes *are* accompanied by changes in chin EMG (increase in amplitude). Isolated increases in chin EMG amplitude without changes in EEG *do not* constitute an arousal "Movement arousal" is defined as a body movement associated with an EEG arousal (increase in alpha wave activity, decrease in wave amplitude, or paroxysmal high-voltage waveforms), and increase in EMG activity. Arousal index is calculated as the number of arousals per hour of sleep.
Awakening	Occurrence of an awake state (alpha, and beta EEG activity, and increase in chin EMG tone) from any state of sleep
Bedtime	Time when a person gets into bed, and attempts to fall asleep
Drowsiness	Period of wakefulness that commonly precedes sleep onset, characterized by diffuse alpha EEG activity with eyes closed
Final wake-up	Time when a person awakens for the final time

Table 2–5. Definitions of polysomnographic parameters—cont'd

Term	Definition
Hypopneas	Reduction of airflow or amplitude of thoraco-abdominal movement by at least 30% from baseline, of at least 10 seconds in duration, and accompanied by oxyhemoglobin desaturation of at least 4% (Medicare criteria) Alternative definition: Reduction of airflow by at least 50% from baseline, of at least 10 seconds in duration (AASM Chicago criteria)
Lights out	Time when sleep recording started
Lights on	Time when sleep recording ended
Movement time	Epochs in which sleep stage scoring is not possible because more than 50% of the epoch is obscured by movement artifact (if it occurs between two epochs of sleep) Note: Epoch is scored as stage wake if it meets criteria for movement time but is between two epochs of wake.
Periodic limb movement index	Number of periodic limb movements per hour of sleep
REM sleep latency	Time in minutes from the onset of sleep to the first epoch of REM sleep; About 60 to 120 minutes in healthy normal adults
Respiratory disturbance index	Number of apneas *plus* hypopneas *plus* respiratory effort related arousal per hour of sleep
Respiratory effort–related arousal	Arousals accompanied by a reduction in airflow (and increasing inspiratory effort) for at least 10 seconds that does not meet the criteria for either apnea or hypopnea, and is not associated with significant oxygen desaturation Identified as a transient flattening of the nasal pressure signal, or increasingly negative deflections on esophageal pressure monitoring (gold standard) followed by a sudden change in pressure to a less negative level, and an arousal
Respiratory arousal index	Number of arousals due to apneas, hypopneas, and respiratory effort related arousals per hour of sleep
Sleep efficiency	Ratio of total sleep time (TST) to time in bed (TIB) or total recording time; (TST × 100)/TIB
Sleep latency	Time from lights out to sleep onset (first epoch of any stage of sleep) Normally < 15–30 minutes; longer sleep latency (> 30 minutes) characterizes sleep-initiation insomnia Longer sleep latency also occurs when sleeping in a new environment ("first-night effect")
Time in bed	Duration of monitoring between lights out to lights on
Total recording time	Time from sleep onset to final awakening (total sleep time *plus* wake time after sleep onset *plus* movement time)
Total sleep episode	Time available for sleep during a study (total sleep time [TST] *plus* wake after sleep onset) Also known as total sleep period or sleep period time
Total sleep time	Sum of all sleep stages (NREM stages 1-4 sleep *plus* REM sleep) in minutes; also: total sleep episode *minus* wake time after sleep onset
Wake time after sleep onset	Time spent awake from sleep onset to final awakening

EEG = electroencephalography; EMG = electromyography.
NREM = non-rapid eye movement; REM = rapid eye movement.

to the first epoch of REM sleep. REM sleep latency usually ranges from 60 to 120 minutes. A sleep-onset REM period is generally defined as the occurrence of REM sleep within 10 to 20 minutes of sleep onset. Factors affecting REM sleep latency and percent REM sleep are described in Tables 2–6 and 2–7, respectively. Polysomnographic characteristics of sleep disorders are summarized in Table 2–8.

Table 2-6.   Factors affecting rapid eye movement sleep latency

Increase in REM latency	Decrease in REM latency	No change in REM latency

Advance in bedtime or first-night effect
Alcohol
Medication use:
  Clonidine
  REM sleep suppressant
    agents (MAOI, SSRI, TCA,
    trazodone, venlafaxine)
  Stimulant agents
    (amphetamine)
	Delay in bedtime
	Depression
	Narcolepsy (sleep onset REM
	  periods)
	Medication use:
	  Bupropion decreases REM sleep
	  latency
	Obstructive sleep apnea syndrome
	  (secondary to sleep deprivation)
	REM sleep deprivation
	Schizophrenia
	Sudden withdrawal of REM-
	  suppressing agents
		Medication use: Mirtazapine, and
		  nefazodone do not change REM
		  sleep latency

MAOI: Monoamine oxidase inhibitors; SSRI: Selective serotonin receptor inhibitors; TCA: Tricyclic antidepressants.

Table 2-7.	Increase in REM sleep	Decrease in REM sleep

Factors affecting percent rapid eye movement (REM) sleep	Bupropion
	Nefazodone
	Reserpine
	Withdrawal of REM-suppressants
	Note: Bupropion, and nefazodone
	  increase REM sleep in depressed
	  patients.
		Alcohol
		Amphetamines
		Benzodiazepines
		Clonidine
		Lithium
		MAOI
		Methylphenidate
		SSRI
		TCA
		Note: MAOIs are the most potent inhibitors of
		  REM sleep; mirtazapine, and trazodone do
		  not change REM sleep.

MAOI: Monoamine oxidase inhibitors; SSRI: Selective serotonin reuptake inhibitors; TCA: Tricyclic antidepressants.

Performing a Polysomnography: An Overview

Understanding the Polygraph Equipment

A polygraph is used to monitor and record several physiologic variables during sleep. It consists of a series of AC and DC amplifiers, and filters.

Table 2–8.	Sleep disorder	Polysomnographic features
Polysomnographic features of sleep disorders	Obstructive sleep apnea	↓ Sleep latency ↓ Sleep efficiency ↑ NREM stage 1 sleep ↓ NREM stages 3, and 4 sleep ↓ REM sleep ↑ Frequency of awakenings, and microarousals
	Narcolepsy	↓ Sleep latency ↓ Sleep efficiency ↑ NREM stage 2 sleep ↑ REM sleep ↓ REM sleep latency (< 20 minutes) ↑ Frequency of awakenings, and microarousals ↑ Wake time after sleep onset *Multiple sleep latency test:* ↓ Sleep latency ↓ REM sleep latency (sleep onset REM periods)
	Periodic limb movements of sleep	↑ NREM stage 1 sleep ↓ NREM stages 3, and 4 sleep ↑ Frequency of awakenings, and microarousals
	Primary insomnia	↑ Sleep latency ↓ Total sleep time ↓ NREM stages 3, and 4 sleep ↓ REM sleep latency ↑ REM sleep ↑ Wake time after sleep onset Note: May be normal

Specifically, AC amplifiers are used to record high-frequency parameters, such as EEG, EOG, EMG, and EKG. Filters are commonly incorporated into AC amplifier systems. High-frequency filters attenuate fast, presumably nonphysiologic, potentials, and low-frequency filters reduce slow potentials that might interfere with proper recording of physiologic parameters.

DC amplifiers, on the other hand, are used to record low-frequency physiologic variables, including oxygen saturation, esophageal pressures, or CPAP levels. DC amplifiers are not equipped with low-frequency filters.

Either AC or DC amplifiers can be used to record airflow and respiratory effort.

Most current polygraph systems convert data into digital signals rather than analog tracings (paper and ink). Digital systems permit multiple leads (EEG, EOG, and chin EMG) to be recorded against a common *referential* electrode. With referential recording, failure of individual electrodes can be easily identified; in contrast, failure of the referential electrode will result in poor signals in all leads. With *bipolar* recording, the voltage difference between two leads is recorded.

Patient Preparation

The polysomnography should, whenever possible, be performed during the patient's customary bedtime. A sleep diary should be completed for 2 weeks before the study. A presleep questionnaire, including measures of sleepiness (eg, Stanford Sleepiness Scale, Epworth Sleepiness Scale), is often completed by the patient prior to the start of the study.

Electrode Application

The quality of the recorded data depends on proper electrode application. Electrode impedances should be low (< 5000 Ω). EEG electrodes are applied according to the International 10–20 System of electrode placement. EOG electrodes are placed (using adhesive and *not collodion*) 1 cm lateral and superior to the outer canthus of one eye (right outer canthus) and 1 cm lateral and inferior to the outer canthus of the other eye (left outer canthus). Chin EMG electrodes are placed in the mental and submental areas.

Each channel should be calibrated properly using the appropriate settings for sensitivity, and high- and low-frequency filters. Typical settings for polysomnography leads are given in Table 2–9. Low filter settings, if set too high (eg, 1 Hz), can reduce the amplitude of delta wave activity in the EEG and amplitude of eye movements in the EOG. Polygraphs also have a 60-Hz notch filter designed to attenuate 60-cycle artifacts resulting from interference by 60-Hz electrical activity from power lines.

Table 2-9. Typical settings for PSG leads

	EEG	EOG	EMG	EKG	Airflow, and respiratory effort
Sensitivity	5 μV/mm	5 μV/mm	5–10 μV/mm	Start at 1 mV/cm	Start at 5–7 μV/mm
High-frequency filter (Hz)	30	30	90	30	15
Low-frequency filter (Hz)	0.3	0.3	10.0	0.3	0.1
Time constant (seconds)[a]	0.4	0.4	0.04	0.12	1

[a]Time constant (in seconds) is determined by the formula, $Fc = 1 / (2\pi / Tc)$, where Fc is the frequency at which the output voltage across a resistor is decreased to 70% of input voltage.

Other devices to measure EKG, airflow, respiratory effort, snore, extremity EMG, body position, and esophageal pressure are applied as previously discussed.

Physiologic Calibrations

Biocalibrations are performed after the electrodes have been applied and the patient has been attached to the polygraph machine. Specific instructions given to the patient are used to check the integrity of the electrodes and amplifiers, including their chosen filter and sensitivity settings (Table 2–10).

Starting and Monitoring the Study

The time when the recording started ("lights out") must be noted. Specific events that occur during the study (eg, unusual behavior or movements, snoring, parasomnias, seizures, bathroom trips,

Table 2–10. Biocalibration instructions

Instructions by sleep technologist	Polysomnographic leads checked
Open eyes, and look straight ahead for 30 seconds	EEG (attenuation of alpha activity)
Close eyes for 30 seconds	EEG (presence of alpha activity) EOG (slow rolling eye movements)
Look right, left, up, and down while keeping head still; slowly blink eyes five times	EOG
Clench teeth	Chin EMG
Breathe in, and breathe out; hold breath for 10 seconds	Airflow Respiratory effort
Move right toe/foot; move left toe/foot	Leg EMG
Extend, and flex right wrist; extend, and flex left wrist	Upper extremity EMG (if present)

or patient complaints) and the time of their occurrence should be noted. Any intervention by the sleep technologist, such as application of CPAP, changes in electrode placement, or alterations in polygraph settings, should also be properly documented.

Artifact Recognition and Troubleshooting

Artifacts can arise from faulty electrode placement or unwanted contamination by physiologic variables and environmental factors. Generalized artifacts affecting several or most channels often indicate a faulty reference electrode common to the affected channels, whereas localized artifacts affecting a single channel suggest a defect with the specific electrode itself. Less commonly, artifacts can be due to problems with monitoring devices or amplifiers. Problems with artifacts are described in Table 2–11.

Ending the Study

The time the study ended should be recorded ("lights out"). Biocalibrations are repeated to ensure the proper functioning of the monitoring devices and electrode leads. Finally, the patient is asked to complete a post-study questionnaire that includes a subjective assessment of sleep quality, latency and duration, and frequency of awakenings.

Indications for Polysomnography

Polysomnography is indicated for diagnosing SRBDs; titrating CPAP for SRBD; determining therapeutic benefits after upper airway surgery or therapy with dental devices for SRBD; monitoring resolution or recurrence of SRBD following significant weight loss or gain, respectively; diagnosing narcolepsy (followed by MSLT); and evaluation of atypical or injurious parasomnias, seizures, suspected periodic limb movements during sleep, or insomnia that persists despite pharmacologic and nonpharmacologic interventions. The AASM recommendations for polysomnography are listed in Box 2–4.

Table 2–11. Polysomnographic artifacts and troubleshooting

Artifact	Description	Correction (if required)
60-Hz interference	Due to interference from 60-Hz electrical activity from power lines, high, and unequal electrode impedance, or lead failure Produces a dense, almost square-shaped EEG tracing	Fix electrode placement or change leads to correct high, and unequal electrode impedance Use 60-Hz filter as a last resort
Bruxism	Episodic increase in chin EMG discharge that can also be noted in the EEG leads	
EKG artifact	Sharp deflections in affected leads synchronous with the electrocardiographic QRS complex	Link two affected reference electrodes (double referencing) to both mastoid electrodes
Electrode popping	Sudden, sharp high-amplitude, "spikelike" deflections due to electrode leads being pulled away from the skin (change in impedance) brought about by body or respiratory movements, or when the patient lies on the electrode itself May also be due to drying out of the electrode gel or to faulty electrodes	Fix electrode placement, or change to an alternate lead May try applying more electrode gel
EMG artifact	Brief discharges generally noted in the frontal (frontalis muscle), and temporal (temporalis muscle) leads	Fix electrode placement or change to an alternate lead
Prosthetic eye ("glass eye" artifact)	Eye movement is absent on one side corresponding to the enucleated eye	
Movement artifact	Discharges occurring with body movements The epoch is scored as movement time when greater than 50% of the epoch is obscured by movement artifacts	
Pulse artifact	Corresponds to cardiac pulsations	Change placement of electrodes, preferably over bony sites
Respiratory artifact	Slowly undulating waves synchronous with respiration	May be eliminated by changing sleep position
Snore artifact	Corresponds to periods of snoring	May be eliminated by repositioning electrodes
Sweat artifact	Slow-frequency undulating movement present in most channels often synchronous with respiration Due to alterations in electrode potentials by salt in sweat May resemble delta waves, and might result in overscoring of NREM stages 3, and 4 sleep	Can be prevented, and minimized by decreasing room temperature

Box 2–4.	
American Academy of Sleep Medicine recommendations for polysomnography	

SLEEP-RELATED BREATHING DISORDERS

The following recommendations apply to attended polysomnography or attended cardiorespiratory sleep study (type 3).

Indications for polysomnography:

1. Diagnosis of sleep-related breathing disorders (SRBD) (standard);

   a. A full-night polysomnography (PSG) is recommended. A second PSG night may be required if the first study is inconclusive in patients with a strong clinical suspicion for SRBD (standard).

   b. An attended cardiorespiratory sleep study (type 3) may be an acceptable alternative to full-night PSG for patients with a high likelihood of having SRBD provided that repeat testing with a full-night PSG is performed for negative cardiorespiratory sleep studies in symptomatic patients (standard).

2. Positive airway pressure (PAP) titration for SRBD (standard);

   a. A full-night PSG with continuous positive airway pressure (CPAP) titration is recommended for SRBD in patients with any of the following (standard):

      i. An RDI ≥ 15 per hour regardless of symptoms; or

      ii. An RDI ≥ 5 per hour, *and* excessive daytime sleepiness

   b. A cardiorespiratory sleep study (type 3) without the ability to perform sleep staging is not recommended for CPAP titration (standard)

   c. A split-night PSG with an initial diagnostic portion followed by CPAP titration on the same night is an acceptable alternative to a full-night PSG with CPAP titration for (standard):

      i. An apnea-hypopnea index (AHI) ≥ 40 during a minimum of 2 hours of diagnostic PSG

      ii. An AHI of 20 to 40 based on clinical judgment such as the presence of repetitive prolonged obstructions or marked oxygen desaturations

      iii. Duration of CPAP titration of greater than 3 hours

      iv. CPAP eliminates or nearly eliminates respiratory events during sleep, including REM sleep in a supine position

      v. A second full-night PSG with CPAP titration is recommended if duration of CPAP titration is less than 3 hours or if CPAP fails to successfully eliminate respiratory events during both NREM, and REM sleep.

3. Evaluation, as part of preoperative clinical work-up, to determine the presence of obstructive sleep apnea (OSA), prior to upper airway surgery for snoring or OSA. An attended cardiorespiratory sleep study (type 3) may also be used (standard).

4. Assessment of nocturnal symptoms suggestive of SRBD, or persistent symptoms despite optimal medical therapy in patients with heart failure (standard);

5. Evaluation of signs, and symptoms suspicious for SRBD in patients with:

   a. Coronary artery disease (guideline)

   b. Significant tachyarrhythmias or bradyarrhythmias (guideline)

   c. History of stroke or transient ischemic attacks (option)

Continued

(continued from page 57)
Box 2–4.

American Academy of Sleep Medicine recommendations for polysomnography

6. Evaluation of sleep-related symptoms that are not adequately diagnosed by other methods in patients with neuromuscular disorders (standard).

Indications for follow-up polysomnography:

1. Assessment of treatment results after good clinical response to oral devices, or after surgical treatment in patients with moderate to severe OSA; or after dental or surgical treatment of OSA if symptoms recur following a good initial therapeutic response. An attended cardiorespiratory sleep study (type 3) may also be used (standard).

2. Assessment of treatment results following significant weight loss in patients on (CPAP) therapy for OSA to determine if changes in CPAP pressures are necessary; following significant weight gain with recurrence of symptoms after an initial success with CPAP therapy for OSA to determine if changes in CPAP pressures are necessary; or with insufficient clinical response or with recurrence of symptoms after an initial success with CPAP therapy for OSA to determine if other sleep disorders are present (standard)

Follow-up polysomnography (or attended cardiorespiratory sleep study (type 3)) is *not* routinely indicated for patients who have become, and remain, symptom-free while on CPAP therapy (option).

A multiple sleep latency test (MSLT) is not routinely indicated for most patients with SRBD (standard).

Polysomnography used for the evaluation of SRBD should include recordings of EEG, EOG, chin EMG, EKG, airflow, respiratory effort, and oxygen saturation. Anterior tibialis EMG may be added to detect periodic limb movements (standard).

A cardiorespiratory sleep study (type 3) should include recordings of EKG (or heart rate), airflow, respiratory effort, and oxygen saturation (standard).

An attended study requires the continuous presence of a person trained to properly monitor both the patient, and polygraph recordings. (guideline)

Oximetry is not an acceptable alternative to PSG or an attended cardiorespiratory sleep study (type 3) for diagnosing SRBD (guideline).

The routine use of unattended polysomnography or cardiorespiratory sleep studies is not recommended. These studies may be used for those with severe symptoms of OSA, when an attended study is not readily available, and treatment is considered urgent (guideline).

The use of clinical models to predict the severity of OSA is not recommended. (option)

OTHER RESPIRATORY DISORDERS (CHRONIC LUNG DISORDERS, AND DISEASES ASSOCIATED WITH CHRONIC ALVEOLAR HYPOVENTILATION, AND HYPOXEMIA)

Polysomnography is *not* routinely indicated for the diagnosis of chronic lung diseases (standard).

Polysomnography is indicated for the evaluation of sleep-related symptoms that are not adequately diagnosed by other methods in patients with neuromuscular disorders (standard).

Nocturnal oximetry may be indicated to assess the level of hypoxemia (standard)

Pulmonary function tests, and arterial blood gases may be indicated to assess the level of respiratory dysfunction (option).

(continued from page 58)
Box 2–4.

American Academy of Sleep Medicine recommendations for polysomnography

NARCOLEPSY

Polysomnography, and an MSLT (performed on the day following PSG) are routinely indicated in the evaluation of patients with suspected narcolepsy (standard).

There are no alternatives to PSG, and MSLT for the diagnosis of narcolepsy (standard).

HLA (human leukocyte antigen) typing should not be used to replace PSG, and MSLT for the diagnosis of narcolepsy (option).

Polysomnography, and MSLT used for the evaluation of narcolepsy should include recordings of EEG, EOG, chin EMG, and EKG (standard).

Cardiorespiratory channels, and anterior tibialis EMG may be added to detect SRBD, and periodic limb movements (option).

Multiple sleep latency test should be performed based on recommended protocols. (standard).

PARASOMNIAS, AND SEIZURE DISORDERS

Indications for polysomnography:

1. Evaluation, with additional EEG derivations, and video recording, of arousals, and sleep disturbances that are presumed to be related to seizures when clinical evaluation, and standard EEG are inconclusive. (option).

2. Evaluation, with additional EEG derivations, and video recording, of sleep-related behaviors that are violent or potentially injurious (option).

3. Evaluation of presumed parasomnias with unusual or atypical features (guideline)

4. Evaluation of cases with forensic implications, either with onsets following trauma, or those associated with injurious behavior (option).

5. Evaluation of presumed parasomnia or seizure disorder that fail to respond to therapy (option)

Polysomnography is not routinely indicated for:

1. Clear diagnosis of typical, uncomplicated, and non-injurious parasomnias (option)

2. Seizure disorders with no signs, and symptoms consistent with a sleep disorder (option)

Polysomnography used for the evaluation of parasomnias or sleep-related seizure disorders should include recordings of EEG (including expanded bilateral montage), EOG, chin EMG, anterior tibialis or extensor digitorum EMG for body movements, audiovisual recording, and technologist observations (option).

Enhanced recognition of seizure activity requires paper speeds of at least 15 mm per second (preferably 30 mm per second), or, in digital EEG systems, sampling rates adequate to identify paroxysmal discharges (option).

Persons experienced or trained in both sleep medicine, and seizure recognition should make interpretations of polysomnography with video, and extended EEG montage (option).

A detailed clinical history (age of onset, time of occurrence during the night, frequency, regularity, and duration of episodes) must be obtained for every case of parasomnia (standard).

(continued from page 59)
Box 2–4.

American Academy of Sleep Medicine recommendations for polysomnography

Clinical evaluation alone is usually sufficient to diagnose uncomplicated, and non-injurious parasomnias (eg, disorders of arousal, nightmares, enuresis, sleep talking, and bruxism) (standard).

Clinical evaluation, neurologic examination, and EEG (awake, and asleep) are usually sufficient to diagnose sleep-related seizure disorder (option).

RESTLESS LEGS SYNDROME, AND PERIODIC LIMB MOVEMENT DISORDER

Polysomnography is indicated for the diagnosis of periodic limb movement disorder (standard).

Polysomnography is *not* routinely indicated for the diagnosis, and treatment of restless legs syndrome (standard).

Polysomnography used for the evaluation of periodic limb movements should include recordings of EEG, EOG, chin EMG, and anterior tibialis EMG. Respiratory effort, airflow, and oximetry may be added to detect SRBD (standard).

More than one PSG may be required to establish the diagnosis of PLMD because of its night-to-night variability (option).

Actigraphy is *not* indicated for the diagnosis of restless legs syndrome or periodic limb movement disorder. Actigraphy may be useful in assessing treatment effects of these disorders (option).

The suggested immobilization test, and forced immobilization test may aid in the diagnosis, and assessment of treatment response of restless legs syndrome (option).

DEPRESSION WITH INSOMNIA

Polysomnography, and MSLT are *not* routinely indicated for the diagnosis of depression (standard).

Interpretation of PSG or MSLT should take into consideration the use of antidepressants, which can affect sleep (guideline).

Antidepressant medications can alter REM sleep, and should be discontinued prior to PSG, and MSLT in patients who are being evaluated for narcolepsy (guideline).

CIRCADIAN RHYTHM SLEEP DISORDERS

Polysomnography is *not* routinely indicated for the diagnosis of circadian rhythm sleep disorders (standard).

Actigraphy may be useful in evaluating circadian rhythm patterns or disturbances in elderly, and nursing home patients; newborns, infants, children, and adolescents; patients with hypertension, depression or schizophrenia; or patients in inaccessible situations (option).

Serum, and urinary melatonin levels, as well as 24-hour core body temperature levels are alternative diagnostic methods used in research settings. (option).

Source: Adapted, and modified from: Kushida CA, Littner MR, Morgenthaler T, et al. Practice parameters for the indications for polysomnography, and related procedures: an update for 2005. Sleep. 2005;28(4):499–521.

A "split-night" polysomnography consists of an initial diagnostic portion during which at least 2 hours of sleep are recorded. This is followed by a CPAP titration to determine the single most effective pressure that eliminates respiratory events in all sleep stages and all sleep positions, corrects oxygen desaturation, and improves sleep quality.

Portable Polysomnography

Several levels of diagnostic sleep studies, both in attended and unattended settings, have been described (Table 2–12). The current standard of practice for the evaluation of patients with sleep-related breathing disorders in the United States is an attended in-laboratory overnight polysomnography.

Table 2-12.   Levels of diagnostic sleep studies

Level of study	Characteristics	Comments
Level 1	Attended in-laboratory full polysomnography (typically consists of EEG, EOG, chin EMG, airflow, respiratory effort, SaO$_2$, EKG, leg EMG, and body position)	Gold standard for the diagnosis of OSA
Level 2 (comprehensive portable polysomnography)	Unattended full polysomnography (monitors same parameters as Level 1 study including EEG, EOG, chin EMG, airflow, respiratory effort, SaO$_2$, EKG, leg EMG, and body position)	Validity of results may be limited by insufficient sleep time, absence of REM sleep, or absence of sleep in the supine position.
Level 3 (cardiorespiratory sleep studies, or modified portable sleep-apnea testing)	Cardiopulmonary studies consisting of 4 or more parameters (eg, airflow, SaO$_2$, respiratory effort, EKG, or body position)	Useful when there is a high pretest likelihood of OSA, Levels 1 or 2 studies are not readily available, and delay in testing is unacceptable. Might be useful for follow-up evaluation following therapy of patients previously diagnosed with OSA
Level 4 (continuous single or dual bioparameter recording)	Monitoring using only one or two parameters (eg, SaO$_2$, airflow or snoring)	Poor specificity, and sensitivity Not recommended for diagnosis of OSA

EEG = electroencephalography; EOG = electro-oculography; EMG = electromyography; EKG = electrocardiography; SaO$_2$ = oxygen saturation.

Portable monitoring utilizing devices that measure from one to several physiologic parameters have been used as a substitute for standard overnight polysomnography to assess patients with suspected OSA. Advantages of portable monitoring over standard overnight polysomnography include greater convenience and accessibility for patients, and lesser cost. Limitations of portable monitoring include the absence of a trained sleep technologist to correct any technical difficulties and attend to any patient needs during the test.

The use of portable monitoring has been proposed for evaluating patients with suspected OSA when standard PSG is not readily available and urgent therapy is required due to the severity of symptoms or when patients are unable to undergo laboratory testing (eg, medically unstable or nonambulatory). Portable monitoring can also be used to follow-up a patient with a prior diagnosis of OSA established by standard overnight polysomnography to determine their response to prescribed therapy. The AASM recommendations for the use of portable monitoring are listed in Box 2–5.

Box 2–5.

American Academy of Sleep Medicine recommendations for the use of portable monitoring devices in the evaluation of adults with suspected obstructive sleep apnea

TYPE 2 PORTABLE MONITORING DEVICES: COMPREHENSIVE PORTABLE POLYSOMNOGRAPHY

Type 2 portable monitoring (PM) devices, in both the attended, and unattended settings, are not recommended in the evaluation of patients with suspected OSA (option).

TYPE 3 PORTABLE MONITORING DEVICES: MODIFIED PORTABLE SLEEP APNEA TESTING

The use of some type 3 PM devices in an attended setting (standard), but not in an unattended setting (guideline), can be used to decrease or increase the probability that a patient has an apnea-hypopnea index (AHI) > 15.

The use of type 3 PM devices in an attended in-laboratory setting (standard), but not in an unattended setting (guideline), can be used to both rule in, and rule out a diagnosis of OSA.

TYPE 4 PORTABLE MONITORING DEVICES: CONTINUOUS SINGLE OR DUAL BIOPARAMETER RECORDING

The use of type 4 PM devices (with oximetry, and at least one other airflow measurement), in an attended setting, is not recommended to decrease or increase the probability that a patient has an AHI > 15 (option).

The use of type 4 PM devices (with oximetry, and at least one other airflow measurement), in an unattended setting, not recommended for the diagnosis of OSA, or establishing that a patient has an AHI > or is < 15 (guideline).

MISCELLANEOUS RECOMMENDATIONS

PM devices are not recommended for screening or diagnosis without knowledge of a patient's sleep-related history, and complaints, or for use in patients with comorbid disorders or secondary sleep complaints.

Review of raw data, manual scorning of data, and interpretation of data by physicians with sleep training, and who are familiar with PM devices are recommended.

Sleep laboratories using PM devices should confirm that studies documenting their performance, and conformity to other devices in their category are present.

Trained personnel should be available to perform technical scoring.

Source: Adapted, and modified from Practice parameters for the use of portable monitoring devices in the investigation of suspected obstructive sleep apnea in adults. A joint project sponsored by the American Academy of Sleep Medicine, the American Thoracic Society, and the American College of Chest Physicians. Sleep. 2003;26(7):907-13.
For a definition of terms , see the notefollowing Box 2-4

Multiple Sleep Latency Test

An MSLT measures a person's physiologic propensity to fall asleep in quiet situations. The indications for an MSLT are listed in Box 2–6. A nocturnal polysomnography during the patient's usual major sleep period should be performed immediately before an MSLT to exclude the presence of other sleep disorders and to ensure an adequate duration of nocturnal sleep (at least 6 hours). An MSLT should not be performed after a split-night sleep study.

Box 2-6. Indications for Multiple Sleep Latency Test	Evaluation of patients with complaints of excessive sleepiness
	Evaluation of patients with suspected narcolepsy or idiopathic hypersomnia
	Evaluation of response to treatment of excessive sleepiness

It consists of four or five nap opportunities, each 20 minutes in duration, performed every two hours. It is usually scheduled between 8:00 to 9:00 AM and 4:00 to 5:00 PM, with the first nap opportunity starting about 1.5 to 3 hours after awakening from the previous night's polysomnography.

Breakfast is provided at least 1 hour before the first nap, and lunch is given immediately after the second nap study. Smoking should be stopped 30 minutes before the start of every test. Bathroom trips, if needed, are scheduled prior to each trial. Caffeinated beverages, unusual bright light exposure, and vigorous physical activity should be avoided during the day of the study. Stimulating activities should be stopped 15 minutes prior to each nap trial. Electrodes should be connected and calibrated 5 minutes before lights out.

The patient is instructed to lie quietly, assume a comfortable position, close his/her eyes and try to fall asleep in a dark, quiet room. Room temperature should be adjusted based on the patient's level of comfort. Lights are then turned off ("lights out") and monitoring started. The EEG (central C3-A2, C4-A1, and occipital 01-A2, 02-A1), EOG, chin EMG and EKG are monitored to determine sleep latency (time from lights out to the onset of sleep) and the occurrence of REM sleep for each nap. Standard biocalibrations are performed before each trial.

The study is terminated if no sleep is recorded for 20 minutes. If sleep is recorded, the test is continued for another 15 minutes to allow REM sleep to develop. The test is stopped after the first epoch of unequivocal REM sleep. If no sleep occurs during a nap, its sleep latency is recorded as 20 minutes.

Between nap opportunities, the patient is asked to get out of bed and to remain awake until the next test. The shorter 4-nap test may be considered if at least two sleep onset REM periods have already occurred during earlier nap opportunities.

Sleep onset for clinical MSLTs is defined as the first epoch of any stage of sleep. Sleep latency (from lights out to the first epoch of sleep [sleep onset]), and the presence of sleep-onset REM periods (SOREMPs), defined as greater than 15 seconds of REM sleep in a 30-second epoch, are determined for each nap. REM latency is the duration from the first epoch of sleep to the beginning of the first epoch of REM sleep.

Sleep deprivation and acute withdrawal of stimulant agents can both influence the test results and should be excluded. An adequate sleep duration and regular sleep-wake schedule, as documented by sleep diaries or actigraphy, must have been maintained for at least 1 to 2 weeks preceding MSLT. Furthermore, medications that can potentially influence sleep latency and REM sleep, such as stimulants, opiates, benzodiazepines, narcotics, and REM suppressants, should be discontinued for at least 2 weeks before the study. A urine drug screen during the study is required to rule out the recent use of opiates, sedatives, hypnotics, and stimulants. OSA, if present, should be appropriately treated before performing an MSLT. In patients using CPAP for OSA, both PSG and MSLT are performed at the usual prescribed CPAP pressure.

Short mean sleep latencies suggest the presence of excessive sleepiness. There appears to be a circadian variability in sleep latencies (shortest during the third and fourth naps occurring at noon and early afternoon, and longest in the late afternoon), and propensity for REM sleep (greatest during the first nap). Some values for mean sleep latencies are given in Table 2–13.

Table 2–13. Mean sleep latencies

Patient group	Mean +/-SD (minutes)
Normal controls, four-nap MSLT[a]	10.4 +/– 4.3
Normal controls, five-nap MSLT[a]	11.6 +/– 5.2
Patients with narcolepsy	3.1 +/– 2.9
Patients with idiopathic hypersomnia	6.2 +/– 3.0

[a]Mean sleep latency values are lower for normal middle-aged adults (30-39 years of age) compared with normal older adults.

The presence of 2 or more SOREMPs has a sensitivity of 0.78 and a specificity of 0.93 for the diagnosis of narcolepsy. SOREMPs can also be seen in other sleep disorders, such as OSA and sleep deprivation. The frequency of SOREMPs is inversely related to mean sleep latency values.

Results of MSLT should be interpreted along with data obtained from clinical evaluation, polysomnography, and other laboratory tests. MSLT parameters are not as well established for children less than 8 years of age.

Recommendations for use of the MLST are listed in Box 2–7.

Maintenance of Wakefulness Test

The Maintenance of Wakefulness Test (MWT) measures a person's ability to remain awake in quiet situations. It consists of four nap opportunities, each 40 minutes in duration, performed at 2-hour intervals, with the patient in a dark, quiet room sitting in bed in a semireclined position with the back and head supported by a bed rest. Room temperature should be adjusted based on the patient's level of comfort. The first nap trial is started about 1.5 to 3 hours after the patient's customary wake time. Whether or not sleep logs are used or if polysomnography is to be performed prior to the test should be individualized as determined by the clinician. The use of tobacco, caffeine, and stimulant agents should be avoided.

A light breakfast is provided 1 hour before the first trial, and lunch is given immediately after the second trial. Bathroom trips, if needed, are scheduled prior to each trial. Standard biocalibrations are performed before each trial.

Patients are instructed to sit still, look directly while avoiding the light, and try to stay awake during the test. Measures to stay awake such as singing are not allowed. EEG (central and occipital leads), EOG, and chin EMG are used to determine the sleep latency (from lights out to the first epoch of sleep [sleep onset]) for each nap. Each nap test is terminated once unequivocal sleep (defined as three consecutive epochs of stage 1 sleep, or one epoch of any other sleep stage) occurs, or after 40 minutes if no sleep is recorded. Drug screening may be considered.

Box 2–7.	**STANDARD**
American Academy of Sleep Medicine (ASAM) recommendation for use of the multiple sleep latency test	

STANDARD

1. The MSLT is an objective measure of an individual's ability or tendency to fall asleep.

2. Appropriate conditions for the test, proper recording techniques, accepted protocols, and interpretation by qualified clinicians are required.

3. The test is indicated for patients suspected of having narcolepsy.

4. Indications for repeat MSLT testing include:

    a. Absence of appropriate study conditions or presence of extraneous factors that might affect the results during the initial testing;

    b. Results are uninterpretable, vague or uncertain;, and

    c. Failure of initial test to confirm the diagnosis of narcolepsy in patients with a high clinical suspicion of narcolepsy.

GUIDELINE

The MSLT is not routinely indicated in the initial evaluation, or follow-up during CPAP therapy, of patients with obstructive sleep apnea.

OPTION

1. The MSLT may be indicated for the evaluation of sleepiness to distinguish between idiopathic hypersomnia, and narcolepsy.

2. The MSLT is not routinely indicated for evaluation of sleepiness secondary to insomnia, circadian rhythm disorders, and medical or neurologic disorders (except narcolepsy).

Source: Adapted, and modified from Standards of Practice Committee of the American Academy of Sleep Medicine (AASM). Practice parameters for clinical use of the multiple sleep latency test, and the maintenance of wakefulness test. Sleep. 2005;28(1):113-121. For a definition of terms , see the notefollowing Box 2-4

Sleep latency correlates with the ability to stay awake. Mean sleep latency of less than 8 minutes on the 40-min MWT is considered abnormal. Staying awake on all trials may provide an appropriate expectation for individuals who require the highest level of alertness for safety. Values greater than 8 minutes but less than 40 minutes are of uncertain significance.

The MWT is less sensitive than MSLT in measuring sleepiness but may be useful for monitoring treatment response to stimulant medications used for excessive sleepiness in narcolepsy or to CPAP therapy for OSA. The AASM recommendations for use of the MWT are listed in Box 2–8.

Actigraphy

Periods of rest/sleep or activity can be discerned using an actigraph, which produces a signal whenever movement is detected. Movements are detected using accelerometers that are typically worn on the wrist. Motion of the wrists generates changes in voltages that are recorded over several days to weeks. Movement data are summed over a specified time interval from 15 seconds to 15 minutes,

Box 2–8.

American Academy of Sleep Medicine recommendations for use of the maintenance of wakefulness test

STANDARD

1. The MWT is an objective measure of an individual's ability to remain awake for a defined time. It is used, in association with clinical history, to assess the ability to maintain wakefulness.

2. Appropriate conditions for the test, proper recording techniques, accepted protocols, and interpretation by qualified clinicians are required.

GUIDELINE

1. The MWT may be indicated to assess response to treatment in patients with excessive sleepiness.

OPTION

1. The MWT 40 minute protocol is recommended in assessing an individual's ability to remain awake or when an inability to remain awake represents a public or personal safety issue.

Source: Adapted, and modified from Standards of Practice Committee of the American Academy of Sleep Medicine (AASM). Practice parameters for clinical use of the multiple sleep latency test, and the maintenance of wakefulness test. Sleep. 2005;28(1):113-121. For a definition of terms , see the notefollowing Box 2-4

with a typical epoch duration of less than 2 minutes when scoring sleep. Each epoch is scored as wake or sleep based on predetermined amplitude or time thresholds for activity counts. Thus, an epoch is considered wake if the summed voltage of an epoch is greater than the set amplitude threshold, or if the duration of an epoch with voltages over a certain level is greater than the set time threshold.

Actigraphy provides estimates of circadian rhythms of sleep and wakefulness. It permits the following data to be obtained: total wake time, total sleep time, sleep latency (if used along with an event monitor to mark the time when the patient desires to fall asleep), frequency of awakenings, and wake time after sleep onset. In addition, it appears to be better at measuring sleep duration than in identifying sleep initiation. There is a higher degree of correlation between polysomnography and actigraphy for total sleep time, total awake time, and sleep continuity among normal sleepers than in patients with insomnia or sleep disturbances. Polysomnography tends to detect more sleep time compared to actigraphy in both normal sleepers and in patients with insomnia. Accuracy of recordings is decreased in persons with periodic limb movements during sleep or other sleep-related movement disorders as well as in those who habitually remain inactive in bed or in a chair while awake.

Because of its portability, actigraphy permits extended monitoring over several days to weeks while the patient maintains regular daytime and nighttime activities, with minimal patient bias or compliance. The precise role(s) of actigraphy in the evaluation of the patient with a sleep complaint remains to be defined. It may provide additional information regarding patterns of sleep and wakefulness in persons whose reported sleep diary may be unreliable. AASM recommendations for the role of actigraphy in the study of sleep are described in Box 2–9.

Box 2-9.

American Academy of Sleep Medicine recommendations for the role of actigraphy in the study of sleep, and circadian rhythms

1. Actigraphy is a reliable, and valid method of detecting sleep in normal, healthy adults (standard).

2. Actigraphy is not indicated for the *routine* diagnosis, assessment of severity, and management of any sleep disorder (guideline).

3. Actigraphy may be useful in the following clinical situations:

    a. Assessing specific aspects of insomnia (ie, sleep variability, sleep phase alterations, and treatment effects) or restless legs syndrome/periodic limb movement disorder (ie, treatment effects) (guideline)

    b. As an adjunct to history, examination, and sleep diary for the diagnosis, and treatment of insomnia, circadian -rhythm disorders, and excessive sleepiness when (option):

        i. Evaluation, and therapy would benefit from additional objective data such as multiday rest-activity patterns, day-to-day timing, amount or patterns of sleep;

        ii. Severity of reported sleep disturbance appears inconsistent with clinical impressions or laboratory data

        iii. Clarification of effects of, and compliance with, therapy is necessary

        iv. Regular sleep assessment methods are not clearly helpful (ie, history cannot be obtained accurately, and polysomnography has either already been done, is considered unlikely to be useful in diagnosis; or is not indicated or immediately available) in symptomatic patients

    c. Assessing daytime sleepiness when more standard techniques, such as the multiple sleep latency test, is not practical (option).

    d. Characterizing, and monitoring patterns or disturbances in circadian rhythm among the elderly, and nursing home residents; children from birth to adolescence; patients with hypertension, depression, or schizophrenia;, and persons in inaccessible locations (option).

    e. Conducting outcome studies in patients with sleep disorders enrolled in interventional trials; healthy adults; children; elderly;, and patients with certain medical, and psychiatric disorders (option).

    f. Determining patterns of rest, and activity as part of portable sleep apnea testing (option).

4. Actigraphy is effective in demonstrating multiday rest-activity patterns, and in estimating sleep-wake patterns when sleep logs or observations cannot provide similar information. Nevertheless, completion of a sleep log during the period of actigraphic testing is useful (option).

5. Actigraphy monitoring should include at least three consecutive 24-hour periods (option).

6. Superiority of one actigraphy placement over others on different parts of the body is not established (guideline).

7. Personnel using actigraphy should inspect the raw data obtained by proper procedures utilizing algorithms validated for the specific actigraphy device used. Automatic scoring is acceptable in addition to manual methods of scoring, as is some preprocessing of movement counts. Epoch lengths up to 1 minute are usually sufficient except for assessment of circadian rhythms (option).

Source: Adapted, and modified from: Standards of Practice Committee of the American Academy of Sleep Medicine (AASM). Practice parameters for the role of actigraphy in the study of sleep, and circadian rhythms: an update for 2002. Sleep. 2003;26(3):337-41. For a definition of terms , see the notefollowing Box 2-4

References

General References

American Academy of Sleep Medicine. *The International Classification of Sleep Disorders: Diagnostic and Coding Manual.* 2nd ed. Westchester, IL: American Academy of Sleep Medicine, 2005.

Bowman TJ. *Review of Sleep Medicine.* Burlington, MA: Butterworth-Heinemann, 2002.

Berry RB. *Sleep Medicine Pearls* (2nd ed.). Philadelphia, PA: Hanley & Belfus, 2002.

Chokroverty S. *Clinical Companion to Sleep Disorders Medicine.* 2nd ed. Butterworth-Heinemann, 2000.

Lavie P, Pillar G, Malhotra A. *Sleep Disorders Handbook.* New York, NY: Taylor & Francis, 2002.

Lee-Chiong TL, ed. *Sleep: A Comprehensive Handbook.* Hoboken, NJ: John Wiley & Sons, 2006.

Lee-Chiong TL, Sateia M, Carskadon M, eds. *Sleep Medicine.* Philadelphia, PA: Hanley & Belfus (Elsevier), 2002.

Perlis ML, Lichstein KL, eds. *Treating Sleep Disorders: Principles and Practice of Behavioral Sleep Medicine.* Hoboken, NJ: John Wiley & Sons, 2003.

Rechtschaffen A, Kales A. *A Manual of Standardized Terminology, Techniques and Scoring System for Sleep Stages of Human Subjects.* Los Angeles, CA: Brain Information Service/Brain Research Institute, University of California, 1968.

Reite M, Ruddy J, Nagel K. *Concise Guide to Evaluation and Management of Sleep Disorders.* 3rd ed. Arlington, VA: American Psychiatric Publishing, April 2002.

Rosen G. Evaluation of the patient who has sleep complaints: a case-based method using the sleep process matrix. *Sleep Medicine. Primary Care: Clinics in Office Practice.* Philadelphia, PA: Elsevier Saunders, 2005.

Sleep Disorders. Medical Clinics of North America. Philadelphia, PA: Elsevier Saunders, 2004.

Sleep Medicine. Primary Care: Clinics in Office Practice. Philadelphia, PA: Elsevier Saunders, 2005.

Sleep Research Society. *SRS Basics of Sleep Guide.* Westchester, IL: Sleep Research Society, 2005.

Sleep History

Lee-Chiong TL, ed. *Sleep: A Comprehensive Handbook.* Hoboken, NJ: John Wiley & Sons, 2006.

Lee-Chiong TL, Sateia M, Carskadon M, eds. *Sleep Medicine.* Philadelphia, PA: Hanley & Belfus (Elsevier), 2002.

Manifestations of Sleep Disorders

Lee-Chiong TL, ed. *Sleep: A Comprehensive Handbook.* Hoboken, NJ: John Wiley & Sons, 2006.

Lee-Chiong TL, Sateia M, Carskadon M, eds. *Sleep Medicine.* Philadelphia, PA: Hanley & Belfus (Elsevier), 2002.

Sleep Diaries

Lee-Chiong TL, ed. *Sleep: A Comprehensive Handbook.* Hoboken, NJ: John Wiley & Sons, 2006.

Lee-Chiong TL, Sateia M, Carskadon M, eds. *Sleep Medicine*. Philadelphia, PA: Hanley & Belfus (Elsevier), 2002.

Sleep Questionnaires

Lee-Chiong TL, ed. *Sleep: A Comprehensive Handbook*. Hoboken, NJ: John Wiley & Sons, 2006.

Lee-Chiong TL, Sateia M, Carskadon M, eds. *Sleep Medicine*. Philadelphia, PA: Hanley & Belfus (Elsevier), 2002.

Physical Examination

Lee-Chiong TL, ed. *Sleep: A Comprehensive Handbook*. Hoboken, NJ: John Wiley & Sons, 2006.

Lee-Chiong TL, Sateia M, Carskadon M, eds. *Sleep Medicine*. Philadelphia, PA: Hanley & Belfus (Elsevier), 2002.

Polysomnography

American Academy of Sleep Medicine Task Force. Sleep-related breathing disorders in adults: recommendations for syndrome definition and measurement techniques in clinical research. *Sleep*. 1999;22:667–689.

Argod J, Pepin JL, Levy P. Differentiating obstructive and central sleep respiratory events through pulse transit time. *Am J Respir Crit Care Med*. 1998;158:1778–1783.

Ayappa I, Norman RG, Rapoport DM. Cardiogenic oscillations on the airflow signal during continuous positive airway pressure as a marker of central apnea. *Chest*.1999;116:660–666.

Berg S, Haight JSJ, Yap V, Hoffstein V, Cole P. Comparison of direct and indirect measurements of respiratory airflow: implications for hypopneas. *Sleep*. 1997;20:60–64.

Boudewyns A, Willeman M, Wagemans M, De Cock W, Van de Heyning P, De Backer W. Assessment of respiratory effort by means of strain gauges and esophageal pressure swings: a comparative study. *Sleep*. 1997;20:168–170.

Cantineau JP, Escourrou P, Sartene R, Gaultier C, Goldman M. Accuracy of respiratory inductive plethysmography during wakefulness and sleep in patients with obstructive sleep apnea. *Chest*. 1992;102:1145–1151.

Chadha TS, Watson H, Birch S, Jenouri GA, Schneider AW, Cohn MA, et al. Validation of respiratory inductive plethysmography using different calibration procedures. *Am Rev Respir Dis*. 1982;125:644–649.

Clark JS, Votteri B, Ariagno RL, Cheung P, Eichhorn JH, Fallat RJ, et al. Noninvasive assessment of blood gases. *Am Rev Respir Dis*. 1992;145:220–232.

Collard P, Aubert G, Rodenstein DO. Value of nocturnal pulse oximetry as a screening tool for sleep apnea-hypopnea syndrome. *Am Rev Respir Dis*. 1992;145:A724.

Cummiskey J, Williams TC, Krumpe PE, Guilleminault C. The detection and quantification of sleep apnea by tracheal sound recordings. *Am Rev Respir Dis*. 1982;126:221–224.

Davies RJO, Vardi-Visy K, Clarke M, Stradling JR. Identification of sleep disruption and sleep disordered breathing from systolic blood pressure profile. *Thorax*. 1993;48:1242–1247.

Epstein LJ, Dorlac GR. Cost-effectiveness analysis of nocturnal oximetry as a method of screening for sleep apnea-hypopnea syndrome. *Chest*. 1998;113:97–103.

Farre R, Montserrat JM, Ballester E, Hernandez L, Rotger M, Navajas D. Importance of the pulse oximeter averaging time when measuring oxygen desaturation in sleep apnea. *Sleep*. 1998;21: 386–390.

Farre R, Montserrat JM, Rotger M, Ballester E, Navajas D. Accuracy of thermistors and thermo-couples as flow-measuring devices for detecting hypopneas. *Eur Respir J*. 1998; 11:179–182.

Gyulay S, Olson LG, Hensley MJ, King MT, Allen KM, Saunders NA. A comparison of clinical assessment and home oximetry in the diagnosis of obstructive sleep apnea. *Am Rev Respir Dis*. 1993;147:50–53.

Hosselet JJ, Norman RG, Ayappa I, Rapoport DM. Detection of flow limitation with a nasal can-nula/pressure transducer system. *Am J Respir Crit Care Med*. 1998;157:1461–1467.

Kesten S, Chapman KR, Rebuck AS. Response characteristics of a dual transcutaneous oxygen/carbon dioxide monitoring system. *Chest*. 1991;99:1211–1215.

Konn K, Mead J. Measurement of the separate volume changes of rib cage and abdomen during breathing. *J Appl Physiol*. 1967;22:407–422.

Kryger MH. Monitoring respiratory and cardiac function. In: Kryger MH, Roth T, Dement WC, eds. *Principles and Practice of Sleep Medicine* (3rd ed.). Philadelphia, PA: W.B. Saunders 2000, 1217–1230.

Loveridge B, Perez-Padilla R, West P, Anthonisen NR, Kryger M. Comparison of the stability of the respiratory inductance plethysmograph versus mercury strain gauges in measuring ventilation. *Am Rev Respir Dis*. 1984;129:A82.

Morielli A, Desjardins D, Brouillette RT. Transcutaneous and end-tidal carbon dioxide pressures should be measured during pediatric polysomnography. *Am Rev Respir Dis*. 1993;148:1599–1604.

Norman RG, Ahmed MM, Walsleben JA, Rapoport DM. Detection of respiratory events during NPSG: nasal cannula/pressure sensor versus thermistor. *Sleep*. 1997;20:1175–1184.

Phillips BA, Anstead MI, Gottlieb DJ. Monitoring sleep and breathing: methodology. Part I: Monitoring breathing. *Clin Chest Med*. 1998;1:203–212.

Pitson DJ, Sandell A, van der Hout R, Stradling JR. Use of pulse transit time as a measure of inspi-ratory effort in patients with obstructive sleep apnoea. *Eur Respir J*. 1995;8:1669–1674.

Sanders MH, Kern NB, Costantino JP, Stiller RA, Strollo PJ, Studniki KA, et al. Accuracy of end-tidal and transcutaneous PCO$_2$ monitoring during sleep. *Chest*. 1994;106:472–483.

Series F, Marc I. Accuracy of breath-by-breath analysis of flow-volume loop in identifying sleep-induced flow-limited breathing cycles in sleep apnoea-hypopnoea syndrome. *Clin Sci*. 1995;88:707–712.

Series F, Marc I. Nasal pressure recording in the diagnosis of sleep apnoea hypopnoea syndrome. *Thorax*. 1999;54:506–510.

Sharp JT, Druz WS, Foster JR, Wicks MS, Chokroverty S. Use of the respiratory magnetometer in diagnosis and classification of sleep apnea. *Chest*. 1980;77:350–353.

Sorkin B, Rapoport DM, Falk DB, Goldring RM. Canopy ventilation monitor for quantitative mea-surement of ventilation during sleep. *J Appl Physiol*. 1980;48:724–730.

Staats BA, Bonekat HW, Harris CD, Offord KP. Chest wall motion in sleep apnea. *Am Rev Respir Dis*. 1984;130:59–63.

Stoohs R, Skrobal A, Harter R, Guilleminault C. Snoring sound level as a predictor of flow limitation. *Am Rev Respir Dis.* 1992;145:A724.

West P, George CF, Kryger MH. Dynamic in vivo response characteristics of three oximeters: Hewlett-Packard 47201A, Biox III, and Nellcor N-100. *Sleep.* 1987;10:263–271.

Whyte KF, Allen MB, Fitzpatrick MF, Douglas NJ. Accuracy and significance of scoring hypopneas. *Sleep.* 1992;15:257–260.

Whyte KF, Gugger M, Gould GA, Molloy J, Wraith PK, Douglas NJ. Accuracy of respiratory inductive plethysmograph in measuring tidal volume during sleep. *J Appl Physiol.* 1991;71:1866–1871.

Yamashiro Y, Kryger MH. Nocturnal oximetry: is it a screening tool for sleep disorders? *Sleep.* 1995;18:167–171.

Yelderman M, New W. Evaluation of pulse oximetry. *Anesthesiology.* 1983;59:349–352.

Sleep-Related Breathing Disorders

American Academy of Sleep Medicine Task Force. Sleep-related breathing disorders in adults: recommendations for syndrome definition and measurement techniques in clinical research. *Sleep.* 1999;22:667–689.

Sleep Staging

Lee-Chiong TL, ed. *Sleep: A Comprehensive Handbook.* Hoboken, NJ: John Wiley & Sons, 2006.

Lee-Chiong TL, Sateia M, Carskadon M, eds. *Sleep Medicine.* Philadelphia, PA: Hanley & Belfus (Elsevier), 2002.

Scoring Sleep in Newborns

Lee-Chiong TL, ed. *Sleep: A Comprehensive Handbook.* Hoboken, NJ: John Wiley & Sons, 2006.

Lee-Chiong TL, Sateia M, Carskadon M, eds. *Sleep Medicine.* Philadelphia, PA: Hanley & Belfus (Elsevier), 2002.

Factors Affecting Sleep Architecture

Lee-Chiong TL, ed. *Sleep: A Comprehensive Handbook.* Hoboken, NJ: John Wiley & Sons, 2006.

Lee-Chiong TL, Sateia M, Carskadon M, eds. *Sleep Medicine.* Philadelphia, PA: Hanley & Belfus (Elsevier), 2002.

Definitions of Common Polysomnographic Parameters

Lee-Chiong TL, ed. *Sleep: A Comprehensive Handbook.* Hoboken, NJ: John Wiley & Sons, 2006.

Lee-Chiong TL, Sateia M, Carskadon M, eds. *Sleep Medicine.* Philadelphia, PA: Hanley & Belfus (Elsevier), 2002.

Performing a Polysomnography: An Overview

Lee-Chiong TL, ed. *Sleep: A Comprehensive Handbook.* Hoboken, NJ: John Wiley & Sons, 2006.

Lee-Chiong TL, Sateia M, Carskadon M, eds. *Sleep Medicine.* Philadelphia, PA: Hanley & Belfus (Elsevier), 2002.

Indications for Polysomnography

Kushida CA, Littner MR, Morgenthaler T, et al. Practice parameters for the indications for polysomnography and related procedures: an update for 2005. *Sleep.* 2005;28(4):499–521.

Portable Polysomnography

Practice parameters for the use of portable monitoring devices in the investigation of suspected obstructive sleep apnea in adults. A joint project sponsored by the American Academy of Sleep Medicine, the American Thoracic Society, and the American College of Chest Physicians. *Sleep.* 2003;26(7):907–13.

Multiple Sleep Latency Test

Lee-Chiong TL, ed. *Sleep: A Comprehensive Handbook.* Hoboken, NJ: John Wiley & Sons, 2006.

Lee-Chiong TL, Sateia M, Carskadon M, eds. *Sleep Medicine.* Philadelphia, PA: Hanley & Belfus (Elsevier), 2002.

Standards of Practice Committee of the American Academy of Sleep Medicine (AASM). Practice parameters for clinical use of the multiple sleep latency test and the maintenance of wakefulness test. *Sleep.* 2005;28(1):113–121.

Maintenance of Wakefulness Test

Lee-Chiong TL, ed. *Sleep: A Comprehensive Handbook.* Hoboken, NJ: John Wiley & Sons, 2006.

Lee-Chiong TL, Sateia M, Carskadon M, eds. *Sleep Medicine.* Philadelphia, PA: Hanley & Belfus (Elsevier), 2002.

Standards of Practice Committee of the American Academy of Sleep Medicine (AASM). Practice parameters for clinical use of the multiple sleep latency test and the maintenance of wakefulness test. *Sleep.* 2005;28(1):113–121.

Actigraphy

Lee-Chiong TL, ed. *Sleep: A Comprehensive Handbook.* Hoboken, NJ: John Wiley & Sons, 2006.

Lee-Chiong TL, Sateia M, Carskadon M, eds. *Sleep Medicine.* Philadelphia, PA: Hanley & Belfus (Elsevier), 2002.

Standards of Practice Committee of the American Academy of Sleep Medicine (AASM). Practice parameters for the role of actigraphy in the study of sleep and circadian rhythms: an update for 2002. *Sleep.* 2003;26(3):337–41.

Insomnia 3

Definition and Clinical Features

Individuals who complain of insomnia report repeated difficulty with either initially falling asleep (sleep onset insomnia) or remaining asleep (sleep maintenance insomnia) despite adequate opportunity, condition, and time for sleep. Their sleep is described as short and inadequate, light and easily disrupted, of poor quality, unrefreshing, unsatisfactory, or nonrestorative. Frequent extended periods of wakefulness or persistent early morning awakenings may be reported. In children, insomnia may present as bedtime resistance or lack of ability to sleep independently. This sleep disturbance is associated with impairment of daytime function.

Most investigators define insomnia as a sleep latency of 30 minutes or more; wake time after sleep onset of 30 minutes or more; sleep efficiency of less than 85%; or total sleep time less than 6 to 6.5 hours, occurring at least 3 nights a week.

Patients with insomnia often report greater subjective sleep disturbance compared to objective polysomnographic parameters. The discrepancy between subjective estimates and objective measures of sleep is believed to be due to persistent sensory processing during non–rapid eye movement (NREM) sleep, which decreases the ability of patients with insomnia to distinguish sleep from wakefulness. Perception of sleep appears to be altered. Persons with insomnia may have a greater tendency to describe, when awakened from sleep, of being awake all along, compared with those without insomnia. In addition, they may overestimate the duration of their sleep latencies.

Demographics

Insomnia is the most common sleep disorder, with about a third of adults reporting occasional insomnia and approximately 10% with chronic insomnia. The prevalence of insomnia is greater among the elderly; in individuals who belong to a low socioeconomic status; in shift workers; and in those who are widowed, divorced, or separated. Women are more likely to be affected than men. In addition, prevalence of insomnia may be greater among substance and alcohol users, in hospitalized or institutionalized persons, and in individuals with an underlying medical or neurologic disorder.

There appears to be a strong correlation between insomnia and psychiatric disorders. Many patients with insomnia have either an underlying psychiatric pathology or an increased risk of developing a new-onset psychiatric illness. A recent stressor increases the risk of developing insomnia.

Consequences

The daytime consequences of insomnia include fatigue, malaise, reduced energy and motivation, cognitive impairment (eg, concentration, memory, reaction time and judgment), diminished performance, decreased productivity at school and work, alterations in mood, and diminished quality of life. Patients may express concerns about the quality of their sleep and its impact on daytime functioning. Although subjective complaints of daytime sleepiness are common, objective tests, such as the Multiple Sleep Latency Test (MSLT), generally fail to demonstrate significant sleepiness. Excessive sleepiness appears to be more common during acute insomnia compared to chronic insomnia. Patients with chronic insomnia commonly describe difficulty falling asleep during the daytime as well.

Insomnia is associated an increased likelihood of accidents at home, in the workplace, and while driving. Alcoholism and illicit drug use may be increased in this population. There is also an increased risk of developing psychiatric disorders (eg, major depression and anxiety). Somatic manifestations such as headaches and gastrointestinal complaints have been described. Several medical disorders, including chronic pain, hypertension and diabetes, may occur more frequently in patients with insomnia. The various consequences of insomnia are listed in Box 3–1.

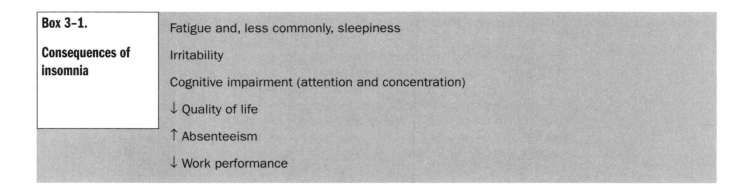

Box 3-1. **Consequences of insomnia**	Fatigue and, less commonly, sleepiness
	Irritability
	Cognitive impairment (attention and concentration)
	↓ Quality of life
	↑ Absenteeism
	↓ Work performance

Health care utilization is increased in individuals with insomnia compared with those without insomnia. Finally, affected individuals may have significant impairment with interpersonal relationships and appear to be at greater risk for job loss and marital difficulties.

Clinical Course

Without effective therapy, chronic insomnia tends to persist. Many patients with chronic insomnia report suffering from disturbed sleep for several years. An estimated 50% of all patients with moderate and severe sleep disturbance have no significant remission of their insomnia over time.

Classification

Insomnia can be divided based on its duration into acute (transient: lasting only a few days or short-term: lasting up to 3 to 4 weeks) or chronic (persisting for more than 1 to 3 months) (Table 3–1). Insomnia can also be classified by severity into mild, moderate, or severe based on the International Classification of Sleep Disorders (ICSD 1) criteria (Table 3–2).. Finally, insomnia can be classified based on temporal profiles into sleep-onset, sleep maintenance, terminal, or nonrestorative sleep, or on etiology into primary or co-morbid (Tables 3–3 and 3–4).

Table 3–1.   Classification of insomnia based on duration

Duration	Characteristics
Acute	Less than one month Transient—lasting a few days Short-term—lasting up to 3 or 4 weeks
Chronic	Persisting for more than 1 to 3 months

Pathophysiology

Several factors are important in the pathophysiology of insomnia. Clearly, misalignment of circadian sleep-wake and body temperature rhythms and desired bedtime and arising times are central

Table 3–2.   Classification of insomnia based on severity

Severity	Occurrence	Impairment of social or occupational functioning
Mild	Almost nightly	Little or none
Moderate	Nightly	Mild or moderate
Severe	Nightly	Marked or severe

Table 3–3.   Classification of insomnia based on temporal profiles

Temporal profile	Characteristics
Sleep-onset insomnia	Difficulty falling asleep
Sleep maintenance insomnia	Frequent or prolonged awakenings
Terminal insomnia (early morning awakening)	Final awakening that is earlier than desired
Nonrestorative sleep	Feeling unrefreshed upon awakening

Table 3–4.   Classification of insomnia based on etiology

Etiology	Characteristics
Primary insomnia	Idiopathic insomnia unrelated to any comorbid medical, neurologic or psychiatric disorder, or medication use or withdrawal effects
Comorbid insomnia	Insomnia that is related to a comorbid medical, neurologic, or psychiatric disorder, or medication use or withdrawal effects

to the different circadian rhythm sleep disorders. Compared to good sleepers, patients with sleep-onset insomnia have a later minimum core body temperature (3:00 vs. 7:00 AM). It is also increasingly apparent that the daytime consequences of insomnia are due not merely to the disturbed nighttime sleep and associated sleep deprivation but also to a state of somatic and cognitive arousal that is present throughout the 24-hour day. Sensory inputs and information processing may persist during sleep and impede sleep initiation and consolidation. Patients with insomnia have higher metabolic rates and greater high-frequency electroencephalographic (EEG) activity during sleep. Finally, maladaptive behavior and dysfunctional beliefs (eg, excessive worry about catastrophic consequences of insomnia and unrealistic concerns about disturbed sleep) and conditioned cortical arousal may perpetuate an acute insomnia that would had otherwise been limited in duration.

Causes of Insomnia

Insomnia is a symptom with numerous and diverse etiologies, and in many individuals, more than one cause may be present. Causes of insomnia include primary sleep disturbances, other sleep disorders, disturbances of the circadian sleep-wake rhythm, medical, neurologic and psychiatric illnesses, behavioral disorders, and medication use or withdrawal. Identifying a specific precipitating cause may be especially difficult when the condition has been present for many years.

It is estimated that psychophysiologic insomnia is responsible for 15% of cases of chronic insomnia. Other specific causes of chronic insomnia include restless legs syndrome (about 12% of cases) as well as alcohol or drug use and abuse (about 12% of cases).

In a proposed model of the genesis and maintenance of insomnia, factors related to insomnia are classified into those that predispose a person to develop insomnia, those that trigger the start of insomnia, and those that sustain the sleep disturbance (often long after the precipitating event has resolved) (Table 3–5).

Table 3–5.   Factors causing and maintaining insomnia

Factors	Characteristics
Predisposing factors	Factors present before the start of insomnia that increase the likelihood of developing insomnia May, if sufficiently severe, independently cause insomnia Includes genetic predisposition, personality traits, physiologic hyperarousal (eg, increased muscle tension, body temperature, metabolic rate and heart rate, and shift in EEG to faster frequencies at sleep onset and during NREM sleep), psychologic arousal (eg, tendency to ruminate, agitation, anxiety, or heightened vigilance), and time of day sleep-wake preference
Precipitating factors	Factors that trigger the start of insomnia Includes stressful events, change of usual habits, abrupt alterations in sleep-wake schedules, environmental disturbances, medication use or withdrawal, substance use; or medical, neurologic, psychiatric or primary sleep disorders
Perpetuating factors	Factors that sustain sleep disturbance and contribute to the persistence of insomnia independent of the precipitating causes Includes poor sleep hygiene, irregular sleep-wake schedules, caffeine or alcohol consumption, ongoing worries, anxiety or unrealistic expectations about sleep, and maladaptive sleep-wake behaviors With acute insomnia, rumination centers around the precipitating stressful event; on the other hand, rumination shifts to the inability to sleep and the possible consequences of poor sleep in patients with chronic insomnia. Over time, insomnia persists because of the cognitive association between the bedroom environment (conditioned stimuli) and psychologic and physiologic hyperarousal (unconditioned stimuli).

Source: Adapted from Spielman AJ, Caruso LS, Glovinski PB. A behavioral perspective on insomnia treatment. Psychiatr Clin North Am. 1987;10:541-553.

Co-Morbid Insomnia

Co-morbid insomnia accounts for a major portion of cases of insomnia, and it is particularly common among older adults. The development of insomnia is more likely in the setting of certain primary disorders (eg, acute and chronic pain, cancer and mood disorders) than in others (eg, asthma or gastroesophageal reflux). In addition, patients with a prior history of insomnia from whatever cause may have a higher risk of developing sleep disturbance associated with a newly diagnosed medical, psychiatric, neurologic, or sleep disorder.

Etiology of Transient Insomnia

Sleep is typically normal prior to the start of sleep disturbance in individuals with transient insomnia. Sleep normalizes with resolution of the inciting event. These individuals appear to have increased central nervous system (CNS) arousal and are more vulnerable to acute stresses (eg, changes in familiar routines or sleep schedules, significant social events, and drug ingestion or withdrawal). As shown in Table 3–6, causes of transient sleep disturbance include adjustment sleep disorder, jet lag, and shift work sleep disorder.

Table 3–6. Causes of transient insomnia

Etiology	Sleep disorders	Characteristics
Acute life stresses, alterations in familiar routines or changes in sleep schedules	Adjustment sleep disorder Jet lag Shift work sleep disorder	Normal sleep prior to and following transient sleep disturbance.

Adjustment Sleep Disorder

Definition

An identifiable acute stressor can elicit a sudden heightened state of arousal that may significantly diminish sleep propensity. Insomnia may also be precipitated by momentous or stressful life events (eg, bereavement, divorce, job loss), a change in the sleeping environment (ie, sleeping in unfamiliar places), or an acute medical disorder or physical illness (eg, hospitalization). The association between the new-onset insomnia and acute stressor is often readily apparent.

Demographics

Adjustment sleep disorder can affect persons of all ages. Prevalence may be greater among women and older adults. Individuals with a previous history of insomnia, stress-related sleep disturbance, or mood disorder may have a higher risk of developing adjustment sleep disorder.

Clinical Course

The course is acute and generally brief. Sleep tends to normalize once the acute stressor decreases or resolves, or if there is an increase in the individual's level of adaptation to the stressor.

Consequences

Adjustment sleep disorder is not typically associated with any major long-term complications. Nevertheless, acute insomnia should be promptly recognized and appropriately treated before learned habits, attitudes, and coping mechanisms incongruous with sleep become established and perpetuate the sleep disturbance.

Evaluation

Polysomnographic features may include increases in sleep latency and frequency of awakenings, as well as decreases in sleep efficiency and total sleep time. NREM stages 1 and 2 sleep may be increased along with decreases in NREM stages 3 and 4, as well as rapid eye movement (REM) sleep.

Differential Diagnosis

Differential diagnosis includes psychophysiologic insomnia, which should be considered if the sleep disturbance persists beyond 1 to 3 months, especially if the initial stressor is no longer present. Unlike adjustment sleep disorder, an identifiable precipitant may not be present in psychophysiologic insomnia.

Jet Lag

Rapid travel across multiple time zones can precipitate insomnia, because the traveler's intrinsic circadian rhythm remains synchronized to the home time zone. A westward flight is associated with increased wakefulness during the early morning hours. The advanced bedtimes following eastward flights result in difficulty falling asleep at night. Symptoms increase in severity with greater amounts and rates of time zone transitions.

Other factors that may contribute to insomnia during prolonged travel include uncomfortable sitting conditions, limited mobility, intermittent brief napping, variable light exposures, ingestion of alcohol and caffeine, and nonspecific complaints (eg, ocular dryness, nasal congestion, gastrointestinal symptoms, or headaches). The elderly appear to be more prone to develop jet lag than younger individuals.

Polysomnography demonstrates a decrease in sleep efficiency and increase in frequency of arousals.

Jet lag typically remits spontaneously after 2 to 3 days, with symptoms generally persisting longer with eastbound travel.

Shift Work Sleep Disorder

Insomnia may develop in persons whose work schedules are outside of the traditional 8:00 AM to 5:00 PM shift. Sleep time is altered and is generally misaligned to environmental and conventional social time cues. Sleep during the morning following night work shift may be associated with prolonged sleep latency. Individuals who have to arise shortly after midnight to start their early morning work may complain of difficulty falling asleep in the early evening. Insomnia is further heightened in shift work sleep disorders compared to jet lag because the conventional time cues of sunlight and social activities are frequently out of phase with the altered sleep time.

In shift work sleep disorder, not only is total daily sleep duration reduced, sleep quality is often decreased as well. Fragmented sleep and increase in frequency of arousals are common polysomnographic findings.

Etiology of Chronic Insomnia

Chronic insomnia may be either primary or co-morbid (secondary). It may be secondary to alterations in circadian rhythms, behavioral disorders, environmental factors, sleep disorders, movements disorders, medical, neurologic and psychiatric disorders, menstruation and pregnancy, and medication use and abuse. Sleep disturbance in patients with chronic insomnia may arise from one or several of these conditions, and each of the various disorders may contribute to a patient's complaint of nonrestorative sleep. The many causes of chronic insomnia are presented in Table 3–7.

Table 3–7. Causes of chronic insomnia

Etiology	Sleep disorders	Characteristics
Primary insomnia	Idiopathic insomnia Paradoxical insomnia (sleep state misperception) Psychophysiologic insomnia	Insomnia is not due to another sleep, medical, neurologic or psychiatric disorder, nor to substance abuse or withdrawal.
Alterations in circadian rhythms	Advanced sleep phase syndrome Delayed sleep phase syndrome Irregular sleep-wake pattern Non–24-hour sleep-wake syndrome	Insomnia is related to disorders of the timing of sleep periods secondary to desynchrony between endogenous circadian rhythms and the environment.
Behavioral disorders	Inadequate sleep hygiene Limit-setting sleep disorder Sleep-onset association disorder Nocturnal eating (drinking) syndrome	Insomnia is associated with behaviors that are arousing and not conducive to sleep.
Environmental factors	Altitude insomnia Environmental sleep disorder Food allergy insomnia Toxin-induced sleep disorder	Insomnia is due to environmental conditions or external factors that are not conducive to sleep.
Sleep disorders	Central sleep apnea Obstructive sleep apnea Parasomnias Confusional arousals Sleep terrors Sleepwalking Rhythmic movement disorder Sleep starts Nocturnal leg cramps Nightmares REM sleep behavior disorder	Insomnia is associated with sleep-related breathing disorders or parasomnias.
Movement disorders	Periodic limb movement disorder Restless legs syndrome	In some individuals, periodic limb movements of sleep (PLMS) may be associated with arousals, awakenings, and sleep disruption. Restless legs syndrome can give rise to sleep-onset insomnia and may coexist with PLMS in many individuals.

Continued

Table 3-7. Causes of chronic insomnia—cont'd

Etiology	Sleep disorders	Characteristics

Medical disorders	Respiratory disorders
	  Asthma
	  Chronic obstructive pulmonary disease
	  Central alveolar hypoventilation
	    syndrome
	Cardiac disorders
	  Nocturnal angina
	  Congestive heart failure
	Pain syndromes
	Gastrointestinal disorders
	  Sleep-related gastroesophageal reflux
	  Peptic ulcer disease
	  Sleep-related abnormal swallowing
	    syndrome
	
	Dermatologic disorders
	  Pruritus
	Cancer
	Infectious disorders
	  Acquired immunodeficiency syndrome
		Insomnia may result from physiologic alterations involving the respiratory, cardiac, gastrointestinal, and musculoskeletal systems.

Neurologic disorders	Cerebral degenerative disorders Dementia Fatal familial insomnia Nocturnal paroxysmal dystonia Parkinson disease Sleep-related headaches Sleep-related seizures	Neurologic disorders can prevent sleep onset and disrupt its continuity.
Psychiatric disorders	Alcoholism Anxiety disorders Mood disorders Panic disorders Personality disorders Psychoses Somatoform disorders	Many persons with insomnia have an underlying psychiatric disorder. Conversely, among this patient group, there is an increased risk of developing a new psychiatric illness within a year of presentation.
Menstruation and pregnancy	Menstrual-associated sleep disorder Pregnancy-associated sleep disorder	Both pregnancy and the menstrual cycle can produce insomnia among women.
Medication and substance use	Alcohol-dependent sleep disorder Hypnotic-dependent sleep disorder Stimulant-dependent sleep disorder	The use and abuse of hypnotic agents, stimulants, and alcohol are important causes of insomnia. The effects of these and other medications are also influenced by the possible development of tolerance, withdrawal symptoms, and drug interactions.

Primary Insomnia

Insomnia is considered primary if it is not due exclusively to another sleep, medical, neurologic or psychiatric disorder, or to the effects of substance use, abuse, or withdrawal. Some polysomnographic features of primary insomnia are listed in Box 3–2. Three subgroups of insomnia are included in the category of primary insomnia, namely *idiopathic insomnia, paradoxical insomnia* (sleep state misperception), and *psychophysiologic insomnia.*

Box 3-2. **Polysomnographic features of primary insomnia**[a]	↑ Sleep latency
	↓ Total sleep time
	↓ NREM stages 3 and 4 sleep
	↑ Wake time after sleep onset
	Note: May be normal

[a] *Compared to good sleepers.*

Psychophysiologic Insomnia

Definition

In psychophysiologic insomnia, maladaptive sleep-preventing behavior develops and eventually progresses to become the predominant factor perpetuating sleep disturbances. Although the onset of insomnia is related to a stressor, sleep disturbance persists long after the stressor abates. Insomnia is associated with distress and daytime functional impairment, and it persists for at least 1 month.

Clinical Features

Insomnia is related to heightened conditioned cognitive and physiologic arousal responses that are incompatible with sleep. It is associated with learned sleep-preventing associations. There is greater somatized tension, such as increased agitation and muscle tone, and mental arousal with persistent intrusive thoughts during bedtime. Thus, patients are unable to both physically relax and cease their rumination in order to permit sleep to occur.

Patients are overly concerned and excessively worry about their inability to sleep, and they are frustrated about not being able to sleep better. Affected individuals are likely to equate events and activities leading to sleep with frustration. Thus, a vicious cycle is created in which they try too hard to sleep and, in so doing, become tense, and more aroused and anxious; this, in turn, diminishes further their propensity to sleep. Interestingly, sleep commences readily when they are not trying too hard to do so or when they are distracted. Conditioned arousal is limited to the person's own bed and bedroom, and they commonly report sleeping better in any room other than their own (including the sleep laboratory [reverse first-night effect]).

Demographics

Psychophysiologic insomnia accounts for approximately 15% of cases of chronic insomnia. It often begins during adolescence and young adulthood, and it seldom affects young children. Women tend to be affected more often than men.

Risk Factors

Many patients with psychophysiologic insomnia have a lifelong history of episodic poor or light sleep. They often demonstrate a preoccupation with their sleep duration and quality as well as the potential consequences of sleep disturbances.

Clinical Course

Onset of insomnia can be either acute or insidious. Its course is commonly chronic, and if left untreated, it may progressively worsen.

Complications

Diminished neurocognitive function (concentration and attention), vigilance, energy and alertness, and increased daytime sleepiness and fatigue may be present. As with other types of chronic insomnia, there is a greater risk of developing depression among persons with psychophysiologic insomnia. Affected individuals may also be more prone to excessive use of hypnotic agents.

Evaluation

Diagnosis of psychophysiologic insomnia relies mainly on clinical history. Polysomnography is not routinely indicated as it seldom provides information that cannot be obtained from clinical history alone. Polysomnography can be entirely normal or may show an increase in sleep latency, decrease in sleep efficiency, frequent awakenings, and increase in wake time after sleep onset. Total sleep time may be reduced. An increase in NREM stage 1 sleep and a decrease in NREM stages 3 and 4 sleep may also be observed. A pattern of alpha intrusion may be appreciated. Both the "first-night effect" (worse sleep than usual during the first night in the sleep laboratory) and the "reverse first-night effect" (better sleep than usual during the first sleep laboratory night) can influence sleep architecture. Subjective reports of sleep time are often less than objective total sleep time determined by polysomnography.

The MSLT demonstrates normal daytime alertness. Actigraphy is less reliable in measuring sleep in this patient group, commonly underestimating wake time and overestimating sleep time.

Differential Diagnosis

Differential diagnosis of psychophysiologic insomnia includes *environmental sleep disorder* (presence of adverse environmental conditions that are not favorable for sleep), *idiopathic insomnia*, *paradoxical insomnia*, and *adjustment sleep disorder* (insomnia is acute and directly related to an identifiable stressor). Unlike adjustment sleep disorder, psychophysiologic insomnia persists even after the precipitating factor has disappeared.

It is also important to distinguish psychophysiologic insomnia from generalized anxiety in which worry and tension pervade other aspects of daily living. In this insomnia, anxiety is limited to issues regarding sleep. In addition, any condition that could cause insomnia, such as an underlying medical, neurologic, or psychiatric disorder, as well as substance use or withdrawal should be excluded.

Paradoxical Insomnia (Sleep State Misperception)

Definition

In paradoxical insomnia, patients complain of chronic severe insomnia but have no polysomnographic evidence of significant sleep disturbance and no impairment of daytime function consistent with subjective reports of extreme sleep loss. Affected individuals are believed to be unable to reliably discern the total time spent asleep, often overestimating sleep latency and underestimating sleep duration compared to objective measures of sleep. Insomnia is present for 1 or more months.

Clinical Features

Patients may report having very little or no sleep during most nights and no daytime napping. This is associated with "consciousness" of the environment or ongoing thought processes during most of the night.

Demographics

Paradoxical insomnia is seen in less than 5% of chronic insomniacs. Onset is generally during early to mid-adulthood. It is less common during childhood and adolescence. Prevalence is higher in women.

Clinical Course and Complications

Course tends to be chronic and complaints of insomnia can persist for several years. Chronic sleep disturbance can give rise to mood disorders, such as depression or anxiety, and excessive use of hypnotic agents.

Evaluation/

Despite subjective reports of little or no sleep during polysomnography, the study demonstrates a normal or near normal sleep latency, quality, and architecture. Total sleep duration typically exceeds 6.5 hours. Similar discrepancies between subjective estimates of sleep duration and objective measures can be noted with actigraphy. The MSLT is either normal or demonstrates mild sleepiness.

Idiopathic Insomnia

Definition

Idiopathic insomnia is characterized by long-standing sleep disturbance that generally starts during infancy or in early childhood and is not associated with any identifiable etiology. Patients with idiopathic insomnia may complain of difficulty with sleep initiation or sleep maintenance, or they may report insufficient sleep duration. Insomnia is associated with distress and impaired daytime functioning.

Clinical Features

Idiopathic insomnia is believed to be due to an underlying defect in the CNS substrate responsible for the sleep-wake cycle, which may also produce subtle impairments in concentration, hyperkinesis or dyslexia.

Demographics

It accounts for less than 10% of patients presenting to sleep clinics with complaints of insomnia. This disorder affects both genders equally.

Clinical Course and Complications

Onset is typically insidious. The course is chronic and relentless, and it persists for life without periods of remission. Insomnia is typically refractory to therapy. Affected individuals may become dependent on hypnotics or alcohol to aid in sleep. Patients may complain of daytime fatigue as well as difficulties with attention and concentration. Risk of developing depression is increased.

Evaluation

The diagnosis of idiopathic insomnia is arrived at by excluding other causes of insomnia such as primary sleep disorders; medical, neurologic, or psychiatric conditions; and circadian rhythm–related sleep disturbances. Typical polysomnographic features include a significantly diminished sleep efficiency, prolonged sleep latency, decreased total sleep time, increase in wake time after sleep onset, increase in NREM stages 1 and 2 sleep, and decrease in NREM stages 3 and 4 sleep.

Disorders of the Circadian Rhythm

Four subgroups of chronic insomnia are related to disorders of the timing of the sleep-wake pattern: (1) delayed sleep-phase syndrome, (2) advanced sleep-phase syndrome, (3) non–24-hour sleep-wake syndrome, and (4) irregular sleep-wake pattern syndrome (Table 3–8). These disorders arise from desynchrony between the endogenous biologic rhythms controlling sleep and wakefulness, and environmental time cues. Although the light-dark cycle has the greatest influence on circadian rhythms, other factors such as social patterns, illnesses and acquired behavior may exert complementary or disruptive effects.

Table 3–8.   Circadian rhythm disorders causing insomnia

Disorder	Characteristics	Sleep disturbance
Delayed sleep-phase syndrome	Major nocturnal sleep period occurs consistently later than the desired bedtime despite voluntary attempts to advance the sleep period. Distinction has to be made between the altered sleep-wake pattern due to an acquired lifestyle and the delayed sleep-phase syndrome that it may resemble.	Habitual late sleep onset with inability to sleep until the early morning hours. No difficulty remaining asleep following sleep onset. Awakening is equally late (late morning to early afternoon). Polysomnography performed during the person's desired bedtime commonly demonstrates an increase in sleep latency.

Table 3–8. Circadian rhythm disorders causing insomnia—cont'd

Disorder	Characteristics	Sleep disturbance
Advanced sleep-phase syndrome	Shift in the major nocturnal sleep episode to an earlier time relative to the desired bedtime, accompanied by an inability to voluntarily delay sleep time. Depression may mimic advanced sleep-phase syndrome with its early morning awakenings.	Habitual early sleep onset accompanied by early morning awakening (arising times often between 1:00 and 3:00 AM). Polysomnography is normal when done during the patient's regular sleep period, but shows short or normal sleep latency with a brief sleep period terminating in an early awakening if it is performed over the patient's desired clock time.
Non–24-hour sleep-wake syndrome	Sleep-wake patterns have no apparent relationship to environmental time cues and appear to rely solely on intrinsic biologic rhythms. Free-running internal rhythms behave with a periodicity of slightly over 24 hours. This condition is rare and the majority of reported cases involved persons who are blind or mentally retarded. Its course is chronic and unrelenting.	Daily progressive delay in sleep onset and arising times. Cyclic pattern of sleep disturbance characterized by recurring periods of insomnia and excessive sleepiness. When polysomnography is recorded at a fixed time daily over several days, sleep latency becomes progressively longer and total sleep time becomes commensurately shorter.
Irregular sleep-wake pattern syndrome	Disorganization of sleep and wake times due to absence of basic circadian rhythmicity Replacement of the major nocturnal sleep period by three or more shorter sleep episodes occurring throughout the 24-hour day Total sleep time over a 24-hour period is normal. It is most frequently encountered in persons with severe brain dysfunction. Normal individuals who repetitively ignore environmentally determined time cues and voluntarily perpetuate the sleep-wake irregularity by indiscriminate napping may likewise acquire this condition. Course tends to be chronic.	Evening insomnia or daytime sleepiness The loss of the normal pattern of sleep and wakefulness is evident during a 24-hour polysomnography. If recordings are continued for several days, the sleep and wake schedules are observed to be variable and disorganized.

Insomnia develops when sleep is attempted at a time the person's circadian clock is promoting wakefulness rather than sleep. As a group, disorders of the circadian sleep-wake rhythm are responsible for approximately 2% or less of cases of chronic insomnia.

Behavioral Disorders

Certain sleep disturbances are rooted in behaviors that are arousing and not conducive to sleep. A variety of behavioral disorders (eg, *inadequate sleep hygiene, limit-setting sleep disorder, sleep-onset association disorder* and *nocturnal eating (drinking) syndrome*) may be responsible for chronic insomnia and nonrestorative sleep.

Inadequate Sleep Hygiene

Definition

Insomnia has its origins in acquired habits that enhance wakefulness or curtail sleep propensity (eg, excessive caffeine ingestion, alcohol intoxication, cigarette smoking, strenuous exercise, excitement, and stimulating mental activities performed too close to bedtime).

Clinical Features

Persons may spend excessive amounts of time in bed and use their beds for non–sleep-related activities (eg, homework, television watching, or telephone conversations). Significant day-to-day variability in bedtimes and rising times, coupled with frequent daytime napping, also contributes to sleep disruption. Disregard for environmental factors that could potentially disrupt sleep (eg, excessive noise from a radio) may be present. These activities and behaviors that are inconsistent with the initiation and maintenance of good sleep can be modified or terminated if the person wishes to do so.

Although poor sleep hygiene may, by itself, lead to insomnia, it is more commonly encountered in association with other causes of sleep disturbance. Inadequate sleep hygiene may, thus, precipitate insomnia by interacting with factors (eg, acute stressors or mood disorders) that by themselves may not be sufficiently severe to independently induce a sleep disorder or may sustain a preexisting sleep difficulty that would otherwise be short lived.

Demographics

Insomnia may begin anytime during childhood or adulthood and is present for at least a month.

Evaluation

Polysomnography reveals a decrease in sleep efficiency, increase in sleep latency, and increase in frequency of arousals.

Limit-Setting Sleep Disorder

Definition

Limit-setting sleep disorder is seen in children who repeatedly refuse to go to sleep when requested to do so and often delay going to bed.

Clinical Features

In order to stay up later, children may take multiple trips to the bathroom, ask to be read a story or to have the lights turned on again, demand food or water, or request permission to watch a few more minutes of television. If the caretaker recognizes the child's attempts to delay his or her bedtime and strictly enforces limits to further activities, sleep comes naturally and quickly.

Demographics

Limit-setting sleep disorder affects an estimated 5% to 10% of children, with a greater prevalence among boys. It is not commonly encountered until children start to develop verbal communications skills, at 2 years of age or older.

Evaluation

Sleep is normal on polysomnography.

Differential Diagnosis

Limit-setting sleep disorder must be differentiated from a variable sleep schedule, childhood fears of darkness or being left alone in their room, delayed sleep-phase syndrome, or enforcement of bedtime at an inappropriately early time, all of which may mimic the disorder.

Sleep-Onset Association Disorder

Definition

The patient with sleep-onset association disorder is incapable of falling asleep without the presence of certain desired conditions.

Clinical Features

This condition is typically seen in a child who is unable to sleep unless a feeding bottle, pacifier or a favorite toy is available.

Demographics

It is estimated to affect 15% to 20% of children 6 months to 3 years of age. Boys appear to be affected more often than girls.

Clinical Course

This disorder commonly remits at 3 to 4 years of age but may persist into adulthood (eg, dependence on a television set or radio.)

Evaluation

Two possible polysomnographic patterns can be expected in patients with sleep-onset association disorder. In the absence of desired circumstances, there is an increase in both sleep latency and frequency of awakenings. Sleep quantity and quality are normal when the required associations are met.

Nocturnal Eating (Drinking) Syndrome

This syndrome is characterized by repetitive nighttime awakenings, which, in many instances, appear to be triggered by learned behavior rather than by real hunger or thirst, with the reestablishment of sleep only after eating or drinking. It may be encountered in persons who have chronic gastrointestinal symptoms such as peptic ulcer disease or gastritis, which are relieved by eating, or who have considerable variability in their sleep-wake and meal times.

This syndrome is seen in approximately 5% of children 6 months to 3 years of age. Obesity may develop in these patients. Polysomnography demonstrates an increase in frequency of awakenings.

Environmental Factors

Environmental factors influence both sleep quality and quantity. Four conditions, *environmental sleep disorder*, *food allergy insomnia*, *toxin-induced sleep disorder*, and *altitude insomnia* are considered environmentally induced.

Environmental Sleep Disorder

Adverse environmental conditions, including excessive noise, noxious odors, bright lights, extremes of ambient temperature, or a snoring bed partner, can disturb sleep. The elderly are more sensitive to environmental disturbances and are, thus, at greater risk of developing this type of insomnia. Sleep normalizes following removal of the causative factor/s.

Polysomnography performed in the sleep laboratory shows normal sleep quality and duration. In contrast, reduced sleep efficiency and diminished total sleep time are seen during ambulatory polysomnography performed in the patient's customary sleep environment.

Food Allergy Insomnia

Ingestion of a particular food or drink may give rise to sleep disturbance with an increase in the frequency of arousals. Both children and adults may suffer from this disorder, although it is seen more frequently in children from infancy to 4 years of age. Other symptoms of allergy, including skin irritation or rashes, gastrointestinal difficulties, and respiratory distress, may also be present. Sleep normalizes following removal of the inciting food allergens.

Polysomnographic recording may demonstrate frequent arousals. Other useful tests include allergy testing and measurement of serum antibodies to suspected dietary constituents.

Toxin-Induced Sleep Disorder

Poisoning with a variety of chemicals and toxins (eg, arsenic, copper, lead, mercury) can produce either insomnia secondary to CNS excitation or hypersomnolence and decreased vigilance due to CNS depression. Polysomnography in patients with toxin-induced insomnia may reveal prolonged sleep latency, diminished sleep efficiency, and repetitive awakenings.

Altitude Insomnia

Sleep disturbance, including insomnia, can develop following ascent to elevations greater than 2000 to 4000 meters. Sleep fragmentation, decrease in sleep efficiency, shortened total sleep time, and reduction of REM sleep can occur. Other symptoms consist of easy fatigability, headaches, and anorexia. Severity is magnified with greater altitudes. Incidence increases in persons with underlying cardiorespiratory disorders or anemia.

The primary cause of sleep disruption is periodic breathing with periods of central apnea during sleep as a result of hypoxia and respiratory alkalosis. Arousals can occur during the hyperpneic phase of periodic breathing. Adverse environmental conditions may also contribute to the complaint of insomnia.

Symptoms resolve with acclimatization or after descent to lower altitudes. Oxygen therapy may decrease periodic breathing but does not significantly improve sleep quality. Acetazolamide, a carbonic anhydrase inhibitor, stimulates respiration via production of metabolic acidosis; it improves sleep quality, hypoxemia and periodic breathing. Benzodiazepines can blunt the respiratory response to hypercapnia and should be avoided.

Movement Disorders

Movement disorders such as *periodic limb movement disorder* or *restless legs syndrome* may be detected during the course of an investigation into the causes of insomnia (Table 3–9). In many cases, periodic limb movements of sleep are merely incidental findings unrelated to the complaint of insomnia. The clinical significance of periodic limb movements of sleep is commonly uncertain and remains so until insomnia improves upon instituting effective pharmacologic therapy for this underlying condition.

Table 3–9. Movement disorders causing insomnia

Disorder	Characteristics	Sleep disturbance
Restless legs syndrome	An uncomfortable sensation involving the lower extremities that becomes apparent whenever the patient sits, lies down, or remains still. This "creepy" or "crawling" uncomfortable sensation is usually worse at night; it extends from the feet and ankle up to the legs, the occasionally involving the, thighs. Leg movements relieve it, either partially or completely, but symptoms recur with cessation of leg motion. It affects approximately 5% to 15% of normal individuals, predominantly among women, with an increased prevalence with pregnancy, uremia, anemia, and rheumatoid arthritis. Many have concurrent periodic limb movements during sleep.	Insomnia may develop when these sensations occur prior to the desired bedtime. Electromyographic (EMG) recordings of the lower extremities can detect limb movements during sleep onset. Polysomnographic features include an increase in sleep latency, decrease in sleep efficiency, and increase in frequency of awakenings.

Continued

Table 3-9. Movement disorders causing insomnia—cont'd

Disorder	Characteristics	Sleep disturbance
Periodic limb movement disorder	Recurrent, almost rhythmic, limb movements, typically involving the toes, feet, ankles and legs, occur during sleep. It has also been reported in the hips and upper limbs.	Periodic limb movements can arouse the patient from sleep. Sleep fragmentation secondary to period limb movement disorder can lead to either insomnia or hypersomnolence. The former may be more common following complete awakenings, whereas increased sleepiness appears to be more frequent as a result of brief and partial awakenings. EMG of the anterior tibialis demonstrates repetitive muscle contractions that last from 0.5 to 5 seconds and commonly recur every 20 to 40 seconds.

Parasomnias

Parasomnias are physical phenomena that occur during, and intrude into, sleep. They manifest as activation of skeletal muscles or the autonomic nervous system during sleep. Sleep disturbance can occur with various parasomnias such as *confusional arousals, sleep terrors, sleepwalking, rhythmic movement disorder, sleep starts, nocturnal leg cramps, nightmares,* and *REM sleep behavior disorder* (Table 3–10.) They may, if sufficiently severe, lead to chronic insomnia.

Medical Disorders

Sleep disturbance may result from physiologic alterations involving the respiratory, cardiac, gastrointestinal, and musculoskeletal systems. Therefore, many medical disorders are responsible for the development of acute and chronic insomnia.

Respiratory Disorders

Respiratory disturbances can affect sleep in various ways. Insomnia can result from obstructive sleep apnea, central sleep apnea, central alveolar hypoventilation syndrome, chronic obstructive pulmonary disease, and sleep-related asthma.

   Apnea is defined as the absence of airflow for ten or more seconds. When airflow is diminished but not absent, the event is termed *hypopnea*. Respiratory events are classified as *central* if respiratory efforts are absent, and as *obstructive* if cessation of airflow is noted despite the presence of respiratory efforts. Respiratory disorders that may result in insomnia are outlined in Table 3–11.

Cardiovascular Disorders

Both ischemic heart disease and congestive heart failure can give rise to sleep disturbance and complaints of insomnia (Table 3–12).

Table 3–10. Parasomnias causing insomnia

Disorder	Characteristics	Sleep disturbance
Confusional arousals	Episodes of confusion may occur following arousals from NREM stages 3 and 4 sleep, usually in the first third of the night. Associated features include disorientation, inappropriate behavior and amnesia for the event.	Repetitive arousals can give rise to significant sleep disruption.
Sleep terrors	During an episode of sleep terror, the individual may bolt upright from bed, crying or yelling. These abrupt awakenings occur out of NREM stages 3 and 4 sleep, often in the first third of the night. Profound fear, confusion, amnesia for the episode, tachycardia, tachypnea, profuse sweating, sleep talking or screaming, and urinary incontinence are common.	Repetitive arousals can give rise to significant sleep disruption.
Sleepwalking	Sleepwalking is seen most commonly during the first third of the night, during NREM stages 3 and 4 sleep. Associated features include diminished arousability, inappropriate behavior and amnesia for the event.	Repetitive arousals can give rise to significant sleep disruption.
Sleep starts or hypnic jerks	Brief asymmetric contractions of the extremities or, less commonly, the head, which can interfere with sleep onset.	Patients may be startled out of sleep by a feeling of "falling" or "dreaming," and the subsequent wakefulness may, at times, be prolonged.
Rhythmic movement disorder	Repetitive, rhythmic, and stereotypic movements of various body areas that precede sleep onset and may continue transiently during early light sleep. It includes head banging, head rolling, body rolling, body rocking, and rhythmic vocalizations.	Sleep-onset insomnia can develop. During polysomnography, rhythmic movements can be demonstrated arising out of all sleep stages, although a majority occurs during early NREM sleep.
REM sleep behavior disorder	REM sleep-related muscular atonia is intermittently disinhibited. Body movements, ranging from simple motions to highly elaborate performances (eg, screaming, punching, kicking, or running), are associated with dreaming.	May lead to repetitive awakenings and sleep fragmentation. Polysomnographic features include increased muscle tone, gross body movements, and complex motor phenomena seemingly related to dream mentation occurring during REM sleep.

Continued

Table 3-10.   Parasomnias causing insomnia—cont'd

Disorder	Characteristics	Sleep disturbance
Nightmares	Frightful dreams can abruptly awaken the sleeper out of REM sleep. The individual is profoundly fearful and anxious, and there is vivid recall of the preceding dream.	Once awakened, the person is fully alert and is generally unable to rapidly return to sleep.
Nocturnal paroxysmal dystonia	Stereotypic and dystonic movements, which are either ballistic or choreoathetoid, follow sudden awakenings from NREM sleep.	Repetitive arousals can give rise to significant sleep disruption. During polysomnography, electroencephalographic arousals are followed almost immediately by dyskinetic movements.
Nocturnal leg cramps	Painful spasms or tightening of the muscles of the calf (gastrocnemius) or foot cause awakenings from sleep. Pain is relieved by forcible dorsiflexion of the foot or by local massage.	Sleep is reestablished only after the painful sensation has been relieved.
Sleep-related painful erections	Painful penile erections occur during REM sleep. There is no apparent penile disorder or pain during sexual erections while awake.	These can lead to repetitive awakenings and insomnia.

Table 3-11.   Insomnia due to respiratory disorders

Disorder	Characteristics	Sleep disturbance
Obstructive sleep apnea syndrome (OSA)	OSA results from repetitive upper airway obstruction resulting from reduced activity of the upper airway dilating muscles.	Episodes of OSA may recur throughout the evening, at times reaching numbers substantial enough to produce sleep fragmentation and insomnia.
	OSA tends to affect middle-aged individuals and is strongly associated with obesity. Other predisposing factors include male gender; hypothyroidism; acromegaly; and structural abnormalities of the head and face, such as macroglossia or micrognathia.	In contrast to obese persons with severe OSA who typically present with excessive sleepiness, those with complaints of insomnia generally have less severe sleep-disordered breathing (lower apnea frequency and duration, and milder oxygen desaturation) and are less likely to be obese. Women with OSA may have a greater predilection for developing insomnia than men.

Table 3-11. Insomnia due to respiratory disorders—cont'd

Disorder	Characteristics	Sleep disturbance
		During polysomnography, the respiratory events are often more frequent, last longer, and associated with more profound oxygen desaturation during REM sleep.
	OSA tends to affect middle-aged individuals and is strongly associated with obesity. Other predisposing factors include male gender; hypothyroidism; acromegaly; and structural abnormalities of the head and face, such as macroglossia or micrognathia.	In contrast to obese persons with severe OSA who typically present with excessive sleepiness, those with complaints of insomnia generally have less severe sleep-disordered breathing (lower apnea frequency and duration, and milder oxygen desaturation) and are less likely to be obese. Women with OSA may have a greater predilection for developing insomnia than men. During polysomnography, the respiratory events are often more frequent, last longer, and associated with more profound oxygen desaturation during REM sleep.
Central sleep apnea syndrome (CSA)	Episodic cessation of airflow during sleep due to a reduction or loss of ventilatory effort Its prevalence increases with age and in persons with cardiac or neurologic disorders, or during ascent to high altitude.	CSA can give rise to insomnia with repeated nocturnal awakenings. During polysomnography, central apneas are most likely to be noted during sleep onset and light NREM sleep.
Central alveolar hypoventilation syndrome	Blood gas disturbances, including hypercapnia and hypoxemia, occur during sleep as a result of sleep-related hypoventilation This syndrome is also referred to as "obesity-hypoventilation" syndrome, a term that emphasizes its strong association with obesity. Persons may also have an idiopathic variety involving nonobese individuals or an acquired form following significant neurologic disorders such as demyelinating illnesses, poliomyelitis, or a brainstem stroke. A defect in the ventilatory chemoreceptors of the medulla is believed to be the cause of the idiopathic type that is most frequently seen in males during adolescence or early adulthood.	Insomnia and sleep fragmentation are common. During polysomnography, recurrent episodes of hypoventilation associated with oxygen desaturation and arousals are noted.

Continued

Table 3-11. **Insomnia due to respiratory disorders—cont'd**

Disorder	Characteristics	Sleep disturbance
Asthma	Worsening of bronchospasm related to circadian changes in airway function or due to the direct effects of sleep itself	Awakenings due to coughing, dyspnea, wheezing, and chest discomfort due to bronchospasm Medications used to treat asthma such as theophylline and beta-agonists may increase nighttime awakenings.
Chronic obstructive pulmonary disease (COPD)	Respiratory and arterial blood gas abnormalities related to either chronic bronchitis or emphysema Hypoxemia can occur in COPD patients, particularly during REM sleep.	Sleep disruption due to nocturnal coughing, dyspnea or respiratory distress may lead to sleep-onset insomnia, frequent nighttime awakenings and non-restorative sleep.

Table 3-12. **Insomnia due to cardiovascular disorders**

Disorder	Characteristics	Sleep disturbance
Nocturnal cardiac ischemia	Left-sided or retrosternal chest pressure, diaphoresis, nausea and palpitation. Consequences include myocardial infarction, congestive heart failure, cardiac arrhythmias, and sudden cardiac death.	Patients can present with a complaint of insomnia.

Gastrointestinal Disorders

Of the numerous gastrointestinal disorders that can give rise to chronic insomnia, three syndromes are noteworthy, namely *sleep-related gastroesophageal reflux, sleep-related abnormal swallowing syndrome*, and *peptic ulcer disease* (Table 3–13).

Table 3-13. **Insomnia due to gastrointestinal disorders**

Disorder	Characteristics	Sleep disturbance
Gastroesophageal reflux disease (GERD)	Repeated epigastric and retrosternal discomfort ("heartburn") caused by regurgitation of gastric material into the esophagus Other features include coughing, choking, and a sour or bitter taste in the mouth.	GERD can be noted during sleep, but most episodes occur during arousals or awakenings from sleep Insomnia may develop with repeated awakenings from sleep due to GERD. GERD-related arousals can be identified during polysomnography with the use of continuous esophageal pH measurements.

Table 3-13. Insomnia due to gastrointestinal disorders—cont'd

Disorder	Characteristics	Sleep disturbance
Sleep-related abnormal swallowing syndrome	Patients have difficulty swallowing their saliva during sleep.	Arousals from sleep occur due to coughing and choking. A "gurgling" sound secondary to pooling of secretions in the oral cavity can be heard preceding each coughing spell.
Peptic ulcer disease	Patients report abdominal pain that is typically dull, burning, steady, or intermittent, and it is localized to the epigastric area. Gastric acid production follows a circadian rhythmicity, with basal acid secretion peaking between 9 o'clock and 12 o'clock in the evening.	Awakenings from sleep by nocturnal epigastric pain occur, often within the first 4 hours of sleep onset.

Pain Syndromes

Insomnia is common among persons with musculoskeletal disorders including osteoarthritis, rheumatoid arthritis, and fibromyalgia (Table 3–14).

Table 3-14. Insomnia due to pain syndromes

Disorder	Characteristics	Sleep disturbance
Fibromyalgia	Patients often complain of chronic fatigue, diffuse muscle discomfort, and muscle tenderness. Onset is typically in early adulthood, and women tend to be affected more often than men.	Sleep is often described as light and nonrestorative. Patients may complain of insomnia. Polysomnography demonstrates an increase in frequency of arousals and a decrease in total sleep time. Greater alpha activity with intrusion of alpha waves into NREM sleep can be present.
Chronic pain syndromes (nocturnal cardiac ischemia, headaches, cancer, musculoskeletal pain, or rheumatologic conditions)	Chronic pain is the primary cause of sleep disturbance in many of the medical disorders that are associated with chronic insomnia. Sleep disturbance in patients with chronic pain syndromes may be made worse by the development of depression.	Chronic insomnia (sleep initiation or sleep maintenance) can arise as a result of pain syndromes. Individuals may awaken during the night or in the early morning when the effects of analgesics diminish. Polysomnographic features include a decrease in sleep efficiency and an increase in frequency of awakenings.

Neurologic Disorders

Given the complex neural network that regulates the states of sleep and wakefulness, it is not difficult to imagine how neurologic disorders such as dementia, parkinsonism, cerebral degenerative disorders, headaches, and seizure disorders can prevent sleep onset and disrupt its continuity (Table 3–15). Other neurologic disorders that can give rise to insomnia include brain tumors, strokes, painful neuromuscular syndromes, and traumatic brain injury. Finally, medications used to treat neurologic diseases can give rise to sleep disturbance.

Table 3–15. Neurologic disorders causing insomnia

Disorder	Characteristics	Sleep disturbance
Dementia	Significant neurocognitive impairment is present. In many patients, there is reversal of the day-night cycle due to abnormalities in circadian rhythms of sleep and wakefulness.	Sleep is often disrupted with repetitive arousals. Nocturnal confusion, agitation, and wandering ("sun downing") further contribute to sleep disruption. Polysomnographic features include decreased sleep efficiency, increased frequency of arousals, and an increase in NREM stage 1 sleep.
Parkinson disease	The clinical triad of muscle rigidity, hypokinesia, and resting tremors defines parkinsonism.	Insomnia is a major complaint of patients with Parkinson disease, and up to 90% of patients may complain of poor sleep. The etiology of sleep disturbance in persons with Parkinson disease is varied and include painful leg cramps, repetitive body movements (eg, tremors, myoclonus, or periodic leg movements), muscle rigidity and immobilty, adverse reactions related to medications prescribed, alterations in the circadian sleep-wake patterns, dementia-related sleep fragmentation, and depression. Parkinson disease may also be associated with different sleep disorders, including obstructive and central sleep apnea, periodic limb movement disorder, and REM sleep behavior disorder. Dopaminergic medications used in the therapy of Parkinson disease are associated with vivid dreams, nightmares, and night terrors. Common polysomnographic features of parkinsonism include increased sleep latency, decreased total sleep time, reduced sleep efficiency, frequent body movements during sleep, atypical sleep architecture, decrease in REM sleep, and episodic tremors occurring throughout the night.

Table 3-15. Neurologic disorders causing insomnia—cont'd

Disorder	Characteristics	Sleep disturbance
Cerebral degenerative disorders (Huntington disease, dystonia, ataxia, olivopontocerebellar and spinocerebellar degeneration, spastic torticollis, and musculorum deformans)	Abnormalities in movement and behavior are present. Muscular contractions and gross body movements are most prominent during NREM sleep stages 1 and 2 sleep.	Sleep efficiency is diminished by numerous and, at times, prolonged awakenings.
Seizure disorders	Some seizures occur more commonly during sleep (nocturnal) rather than during wakefulness (diurnal), and others may occur during both sleep and wakefulness (random seizures). About 25% to 30% of patients with epilepsy have their seizures mostly restricted to sleep. Certain seizure types have a tendency to occur during sleep, including tonic-clonic seizures, partial seizures with motor symptomatology and partial seizures with complex symptomatology.	Insomnia due to sudden nighttime awakenings may result in instances when repetitive seizures occur during sleep.
Sleep-related headaches	Several headaches commonly have their onset during sleep, including migraines, cluster headaches, and chronic paroxysmal hemicrania.	Headaches may either cause awakenings during the night or be experienced upon awakening.

Fatal Familial Insomnia

Definition

Familial fatal insomnia (FFI) is an autosomal dominant disorder secondary to a prion disease (an amino acid substitution in the prion protein related to a point mutation at codon 178 of the prion protein gene, with coding for methionine by codon 129 on the mutated allele). It is a rare disorder characterized by sleep disturbances, including relentlessly progressive insomnia, autonomic dysregulation, and neurologic abnormalities. Sleep loss eventually becomes total, terminating in stupor, coma, and death, generally within 12 months to a few years after its onset.

Clinical Features

Clinical features of FFI include disrupted sleep (eg, vivid dreaming and increasingly frequent spontaneous lapses into a dreamlike (oneiric) state with motor activity as the disease progresses), hallucinations, tremors, myoclonus, dystonia, ataxia, dysarthria, autonomic hyperactivity, generalized body wasting, dyspnea and tachypnea, tachycardia, hypertension, hyperthermia, and excessive sweating and salivation. A positive Babinski sign may be present.

There is loss of circadian rhythms of body temperature, hemodynamic parameters (eg, blood pressure, heart rate, and respiratory rate), and endocrine hormones (eg, adrenocorticotropic hormone, follicle-stimulating hormone, luteinizing hormone, growth hormone, and prolactin).

Demographics

FFI typically has its onset in adulthood, often during the fifth or sixth decade. Both genders are affected equally.

Pathophysiology

Similar to other human prion diseases, FFI is caused by a misfolded variation of a prion, an intracellular protein structure. The hereditary form results from a point (GAC to AAC) mutation (substitution of aspartic acid with asparagine) at codon 178 of the prion gene PRNP located on chromosome 20, and it is transmitted in an autosomal dominant fashion. (Note: Interestingly, the familial form of Creutzfeldt-Jakob disease, another prion disease, results from a similar mutation at codon 178 with coding for valine by codon 129 on the mutated allele.)

The point mutation at codon 178 cosegregates with a methionine polymorphism at codon 129. As shown in Table 3–16, a shorter disease course with a survival generally less than 12 months is seen in patients who are methionine homozygous at codon 129, whereas those who are methionine-valine heterozygous at codon 129 have a longer disease course of 1 to 6 years. Sporadic cases do not demonstrate the PRNP mutation at codon 178 but possess the codon 129-methionine polymorphism on both alleles.

Table 3–16. Classification of fatal familical insomnia based on methionine polymorphism at codon 129

Type	Disease course	Duration of survival
Methionine homozygous	Short	< 12 months
Methionine-valine heterozygous	Longer	1 to 6 years

Pathology reveals degeneration as well as reactive gliosis of thalamic nuclei (anterior ventral and dorsomedial) and inferior olivary nucleus, along with grey matter deposition of prion protein type 2. Involvement of the striatum and cerebellum has also been described. There is no associated inflammation. Thalamic hypometabolism has been demonstrated using positron emission tomography scanning.

Complications

Complications of FFI include respiratory and urinary tract infections, dysphagia, and ulcerations.

Clinical Course

Course and prognosis of FFI is influenced by the type of substitution, either methionine (more severe and shorter duration type) or valine (less severe and longer duration type) in codon 129 on the non-mutated allele.

Evaluation

Polysomnographic features vary depending on the stage of the disease. The EEG may be normal or show alternating periods of wakefulness and EEG desynchronization, with bursts of REM activity and loss of muscle tone, in early stages of the disease. This pattern changes to a monomorphic flat activity with occasional 1-to 2-Hz sharp waves, absent sleep spindles, K complexes, and delta activity, as well as reduced and fragmented REM sleep. REM sleep may occur without muscle atonia, reminiscent of REM sleep behavior disorder. Myoclonic tremors may be observed. Progressive flattening and nonreactivity of the EEG characterize the terminal stages of the disease.

Differential Diagnosis

Differential diagnosis of FFI includes other prion diseases (eg, familial Creutzfeldt-Jakob disease), schizophrenia, delirium tremens, and advanced dementia.

Therapy

There is no known specific treatment for FFI.

Psychiatric Disorders

There is a strong correlation between insomnia and psychiatric disorders. Many persons with insomnia have an underlying psychiatric pathology. Conversely, there is an increased prevalence of insomnia among patients with psychiatric disorders.

Insomnia, which is present for at least a month, causes distress and requires independent therapy in addition to that directed at the underlying psychiatric disorder. Onset of insomnia is temporally associated with the psychiatric disorder, and its clinical course parallels that of the latter. *Mood disorders, anxiety disorders, panic disorders, post-traumatic stress disorder, psychoses, eating disorders, alcoholism, somatoform disorders,* and *personality disorders* can all give rise to chronic insomnia (Table 3–17). In addition, medications used to treat psychiatric disorders can also precipitate sleep disturbance or exacerbate an existing complaint of insomnia.

In general, insomnia due to psychiatric disorders is characterized by prolonged sleep latency, sleep fragmentation, frequent arousals during the night, shortened total sleep time, and reduced sleep efficiency. Polysomnographic abnormalities (Box 3–3) may persist even after remission of the psychiatric disorder.

Pregnancy and Menstruation

Both pregnancy and the menstrual cycle can produce insomnia among women (*menstrual-associated sleep disorder* and *pregnancy-associated sleep disorder*) (Table 3–18).

Table 3-17. Psychiatric disorders causing insomnia

Disorder	Sleep disturbance
Mood disorders (major depressive, bipolar, dysthymic, and cyclothymic disorders)	Insomnia is common in mood disorders, including major depression and bipolar disorders. The risk of acquiring a new major depression is greater among patients with insomnia for at least 1 year than in those without sleep disturbances. There is a correlation between the severity of the mood disorder and insomnia in most patients. Patients with major depression commonly complain of frequent nighttime awakenings and spontaneous early morning awakenings. Difficulty with sleep onset and decreased requirements for sleep can be striking during the manic phase of a bipolar disorder. Conversely, sleep loss in patients with bipolar disorder can increase the likelihood of developing mania Polysomnographic features: ↓ Sleep efficiency ↓ Total sleep time ↑ Frequency of arousals ↓ NREM stages 3 and 4 sleep ↓ REM sleep latency (depression) ↑ First REM period duration ↑ REM sleep ↑ REM density Therapy of depression with selective serotonin reuptake inhibitors may exacerbate insomnia.
Anxiety disorders	Sleep-onset insomnia, frequent nighttime awakenings, or recurring anxiety dreams or nightmares can occur. Polysomnographic features: ↓ Sleep efficiency ↑ Sleep latency ↓ REM sleep
Panic disorder	Insomnia, abrupt awakenings with sustained wakefulness, or sleep-related panic attacks have been described. Panic attacks generally arise from NREM stages 2 and 3 sleep. Nocturnal panic attacks can decrease sleep efficiency and prolong sleep latency.
Post-traumatic stress disorder	Frequent sleep-related complaints include sleep-initiation and sleep-maintenance insomnia, restless sleep and daytime fatigue. Flashbacks (eg, anxiety dreams or nightmares) may occur during sleep. Dream recall is reduced. Polysomnographic features: ↓ Total sleep time ↑ Frequency of awakenings ↓ or ↑ REM sleep latency ↓ or ↑ REM sleep ↑ REM density ↑ REM sleep phasic events (e.g., twitches)
Psychoses	Insomnia is a common feature of acute psychotic decompensation. Wakefulness may be maintained for prolonged periods and terminated only by exhaustion. Increased sleep disruption, reversal of day-night sleep patterns, polyphasic sleep episodes, and alternating phases of sleeplessness and hypersomnolence have been described.

Table 3–17. Psychiatric disorders causing insomnia—cont'd

Disorder	Sleep disturbance
Eating disorders	Sleep disorders, including insomnia and repetitive nighttime awakenings, can develop in persons with eating disorders (eg, anorexia nervosa, bulimia, or binge eating).
Alcoholism	Consumption of alcohol close to bedtime decreases wakefulness during the first several hours of sleep; however, the frequency of awakenings increases during the last 2 to 3 hours of sleep as alcohol is metabolized and its serum levels fall.
	Alcohol consumption may intensify snoring and worsen obstructive sleep apnea. Anxiety dreams, enuresis, sleep terrors, and sleepwalking may increase.
	Persons may experience frequent awakenings with chronic alcohol use or during early abstinence.

Box 3–3. **Polysomnographic features of psychiatric disorders**	↓ Sleep efficiency ↑ Sleep latency ↑ Frequency of arousals and awakenings ↑ NREM stages 1 and 2 sleep ↓ NREM stages 3 and 4 sleep

Table 3–18. Sleep disorders due to pregnancy and menstruation

Disorder	Sleep disturbance
Menstrual-associated sleep disorder	Sleep disruption and insomnia can develop during the premenstrual period. The cause of menstrual-associated sleep disorder is unknown.
Pregnancy-associated sleep disorder	Sleep quality and duration differ significantly across the various trimesters of pregnancy.
	Sleeplessness and nighttime awakenings increase during the second trimester reaching their peak in the last trimester. Sleep normalizes shortly after delivery in most women.

Medications and Substances That Can Cause Insomnia

Numerous agents, both prescription medications and recreational drugs, as well as alcohol, are associated with insomnia (Box 3–4). Sleep disturbance can develop during drug use, intoxication, dependency, or discontinuation, or as a result of an adverse reaction to the medication. Insomnia is present for at least 1 month.

Box 3–4.	Alcohol
Medications that can cause insomnia	Anorectic agents

Anticholinergics (ipratropium bromide)

Anticonvulsants (lamotrigine, phenytoin)

Antidepressants (bupropion, fluoxetine, phenelzine, protriptyline, tranylcypromine, venlafaxine)

Antihypertensives (beta-blockers, calcium-channel blockers, clonidine, methyldopa, reserpine)

Antineoplastics (daunorubicin, goserelin, interferon-α, leuprolide)

Antiparkinsonian drugs

Bronchodilators (albuterol, metaproterenol, salmeterol, terbutaline)

Contraceptives (oral)

Corticosteroids

Cough and cold medications/decongestants (phenylpropanolamine, pseudoephedrine)

Diuretics (thiazides)

Hormones (progesterone, thyroid hormones)

Hypolipidemics

Nicotine

Quinidine

Stimulants (caffeine, cocaine, dextroamphetamine, methamphetamine, methylphenidate, modafinil, pemoline)

Theophylline

Polypharmacy using various combinations of these agents is not unusual. Therefore, it may be extremely difficult, in certain instances, to accurately define the contribution of each drug to the complaint of insomnia. The effects of these medications are also influenced by the possible development of tolerance, withdrawal symptoms, or drug interactions (synergistic or antagonistic).

The use and abuse of hypnotic agents, stimulants, and alcohol are major causes of insomnia (*hypnotic-dependent sleep disorder, stimulant-dependent sleep disorder* and *alcohol-dependent sleep disorder*, respectively) (Table 3–19).

Table 3–19.   Insomnia due to hypnotics, stimulants, or alcohol

Disorder	Sleep disturbance

Hypnotic-dependent sleep disorder	Abrupt cessation following chronic use of hypnotic agents can lead to severe insomnia.
	Hypnotics (eg, benzodiazepines) may also precipitate or aggravate sleep-disordered breathing.
	Polysomnographic features of chronic use of benzodiazepines:
	  ↑ Alpha and beta activity
	  ↓ K-complexes
	  ↓ Delta activity
	  ↓ NREM stages 1 sleep
	  ↓ NREM stages 3 and 4 sleep
	  ↓ REM sleep
	  ↓ REM sleep eye movements

Stimulant-dependent sleep disorder	Insomnia may develop whenever stimulant therapy is begun, especially when the medication is taken close to bedtime, or its dosage is increased. Sleep improves following the development of tolerance to the stimulant drugs.
	Polysomnographic features:
	During stimulant use
	  ↑ Sleep latency
	  ↑ Frequency of arousals
	  ↓ Total sleep time
	  ↑ REM sleep latency
	  ↓ REM sleep
	
	During stimulant withdrawal
	  ↓ Sleep latency
	  ↑ Total sleep time
	  REM sleep rebound
	  ↓ Daytime sleep latency on Multiple Sleep Latency Test

Alcohol-dependent sleep disorder	Habitual pre-bedtime self-prescribed use of alcohol in an effort to ensure sleep onset and maintain sleep continuity can paradoxically give rise to insomnia.
	Alcohol consumed prior to anticipated bedtime can produce drowsiness; however, as serum levels of alcohol decline in the latter half of the night, persons may awaken repeatedly with headaches and diaphoresis. Frequent sleep-stage transitions are often seen.
	Abrupt termination of alcohol use can precipitate profound insomnia with frequent awakenings and vivid, disturbing dreams.
	Sleep fragmentation may persist during abstinence among chronic heavy alcohol users.
	Polysomnographic features:
	During alcohol use
	  ↓ NREM stages 3 and 4 sleep
	  ↓ REM sleep
	  REM-sleep fragmentation
	During alcohol withdrawal:
	  ↑ REM sleep (rebound)

Evaluation of Insomnia

Evaluation of insomnia relies primarily on a careful history obtained from patients and their bed partners or roommates, often aided by a well-kept sleep diary. See Box 3–5 for details. In some patients, polysomnography may uncover causes otherwise unsuspected from clinical history.

Box 3–5. **Evaluation of insomnia**	Clinical history

Clinical history

  Sleep complaints (duration of insomnia and timing of sleep disturbance)

  Sleep history

  Medical, surgical, neurologic and psychiatric history

  Family history

  Habits

  Medication use

  Nighttime activities

  Response to previous therapy of insomnia

Questionnaires (including psychologic assessments)

  Beck Anxiety Inventory–evaluation of anxiety

  Beck Depression Inventory–evaluation of depression

  Beliefs and Attitudes about Sleep Scale–evaluation of sleep

  Epworth Sleepiness Scale–evaluation of sleepiness

  Hamilton Rating Scale for Depression–evaluation of depression

  Insomnia Severity Index–evaluation of insomnia

  Multidimensional Fatigue Inventory–evaluation of fatigue

  Penn State Worry Questionnaire–evaluation of anxiety

  Pittsburgh Sleep Quality Index–evaluation of sleep

  Rochester Sleep Continuity Inventory–evaluation of sleep

  State-Trait Anxiety Inventory–evaluation of anxiety

Sleep diaries

Actigraphy (not routinely indicated)

Polysomnography (not routinely indicated)

Laboratory evaluation (not routinely indicated)

Medical Interview

History alone is often sufficient to determine the etiology and severity of insomnia. Sleep duration, quality, and continuity should be assessed. It is useful to inquire about the onset and duration of insomnia; consequences of insomnia; timing of sleep disturbance during the evening; history of medical, surgical, or psychiatric conditions; family history; use of caffeinated beverages, alcohol, tobacco products, illicit drugs, or medications; nighttime activities; any precipitating or perpetuating factors; and response to previous therapy for insomnia.

Onset of Insomnia

One should search for specific acute stressor(s) for cases of insomnia that have a sudden onset.

Duration of Insomnia

Transient insomnia may develop with jet lag, shift work, or acute stressors (eg, pain, anxiety, bereavement, or illness). Chronic insomnia may be secondary to psychophysiologic insomnia, idiopathic insomnia, circadian rhythm disturbances, parasomnias, or underlying medical, neurologic, or psychiatric disorders.

Timing of Sleep Disturbance

Sleep-onset insomnia may be due to delayed sleep-phase syndrome, restless legs syndrome, or anxiety. Recurrent awakenings throughout the night, on the other hand, can be encountered with periodic limb movement disorder, obstructive sleep apnea, excessive alcohol ingestion close to bedtime, or an underlying medical condition. Advanced sleep-phase syndrome or depression may be responsible for early morning awakenings.

Consequences of Insomnia

Patients should be asked about *daytime* consequences of insomnia, including impaired performance, fatigue, sleepiness, accidents, and mood changes.

History of Medical, Surgical, or Psychiatric Conditions

Medical disorders such as pain from degenerative joint disease, muscle spasm or malignancy, epigastric and retrosternal discomfort from gastroesophageal reflux, frequent urination from prostatic or bladder disorders, or dyspnea from poorly controlled asthma can each be sufficiently severe to cause insomnia.

Surgical conditions, including trauma, can likewise disrupt sleep and should not be overlooked in the interview. Any oropharyngeal surgery or trauma to the face and cervical area may contribute to the genesis of obstructive sleep apnea.

Patients should be encouraged to describe their mood. Common complaints among insomniacs include increased irritability, apathy, melancholy, or depression. Patients may volunteer stressful events or relationships. If the stressors are of a recurring or chronic nature, patients should be asked how they have coped with them. Any past psychiatric history of mood disorders, anxiety, psychosis, or schizophrenia may provide insights into the nature of the patient's insomnia.

History of Sleep Disorders

Insomnia can develop in patients with sleep-related breathing disorders (obstructive or central sleep apnea), restless legs syndrome, periodic limb movement disorder, and circadian rhythm sleep disorders.

Habits

Coffee and other caffeine-containing beverages such as tea, and cola sodas are powerful stimulants. The number of drinks typically consumed each day, the amount of caffeine in each drink, and the time during the day when they are consumed, particularly if during the late afternoon or evening hours, are all important. Patients should also be asked if their coffee consumption is increasing or decreasing, or if it has remained stable for the past couple of years.

Other pertinent areas in the social history include the use of alcohol or tobacco products and exercise habits. Excessive smoking and alcohol ingestion close to bedtime may interfere with subsequent sleep quality. Similarly, strenuous exercise performed late in the evening may be sufficiently stimulating to prevent sleep onset. Finally, irregular bedtimes and awakening times, as well as frequent napping can contribute to nighttime sleep disturbance.

Medication Use

Many drugs, including theophylline, beta-adrenergic bronchodilators, beta-blockers, and diuretics are recognized causes of insomnia. Chronic use of hypnotic drugs can produce rebound insomnia with worsening sleep complaints upon its discontinuation. Frustrated with their sleep difficulties and poor daytime performance, patients may attempt to treat themselves with over-the-counter sleeping "aids" such as antihistamines, melatonin, and botanical compounds. The possibility of such use, and its frequency and efficacy should be addressed.

Response to Previous Therapy for Insomnia

It is useful to document the benefit or lack thereof of previous pharmacologic and nonpharmacologic therapy for insomnia. In addition, it is important to ask about the patient's preference for treatment and prior adherence to therapy.

Sleep Diary

A sleep log is useful not only for determining the cause of insomnia (eg, circadian sleep disorders or poor sleep hygiene) but also in monitoring the efficacy of the chosen treatment regimen (Table 3–20).

Polysomnography

Polysomnography is not routinely indicated in the evaluation of transient or chronic insomnia and should not be used as a substitute for a carefully obtained clinical history. Polysomnography may be used when there is strong evidence based on clinical history for insomnia to be due to periodic limb movement disorder or sleep-related breathing disorder. It may also be useful if insomnia is severe and persists despite an adequate trial of behavioral therapy, sleep hygiene, and pharmacologic intervention.

Table 3-20.   American Academy of Sleep Medicine (AASM) recommendations regarding the evaluation of insomnia

Standard
Screening for insomnia should be part of regular health examinations.
A sleep history is essential in determining the cause of insomnia. A physical examination is important for patients with medical symptoms.
Polysomnography (PSG) is not routinely indicated for evaluating insomnia.

Guideline
The following instruments are helpful in evaluating insomnia:
   Self-administered questionnaires
   Sleep logs
   Checklist of symptoms
   Psychological screening tests
   Bed partner interviews
The Multiple Sleep Latency Test (MSLT) is not routinely indicated for evaluating insomnia.
Note: No recommendations were provided due to insufficient evidence regarding portable sleep studies, actigraphy, and static charge sensitive beds in the evaluation of insomnia.

Adapted and modified from Chesson A Jr, Hartse K, Anderson WM, Davila D, Johnson S, Littner M, Wise M, Rafecas J. Practice parameters for the evaluation of chronic insomnia. An American Academy of Sleep Medicine report. Standards of Practice Committee of the American Academy of Sleep Medicine. Sleep. 2000 Mar 15;23(2):237-41.

AASM Definition of Terms

Standard	Generally accepted practice with a high level of clinical certainly
Guideline	Practice associated with a moderate degree of clinical certainty
Option	Practice of uncertain clinical use

Polysomnographic features of insomnia include a prolonged sleep latency, reduced sleep efficiency, decreased total sleep time, and increased awakenings (Table 3–21). A "first-night" effect may occur, with further worsening of the severity of sleep disturbance. On the other hand, sleep duration and quality in the sleep laboratory may be better than usual in patients with psycho-physiologic insomnia.

Table 3-21.   Polysomnographic features of insomnia

General features	↑ Sleep latency ↓ Sleep efficiency ↓ Total sleep time ↑ Frequency of awakenings ↓ NREM stages 3 and 4 sleep ↓ REM sleep
Due to depression	↓ REM sleep latency
Due to dementia	↓ NREM stages 3 and 4 sleep ↓ REM sleep latency ↓ REM sleep
Due to fibromyalgia	Intrusion of alpha waves into NREM stages 3 and 4 sleep
Due to paradoxical sleep	Normal sleep quality and quantity

Less specific abnormalities due to secondary causes of insomnia (eg, depression, dementia, or fibromyalgia) may be present as well. Finally, other sleep disorders, such as sleep apnea, restless legs syndrome, or periodic limb movement disorder, may be detected during polysomnography.

For the AASM recommendations for polysomnography in the evaluation of insomnia, see Table 3–22.

Table 3–22. American Academy of Sleep Medicine recommendations for polysomnography in the evaluation of insomnia

Standard	1. Insomnia requires accurate diagnosis and effective treatment.
	2. Diagnosis of insomnia is made primarily by clinical evaluation.
	3. Polysomnography is indicated for suspected sleep-related breathing disorders or periodic limb movement disorder.
Guideline	1. Polysomnography is indicated when
	Diagnosis is uncertain
	Prescribed therapy fails
	Associated with violent or injurious behavior
	2. Polysomnography is not indicated for routine evaluation of:
	Transient or chronic insomnia
	Insomnia due to psychiatric disorders
	3. Polysomnography is not useful in:
	Distinguishing insomnia associated with dementia
	Diagnosing insomnia in patients with fibromyalgia or chronic fatigue syndrome because the alpha-delta sleep pattern is a nonspecific finding.

Source: Adapted and modified from Standards of Practice Committee of the American Academy of Sleep Medicine. Practice parameters for using polysomnography to evaluate insomnia: an update for 2002. Sleep. 2003;26(6):754-60.
For an AASM definition of terms, see Table 3-20.

Quantitative Electroencephalography

Quantitative EEG may demonstrate an increase in high-frequency beta (14 to 45 Hz) activity both at sleep onset and during NREM sleep in patients with primary insomnia. Insomnia related to major depression may be accompanied by reductions in NREM stages 3 and 4 sleep.

Multiple Sleep Latency Testing

An increase, compared to good sleepers, in sleep latency, indicating higher levels of arousal is typically present during multiple sleep latency testing.

Actigraphy

By monitoring motion as a surrogate measure of sleep and waking, actigraphy conducted over several days has been utilized, with sleep diaries, in the diagnosis of insomnia. It may be most useful as an adjunct to other assessments in the evaluation of paradoxical insomnia or sleep disturbance secondary to circadian rhythm disorders.

Differential Diagnosis of Insomnia

A short sleeper, despite voluntary attempts to lengthen sleep, has a habitual sleep duration that is persistently less than is customary for a similarly aged person. This condition is not associated with any daytime symptoms. Polysomnography confirms the presence of reduced total sleep time. Its course is chronic.

Therapy for Insomnia

The goals of therapy for insomnia include alleviation of nighttime sleep disturbance as well as relief of its daytime consequences. Therapy involves both pharmacotherapy and nonpharmacologic interventions such as proper sleep hygiene practices.

Insomnia may result from many causes. Therefore, one should attempt to identify any factors that may have precipitated or perpetuated the complaints and initiate appropriate corrective measures. Any underlying co-morbid causes of insomnia, such as obstructive sleep apnea, restless legs syndrome, chronic pain syndromes or mood disorders, should be identified and managed accordingly.

General Measures

Many cases of chronic insomnia have their origins in transient disruptions of sleep that have taken root. It is essential that short-term insomnia be promptly recognized and appropriately treated before learned habits, attitudes, and coping mechanisms incongruous with sleep become established and perpetuate the sleep disturbance. Recovery may be more elusive once maladaptive patterns become established.

The treatment of co-morbid insomnia due to a primary sleep, medical, neurologic, or psychiatric illness should, ideally, be directed at the correction of its underlying cause. Therefore, patients with obstructive sleep apnea may benefit from weight reduction if obesity is present; continuous positive airway pressure therapy; dental appliances; or a variety of surgical procedures, including uvulopalatopharyngoplasty, when appropriate. Dopaminergic agents (carbidopa-levodopa), dopamine agonists (pramipexole or ropinirole), benzodiazepines, anticonvulsants, and opioids may be tried in patients with significant restless legs syndrome or periodic limb movement disorder during sleep; iron supplementation should be considered in patients whose serum ferritin levels are less than 50 µg. In patients with mood disorder, anxiety, or psychosis, noticeable improvement in sleep may occur following psychopharmacotherapeutic intervention or counseling. Finally, specific treatment for medical conditions associated with insomnia, such as gastroesophageal reflux disease, cardiac angina, or nocturnal asthma, may alleviate many sleep complaints without having to resort to the use of hypnotic agents.

A referral to a sleep disorder center should be considered for intractable insomnia or for cases with atypical features.

Nonpharmacologic Therapy for Insomnia

Nonpharmacologic therapies for insomnia consist of (1) sleep hygiene (2) relaxation techniques; (3) stimulus control; (4) sleep restriction; (5) cognitive therapy; and (6) paradoxical intention.

Sleep Hygiene

Poor sleep hygiene can, by itself, lead to the development of insomnia. More importantly, it can interact with other etiologies of insomnia resulting in further deterioration of sleep quality.

Promotion of sleep hygiene is, therefore, of paramount importance in the management of patients complaining of poor sleep.

Sleep hygiene involves education to increase activities and behaviors that enhance sleep, and elimination of those that curtail sleep propensity. A regular bedtime and arising time should be established. Patients must adhere strictly to this sleep schedule, even during weekends or vacations. Patients should be instructed to avoid taking prolonged naps during the day, which may have a profound influence on the subsequent night's sleep. Napping in the late afternoon or early evening is especially prone to interfere with nocturnal sleep. Patients should also avoid spending excessive time while awake in bed.

A variety of commonly used substances such as alcohol, caffeine, and nicotine in cigarette smoke can interfere with sleep and are best avoided.

1.   Patients suffering from insomnia may ingest alcohol prior to bedtime in a misguided attempt to improve sleep onset. Unfortunately, the subsequent metabolism of alcohol and the decline in its blood level can produce a sympathetic activation leading to awakenings. Alcohol is metabolized at a rate of approximately one drink per hour (equal to 12 ounces of beer, 5 ounces of wine, 1.5 ounces of vodka or gin, or 1 ounce of 100-proof whiskey). However, alcohol-induced sympathetic hyperactivity may persist for a couple of hours after the blood alcohol level has normalized.

2.   Caffeinated drinks such as coffee, tea, and soda can disrupt sleep and increase the frequency of nighttime awakenings. Caffeine competes with the inhibitory neurotransmitter adenosine for its receptors and the resulting central nervous system arousal can persist for several hours following ingestion. Patients who consume large quantities of caffeine should be encouraged to refrain from further consumption by early or mid-afternoon. Intake of more than 500 mg of caffeine (e.g., five average-sized cups of coffee or seven to ten cans of cola drinks) daily should be avoided.

3.   Smoking can also interfere with sleep. Whereas low blood levels of nicotine can produce mild relaxation, high blood levels have an arousing effect.

Medications that can cause insomnia should be identified. Selecting an alternative drug with lesser impact on sleep, or altering the time of administration from bedtime to late afternoon or early evening can minimize drug-related insomnia.

It is important to avoid stimulating activities late in the evening. Strenuous exercise, challenging mental tasks, and intense arguments all have an arousing effect. Allowing a few minutes each evening to write down the various ongoing worries and concerns and to schedule activities for the following day is an effective way of putting an "end" to the extended work day. Regular exercise during the day may be beneficial, but should not be performed within 3 to 5 hours of bedtime.

Environmental control is often overlooked. Bright lights (eg, from a television set or hallway fixtures) may disrupt sleep. Although most patients prefer the bedroom to be kept as dark as possible, others, especially those fearful of the dark, may find solace in a dim light in the bedroom. Needless to say, the bedroom should be kept quiet and its temperature adjusted to fit individual tastes. If excessive bright light or noise cannot be avoided such as in cases involving nearby street traffic or sunlight for shift workers trying to sleep during the daytime, earplugs and eye masks may be tried.

Some people find that light reading or contemplative meditation is useful.

"Clock watchers," who become increasingly distressed and alarmed as they see the seconds and minutes ticking away while they remain awake, should be told to remove the clock from the bedroom. On the other hand, looking at the clock and realizing that a considerable amount of time has passed while the patient has been asleep can quell the anxiety among those who awaken frequently during the night.

Concerns about safety should be addressed prior to bedtime by properly securing door locks, making certain that children or pets are safe, and that any other potential hazards have been attended to. Pets that jump onto the bed, thereby awakening the patient in the middle of the night, should be kept away from the bedroom.

Activities in bed should be restricted to those that enhance sleep propensity. Because sexual activity can be either stimulating or relaxing, its performance close to bedtime should be individualized.

Ingestion of liquids at bedtime should be limited. However, patients should avoid going to bed hungry or thirsty.

In summary, educating patients with insomnia on proper sleep hygiene is a necessary component of therapy and complements other behavioral interventions. However, it is rarely sufficiently effective by itself to reverse the symptoms of sleep disturbance.

Light Therapy

Circadian rhythm sleep-wake disturbances are generally amenable to light treatment (ie, exposure to light in the early morning in persons with delayed sleep-phase syndrome, or in the late evening in cases of advanced sleep-phase disorder). Light treatment should be complemented by appropriate light restriction at either the start or end of the sleep period. The duration and frequency of sessions should be tailored to individual needs. For more information about light therapy, see Table 3–23.

Table 3-23. Effect of bright light therapy

Morning exposure for sleep-onset insomnia	Evening exposure for early morning awakenings
Produces a phase advance in circadian sleep-wake, core body temperature and melatonin rhythms	Produces a phase delay in circadian sleep-wake, core body temperature and melatonin rhythms
Shortens sleep latency	Increases sleep efficiency
Increases total sleep time	Increases total sleep time
Causes earlier final awakening time	Causes later final awakening time

It is reasonable to schedule an ophthalmologic examination prior to the initiation of light therapy since retinopathy is a contraindication to this form of therapy. Persons with glaucoma or cataracts should be followed closely, and light treatment should be promptly discontinued if any adverse reactions should occur.

Table-mounted lights or visor lamps that provide 2,500 to 10,000 lux illumination are commercially available. Because of the dangers of excessive irradiation with resulting damage to the eyes, it is inadvisable to use makeshift devices that may not provide the desired intensity and spectrum of light.

Behavioral Treatment for Insomnia

Behavioral therapy is designed to curtail physical and psychic influences that may disrupt sleep onset and maintenance, promote activities that are conducive to sleep, and regularize sleep-wake schedules. It is appropriate as initial treatment of primary insomnia (eg, psychophysiological insomnia) as well as adjunctive therapy for co-morbid insomnia. Several behavioral interventions have been described. Selection among the various therapies must be individualized; it is common to combine several approaches, with or without concurrent use of hypnotic agents, in the management of patients with chronic insomnia. Approaches used in the behavioral therapy of insomnia are listed in Box 3–6.

Box 3-6. **Behavioral therapy of insomnia**	Relaxation techniques
	Stimulus control
	Temporal control
	Cognitive therapy
	Sleep restriction
	Paradoxical intention
	Cognitive behavioral therapy

Several treatment approaches for behavioral therapy have been described, including self-help programs (books or audiovisual presentations), therapist-guided individual sessions, and group therapy. Whether any treatment format is superior over others or whether therapist-driven protocols are better than those that do not require active therapist intervention needs further study. Some therapies, such as sleep restriction, stimulus control, and temporal control, require more sessions than others, such as relaxation techniques and cognitive therapy. The AASM recommendations concerning behavioral therapy in insomnia are listed in Box 3–7.

Box 3-7 **American Academy of Sleep Medicine recommendations regarding the behavioral therapy of insomnia**	1. The following therapies are effective in the treatment of chronic insomnia:
	  a. Stimulus control (standard)
	  b. Progressive muscle relaxation (guideline)
	  c. Biofeedback (guideline)
	  d. Paradoxical intention (guideline)
	  e. Sleep restriction (option)
	  f. Multicomponent (cognitive) behavioral therapy (option)
	2. No recommendations were provided for the following approaches as single therapy for chronic insomnia due to insufficient evidence:
	  a. Sleep hygiene education
	  b. Imagery training
	  c. Cognitive therapy

Source: Adapted and modified from Chesson et al. Practice parameters for the nonpharmacologic treatment of chronic insomnia. Sleep, 1999; 22(8).
For a definition of terms , see the notefollowing Table 3-20

A majority of patients (between 50% and 80%) with insomnia benefit from behavioral therapy, with improvements in sleep quality and duration (Box 3–8). Compared with hypnotic medications that can improve sleep shortly after administration, gains in sleep quality and duration are often not immediately apparent, and it may take several weeks for therapy to produce meaningful benefits. The therapeutic benefits of pharmacologic and behavioral therapy are comparable at 1 to 2 months. Improvements in sleep parameters following behavioral therapy appear to be sustained over time (ie, at least 6 months), unlike pharmacotherapy, which does not retain any significant benefits upon its discontinuation.

Nonetheless, the magnitude of treatment response varies among patients, and not everyone who benefits from therapy becomes a good sleeper. Furthermore, improvements in nighttime sleep with behavioral therapy may not give rise to corresponding positive changes in daytime symptoms.

Box 3–8.	Decrease in insomnia symptoms

Benefits of behavioral therapy for insomnia	Increase in sleep quality
	Improvement in sleep architecture
	   Decrease in sleep latency
	   Increase in sleep duration
	   Decrease in frequency of awakenings
	   Decrease in duration of nocturnal awakenings
	   Decrease in wake time after sleep onset
	Decrease in use of hypnotic medications
	Decrease in associated symptoms (eg, depression or anxiety)
	Decrease in health care utilization

Finally, subjective reports of improvements in sleep may be greater than objective measures obtained with polysomnography.

Relaxation Techniques Relaxation techniques include progressive relaxation, EMG biofeedback, meditation, and guided imagery. Relaxation targets the somatic and psychic-cognitive stressors that perpetuate insomnia. Progressive relaxation has been shown to shorten sleep latency, decrease wake time after sleep onset, increase total sleep time, and improve sleep quality.

Relaxation techniques are often employed for patients with insomnia who are considered to have heightened cognitive and somatic arousal. Patients are taught how to use progressive muscle relaxation (exercises that sequentially tense and relax various muscle groups throughout the body) or biofeedback (method of muscle relaxation aided by EMG feedback) to reduce somatic arousal. The latter consists of immediate feedback using EMG recording during attempted relaxation techniques that enable participants to distinguish between behaviors that increase tension from those that promote relaxation and assists them in refocusing their behavioral patterns towards the latter.

Psychic-cognitive stressors may be minimized by meditation or guided imagery in which thoughts are redirected toward pleasant or neutral subjects. Sensory motor rhythm biofeedback uses EEG recordings to instruct patients on how to enhance their ability to generate sleep spindles. Thought blocking (ie, stopping racing thoughts) to decrease cognitive arousal is also used.

Stimulus Control Stimulus control therapy aims to strengthen the association of the bedroom and bedtime to a conditioned response for sleep rather than with insomnia, arousal, and anxiety. Patients are encouraged to use the bedroom only for sleep and sexual activity. They are instructed to get into bed intending to sleep only when sleepy and to refrain from engaging in activities in bed that are not compatible with sleep, such as eating, watching television, or working. If unable to sleep or return to sleep after awakenings within a reasonable time (eg, after 15 to 20 minutes in bed), patients are taught to leave the bedroom and return only when drowsy. In the interim, they are allowed to engage in restful, nonstimulating and sleep-promoting activities such as reading with a dim light. Maintaining a consistent arising time in the morning and avoiding daytime napping are important. Studies have reported that stimulus control improves sleep onset and sleep maintenance insomnia and decreases both sleep latency and wake time after sleep onset.

Temporal Control Temporal control therapy is designed to enhance sleep efficiency. The constancy of the sleep-wake schedule is promoted by having the patient get out of bed at the same time each day regardless of the quality and quantity of the preceding evening's sleep. Daytime naps are eliminated.

Cognitive Therapy

Cognitive Therapy Cognitive therapy addresses unrealistic expectations about sleep and the consequences of insomnia. It focuses on reversing these dysfunctional attitudes and beliefs about sleep. Techniques may include attention shifting, decatastrophizing, and reappraisal.

Sleep Restriction

Sleep Restriction Sleep restriction consists of limiting the amount of time a patient with insomnia spends in bed, matching the latter with the actual duration of total sleep time. By creating a state of sleep deprivation, this method is designed to decrease sleep latency, increase sleep efficiency, and decrease wake time after sleep onset. Percentage of NREM stages 3 and 4 sleep may increase. This approach is particularly helpful in persons who spend considerable time in bed awake, frustrated and agitated. Sleep restriction involves increasing homeostatic sleep drive by reducing time in bed; time in bed is subsequently increased once sleep efficiency improves.

Time spent in bed is limited to actual sleeping only. For instance, in an individual with a subjective report of 6 hours of sleep but who spends 9 hours in bed, the initial recommended time in bed would be 6 hours from bedtime to arising time by delaying bedtime. Wake up time is kept constant. Time allowed in bed should be at least 4.5 to 5 hours per night and is adjusted periodically depending on the calculated sleep efficiency (the percentage of time in bed spent sleeping [total sleep time/time in bed × 100%]) until a desired sleep duration is attained. Time in bed is increased or decreased by 15 to 30 minutes at the start of each evening's sleep when sleep efficiency is greater than 90% or lower than 80%, respectively. No change in allowable bedtime is made if sleep efficiency is between 80% and 90%. Naps are not allowed.

Paradoxical Intention

Paradoxical Intention Patients with insomnia often display performance anxiety over their ability to fall asleep. Paradoxical intention involves instructing patients with insomnia to go to bed and to try to stay awake as long as they possibly can at night. By persuading the patient with insomnia to remain awake at night rather than trying to sleep, paradoxical intention attempts to decrease the performance anxiety associated with efforts to fall asleep.

Paradoxical insomnia might reduce sleep latency. Specific subsets of patients with insomnia who would respond to this therapy have not been defined.

Cognitive-Behavioral Therapy

Cognitive-Behavioral Therapy Cognitive-behavioral therapy (CBT) is a multimodality therapy, often including sleep hygiene education, relaxation techniques, stimulus control therapy, sleep restriction therapy, and cognitive therapy. It focuses on reversing unrealistic beliefs and attitudes, unreasonable fears, and maladaptive behavior about sleep and sleep loss. Patients are also instructed on proper sleep habits. Improvements in wake time after sleep onset have been described following CBT.

CBT may be used as a single treatment modality or combined with pharmacologic therapy (indications for combined therapy are not established). Alternative approaches to individualized therapy include group sessions, brief office encounters, phone consultations, and self-help programs.

CBT may benefit patients with either primary or co-morbid insomnia. Short-term benefits are generally comparable to pharmacologic therapy, and beneficial effects are sustained over time after the initial treatment period. The effects of CBT on sleep architecture are presented in Box 3–9. Treatment response is noted in about 70% to 80% of patients with insomnia; however, treatment responsiveness does not necessarily result in complete normalization of sleep.

Box 3–9.	↓ Sleep latency
Effects of cognitive behavioral therapy on sleep architecture	↑ Total sleep time ↓ Frequency of awakenings ↓ Wake time after sleep onset

Pharmacologic Therapy for Insomnia

Hypnotic agents enhance drowsiness and facilitate the onset of sleep. They are primarily indicated for the treatment of transient sleep disruption such as those caused by jet lag, shift work, or acute stress, but they may also be used in selected persons with chronic insomnia (primary insomnia that has failed to respond to behavioral therapy, or co-morbid insomnia that has not improved with treatment of the underlying condition).

Medications used in the treatment of insomnia include the benzodiazepines; nonbenzodiazepine benzodiazepine receptor agonists (NBBRAs); antidepressants; melatonin receptor agonists; and the nonprescription hypnotic agents, such as histamine antagonists, melatonin, and herbal compounds. The selection of a particular hypnotic agent among the numerous available compounds should be done cautiously with consideration of its hypnotic efficacy, absorption and elimination profile, onset and duration of action, effect on sleep stages, risks of tolerance, dependency and withdrawal, abuse potential, possible drug interactions, and cost. It is advisable to select an agent with minimal risk of daytime residual effects. Specific characteristics of the patient, including the presence of medical or psychiatric illnesses, age, pregnancy or lactation, occupation, other medications used, and any prior history of polydrug dependence and abuse, should also be taken into account.

It is generally recommended that sedative-hypnotic therapy be limited to short-term use at the lowest effective dose. Whenever sedative-hypnotics are used for longer periods, consideration should be given to intermittent usage, and indications should be reassessed on a regular basis. Monitoring for effectiveness of the drug, adverse reactions, self-escalation of the medication dose, and alterations in medical or psychiatric status must occur. Patients should be informed of the benefits and risks of hypnotic use.

It is recommended that hypnotic agents be taken immediately prior to bedtime when the patient is preparing to sleep, rather than earlier in the evening, with the hope that sleep will occur immediately once the patients gets into bed. Although hypnotic agents may enhance sleep, they often do not improve daytime performance. There appears to be no long-term beneficial effects on sleep following discontinuation of hypnotic agents.

Caution should be exercised when using hypnotic agents in patients with significant respiratory, renal, and hepatic impairment. They are best avoided during pregnancy. In addition, hypnotic agents should not be taken with alcohol.

Characteristics of Sedative Hypnotics

Rate of drug absorption and distribution in the CNS as well as receptor affinity determine the onset and potency of action. The dose administered, elimination half-life, and rate of metabolism influence the drug's duration of action. Sedative-hypnotics differ in their pharmacokinetic profiles with regards to *Tmax* (time to peak plasma concentration), which alters sleep latency, and *biological half-life*, which influences sleep maintenance.

Tmax   Most, if not all, sedative-hypnotics possess a Tmax of less than 1 to 2 hours. An agent with a Tmax of < 1.5 hours reduces sleep latency.

Biological Half-Life   The duration of action of a drug is determined by both the dose administered and its elimination half-life. Generally, a greater dose or a longer half-life results in a longer duration of action. Drugs with shorter half-lives are associated with less residual effects. Conversely, longer half-lives are associated with greater residual effects. Drugs with half-lives greater than 4 hours are generally required for therapy of sleep maintenance insomnia. The half-lives of hypnotic agents are listed in Table 3–24.

Table 3–24.	Agent	Half-life(hours)
Elimination half-lives of hypnotic agents	Zaleplon	1–1.5
	Indiplon	1
	Zolpidem	1.5–4
	Triazolam	2–5
	Temazepam	4–18
	Estazolam	14–24
	Flurazepam	40–250
	Quazepam	40–250

Older Hypnotic Agents

Older hypnotic agents (eg, barbiturates, chloral hydrate, glutethimide, meprobamate, methyprylon, and paraldehyde) have been replaced by newer, more effective, and safer agents. Use of barbiturates is associated with the development of psychologic and physical dependency, and overdoses are ever-present dangers. Furthermore, barbiturates can interact with numerous medications via their induction of liver enzymes. Chronic ingestion of chloral hydrate can be complicated by the rapid development of tolerance as well as the occurrence of rashes, gastric discomfort, and hepatic toxicity.

Benzodiazepines

Benzodiazepines and NBBRAs bind to the supramolecular gamma-aminobutyric acid (GABA)-benzodiazepine (GABA-BZ) receptor complex.

GABA is a CNS inhibitory neurotransmitter. $GABA_A$, the major GABA receptor, is a membrane chloride channel. It consists of five subunits (often 2 alpha, 2 beta, and 1 gamma), each with several subtypes. Binding of benzodiazepine agonists to benzodiazepines receptors at the alpha-gamma subunit of the GABA complex leads to allosterical enhancement of GABA and an increase in the chloride current at the GABA receptor site. The various GABA-BZ receptor subunits (BZ1, BZ2, and BZ3) differ in their action. The hypnotic (soporific) and amnestic actions of the agent are related primarily to BZ1 receptors, whereas BZ2 and BZ3 receptors are believed to be responsible for its effect on memory and cognitive functioning, muscle relaxation, and antiseizure and antianxiety properties.

Benzodiazepines bind nonselectively to the different GABA-BZ receptor subunits. Therefore, in addition to their hypnotic properties, benzodiazepines are potent anxiolytics, myorelaxants, and anticonvulsants. In contrast, NBBRAs preferentially bind to the GABA-benzodiazepine-1 receptor subunit (BZ1).

Duration of Action   Duration of action differs among the various benzodiazepine preparations and this distinction has been used to select the appropriate agent for the different timing of insomnia. Based on duration of action, benzodiazepines can be classified into short-acting (half-life of less than 3–4 hours), intermediate-acting (half-life of 8–24 hours), and long-acting (half-life of greater than 24 hours) agents (Table 3–25).

Table 3–25.	Duration of action	Agents
Duration of action of benzodiazepines	Short-acting agents	Triazolam (Halcion)
	Intermediate-acting agents	Estazolam (ProSom) Temazepam (Restoril)
	Long-acting agents	Flurazepam (Dalmane) Quazepam (Doral)

Short-acting agents such as triazolam are helpful for patients who have difficulty falling asleep. Their brief elimination half-life of 2 to 5 hours substantially minimizes any residual sedation the following morning.

Intermediate-acting agents such as temazepam and estazolam are helpful for patients with both sleep-onset and maintenance insomnia. Patients with frequent awakenings during the evening often find temazepam's extended duration of action of 6 to 8 hours helpful.

Long-acting compounds including flurazepam and quazepam, with elimination half-lives of 36 to 120 hours, are indicated for patients with both early morning awakenings and daytime anxiety.

Onset of Action   Timing of drug administration is determined chiefly by its onset of action. Agents that are rapidly absorbed from the gastrointestinal track have a quick onset of action and can be given at bedtime. These drugs include clorazepate, diazepam, flurazepam, and quazepam. On the other hand, benzodiazepines such as temazepam, whose action is delayed following ingestion, may need to be taken slightly earlier than the desired bedtime.

Adverse Effects of Benzodiazepines   Benzodiazepines are associated with several adverse effects. Short-acting agents may cause rebound daytime anxiety and greater amnesia, as well as more withdrawal symptoms (including rebound insomnia) following cessation of their use. The effect of agents with long elimination half-lives may persist into the following day, producing daytime sleepiness, poor motor coordination, delayed reaction times, and cognitive impairment. Other adverse consequences of benzodiazepines include amnesia, confusion, rebound insomnia, development of tolerance and withdrawal symptoms, and the risk of dependency and abuse.

1. *Impairment of cognition*—Memory impairment appears to be directly correlated to the agent's affinity for the benzodiazepine-GABA receptor. For instance, triazolam, which has increased

affinity for its receptor, also has a high potential for inducing amnesia. Anterograde amnesia, or the inability to register new memory after drug ingestion, is also partially influenced by the sedative properties of the medication. Confusion may develop among older adults.

2. *Relapse*—Recurrence of insomnia is common following discontinuation of benzodiazepines.

3. *Rebound insomnia*—Subjective and objective worsening of sleep (compared with baseline pretreatment levels) and daytime well-being can develop for several days after drug discontinuation. This is more likely to occur with short-acting and intermediate-acting agents. The duration of sleep deterioration can be protracted. Although rebound insomnia can develop following short-term therapy with benzodiazepines, it is particularly prominent after chronic treatment. Rebound insomnia can be minimized by intermittent use of hypnotic agents and by gradual reduction of the dose administered.

4. *Withdrawal symptoms after abrupt drug discontinuation*—Following chronic use of benzodiazepines, abrupt discontinuation can also give rise to anxiety, irritability, restlessness, and tremulousness.

5. *Risk of dependency*—These medications generally have a low risk of dependency, and persons with insomnia typically do not self-escalate the frequency or dose of drug use. Dependency, nevertheless, can occur with long-term use, especially in individuals with a prior history of dependency to similar or related compounds.

6. *Development of tolerance*—Patients typically develop tolerance rapidly to these agents, and their sleep duration and quality may begin to deteriorate and possibly reach baseline levels within several weeks of drug administration. With chronic use, increasingly higher dosages are required to achieve similar therapeutic benefits.

7. *Drug overdose*—Benzodiazepines have a relatively good safety profile following overdose. Lethality with overdose of benzodiazepines, when ingested alone, is low but rises with co-ingestion of other compounds such as alcohol and other CNS depressants.

8. *Safety issues*—The risk of car accidents may be increased among chronic benzodiazepine users. Patients should be cautioned against operating motor vehicles or performing tasks that require vigilance and alertness when using these drugs.

9. *Psychomotor impairment*—Duration of psychomotor impairment (eg, increase in errors, slowing of response times) is related to the dose and half-life of the medication.

10. *Respiratory depression* and *worsening of obstructive sleep apnea.*

11. *Increase in falls*—The frequency of falls *may* increase among older adults.

Use during Pregnancy and Lactation

Benzodiazepines should be avoided in pregnant women and in breast-feeding mothers because they can cross the placenta and are secreted in breast milk.

Use in Persons with Medical Disorders

Doses should be adjusted in patients with significant renal or hepatic impairment. Due to the potential danger of respiratory depression, benzodiazepines should be given cautiously, if at all, to patients with untreated obstructive sleep apnea or profound obstructive and restrictive ventilatory impairment (eg, severe emphysema and obesity-hypoventilation syndrome).

Use in Older Adults

Older adults are particularly susceptible to the hypnotic effects of benzodiazepines. The presence of preexisting memory impairment, reduced clearance of the agent and, possibly, increased CNS sensitivity may increase the risk of confusion and falls among older patients. When prescribing hypnotic agents to older adults, one should start at reduced doses and monitor their effects closely.

Changes in Polysomnographic Features Related to Use of Benzodiazepines

Benzodiazepines typically reduce sleep latency, increase total sleep time, and decrease the frequency of awakenings in patients with insomnia. They also increase NREM stage 2 sleep (more sleep spindles), decrease NREM stages 3 and 4 sleep, and decrease REM sleep.

Nonbenzodiazepine Benzodiazepine Receptor Agonists

As described earlier, NBBRAs (eg, zolpidem, zaleplon, zopiclone, and eszopiclone) selectively bind to the GABA-benzodiazepine-1 receptor subunit (BZ1). Their hypnosedative action is comparable with that of the benzodiazepines. The NBBRAs decrease sleep latency. Total sleep time is either increased or remains unchanged. There is no reduction in NREM stages 3 and 4 sleep or REM sleep.

Compared with conventional benzodiazepines, NBBRAs do not possess myorelaxant, antianxiety, or antiseizure properties, are less likely to cause significant rebound insomnia or tolerance, and are associated with minimal abuse liability. However, risk of abuse remains a concern, particularly among patients with a history of abuse or dependency of alcohol or other drugs, and those with psychiatric disorders. In addition, most of these agents are less likely than benzodiazepines to impair daytime performance and memory due to their relatively short duration of action and their low potential for residual effect. They are relatively safe and are seldom lethal even with over dosage.

The effects of benzodiazepine receptor agonists on sleep architecture are presented in Box 3–10. The half-lives of nonbenzodiazepine benzodiazepine receptor agonists are given in Table 3–26.

Box 3-10. **Effects of benzodiazepine receptor agonists**[a] **on sleep architecture**	↓ Sleep latency ↓ Frequency of awakenings ↑ Total sleep time ↑ NREM stages 3 and 4 sleep (benzodiazepines) ↓ REM sleep (benzodiazepines)

[a] *Benzodiazepine and non-benzodiazepine benzodiazepine receptor agonists*

Zolpidem   Zolpidem is a nonbenzodiazepine imidazopyridine that binds preferentially to the BZ1 subtype of benzodiazepine receptors. In contrast to the benzodiazepines, it possesses no anticonvulsant or muscle relaxant activity. It is rapidly absorbed from the gastrointestinal tract and has a quick onset of action. Zolpidem has a short half-life of approximately 2.4 hours. Its metabolites are inactive and readily excreted. Its effects can be reversed with flumazenil.

The advantages of zolpidem as a hypnotic agent include its relative lack of any appreciable withdrawal symptoms, tolerance, risk of addiction, rebound insomnia, or daytime psychomotor impairment. Compared with the benzodiazepines, it is less likely to disrupt normal sleep architecture.

Table 3-26.   Half-lives of nonbenzodiazepine benzodiazepine receptor agonists

Agent	Half-life (hours)
Zaleplon	1–1.5
Zolpidem	1.5–4
Eszopiclone	4–6

It does not decrease NREM stages 3 and 4 sleep. Side effects are generally mild and include headaches, dizziness, drowsiness, and nausea. Occasionally, patients may experience nightmares or agitation.

The dose of zolpidem is commonly 5 to 10 mg at bedtime. The lower dose is recommended for elderly patients and individuals who have underlying medical disorders. A sustained release form of the agent is also available and is given at a dose of 6.25 to 12.5 mg at bedtime.

Zopiclone   Zopiclone is a cyclopyrrolone agent that potentiates GABA-mediated neuronal inhibition. It has a rapid onset of action and a short half-life. Zopiclone is well tolerated; possesses minimal tolerance potential; and is associated with a low risk of residual daytime effects, rebound insomnia, and withdrawal reactions. It has minimal effects on sleep stages. Zopiclone is not available in the United States.

Eszopiclone   Eszopiclone is a cyclopyrrolone nonbenzodiazepine agent that has received U.S. Food and Drug Administration (FDA) approval without a restriction to short-term usage. Long-term pharmacologic treatment of chronic primary insomnia using eszopiclone does not appear to be associated with drug tolerance. Improvements in sleep latency, wake time after sleep onset, frequency of awakenings, number of nights with awakenings per week, total sleep time, quality of sleep, daytime function, alertness, and sense of physical well-being have been described.

Zaleplon   Zaleplon has a rapid onset of action and an ultrashort duration of action with a half-life of only about 1 hour. Except for a shortened sleep latency, it is associated with minimal effects on sleep architecture. There is no tolerance to its sleep-promoting effects and no rebound insomnia upon its discontinuation.

Zaleplon is administered at a dose of 5 to 10 mg at bedtime. Doses should start at 5 mg in elderly patients. It may also be given during prolonged middle-of-the-night awakenings as long as there is at least 4 hours remaining prior to rising time.

Sedating Antidepressants

Sedating antidepressants have been increasingly prescribed as off-label agents for the treatment of insomnia over the past several years. However, despite their widespread use to aid sleep, data on their appropriate use among persons with insomnia, particularly in patients without mood disorders, is limited. The therapeutic efficacy and safety of sedating antidepressants used as hypnotics for patients with insomnia are incompletely understood. In general, serotonin-specific antidepressants have fewer adverse effects than the older tertiary tricyclics. The effects of sedating antidepressants on sleep architecture are presented in Box 3–11.

Box 3-11.	↓ Sleep latency
Effects of sedating antidepressants on sleep architecture	↓ Frequency of awakenings
	↑ Total sleep time
	↑ Sleep efficiency

Trazodone   A 5-HT (2) and alpha (1) receptor antagonist, trazodone possesses both anxiolytic and sedative properties, which make it one of the most commonly prescribed medications for the therapy of insomnia. Trazodone increases sleep efficiency, total sleep time, and NREM stages 3 and 4 sleep, and decreases NREM stage 2 sleep. It may or may not increase REM sleep latency and decrease REM sleep. Although it is widely prescribed for chronic primary insomnia, there is minimal published data supporting its use for this purpose. Its effectiveness for this indication has not been conclusively established.

Trazodone does not appear to possess any significant potential for tolerance or dependency. Compared with the tricyclic antidepressants such as amitriptyline, trazodone has less anticholinergic action and a shorter half-life. Side effects include cardiac arrhythmias, orthostatic hypotension, priapism (painful erection) in males, and painful clitoral engorgement in females. Concurrent administration with other serotonin-specific agents can give rise to the serotonin syndrome.

Hypnotic doses of trazodone range from 25 to 100 mg given at bedtime. It has a short half-life.

Nefazodone   Nefazodone is a sedating serotonin receptor blocker and mild serotonin reuptake inhibitor. Polysomnographic features associated with its use include either no change in REM sleep parameters or a decrease in REM sleep latency and increase in REM sleep (particularly in patients with depression). Adverse effects include rare liver toxicity.

Mirtazapine   Mirtazapine is a noradrenergic and serotonergic antidepressant. It acts by antagonizing central alpha 2-adrenergic and 5-HT (2) and 5-HT (3) receptors. Changes in sleep architecture during mirtazapine administration consist of a decrease in sleep latency, increase in sleep efficiency, decrease in wake time after sleep onset, and increase in NREM stages 3 and 4 sleep. There are inconsistent changes in REM sleep, with either an increase or no change in REM sleep latency, and a decrease or no change in REM sleep duration. Side effects include weight gain and nausea.

Tricyclic Antidepressants   Sedating tricyclic antidepressants include amitriptyline, doxepin, nortriptyline, and trimipramine. As a group, they have a low risk of abuse. Doxepin acts by blocking uptake of serotonin and norepinephrine. It increases REM sleep latency and decreases REM sleep.

Adverse effects include anticholinergic actions (eg, constipation or dry mouth), abnormalities in cardiac conduction, orthostatic hypotension, and exacerbation of symptoms of restless legs and periodic limb movements of sleep. Sedating tricyclic antidepressants should be used with caution in patients with glaucoma, seizures, or cardiac conduction disorders.

Ramelteon

This agent is a melatonin receptor agonist that is highly selective for ML1 receptors located mainly in cells of the suprachiasmatic nucleus, and has less affinity for other ML receptor subtypes, including ML2. It has clinically relevant sleep-promoting effects, including a decrease in latency to persistent sleep, increase in sleep efficiency, and increase in total sleep time.

Other Prescription Agents

Quetiapine, an atypical antipsychotic with anti-histaminergic, anti-dopaminergic, and anti-adrenergic properties, has been used as a sleep aid for patients with psychiatric illness, although its effectiveness for this indication has not been established. Polysomnographic features include an increase in total sleep time, sleep efficiency, NREM stage 2 sleep and subjective sleep quality.

Finally, antipsychotic agents (eg, chlorpromazine, haloperidol, olanzapine, and risperidone), buspirone, carbamazepine, clonidine, cyproheptadine, divalproex, gabapentin, and oxcarbazepine possess sedative properties and have been used to treat patients presenting with complaints of insomnia. Data on their efficacy and safety for the therapy of insomnia is either limited or absent.

Nonprescription Hypnotic Agents

Patients with insomnia commonly self-administer nonprescription sleep agents, including alcohol, to manage their sleep disturbances. Other commonly used nonprescription products include histamine antagonists, melatonin, and botanical compounds.

Histamine Antagonists

Antihistamines comprise a majority of the over-the-counter hypnotic agents. Aside from their actions on histamine H1 receptors, these agents may also act on serotonergic, cholinergic, and central alpha-adrenergic receptors.

Despite their popularity, there are few published data on the efficacy of antihistamines as sleep aids for insomnia, and their effectiveness in treating chronic insomnia is not well demonstrated. By virtue of their ability to cross the blood–brain barrier, first-generation histamine H1 antagonists (eg, diphenhydramine, doxylamine, promethazine, and chlorpheniramine) can induce sedation. Administration of diphenhydramine decreases sleep latency and increases sleep duration. Second-generation agents (eg, loratadine and fexofenadine) are less likely to cause sedation.

Tolerance to the hypnotic effects of antihistamines can develop rapidly. Many agents possess long half-lives, and daytime sedation can develop following their use. Other adverse effects of histamine antagonists include confusion, delirium, dizziness, blurring of vision, dry mouth, urinary retention, and constipation.

Melatonin

Melatonin, a neurohormone produced in the pineal gland during darkness under the control of the suprachiasmatic nuclei, has been used primarily for the therapy of insomnia secondary to circadian rhythm sleep disturbances (eg, delayed sleep phase syndrome, non–24-hour sleep wake cycles in blind individuals, jet lag or shift work sleep disorder), and for older individuals with reduced levels of endogenous melatonin. The FDA has not approved it for these purposes.

Melatonin has been reported to increase sleep propensity when taken in the evening. Its short half-life of 20 to 30 minutes limits its usefulness to sleep initiation insomnia. Melatonin can also produce a phase delay when administered in the morning. However, its phase shifting effects are less than that of light exposure, and it is incapable of counteracting the phase delaying and phase advancing effects of light exposure during the evening and early morning, respectively. Although high doses have hypnotic effects, published studies on the use of melatonin for primary insomnia are limited. Caution is recommended when using it for children or pregnant women.

Botanical Compounds   Self-medication with herbal preparations (eg, kava, valerian, and passionflower) is a common practice, but there are very few studies evaluating their efficacy in the management of both transient and chronic insomnia.

Limited published data are available on the efficacy of kava (Piper methysticum) for the therapy of insomnia. Kavapyrones, the active constituents of kava, might possibly have an effect on GABA receptors and possess some antianxiety properties. Adverse effects include dizziness, gastrointestinal disturbances, and skin reactions, including a scaly dermatitis known as kava dermopathy. As a result of concerns about hepatotoxicity, this agent has been removed from the market in a number of countries.

Although valerian is a popular botanical sleep remedy and is often found as one of the ingredients of herbal compounds marketed for the therapy of insomnia, there is inconclusive evidence for the efficacy of valerian as a treatment for insomnia. The sedative properties of valerian (Valeriana officinalis) have been ascribed to the possible interaction of its valepotriate and sesquiterpene constituents with GABA, adenosine, or barbiturate receptors. Polysomnography conducted after administration of valerian has demonstrated a decrease in NREM stage 1 sleep and increase in NREM stages 3 and 4 sleep. A subjective decrease in sleep latency and reduction in wake time after sleep onset have been described.

Overdoses of valerian can result in abdominal pain, chest tightness, tremor, and lightheadedness.

No clinical trials on the use of the other natural products (eg, passionflower (Passiflora incarnata) and skullcap (Scutellaria laterifolia) that have been used as mild sedatives for insomnia have been published in the medical literature.

Newer Agents

Indiplon, a nonbenzodiazepine GABA$_A$ receptor modulator, has been shown to improve sleep latency to persistent sleep, increase sleep efficiency, and decrease wake time after sleep onset in patients with primary insomnia.

Discontinuing Long-Term Use of Hypnotic Agents

The long-term use of hypnotic agents for chronic insomnia, although not recommended, is a clinical reality. Patients receiving hypnotic agents chronically should be informed that, for most agents, this practice constitutes an FDA "off-label" use of the medications. Such long-term use is common in both primary insomnia, when conservative and nonpharmacologic treatments have been unsuccessful, unavailable, or simply ignored, as well as in co-morbid insomnia, as an adjunct to treatment of the primary condition or when such treatment has failed to correct the insomnia.

There is little literature that establishes the effectiveness of chronic benzodiazepine administration for insomnia. Some NBBRAs (eg, eszopiclone) may maintain long-term effectiveness without significant safety problems.

The usual clinical protocol for withdrawing from chronic benzodiazepine use includes gradual tapering over several days or weeks. A combination of CBT and benzodiazepine tapering may be superior to tapering alone.

Summary

The management of insomnia should address not only the perceived difficulty with nighttime sleep but also its daytime consequences. The sleep disturbance related to insomnia may be due to many causes. One should, therefore, attempt to identify any factor(s) that may precipitate or perpetuate these complaints and initiate appropriate corrective measures. It is of paramount importance to prevent the progression of transient sleep disturbance into chronic, unrelenting insomnia. Most patients benefit from a combination of sleep hygiene counseling, behavior modification, and the judicious administration of hypnotic agents.

Pharmacotherapeutic management is generally effective for transient insomnia due to jet lag or acute stressors. It may also be used intermittently in patients with more chronic complaints. The selection of a particular hypnotic medication should be based on the characteristics of the patient, duration and timing of insomnia, the pharmacologic profile of the agent (onset of action and rates of absorption and elimination), abuse potential of the agent, and possible drug interactions. It is advisable to use the lowest effective dose and to monitor carefully both the therapeutic response to the medication as well as its side effects.

References

General References

American Academy of Sleep Medicine. *The International Classification of Sleep Disorders: Diagnostic and Coding Manual.* 2nd ed. Westchester, IL: American Academy of Sleep Medicine, 2005.

Bowman TJ. *Review of Sleep Medicine.* Burlington, MA: Butterworth-Heinemann, 2002.

Berry RB. *Sleep Medicine Pearls.* 2nd ed. Philadelphia, PA: Hanley & Belfus, 2002.

Chokroverty S. *Clinical Companion to Sleep Disorders Medicine.* 2nd ed. Butterworth-Heinemann, 2000.

Lavie P, Pillar G, Malhotra A. *Sleep Disorders Handbook.* New York, NY: Taylor & Francis, 2002.

Lee-Chiong TL, ed. *Sleep: A Comprehensive Handbook.* Hoboken, NJ: John Wiley & Sons, 2006.

Lee-Chiong TL, Sateia M, Carskadon M, eds. *Sleep Medicine.* Philadelphia, PA: Hanley & Belfus (Elsevier), 2002.

Neubauer D. Insomnia. *Sleep Medicine.* Primary Care: Clinics in Office Practice. Elsevier Saunders, 2005.

Perlis ML, Lichstein KL, eds. *Treating Sleep Disorders: Principles and Practice of Behavioral Sleep Medicine.* Hoboken, NJ: John Wiley & Sons, 2003.

Rechtschaffen A, Kales A. *A Manual of Standardized Terminology, Techniques and Scoring System for Sleep Stages of Human Subjects.* Los Angeles, CA: Brain Information Service/Brain Research Institute, University of California, 1968.

Reite M, Ruddy J, Nagel K. *Concise Guide to Evaluation and Management of Sleep Disorders.* 3rd ed. Arlington, VA: American Psychiatric Publishing, April 2002.

Sateia MJ, Pigeon WR. Identification and management of insomnia. *Sleep Disorders.* Medical Clinics of North America. Philadelphia, PA: Elsevier Saunders, 2004.

Sleep Disorders. Medical Clinics of North America. Philadelphia, PA: Elsevier Saunders, 2004.

Sleep Medicine. Primary Care: Clinics in Office Practice. Philadelphia, PA: Elsevier Saunders, 2005.

Sleep Research Society. *SRS Basics of Sleep Guide.* Westchester, IL: Sleep Research Society, 2005.

Definition and Clinical Features

Lee-Chiong TL, ed. *Sleep: A Comprehensive Handbook.* Hoboken, NJ: John Wiley & Sons, 2006.

Lee-Chiong TL, Sateia M, Carskadon M, eds. *Sleep Medicine.* Philadelphia, PA: Hanley & Belfus (Elsevier), 2002.

Demographics

Ford DE, Kamerow DB. Epidemiologic study of sleep disturbances and psychiatric disorders. *JAMA*. 1989;262:1479–1482.

Ohayon M. Epidemiological study on insomnia in the general population. *Sleep*. 1996;19(3):S7–15.

Consequences

Lee-Chiong TL, ed. *Sleep: A Comprehensive Handbook*. Hoboken, NJ: John Wiley & Sons, 2006.

Lee-Chiong TL, Sateia M, Carskadon M, eds. *Sleep Medicine*. Philadelphia, PA: Hanley & Belfus (Elsevier), 2002.

Clinical Course

Lee-Chiong TL, ed. *Sleep: A Comprehensive Handbook*. Hoboken, NJ: John Wiley & Sons, 2006.

Lee-Chiong TL, Sateia M, Carskadon M, eds. *Sleep Medicine*. Philadelphia, PA: Hanley & Belfus (Elsevier), 2002.

Classification

American Sleep Disorders Association. *International Classification of Sleep Disorders, Revised: Diagnostic and Coding Manual*. Rochester, MN: American Sleep Disorders Association, 1997.

Pathophysiology

Lee-Chiong TL, ed. *Sleep: A Comprehensive Handbook*. Hoboken, NJ: John Wiley & Sons, 2006.

Lee-Chiong TL, Sateia M, Carskadon M, eds. *Sleep Medicine*. Philadelphia, PA: Hanley & Belfus (Elsevier), 2002.

Causes of Insomnia

American Psychiatric Association. *Diagnostic and Statistical Manual of Mental Disorders*. 4th ed. Washington, DC: American Psychiatric Association, 1994.

American Sleep Disorders Association. *International Classification of Sleep Disorders, Revised: Diagnostic and Coding Manual*. Rochester, MN: American Sleep Disorders Association, 1997.

Benca RM. Sleep in psychiatric disorders. *Neurol Clin*. 1996;14:739–764.

Bliwise DL. Sleep in normal aging and dementia. *Sleep*. 1993;16:40–81.

Bonnet MH, Arand DL. Physiological activation in patients with

sleep state misperception. *Psychosom Med*. 1997;59(5):533–40.

Cartwright RD, Wood E. Adjustment disorders of sleep: the sleep effects of a major stressful event and its resolution. *Psychiatry Res*. 1991;39:199–209.

Cortelli P, Gambetti P, Montagna P, Lugaresi E. Fatal familial insomnia: clinical features and molecular genetics. *J Sleep Res*. 1999 Jun;8 Suppl 1:23–9.

D'Ambrosio CM, Mohsenin V. Sleep in asthma. *Clin Chest Med.* 1998;19:127–137.

Douglas NJ. Sleep in patients with chronic obstructive pulmonary disease. *Clin Chest Med.* 1998;19:115–125.

Fogel RB, White DP. Obstructive sleep apnea. *Adv Intern Med.* 2000;45:351–389.

Ford DE, Kamerow DB. Epidemiologic study of sleep disturbances and psychiatric disorders. *JAMA.* 1989;262:1479–1482.

Guilleminault C, Robinson A. Central sleep apnea. *Neurol Clin.* 1996;14:611–628.

Harding SM. Sleep in fibromyalgia patients: subjective and objective findings. *Am J Med Sci.* 1998;315:367–376.

Haskell SG, Fiebach NH. Clinical epidemiology of nocturnal leg cramps in male veterans. *Am J Med Sci.* 1997;313:210–214.

Lowe AD. Sleep in Parkinson's disease. *J Psychosom Res.* 1998;44:613–617.

Lugaresi E, Cirignotta F, Montagna P. Nocturnal paroxysmal dystonia. *Journal of Neurology, Neurosurgery & Psychiatry.* 1986;49:375–380.

Mahowald MW, Schenck CH. NREM sleep parasomnias. *Neurol Clin.* 1996;14:675–696.

Malow BA. Sleep and epilepsy. *Neurol Clin.* 1996;14:765–789.

Manni R, Ratti MT, Tartara A. Nocturnal eating: prevalence and features in 120 insomniac referrals. *Sleep.* 1997;20:734–738.

Miller JC, Horvath SM. Sleep at altitude. *Aviation Space & Environmental Medicine.* 1977;48:615–620.

O'Keeffe ST. Restless legs syndrome. A review. *Arch Intern Med.* 1996;156:243–248.

Pagel JF. Nightmares and disorders of dreaming. *Am Fam Physician.* 2000;61:2037–2042,2044.

Perlis ML, Giles DE, Mendelson WB, Bootzin RR, Wyatt JK. Psychophysiological insomnia: the behavioural model and a neurocognitive perspective. *J Sleep Res.* 1997;6:179–188.

Polnitsky CA. Fatal familial insomnia. In: Lee-Chiong T, ed. *Encyclopedia of Sleep Medicine.* New York, NY: John Wiley & Sons, 2006. pp 111–115.

Sahota PK, Dexter JD. Sleep and headache syndromes: a clinical review. *Headache.* 1990;30:80–84.

Salin-Pascual RH, Roehrs TA, Merlott LA, Zorick F, Roth T. Longterm

study of the sleep of insomnia patients with sleep-state misperception

and other insomnia patients. *Am J Psychiatry.* 1992;149:904–8.

Schenck CH, Mahowald MW. REM sleep parasomnias. *Neurol Clin.* 1996;14:697–720.

Tabernero C, Polo JM, Sevillano MD, Munoz R, Berciano J, Cabello A, Baez B, Ricoy JR, Carpizo R, Figols J, Cuadrado N, Claveria LE. Fatal familial insomnia: clinical, neuropathological, and genetic description of a Spanish family. *Journal of Neurology, Neurosurgery & Psychiatry.* 2000;68:774–777.

Trenkwalder C, Walters AS, Hening W. Periodic limb movements and restless legs syndrome. *Neurologic Clinics.* 1996;14:629–650.

Wagner DR. Disorders of the circadian sleep-wake cycle. *Neurol Clin.* 1996;14:651–670.

Zarcone V. Alcoholism and sleep. *Adv Biosciences.* 1978;21:29–38.

Evaluation of Insomnia

Chesson A Jr, Hartse K, Anderson WM, Davila D, Johnson S, Littner M, et al. Practice parameters for the evaluation of chronic insomnia. An American Academy of Sleep Medicine report. Standards of Practice Committee of the American Academy of Sleep Medicine. *Sleep*. 2000;23:237–41.

Domino G, Blair G, Bridges A. Subjective assessment of sleep by sleep questionnaire. *Percept Mot Skills*. 1984;59(1):163–70.

Edinger JD, Holescher TJ, Webb MD, et al. Polysomnographic assessment of DIMS: empirical evaluation of its diagnostic value. *Sleep*. 12:315–322, 1989.

Hauri PJ, Wisbey J. Wrist actigraphy in insomnia. *Sleep*. 1992;15(4):293–301.

Kales A, Bixler EO, Soldatos CR, et al. Biopsychobehavioral correlates of insomnia, part I: role of sleep apnea and nocturnal myoclonus. *Psychosomatics*. 1982;23:589–600.

Reite M, Buysse D, Reynolds C, Mendelson W. The use of polysomnography in the evaluation of insomnia. *Sleep*. 1995;18(1):58–70.

Sateia MJ, Doghramji K. Hauri PJ. Morin CM. Evaluation of chronic insomnia. An American Academy of Sleep Medicine review. *Sleep*. 2000;23:243–308.

Zorick FJ, Roth T, Hartze KM, et al. Evaluation and diagnosis of persistent insomnia. *Am J Psychiatry*. 1981;138:769–773.

Differential Diagnosis of Insomnia

Lee-Chiong TL, ed. *Sleep: A Comprehensive Handbook*. Hoboken, NJ: John Wiley & Sons, 2006.

Lee-Chiong TL, Sateia M, Carskadon M, eds. *Sleep Medicine*. Philadelphia, PA: Hanley & Belfus (Elsevier), 2002.

Nonpharmacologic Therapy of Insomnia

Chesson AL Jr, Anderson WM, Littner M, Davila D, Hartse K, Johnson S, Wise M, et al. Practice parameters for the nonpharmacologic treatment of chronic insomnia. An American Academy of Sleep Medicine report. Standards of Practice Committee of the American Academy of Sleep Medicine. *Sleep*. 1999 Dec 15;22(8):1128–33.

Lee-Chiong TL, ed. *Sleep: A Comprehensive Handbook*. Hoboken, NJ: John Wiley & Sons, 2006.

Lee-Chiong TL, Sateia M, Carskadon M, eds. *Sleep Medicine*. Philadelphia, PA: Hanley & Belfus (Elsevier), 2002.

Morin CM, Hauri PJ, Espie CA, Spielman AJ, Buysse DJ, Bootzin RR. Nonpharmacologic treatment of chronic insomnia. An American Academy of Sleep Medicine review. *Sleep*. 1999 Dec 15;22(8):1134–56.

Pharmacologic Therapy of Insomnia

Bélanger L, Morin CM, Bastien CH, Guay B, Leblanc J, Vallières A, et al. Benzodiazepine discontinuation in chronic insomnia: a survival analysis over a 24-month follow-up [abstract]. *Sleep*. 2003;26(suppl):A308–A309.

Chesson AL Jr, Anderson WM, Littner M, Davila D, Hartse K, Johnson S,et al. Practice parameters for the nonpharmacologic treatment of chronic insomnia. An American Academy of Sleep Medicine report. Standards of Practice Committee of the American Academy of Sleep Medicine. *Sleep.* 1999;22:1128–33.

Dingemanse J. Pharmacology of insomnia: practice and prospects. *Pharm World Sci.* 17:67–75, 1995.

Donath F, Quispe S, Diefenbach K, Maurer A, Fietze I, Roots I. Critical evaluation of the effect of valerian extract on sleep structure and sleep quality. *Pharmacopsychiatry.* 2000 Mar;33(2):47–53.

Erman M, Seiden D, Zammit G. Phase II study of the selective ML-1 receptor agonist TAK-375 in subjects with primary chronic insomnia [abstract]. *Sleep.* 2003;26(suppl):A298.

Fugh-Berman A, Jerry M. Cott J. Dietary supplements and natural products as psychotherapeutic agents. *Psychosomatic Medicine.* 1999;61:712–728.

Garfinkel D, Laudon M, Nof D, et al. Improvement of sleep quality in elderly people by controlled-release melatonin. *Lancet.* 1995;346:541–544.

Hajak G, Muller WE, Wittchen HU, Pittrow D, Kirch W. Abuse and dependence potential for the non-benzodiazepine hypnotics zolpidem and zopiclone: a review of case reports and epidemiological data. *Addiction.* 2003;Oct;98(10):1371–8.

Hartmann PM. Drug treatment of insomnia: indications and newer agents. *Am Fam Physician.* 1995;51:191–194.

Jindal RD, Buysse DJ, Thase ME. Maintenance Treatment of Insomnia: what Can We Learn From the Depression Literature? *Am J Psychiatry.* 2004;161:19–24.

Krystal AD, Walsh JK, Laska E, Caron J, Amato DA, Wessel TC, et al. Sustained efficacy of eszopiclone over 6 months of nightly treatment: results of a randomized, double-blind, placebo-controlled study in adults with chronic insomnia. *Sleep.* 2003 Nov 1;26(7):793–9.

Kupfer DJ, Reynolds CF. Management of insomnia. *N Engl J Med.* 1997;336:341–346.

Mendelson WB, Roth T, Cassella J, Roehrs T, Walsh JK, Woods JH, et al. The treatment of chronic insomnia: drug indications, chronic use and abuse liability. Summary of a 2001 New Clinical Drug Evaluation Unit Meeting Symposium.. 2004;8(1):7–17.

Montplaisir J, Hawa R, Moller H, Morin C, Fortin M, Matte J, et al. Zopiclone and zaleplon vs benzodiazepines in the treatment of insomnia: Canadian consensus statement. *Hum Psychopharmacol.* 2003;Jan;18(1):29–38.

Morin CM, Hauri PJ, Espie CA, Spielman AJ, Buysse DJ, Bootzin RR. Nonpharmacologic treatment of chronic insomnia. An American Academy of Sleep Medicine review. *Sleep.* 1999;22:1134–56.

Neubauer DN. Pharmacologic approaches for the treatment of chronic insomnia. *Clin Cornerstone.* 2003;5(3):16–27.

Noble S, Langtry HD, Lamb HM. Zopiclone. An update of its pharmacology, clinical efficacy and tolerability in the treatment of insomnia. *Drugs.* 1998;Feb;55(2):277–302.

Pary R, Tobias CR, Webb WK, et al. Treatment of insomnia. Getting to the root of sleeping problems. *Postgrad Med.* 1996;100:195–210.

Roehrs T, Roth T. Hypnotics: an update. *Curr Neurol Neurosci Rep.* 2003;Mar;3(2):181–4.

Roth T, Walsh J. Phase II study of the selective ML-1 receptor agonist TAK-375 in a first night effect model of transient insomnia [abstract]. *Sleep.* 2003;26(suppl):A294.

Schweizer E, Rickels K. Benzodiazepine dependence and withdrawal: a review of the syndrome and its clinical management. *Acta Psychiatr Scand Suppl.* 1998;393:95–101.

Stevinson C, Ernst E. Valerian for insomnia: a systematic review of randomized clinical trials. *Sleep Medicine.* 1389–9457. 2000(Apr 1);1(2):91–99.

Terzano MG, Rossi M, Palomba V, Smerieri A, Parrino L. New drugs for insomnia: comparative tolerability of zopiclone, zolpidem and zaleplon. *Drug Saf.* 2003;26(4):261–82.

Walsh JK, Lankford DD, Krystal A, Roth T, Jochelson P, Garber M, et al. Efficacy and tolerability of four doses of indiplon (NBI-34060) modified-release in elderly patients with sleep maintenance insomnia [abstract]. *Sleep.* 2003;26(suppl):A78.

Walsh JK, Vogel GW, Scharf M, Erman M, William Erwin C, Schweitzer PK, et al. A five week, polysomnographic assessment of zaleplon 10 mg for the treatment of primary insomnia. *Sleep Medicine.* February 2000;1(1):41–49.

Winokur A, DeMartinis NA III, McNally DP, Gary EM, Cormier JL, Gary KA. Comparative effects of mirtazapine and fluoxetine on sleep physiology measures in patients with major depression and insomnia. *J Clin Psychiatry.* Oct 2003;64(10):1224–9.

Discontinuing Long-Term Use of Hypnotic Agents

Baillargeon L, Landreville P, Verreault R, Beauchemin JP, Gregoire JP, Morin CM. Discontinuation of benzodiazepines among older insomniac adults treated with cognitive-behavioural therapy combined with gradual tapering: a randomized trial. *CMAJ.* 2003 Nov 11;169(10):1015–20.

Curran HV, Collins R, Fletcher S, Kee SC, Woods B, Iliffe S. Older adults and withdrawal from benzodiazepine hypnotics in general practice: effects on cognitive function, sleep, mood and quality of life. *Psychol Med.* 2003;Oct;33(7):1223–37.

Excessive Sleepiness 4

Definition

Persons are considered excessively sleepy if they are unable to consistently achieve and sustain wakefulness and alertness to accomplish the tasks of daily living. Sleep occurs unintentionally or at inappropriate times or places. In children, sleepiness may manifest as hyperactivity.

Excessive sleepiness can be defined using either clinical or Multiple Sleep Latency Test (MSLT) criteria, namely hypersomnolence occurring almost daily for at least 3 months, and mean sleep latency of less than 8 minutes, respectively. Although the likelihood of falling asleep is greater during inactive monotonous situations, severe sleepiness can manifest precipitously as sleep attacks, recurrent episodes of microsleep, or automatic behavior during which there is no memory of semiconscious activities. It is important to distinguish excessive sleepiness from fatigue, exhaustion, tiredness, weariness, listlessness or weakness, which may closely mimic it.

Demographics

Excessive sleepiness is estimated to affect 5% of the general population. Occasional excessive daytime sleepiness may be present in up to a third of the general adult population. Prevalence is greater among adolescents and older adults. Both genders appear to be affected equally.

Among young adults, hours of weekday sleep predict daytime sleepiness, as do snoring, depression, marital status (those who are single are more likely to develop daytime sleepiness than married individuals), and employment status (sleepiness is more prevalent among persons employed full-time compared with those who are employed part-time or unemployed).

Classification of Excessive Sleepiness

Classification of sleepiness on the basis of clinical severity is presented in Table 4–1. The severity of sleepiness based on the Epworth Sleepiness Scale is rated in Table 4–2.

Consequences of Excessive Sleepiness

Consequences of excessive sleepiness include a greater risk of accidents (vehicular, industrial, or household), increased absenteeism, reduced work productivity, poor academic performance, mood disorder (depression or irritability), and impaired interpersonal relationships.

Etiology of Excessive Sleepiness

Inadequate sleep duration is, by far, the most important cause of excessive sleepiness. In others, sleep duration may be sufficient but sleep continuity is disrupted by frequent awakenings. Pathology

Table 4–1. Classification of sleepiness based on severity

Severity of sleepiness	Characteristics
Mild	Sleepiness occurs during times of rest or when little attention is required (eg, reading or watching television) Sleepiness is associated with minor impairment of social and occupational functioning
Moderate	Sleepiness occurs daily and during mild physical activities that involve some degree of attention (eg, group meetings) Sleepiness is associated with moderate impairment of social or occupational functioning
Severe	Sleepiness occurs daily and during physical activities that involve mild to moderate degree of attention (eg, conversation, eating or driving) Sleepiness is associated with marked impairment of social or occupational functioning

Source: American Sleep Disorders Association. International classification of sleep disorders, revised: Diagnostic and coding manual. Rochester, MN: American Sleep Disorders Association, 1997.

Table 4–2. Severity of sleepiness based on Epworth Sleepiness Scale

Severity of sleepiness	Epworth score
Mild	10–12
Moderate	13–17
Severe	> 17

of the central nervous system sleep-wake apparatus is another factor. A disturbance of the endogenous circadian rhythm influencing the timing of wakefulness and sleep can also produce excessive sleepiness. Finally, injudicious use of medications that possess hypnotic properties can lead to unintended sleepiness. Common causes of excessive sleepiness are presented in Table 4–3.

Narcolepsy

Definition

Narcolepsy is a neurologic disorder characterized by excessive sleepiness, and manifestations of rapid eye movement (REM) sleep physiology during wakefulness (eg, cataplexy, sleep paralysis, and hypnagogic hallucinations).

Demographics

Narcolepsy affects an estimated 0.05% of the general population in the United States. The prevalence of narcolepsy in the United States and some other countries is given in Table 4–4. Onset is

Table 4–3.   Common causes of excessive sleepiness

Cause	Description
Inadequate sleep duration	Acute sleep deprivation Chronic sleep deprivation Insufficient sleep syndrome
Frequent awakenings and fragmented sleep	Obstructive sleep apnea syndrome Upper airway resistance syndrome Periodic limb movement disorder Environmental sleep disorder

Pathology of the central nervous system sleep-wake apparatus	Narcolepsy
	  With cataplexy
	  Without cataplexy
	  Due to a medical condition
	Idiopathic hypersomnia
	  With long sleep time
	  Without long sleep time
	Post-traumatic hypersomnia
	Recurrent hypersomnia
	  Kleine-Levin syndrome
	  Menstrual-related hypersomnia

Disturbance of the endogenous circadian rhythm influencing the timing of wakefulness and sleep	Jet lag (time zone change syndrome) Shift work sleep disorder Delayed sleep-phase syndrome Advanced sleep-phase syndrome Non–24-hour sleep-phase disorder Irregular sleep-wake pattern
Drug or substance use	Administration of hypnotic and sedating medications Withdrawal from stimulant agents Adverse effects of medications
Other conditions	Medical disorders (sleeping sickness) Neurologic disorders (brain tumors, meningoencephalitis) Psychiatric disorders (depression)

Table 4–4.   Prevalence of narcolepsy

United States	2-18/10,000 (0.02% to 0.18%)
Israel	1/50,000 (0.002%)
Japan	1/600 (0.17% to 0.18%)
North America and Europe	1/4,000 (0.025%)
Finland	26/100,000 (0.026%)

often during adolescence or early adulthood (in the second decade of life), but cases involving onset in patients younger than 10 years of age or older than 50 years of age have been described. Narcolepsy with cataplexy appears to affect men slightly more frequently than women.

Excessive sleepiness is usually the presenting symptom, followed months to years later by cataplexy, sleep paralysis, and hypnagogic hallucinations. Course is typically chronic, and symptoms persist lifelong.

Genetics

Although most cases of narcolepsy are sporadic, there is a clear familial tendency in up to one-third of patients. About 40% of patients have at least a relative with excessive sleepiness, and 3% have a first-degree relative with cataplexy and excessive sleepiness. The risk of developing the disorder is increased by 10 to 40 times among first-degree relatives of narcoleptic individuals compared with the general population. Twin studies have described discordance in most monozygotic pairs; only about 25% to 30% of monozygotic twins are concordant (ie, when narcolepsy affects one twin, the other twin has narcolepsy only one-fourth to one-third of the time).

Clinical Features of Narcolepsy

The classic clinical tetrad of narcolepsy consists of excessive sleepiness, cataplexy, sleep paralysis, and sleep hallucinations. However, only approximately 10% to 15% of patients demonstrate this full tetrad. The clinical manifestations of narcolepsy are listed in Box 4–1. The prevalence of these features is given in Table 4–5.

Box 4–1.
 	
Clinical features of narcolepsy
	Excessive sleepiness
	
	Sleep attacks
	
	Cataplexy
	
	Sleep paralysis
	
	Sleep hallucinations
	
	Automatic behavior
	
	Nocturnal sleep disturbance
	
	Visual changes (blurred vision, diplopia, ptosis)
	
	Memory lapses
	
	Associated sleep disorders
	
	    Obstructive sleep apnea
	
	    REM sleep behavior disorder
	
	    Periodic limb movement disorder

Table 4–5. Prevalence of clinical features associated with narcolepsy

Clinical feature	Prevalence
Excessive sleepiness	≈ 100%
Cataplexy	≈ 70% to 80%
Hypnagogic/hypnopompic hallucinations	≈ 8% to 70%
Sleep paralysis	≈ 5% to 65%

Excessive Sleepiness

Excessive daytime sleepiness is typically the first, primary, and most disabling manifestation of narcolepsy. Excessive sleepiness is chronic and may manifest as pervasive drowsiness and subwakefulness, frequent napping, microsleep episodes, and unexpected and overpowering sleep attacks occurring almost daily for at least 3 months. Patients with narcolepsy may describe waxing and waning periods of alertness. Although lapses into sleep are more likely to occur during periods of inactivity, abrupt and unexpected sleep attacks can befall the individual at any time. Brief naps, lasting 10 to 20 minutes and seldom over on hour, occur repeatedly from 1 to 8 times throughout the day. Sleepiness is transiently relieved after awakening from a short nap only to gradually increase again within 2 to 3 hours.

Sleepiness may be related to the loss of hypocretin neurons that stimulate arousal processes involving the laterodorsal tegmental and pedunculopontine nuclei (cholinergic) and tuberomamillary nuclei (histaminergic).

Although nocturnal sleep may be characterized by frequent arousals and awakenings, it is commonly normal in duration. There is an increased tendency for REM sleep to rapidly occur during both nocturnal sleep and daytime naps. Excessive sleepiness increases the risk of accidental injuries and impairs social functioning as well as school and work performance.

Sleep Attacks

A person may have sudden, irresistible periods of sleepiness, with sleep occurring during inappropriate places or circumstances. Sleep attacks can be preceded by a period of drowsiness, but they can also occur abruptly without warning. Although the risk of sleep attacks is greater during periods of rest or boredom, they can develop during physical activity.

Cataplexy

Cataplexy is characterized by abrupt, transient, and bilateral loss or reduction of postural muscle tone occurring during wakefulness. It is precipitated by intense emotion such as laughter, anger, fright, surprise, excitement, or embarrassment. Cataplexy may also be triggered by stress, fatigue, or medications (alpha-1 adrenergic blockers or the switch to modafinil from amphetamines). Alternatively, it may occur spontaneously without apparent provocation. Although recovery is generally immediate and complete, prolonged episodes of cataplexy may give rise to REM sleep with hypnagogic hallucinations and dreaming.

Episodes of muscular atonia or hypotonia vary in:

• Duration (lasting from a few seconds to several minutes [generally < 2 minutes in duration])

• Progression (severity being maximal at the start of the attack or worsening over several seconds or minutes)

• Severity (ranging from mild weakness, such as drooping of the eyelids or sagging of the jaw, to complete lack of postural tone with a collapse to a chair or the ground)

• Frequency (from once or twice yearly to as often as several times each day)

• Body area affected (regionally affecting the face, neck, and extremities, or entire body)

Respiratory and oculomotor muscles are spared, and memory and consciousness are unaffected. Blurring of vision may occur.

Status cataplecticus describes repetitive episodes of cataplexy occurring in succession that may last from several minutes to an hour; this may occur following abrupt withdrawal of REM sleep suppressants.

Cataplexy generally first develops several months or years after the onset of excessive sleepiness, but may, occasionally, be the presenting complaint of patients with narcolepsy. Cataplexy may present up to 1 year before the development of sleep-onset REM periods on MSLT. Frequency of cataplexy may decrease over time.

Cataplexy can be considered an intrusion of REM sleep-related muscle atonia during wakefulness. However, it appears that the mechanisms responsible for cataplexy may not be identical to those associated with REM sleep. Cataplexy is produced by inhibition of lower motor neurons, deep tendon reflexes and H reflexes by cholinergic areas of the pons and basal forebrain. It is believed that cataplexy results from a loss of hypocretin-induced excitation of the locus ceruleus (noradrenergic) and dorsal raphe (serotonergic) that inhibit cholinergic neurons located in the laterodorsal tegmental and pedunculopontine nuclei. The "uninhibited" laterodorsal tegmental and pedunculopontine nuclei, in turn, stimulate the nucleus gigantocellularis, leading to a glycine-mediated hyperpolarization of the anterior horn cells of the spinal cord.

During episodes of cataplexy, neurologic examination demonstrates muscle flaccidity, reduction or absence of deep tendon reflexes, loss of pupillary light response, and, occasionally, a positive Babinski sign. Polysomnography demonstrates wakefulness during brief attacks and REM sleep during more prolonged attacks.

Up to 70% to 80% of narcoleptics have cataplexy. Cataplexy is the only pathognomonic symptom of narcolepsy, because normal individuals may occasionally experience sleep paralysis and/or hypnagogic hallucinations. However, the absence of cataplexy does not exclude a diagnosis of narcolepsy.

Cataplexy should be distinguished from syncope, epilepsy (partial complex, atonic or absence seizures), orthostatic hypotension, transient ischemic attack, neuromuscular weakness, vestibular dysfunction, psychosis, conversion disorder, or malingering. Cataplexy can also be seen in association with midbrain tumors, Niemann-Pick disease (type C), and Norrie's disease.

Sleep Paralysis

Sleep paralysis involves a transient loss of the ability to move occurring at sleep onset (hypnagogic) or upon awakening (hypnopompic). It occurs in approximately 25% to 80% of persons with narcolepsy. Less frequently, it can be seen either in an isolated form or in normal persons during sleep deprivation. Recurrent sleep paralysis can affect about 4% of the normal population.

Sleep paralysis involves all voluntary muscles with sparing of the respiratory and ocular muscles; lasts from several seconds to a few minutes; and is frequently accompanied by hypnagogic

Box 4–2.

Medical conditions causing narcolepsy

Narcolepsy with cataplexy

    Brainstem lesions

        Degenerative

        Infectious

        Inflammatory

        Neoplastic (craniopharyngioma, gliomas, pituitary, and hypothalamic tumors)

        Vascular (stroke or arteriovenous malformations)

    Cerebellar ataxia

    Coffin-Lowry syndrome (possible)

    Hydrocephalus secondary to space-occupying lesions

    Multiple sclerosis (hypothalamic)

    Neiman-Pick type C disease

    Norrie's disease

    Paraneoplastic syndrome (associated with anti-Ma2 antibodies)

    Sarcoidosis (hypothalamic)

    Tumors (hypothalamic)

    Viral illness (unspecified)

Narcolepsy without cataplexy

    Head trauma

    Multiple sclerosis

    Multiple system atrophy

    Myotonic dystrophy

    Parkinson disease

    Prader-Willi syndrome

Narcolepsy and sleep apnea[a]

    Myotonic dystrophy

    Prader-Willi syndrome

[a] *Sleep onset REM periods and excessive sleepiness persist after adequate therapy of sleep apnea.*

hallucinations, dyspnea, and a sensation of dread. Sensorium is generally unaffected. Recovery, either spontaneously or following external stimulation (being touched or spoken to), is immediate and complete. It often develops several months to years following the onset of excessive sleepiness. The differential diagnosis includes both isolated and familial (transmitted as an X-linked dominant trait) sleep paralysis and transient (hyperkalemic or hypokalemic) paralysis.

Sleep Hallucinations

Sleep hallucinations are common experiences among persons with narcolepsy and are present in about 30% of cases in this disorder. They are not pathognomonic for narcolepsy, and have been described in normal persons as well. Recurrent sleep hallucinations can be seen in about 4% of the normal population.

Hallucinations may occur during wakefulness at sleep onset (hypnagogic) or on awakening (hypnopompic). Hallucinatory phenomena often last a few seconds or minutes and can be visual (seeing a stranger or object in the room), auditory (being spoken to), tactile (a touch or a sensation of warmth or cold) or kinetic (a sensation of movement). Often the experience has a fearful quality such as being attacked or escaping from danger, and this can be accompanied by sleep paralysis. Sleep hallucinations often begin several months to years after the onset of excessive sleepiness.

Automatic Behavior

Automatic, seemingly meaningless, behavior (eg, driving or writing) during sleep episodes can occur in about 20% to 40% of persons with narcolepsy. There is no recall of the event. It should be differentiated from parasomnias such as sleepwalking or REM sleep behavior disorder, seizures (especially partial complex), fugue-like states, and malingering.

Sleep Disturbance

Disruption of nighttime sleep with repetitive awakenings and poor sleep quality can be seen in up to 70% to 80% of persons with narcolepsy. Affected patients may complain of sleep-maintenance insomnia.

Associated Features

Other common features include a greater prevalence of REM sleep behavior disorder, periodic limb movements of sleep, and sleep apnea (the latter possibly related to a greater tendency for excess body weight). REM sleep behavior disorder can be precipitated or aggravated by therapy of cataplexy with tricyclic antidepressants (TCAs) and stimulant agents. Memory impairment, behavioral problems, decreased performance, headaches, sleep drunkenness, diplopia, visual blurring, irritability, and depression have also been described. There appears to be a high prevalence of psychopathology on the Minnesota Multiphasic Personality Inventory (MMPI). In attempting to reduce or avoid cataplexy, patients may develop a lack of emotional responsiveness. Sleep apnea, both obstructive and central, can occur in about 30% of persons with narcolepsy, and can contribute to the severity of excessive sleepiness. Compared with normal controls, patients with narcolepsy have greater excess body weight and may have a higher risk of developing obstructive sleep apnea (OSA). This is believed to be due to a lower metabolic rate, possibly influenced by hypocretin, which affects feeding and metabolism, and a sedentary lifestyle. Sleep drunkenness, defined by confusion and diminished alertness immediately following an awakening, is observed in approximately 10% of persons with narcolepsy. Finally, there is a possible association between narcolepsy and tumor necrosis factor (TNF)-α and TNF receptor-2 genes.

Clinical Course

Onset of narcolepsy is generally during adolescence and early adulthood (between 15 and 25 years of age). Excessive sleepiness is often the first symptom to appear, followed one to several years later by cataplexy, sleep paralysis, and sleep hallucinations. (Note: The diagnosis of "narcolepsy without cataplexy" is often difficult to make during adolescence because cataplexy may develop later.) Excessive sleepiness is generally persistent and unrelenting, whereas the severity of cataplexy and other manifestations of abnormal REM sleep regulation may wax and wane over time. Patients with narcolepsy may have a greater risk of developing depression and type 2 diabetes mellitus.

Pathophysiology

Animal Models

Animal models of narcolepsy have included canine mutations of hypocretin receptor-2 gene (Hcrt-2) in lateral hypothalamic neurons, and hypocretin knockout rodents with null mutation of the preprohypocretin gene. Mode of inheritance of narcolepsy appears to be recessive in canine narcolepsy (Labrador retrievers and Doberman pinchers).

In dogs, cataplexy is worsened by administration of α1-receptor antagonists (eg, prazosin) and improved by α1-agonists (eg, methoxamine). Cholinergic agonists (physostigmine) also worsen cataplexy, whereas anticholinergics (muscarine blockers such as atropine and scopolamine) decrease cataplexy. Increase in pontine cholinergic M2 muscarinic receptors and basal ganglia and amygdala M1 receptors have been reported in narcoleptic dogs.

Human Studies

Abnormalities involving the hypocretin, cholinergic, monoamine, and dopaminergic systems have been described among patients with narcolepsy.

1. Hypocretin system. Loss of hypocretin (also known as orexin) neurons in the lateral hypo-thalamus appears to be the major underlying mechanism responsible for narcolepsy. Hypocretins are neuropeptides that appear to have multiple functions, including regulation of sleep-wake cycle, appetite, body temperature, and blood pressure. The hypocretin neurotransmitter system is located in the perifornical area of the hypothalamus, with wide projections to several wake promoting areas of the central nervous system (locus ceruleus, medullary reticular formation, raphe nuclei, and thalamus). There are two types of hypocretin receptors (Hcrt), Hcrt-1 and 2. A majority of patients with narcolepsy have decreased levels of Hcrt-1. Low cerebrospinal fluid (CSF) levels of hypocretin in patients with narcolepsy with cataplexy have been described.

2. Cholinergic system. A defective cholinergic system regulating REM sleep (ie, muscarinic super-sensitivity) appears to contribute to the symptoms of narcolepsy.

3. Monoamine system. Noradrenergic and serotonergic cells modulate the cholinergic system during REM sleep. The monoamine system receives excitatory input from the hypocretin system. Noradrenergic "REM-off" cells in the locus ceruleus are inactive during REM sleep. There appears to be a defect in the monoamine system regulation of REM sleep in patients with narcolepsy.

Table 4–6.   Clinical subtypes of narcolepsy

Subtype	Characteristics
Narcolepsy with cataplexy with normal hypocretin-1 levels in the CSF	Normal CSF hypocretin-1 levels are present in up to 10% of cases
Narcolepsy without cataplexy with low hypocretin-1 levels in the CSF	Low CSF hypocretin-1 levels (< 110 pg/mL) are present in up to 10% to 20% of cases of HLA DQB1*0602-positive narcolepsy without cataplexy HLA DQB1*0602-negative narcolepsy without cataplexy patients generally have normal CSF hypocretin-1 levels
Narcolepsy with cataplexy-like or atypical episodes	Low CSF hypocretin-1 levels (< 110 pg/ml) are present in up to 20% of cases
Isolated cataplexy	Rare familial cases with early onset
Hypocretin gene mutations	A case of early-onset (6 months of age) narcolepsy with cataplexy due to a preprohypocretin mutation has been described

Cataplexy is exacerbated by α1-receptor antagonists (prazosin) and α2-receptor agonists; and reduced by α2-receptor antagonists (yohimbine). Stimulants that increase the availability of norepinephrine at the synaptic junction are effective in decreasing sleepiness and enhancing alertness. Raphe serotonergic cells are also REM-off cells. TCAs and selective serotonin reuptake inhibitors (SSRIs) increase the availability of serotonin and are useful in treating cataplexy.

4.   Dopamine system. Narcolepsy may also be affected by an impairment of the dopamine system. CSF levels of dopamine are decreased in patients with narcolepsy.

Narcolepsy Secondary to Medical Disorders

Narcolepsy can also result from an underlying medical or neurologic disorder (referred to as secondary narcolepsy). Diagnosis requires documentation of narcolepsy either clinically (eg, presence of chronic excessive sleepiness for at least 3 months, or cataplexy) or objectively (MSLT demonstrating short mean sleep latency less than 8 minutes and at least 2 sleep onset REM periods) and a coexisting medical condition that is responsible for sleepiness. Sleep may either be normal or moderately disrupted during polysomnography. CSF levels of hypocretin-1 are low (< 110pg/ml or 30% of normal control values). Medical Conditions that may lead to narcolesdy are listed in Box 4–2.

Narcolepsy without Cataplexy

This form of narcolepsy is not associated with cataplexy; however, cataplexy-like symptoms may be described, including prolonged episodes of tiredness or muscle weakness related to atypical triggers (exercise, stress, or sex). It accounts for about 10% to 50% of cases of narcolepsy. Most patients have normal levels of CSF hypocretin-1. Some cases of narcolepsy without cataplexy are associated with loss of hypocretin-containing hypothalamic neurons (but to a lesser degree than that seen in narcolepsy with cataplexy). The types of narcolepsy are described in Table 4–6.

Table 4–7. Polysomnographic and MSLT features of narcolepsy

Polysomnography	Multiple sleep latency test

↓ Sleep latency
↓ Total sleep time
↑ Frequency of arousals
↑ Body movements
↓ NREM stages 3 and 4 sleep
↓ REM sleep latency (sleep onset REM periods in about 50% of cases)
Associated conditions:
   Obstructive sleep apnea
   Central sleep apnea
   REM sleep behavior disorder
   Periodic limb movements of sleep
	↓ Sleep latency (< 8 minutes)
	Two or more sleep onset REM periods

Evaluation

Narcolepsy with cataplexy can be diagnosed by clinical history alone. A thorough evaluation of medication and substance use as well as sleep, medical, neurologic and psychiatric history is mandatory. Polysomnography followed by MSLT is indicated when cataplexy is absent, atypical or equivocal.

Polysomnography

Polysomnographic features include sleep fragmentation and repetitive awakenings. A short sleep latency (< 10 minutes) and sleep-onset REM period (SOREMP; decreased REM sleep latency of ≤ 20 minutes) may be present. SOREMPs during nocturnal polysomnography have been described in up to 25% to 50% of patients. NREM stage 1 sleep is increased. Total sleep time and % REM sleep are often normal. OSA and periodic limb movements of sleep may be observed.

Multiple Sleep Latency Test

The MSLT measures a person's physiologic propensity to fall asleep in quiet situations. A nocturnal polysomnography should be performed immediately before an MSLT to exclude the presence of other sleep disorders and to ensure an adequate duration of nocturnal sleep (at least 6 hours). OSA, if present, should be appropriately treated before performing an MSLT. MSLT is usually performed between 8:00 to 9:00 AM and 5:00 to 6:00 PM, with the first nap opportunity performed about 2 hours after awakening from the previous night's polysomnography.

Characteristic MSLT features include a mean sleep latency of equal to or less than 8 minutes (present in 90% of cases) with at least two SOREMPs (Table 4–7). (MSLT parameters are not as well

Table 4–8. Prevalence of DR2 in subjects with narcolepsy

Japanese	100%
Caucasians	90–95%
African Americans	60%

established for children less than 8 years of age.) Healthy subjects usually have mean sleep latencies of more than 10 to 11 minutes. However, these combined MSLT findings are neither entirely sensitive nor specific for narcolepsy, being present in only about 60% to 85% of cases. Multiple SOREMPs are more specific for narcolepsy than short sleep latency, but they can also be present in patients with significant sleep disruption such as OSA (up to 5%), circadian sleep disorders, insufficient sleep, abrupt withdrawal from REM sleep suppressing agents, and in about 1% to 3% of normal healthy adults. A short sleep latency can be present in up to 16% to 30% of normal individuals.

Sleep deprivation, delayed sleep phase syndrome, and acute withdrawal of stimulant agents can all decrease sleep latency and should be excluded. An adequate sleep duration and regular sleep-wake schedule, as documented by sleep diaries or actigraphy, must have been maintained for at least 1 to 2 weeks preceding MSLT. Furthermore, medications that can potentially influence sleep latency and REM sleep, such as opiates, benzodiazepines, narcotics, and REM suppressants, should be discontinued for at least 15 days before the study. A urine drug screen during the study is required to rule out the recent use of opiates, sedatives, hypnotics, and stimulants.

Table 4–9. Differential diagnosis of sleepiness and cataplexy

Sleepiness	Cataplexy
Environmental sleep disorder	Akinetic seizures
Circadian rhythm sleep disorders	Conversion disorder (pseudocataplexy)
Idiopathic hypersomnia	Hypotension
Inadequate sleep hygiene	Malingering
Insufficient sleep syndrome	Neuromuscular disorders
Malingering	Sleep paralysis
Medication use, abuse or withdrawal	Transient ischemic attacks
Obstructive sleep apnea	Vestibular disorders
Periodic limb movement disorder	
Recurrent hypersomnia	

Maintenance of Wakefulness Test

The Maintenance of Wakefulness Test (MWT) measures a person's ability to remain awake in quiet situations. It might be useful for monitoring treatment response to stimulant medications used for excessive sleepiness.

Cerebrospinal Fluid Hypocretin-1

CSF hypocretin-1 level < or equal to 110 pg/ml (or < one-third of mean normal control values) is highly specific and sensitive for narcolepsy with cataplexy but is less commonly present in cases without cataplexy. In addition, a normal test does not exclude the diagnosis of narcolepsy with cataplexy (CSF hypocretin-1 levels are normal in up to 10% of cases). Measuring CSF hypocretin-1 levels may be useful if patients are taking medications (stimulants or REM sleep suppressants) that may interfere with proper interpretation of MSLT results, if patients are too young to undergo MSLT, or during the early course of the disease prior to the development of cataplexy.

HLA Typing

Narcolepsy is associated with certain human leukocyte antigens (HLA), namely DR2 (particularly the subtype DR15) and DQ1 (in particular DQ6 [DQB1*0602]). Most multiplex family cases

Table 4-10. Pharmacologic therapy of narcolepsy

Excessive sleepiness and sleep attacks	Cataplexy, sleep paralysis and sleep hallucinations	Sleep disruption
Dextroamphetamine	Carbamazepine	γ-hydroxybutyrate
Mazindol	Clomipramine	Hypnotic agents
Methamphetamine	Clonidine	
Methylphenidate	Desipramine	
Modafinil	Fluoxetine	
Pemoline	γ-hydroxybutyrate	
	Imipramine	
	Nortriptyline	
	Paroxetine	
	Protriptyline	
	Sertraline	
	Venlafaxine	
	Viloxazine	

(multiple members of the family with narcolepsy) are HLA DQB1*0602 positive. The prevalence of DR2 in individuals with narcolepsy is given in Table 4–8.

HLA DQB1*0602 is present in most patients with narcolepsy with cataplexy (90%) and in about 40% to 60% of those with narcolepsy without cataplexy. HLA DRB1*1501 is also common among Asians and Caucasians with narcolepsy with cataplexy, whereas DQB1 *0602 is more specific among African Americans with narcolepsy.

DQB1*0602 appears to be associated with both the frequency and severity of cataplexy. Other HLA subtypes are also important, either increasing the susceptibility to developing narcolepsy (DQB1*0301) or protecting against it (DQB1*0501 and DQB1*0601).

However, HLA typing has limited diagnostic utility. Because persons positive for HLA DQB1*0602 may not have narcolepsy (HLA DQB1*0602 is also present in about 12%, 25% and 38% of normal Japanese, Caucasian, and African-American subjects, respectively), and because a negative result does not exclude the diagnosis of narcolepsy, HLA typing is rarely useful in the evaluation of narcolepsy.

Box 4-3. **Behavioral therapy for narcolepsy**	Avoidance of sleep deprivation
	Proper sleep hygiene
	Maintenance of regular sleep-wake schedules, and avoidance of shifts in circadian sleep-wake rhythms (eg, shift work)
	Avoidance of prolonged inactivity during the daytime
	Regular schedule of daytime naps (≈ 15 minutes in duration)
	Appropriately timed use of physical activities and caffeinated beverages to improve alertness and maintain wakefulness
	Maintenance of optimum weight
	Avoidance of stress

Box 4-4.	Reduction of excessive daytime sleepiness
Effects of stimulant medications in patients with narcolepsy	Increase in alertness
	Improvement in quality of life
	Enhanced daytime performance (eg, reaction time)

Differential Diagnosis

The differential diagnosis of narcolepsy includes other causes of excessive sleepiness such as insufficient sleep syndrome; chronic sleep deprivation; OSA; idiopathic hypersomnia; medication, alcohol, and substance use; recurrent hypersomnia; circadian sleep disorders; and medical, neurologic, and psychiatric conditions. Causes of sleepiness are given in Table 4–9.

Table 4-11. Dosing of stimulant medications

Agent	Recommended dosages
Modafinil	100 to 400 mg/day
Dextroamphetamine	5 to 60 mg/day in 2 to 3 divided doses
Methylphenidate	5 to 15 mg 2 to 3 times a day

Therapy

Therapy of narcolepsy consists of pharmacologic therapy for sleep disruption and excessive sleepiness (stimulants such as amphetamines, methylphenidate, and modafinil) as well as prevention of cataplexy and other REM sleep phenomena (TCAs and SSRIs) (Table 4–10). Behavioral modification, education, and support are equally important. Therapy is commonly required for life.

General Measures

Sleep hygiene must be optimized with adequate nocturnal sleep and maintenance of a regular sleep-wake schedule. Some patients find brief naps (30 minutes) scheduled throughout the day beneficial. However, naps are rarely sufficient as primary therapy. Scheduled daytime naps are most likely to benefit patients with severe daytime sleepiness who are unable to maintain alertness during the day. Nonetheless, the benefits in alertness are transient with sleepiness gradually worsening again after a few hours.

Education about the clinical features of narcolepsy, its therapy, and required lifestyle changes should be provided to patients, and their families, school and employers. For information about the behavioral aspects of therapy for narcolepsy, see Box 4–3. Patients should be cautioned against driving or performing other activities that may be potentially dangerous whenever drowsy. They should be counseled regarding career choices such as avoiding jobs that require shift work or irregular work schedules. Regular follow-up is essential to determine treatment efficacy, medication adverse effects, and the development of other sleep disorders.

Treatment of Excessive Sleepiness

Therapy of excessive sleepiness generally involves proper sleep hygiene practices and judicious use of stimulant agents. Effects of stimulant medications in patients with narcolepsy are given in Box 4–4. Low to moderate doses of stimulant agents enable about 40% to 50% of treated patients with

---

Box 4–5.

American Academy of Sleep Medicine recommendations for the treatment of narcolepsy

GENERAL MEASURES

Standard

1. A diagnosis of narcolepsy must be established.

2. Goals of therapy should be established for each patient.

3. Regular follow-up is necessary to monitor response to treatment and address adverse effects of medications.

   a. A health care provider should evaluate a patient stabilized on stimulant medication at least annually (preferably once every 6 months) to determine any adverse effects to the medication.

   b. Follow-up is necessary to assess treatment adherence, efficacy, and safety, as well as to assist the patient with occupational and social difficulties.

   c. Until sleepiness is appropriately controlled by stimulants, patients should be advised to avoid potentially dangerous activities, including operating a motor vehicle.

   d. Amphetamines, especially at high doses, are the most likely of the stimulants used for narcolepsy to lead to tolerance.

   e. Failure to respond to adequate doses of stimulants should prompt assessment for other sleep disorders that may contribute to excessive sleepiness.

   f. Clinicians are advised to refer to appropriate sources for up-to-date information on treatments useful for narcolepsy, including their adverse effects, dosage ranges, and use in pregnancy and by nursing mothers.

   g. Methylphenidate appears relatively safe for the treatment of narcolepsy in children between 6 and 15 years of age. Caution must be exercised regarding the use of other medications for narcolepsy in this age group.

   h. Patients should be provided assistance for specific narcolepsy-related disabilities.

   i. Repeat polysomnography is indicated if there is a significant increase in sleepiness or if new or increased sleep abnormalities (eg, OSA or periodic limb movement disorder) are suspected.

Guideline

1. Scheduled naps are useful to combat sleepiness but are seldom sufficient as primary therapy.

Medications for narcolepsy

The following medications are effective treatments for patients with narcolepsy:

Standard

1. Modafinil for daytime sleepiness

Guideline

1. Amphetamine, methamphetamine, dextroamphetamine, and methylphenidate for daytime sleepiness

2. Selegiline for all narcoleptic symptoms

3. Tricyclic antidepressants and fluoxetine for cataplexy, sleep paralysis, and hypnagogic hallucinations

Option

1. Combinations of long- and short-acting stimulants may be effective for some patients

2. Pemoline for daytime sleepiness (Note: Pemoline has been withdrawn from the market due to concerns regarding hepatotoxicity)

Modified and adapted from Littner, et al. Practice parameters for the treatment of narcolepsy: an update for 2000. Sleep, 2001; 24(4).

Definition of Terms	
Standard	Generally accepted practice with a high level of clinical certainly
Guideline	Practice associated with a moderate degree of clinical certainty
Option	Practice of uncertain clinical use

narcolepsy to achieve acceptable wakefulness throughout the day (Table 4–11). Patients who continue to have significant daytime sleepiness despite optimal use of stimulant agents should be evaluated for insufficient nighttime sleep and other untreated sleep disorders that could be contributing to sleep disturbance.

Treatment of Sleep Fragmentation

γ-Hydroxybutyrate or a hypnotic agent can be used to treat nocturnal sleep disturbance and consolidate nocturnal sleep. γ-Hydroxybutyrate (sodium oxybate), a gamma-aminobutyric acid (GABA) precursor, increases sleep continuity and decreases the frequency of cataplexy in persons with narcolepsy. Gradual and mild improvement in daytime sleepiness has also been reported with chronic use. Adverse effects include headaches, dizziness, and nausea. Overdosage can result in respiratory depression, seizures, coma, or death.

γ-Hydroxybutyrate has a U.S. Food and Drug Administration (FDA) Schedule III rating and is associated with potential for abuse. It has a short half-life and has to be administered at bedtime and several hours later.

Treatment of Cataplexy, Sleep Paralysis, and Sleep Hallucinations

Medications capable of suppressing REM sleep (eg, SSRIs, nontricyclic serotonin-norepinephrine reuptake inhibitor [venlafaxine] and TCAs) are generally used to treat cataplexy, sleep paralysis, and sleep hallucinations. Other medications that can be tried for persistent cases of cataplexy include carbamazepine, clonidine, γ-hydroxybutyrate, monoamine oxidase (MAO) inhibitors, and viloxazine.

The SSRIs inhibit the processes that generate REM sleep. TCAs inhibit adrenergic uptake and the descending cholinergic pathways responsible for the production of cataplexy.

Sedating medications (eg, desipramine or imipramine) can be taken at bedtime, whereas stimulating agents (eg, fluoxetine) are best taken in the morning.

TCAs (eg, clomipramine, imipramine or protriptyline) are associated with anticholinergic adverse effects, such as constipation, urinary retention, dry mouth, blurred vision, tachycardia and other arrhythmias, and orthostatic hypotension, and they are less well tolerated than SSRIs. Other adverse effects include tremors, sexual dysfunction, and weight gain. TCAs, as well as SSRIs, can also precipitate periodic limb movements of sleep.

Sudden discontinuation of medications used for treating cataplexy can give rise to status cataplecticus (continuous attack of cataplexy).

A summary of the American Academy of Sleep Medicine recommendations for the treatment of narcolepsy are given in Box 4–5.

Idiopathic Hypersomnia

Definition

In this disorder, sleepiness occurs after sufficient or even increased amounts of nighttime sleep and without any identifiable cause.

Clinical Features

Excessive sleepiness is generally severe and constant. Sleepiness, manifesting as normal or extended major sleep episodes (often lasting over 8 hours with few or no awakenings) and naps (up to 1 to 2 hours of non–rapid eye movement [NREM] sleep), protracted periods of daytime drowsiness, and paroxysmal sleep attacks, is present almost daily for at least 3 months. It is associated with impairment of daytime function.

Unintended naps are longer compared with those of narcolepsy and OSA, and unlike narcolepsy, they are typically unrefreshing. Affected individuals often report difficulty awakening from sleep. Disorientation and confusion on awakening (ie, sleep drunkenness), automatic behavior, headaches, syncope, orthostatic hypotension, and Raynaud-type vascular symptoms may be present as well. Cataplexy is distinctively absent.

Types of Idiopathic Hypersomnia

Idiopathic hypersomnia may or may not be associated with a long sleep time (Table 4–12).

Demographics and Clinical Course

Idiopathic hypersomnia has a prevalence of approximately 0.002% to 0.005%, and it accounts for about 1% to 10% of patients referred to sleep clinics for excessive sleepiness. Excessive sleepiness usually begins insidiously during adolescence or early adulthood (onset often before

Box 4-6.

Polysomnographic features of idiopathic hypersomnia

Nocturnal polysomnography

↓ Sleep latency (often < 10 minutes)

↑ Sleep efficiency (>85%)

↑ or normal Total sleep time

↓ Frequency of arousals

↑ NREM stages 3 and 4 sleep (in some)

No change in REM sleep latency

Multiple sleep latency test

↓ Mean sleep latency (< 8 minutes)

< 2 sleep onset REM periods

24-hour continuous polysomnography

↑ Duration of sleep over 24 hours (> 11 to 12 hours)

↑ Duration of major sleep episode (> 10 hours)

↑ Daytime sleep periods (at least 1 nap of > 1 hour)

25 years of age). In some cases, onset may be heralded by a viral illness (mononucleosis or hepatitis). It affects males and females equally. Course is typically chronic. After an initial period of progressive worsening of sleepiness, the latter may either become stable or continue to worsen throughout life.

Genetics

Some cases of idiopathic hypersomnia may be familial with an autosomal dominant inheritance pattern. Although there is no obvious association with specific HLAs, a high frequency of HLA-Cw2 has been described for some familial cases of the disorder.

Pathophysiology

The etiology of idiopathic hypersomnia is unknown, but it is presumed to be related to an abnormality of central nervous system mechanisms controlling sleep and wakefulness. This results in failure of the wake processes to inhibit NREM sleep.

Table 4-12. Types of idiopathic hypersomnia

Type	Characteristics
Idiopathic hypersomnia with long sleep time	Excessive amounts of sleep with long nighttime sleep episode and at least one daytime nap lasting more than 1 hour Prolonged nocturnal sleep duration (at least 10 hours, often 12 to 14 hours)
Idiopathic hypersomnia without long sleep time	Nocturnal sleep of normal or slightly prolonged duration (greater than 6 hours but less than 10 hours)

Evaluation

Other causes of excessive sleepiness should be excluded. These include insufficient sleep syndrome, sleep-disordered breathing, narcolepsy, periodic limb movement disorder, medication use, post-traumatic hypersomnia, recurrent hypersomnia, mood disorder, and medical disorders (eg, encephalitis).

Neurologic examination is usually normal. CSF levels of hypocretin-1 are normal. Polysomnography and MSLT are essential for the diagnosis of idiopathic hypersomnia. Monitoring esophageal or nasal pressures during sleep to rule out the presence of mild OSA or upper airway resistance syndrome is recommended.

Polysomnographic features include a normal sleep architecture, decreased sleep latency and increased or normal total sleep time (Box 4–6). No specific sleep disorders or repeated awakenings are present. On MSLT, mean sleep latency is reduced (approximately 3 to 9 minutes), without sleep onset REM periods.

Differential Diagnosis

Differential diagnosis of idiopathic hypersomnia includes conditions that are associated with excessive sleepiness, such as insufficient sleep syndrome; narcolepsy; OSA (including upper airway resistance syndrome); medication or substance use; post-traumatic hypersomnia; medical (encephalitis), neurologic (hydrocephalus or brain tumors), or psychiatric (mood disorder particularly depression) disorders; and long sleeper. Although both narcolepsy and idiopathic hypersomnia are associated with excessive daytime sleepiness, there are distinct differences in clinical presentation between the two disorders (Table 4–13).

Therapy

Treatment of idiopathic hypersomnia requires the use of stimulant agents. Unlike narcolepsy, response to stimulant agents is generally less favorable and unpredictable. Good sleep hygiene,

Table 4–13. Comparison between narcolepsy and idiopathic hypersomnia

Characteristics	Narcolepsy	Idiopathic hypersomnia
Cataplexy	May be present	Absent
Sleep paralysis and hypnagogic hallucinations	May be present	May be present
Daytime napping	Transiently refreshing	Not refreshing
Nighttime sleep	Sleep disturbance common Short sleep latency Short REM sleep latency	May be normal or prolonged in duration Normal sleep architecture
Multiple sleep latency test	Short sleep latency Sleep onset REM periods present	Short sleep latency Sleep onset REM periods generally absent
HLA typing	DQB1*0602	CW2
Response to stimulant therapy	More predictable improvement	Less predictable improvement

with obtaining a sufficient amount of nighttime sleep and avoidance of irregular sleep schedules, is important.

Insufficient Sleep Syndrome

Definition

Insufficient sleep syndrome is a chronic voluntary but unintentional failure to obtain nighttime sleep that is sufficient in duration to achieve and maintain normal alertness while awake. If desired, individuals have no difficulty sleeping longer. This sleep pattern is present almost daily for at least 3 months. Insufficient sleep is the most common cause of excessive sleepiness.

Demographics

Habitual sleep insufficiency is more common during adolescence and among men.

Clinical Features

The disparity between actual sleep obtained each night and the need for sleep may be due to occupational demands, school or social activities, acquired lifestyle, or inadequate consideration of sleep requirements. Duration of sleep is commonly extended during weekends or vacations compared to weekdays.

Consequences

There are differences in susceptibility to sleep deprivation. Nonetheless, significant sleep insufficiency can give rise to excessive sleepiness, fatigue, malaise, increase risk of accidents, and neurocognitive impairment. Insufficient sleep can worsen preexisting sleepiness due to other primary sleep disorders such as OSA or narcolepsy.

Evaluation

History, sleep logs, and actigraphy confirm a habitual sleep duration that is shorter than is normal for age-matched controls. There is often a significant difference in nighttime sleep duration between weekdays and weekends. Resolution of excessive sleepiness generally occurs during a trial of longer nighttime sleep duration. Polysomnography is not required for the diagnosis of insufficient sleep syndrome. If performed, it demonstrates features consistent with inadequate sleep, including a reduced sleep latency and increased sleep efficiency and duration (Table 4–14).

Table 4–14. Polysomnographic and multiple sleep latency test features of insufficient sleep syndrome

Polysomnography	Multiple sleep latency test
↓ Sleep latency (< 10 minutes) ↑ Sleep efficiency (> 90%) ↑ Total sleep time (when sleep is permitted to continue *ad lib*) ↑ NREM stages 3 and 4 sleep ↑ REM sleep	↓ Sleep latency NREM stages 1 and 2 can be observed Note: Ideally, MSLT should be performed after several days of adequate amounts of nocturnal sleep

Therapy

Therapy involves extending nighttime sleep until alertness and neurocognitive function improves and normalizes.

Post-traumatic Hypersomnia

Central nervous system trauma, especially those involving the lateral and posterior hypothalamus, basal forebrain, third ventricle, posterior fossa, midbrain and pons, can lead to excessive sleepiness. The degree of sleepiness usually correlates with severity of head trauma.

Hypersomnia, consisting of prolonged nocturnal sleep and frequent daytime napping, is not present before the trauma. It typically begins immediately after head trauma, and may be accompanied by fatigue, headaches, and cognitive impairment (memory and concentration). No cataplexy or other REM sleep-related phenomena are present.

Symptoms may transiently worsen before gradually resolving over several weeks to months. In some patients, lingering sleep disturbances and sleepiness may be evident. Differential diagnosis consists of seizure disorder, subdural hematoma, progressive hydrocephalus, meningitis, or encephalitis.

Neurologic evaluation, including electroencephalography (EEG), imaging studies and, occasionally, Doppler tests of cerebral blood flow, is indicated. Polysomnography reveals normal sleep duration and quality. There is no specific treatment.

Recurrent Hypersomnia

Recurrent hypersomnia can manifest in two forms: hypersomnia only (monosymptomatic type) or hypersomnia accompanied by binge eating and hypersexuality (Kleine-Levin syndrome). Periods of hypersomnia, during which daily sleep duration may exceed 16 to 18 hours, last from a few days to several weeks (typically 2 days to 4 weeks) and recur 1 or more times annually. This may be associated with impaired cognition, disinhibited behavior, and weight gain (Kleine-Levin type). Patients may awaken only to eat and void. A prodrome with headaches and fatigue may precede these episodes. Other clinical manifestations occurring during episodes of sleepiness include hyperphagia (binge eating), hypersexuality, confusion, memory impairment, hallucinations, depersonalization, irritability, impulsiveness, aggression, depression, and polydipsia. The episodes terminate with transient insomnia, excitement, hyperactivity, and amnesia. Between episodes, sleep, alertness, behavior, and cognitive function are normal.

Characteristically, recurrent episodes of somnolence begin during early adolescence. Episodes can be triggered by an acute febrile illness (eg, viral infections), strong emotions, physical stress, alcohol use, anesthesia, or head trauma. Kleine-Levin syndrome is rare and affects mostly males. The etiology is unknown but is suspected to involve dysfunction of the hypothalamic and limbic systems. There is an increased frequency of HLA DQB1*02 in patients with Kleine-Levin syndrome. The differential diagnosis includes menstrual-related hypersomnia, non–24-hour circadian sleep-phase disorder, and psychiatric conditions such as seasonal affective disorder, bipolar disorder, psychosis, and somatoform disorder.

Polysomnographic features include decreased sleep efficiency, sleep latency and REM sleep latency, and diminished stages 3 and 4 of NREM sleep (Table 4–15).

Course is usually self-limited. The frequency, severity, and duration of episodes may decrease over time. Therapy with lithium or valproic acid has been described. Counseling regarding safety issues is recommended. Consequences of Kleine-Levin syndrome include significant weight gain as well as social and academic/occupational impairment.

Menstrual-related Hypersomnia

Recurrent and transient sleepiness can develop during the premenstrual period. Daytime alertness normalizes following menses. Etiology remains uncertain. Polysomnography performed during periods of hypersomnolence demonstrates a decrease in NREM stages 3 and 4 sleep. Patients with disabling hypersomnia related to menstruation may benefit from oral contraceptives used to inhibit ovulation.

Idiopathic Recurrent Stupor

This is an apparently rare disorder characterized by recurrent episodes of stupor unrelated to any underlying central nervous system dysfunction. Individual episodes of stupor may last from 2 to 120 hours and can recur several times each year. EEG may demonstrate diffuse, nonreactive 14 to 16 Hz rhythms. Symptoms are reversed by administration of flumazenil, which antagonizes benzodiazepine receptors.

Subwakefulness Syndrome

Subwakefulness syndrome is a rare and chronic condition in which the subjective sensation of constant daytime sleepiness occurs in the absence of any objective evidence of excessive sleepiness. There is no history of frequent napping. Nocturnal polysomnography is normal; however, continuous daytime polysomnography may demonstrate intermittent episodes of NREM stage 1 sleep.

Miscellaneous Disorders

Selected behavioral disorders that affect sleep are presented in Table 4–16 and circadian rhythm disorders that affect sleep are presented in Table 4–17. Features of sleep disorders are outlined in Table 4–18.

Medical Disorders

Sleepiness may be directly caused by an underlying medical disorder (eg, hypothyroidism, Addison disease, chronic renal failure, hepatic encephalopathy, and toxic encephalopathy (Table 4–19). Cataplexy is absent. Polysomnography may either be normal or show disturbed sleep. The MSLT demonstrates a decrease in mean sleep latency (< 8 minutes) and less than two sleep onset REM periods.

Neurologic Disorders

A number of neurologic disorders are associated with excessive sleepiness (Table 4–20). These include meningitis, encephalitis, head trauma, stroke, seizures, myotonic dystrophy, neoplasms, neurodegenerative conditions and genetic syndromes (eg, fragile X syndrome, Moebius syndrome, Niemann Pick type C disease, Norrie disease, and Prader-Willi syndrome).

Psychiatric Disorders

Excessive sleepiness (prolonged nighttime sleep duration and frequent napping) can develop in a number of psychiatric disorders, namely mood disorders, psychosis, alcoholism, adjustment

Table 4–15.   Polysomnographic and MSLT features of recurrent hypersomnia during symptomatic periods

Polysomnography	24-hour polysomnography	Multiple sleep latency test
↓ Sleep latency ↓ Sleep efficiency ↑ Wake time after sleep onset ↓ NREM stages 3 and 4 sleep ↓ REM sleep latency Note: General slowing of background EEG activity with generalized bursts of moderate- to high-voltage 5 Hz to 7 Hz waves	↑ Total sleep time (18 hours or more)	↓ Sleep latency (< 10 minutes)

Table 4–16.   Behavioral disorders

Disorder	Characteristics
Adjustment sleep disorder	Daytime sleepiness secondary to sleep disruption related to acute stress or unfamiliar sleep environments
Limit-setting sleep disorder	Sleep onset disruption resulting in a decrease in total sleep time and excessive sleepiness.
Inadequate sleep hygiene	Excessive sleepiness resulting from acquired habits that are incongruous with sleep

Table 4–17.   Circadian rhythm disorders

Disorder	Characteristics
Delayed sleep-phase syndrome	An inability to arise until late morning or early afternoon is typical. Morning sleepiness develops if a person attempts to arise at times closer to socially accepted norms.
Advanced sleep-phase syndrome	There is a severe inability to delay sleep time beyond 6 to 8 PM. Excessive sleepiness may develop in the early evening hours if the person is forced to stay awake beyond the customary bedtime.
Irregular sleep-wake pattern	Disorganization of sleep and wake times, with three or more short "naps" constituting the fragmentary remnants of the major sleep episode, can lead to excessive daytime sleepiness.

Table 4–17. Circadian rhythm disorders—cont'd

Disorder	Characteristics
Non–24-hour sleep-phase disorder	Sleep-wake patterns are entirely dependent on intrinsic biologic rhythms. Because free-running internal rhythms have a periodicity of slightly over 24 hours, the person's sleep onset and arising times are delayed by about 1 hour or more each day. Desynchrony between the external 24-hour world and internal rhythms can give rise to excessive daytime sleepiness.
Jet lag	Excessive sleepiness can develop following rapid travel across multiple time zones. Delay in nighttime sleep after a westward flight and the earlier-than-customary arising times following eastward flights can result sleep deprivation and diminished daytime alertness.
Shift work sleep disorder	Mismatch between the requirements of nighttime work and the demands for sleep, as well as the decreased efficiency of sleep taken during the daytime, produces excessive sleepiness and diminished vigilance among shift workers.

Table 4–18. Sleep disorders

Disorder	Characteristics
Obstructive sleep apnea syndrome	Respiratory events and arousals can recur throughout the evening, at times reaching numbers substantial enough to produce sleep fragmentation and subsequent daytime sleepiness. Naps are generally unrefreshing.
Central sleep apnea syndrome	Persons can present with complaints of daytime sleepiness and cognitive impairment.
Central alveolar hypoventilation syndrome	Hypoventilation during sleep leads to arterial blood gas abnormalities (hypercapnia and hypoxemia), repetitive arousals, sleep fragmentation and, possibly, excessive daytime sleepiness.
Restless legs syndrome	When sufficiently severe, restless legs syndrome can increase sleep onset latency and cause sleep disruption, which can, in turn, lead to excessive daytime sleepiness.
Periodic limb movement disorder	Sleep fragmentation from repetitive limb movement-related arousals can result in excessive sleepiness. Diagnosis requires polysomnographic evaluation.

disorder, conversion disorder (pseudohypersomnia), personality disorder, seasonal affective disorder, schizoaffective disorder, somatoform disorder, and psychosis (Table 4–21). In each of these disorders, sleepiness is temporally related to the underlying condition. There is often considerable time spent in bed but with poor sleep consolidation. Polysomnography demonstrates an increase in sleep latency, decrease in sleep efficiency, and increase in frequency of awakenings. The MLST is often normal but may reveal a short mean sleep latency.

Table 4–19.   Medical disorders

Disorder	Characteristics
Addison disease (hypoadrenalism)	Inadequate secretion of adrenal steroid hormones can result in fatigue and sleepiness.
Chronic fatigue syndrome	In addition to sleepiness, symptoms can include fatigue, exhaustion, headaches, cold intolerance, arthralgias, myalgias, muscle weakness, irritable bowel, depression, anxiety and cognitive impairment. Prevalence is greater among women. Polysomnographic features may include an increase in sleep latency, decrease in sleep efficiency, and frequent arousals. An alpha-delta electroencephalographic (EEG) pattern has been described. Multiple Sleep Latency Test (MSLT) is normal.
Hypothyroidism	Hypothyroidism can directly give rise to excessive sleepiness or indirectly as a result of obstructive sleep apnea.
Sleeping sickness	It is caused by the protozoan *Trypanosoma brucei* and is endemic in certain regions of tropical Africa. Following the bite of an infected tsetse fly, affected persons develop lymphadenopathy, fever, headaches, and progressive sleepiness and inactivity secondary to leptomeningitis, cerebritis and panencephalitis. It culminates in coma and death if left untreated. Recurrent microarousals and loss of sleep spindles, K-complexes and vertex sharp transients may be noted during polysomnography.

Table 4–20.   Neurologic disorders

Disorder	Characteristics
Dementia	Excessive sleepiness and decreased daytime vigilance secondary to sleep fragmentation, repetitive arousals, and reduced sleep efficiency can develop "Sun-downing" with confusion, agitation, and wandering can further contribute to sleep disruption.
Sleep-related seizures	Seizures occurring during sleep can give rise to sleep fragmentation and excessive daytime sleepiness.
Parkinsonism	Sleep disruption may give rise to significant daytime sleepiness.
Fragmentary myoclonus	Asynchronous, asymmetric contractions of the muscles of the face and extremities appear at sleep onset, last from 10 minutes to over an hour, occur predominantly in NREM sleep, and persist into REM sleep. Affected individuals are generally unaware of these movements. This rare disorder has its onset in adulthood, predominantly among males. Its course is generally benign, although excessive sleepiness secondary to sleep disruption may develop in some patients. Polysomnography demonstrates repetitive, brief electromyographic (EMG) potentials.
Sleep-related neurogenic tachypnea	Sustained tachypnea starts at sleep onset and persists throughout sleep. Marked sleep fragmentation may ensue, in turn, leading to excessive sleepiness. This is a rare condition, occurring either in an idiopathic form or in association with lesions in the central nervous system.

Table 4–21. Psychiatric disorders

Disorder	Characteristics
Mood disorders	Persons with mild, atypical, bipolar, or seasonal depression may complain of excessive daytime sleepiness. MSLT results are generally normal.
Psychoses	Excessive sleepiness with increased sleep efficiency occurs during the waning phase of schizophrenia or during residual schizophrenia.
Alcoholism	Sleepiness can develop for several hours after acute consumption of alcohol. Profound sleeplessness may accompany delirium tremens.
Other psychiatric disorders	Excessive sleepiness can develop in persons with adjustment, conversion, personality, schizoaffective and somatoform disorders.

Menstrual and Pregnancy-Related Disorders

Menstrual- and pregnancy-related sleep disorders are described in Table 4–22.

Environmental Factors

Environmental sleep disorders are described in Table 4–23.

Use of Medications or Substances

Sleepiness can be due to the use, abuse, adverse effects, prior prolonged use, or recent withdrawal of medications and substances (Table 4–24).

Differential Diagnosis

Sleepiness should be differentiated from fatigue (sensation of exhaustion or lack of energy) secondary to Addison disease, anemia, cancer, chronic fatigue syndrome, depression, fibromyalgia, hypothyroidism, and infections.

Sleep duration in a *long sleeper* is longer than is typical for the person's age and is often greater than 10 hours during a 24-hour period for a young adult. Excessive sleepiness develops if less than the required amount of sleep is obtained. Polysomnography and MSLT are normal. Its course is chronic and unrelenting.

Table 4–22. Menstrual and pregnancy-related sleep disorders

Disorder	Characteristics
Menstrual-associated sleep disorder	Menses may be associated with excessive sleepiness. Neither etiology, prevalence, nor course of the disease is known. Polysomnography reveals normal sleep.
Pregnancy-associated sleep disorder	Increased sleepiness is common during pregnancy.

Table 4–23. Environmental factors

Disorder	Characteristics
Environmental sleep disorder	Adverse environmental conditions can affect sleep and lead to excessive daytime sleepiness.
Toxin-induced sleep disorder	Ingestion of toxins can produce sleepiness due to CNS depression.

Table 4–24. Pharmacologic factors

Disorder	Characteristics
Alcohol-dependent sleep disorder	Acute ingestion of alcohol can result in sleepiness, especially in those with an underlying sleep deprivation.
Hypnotic-dependent sleep disorder	Habitual use of hypnotic and sedative agents may give rise to excessive daytime sleepiness if large doses are taken, long-acting agents are used, medications are taken close to awakening time, or dose escalation is occuring.
Stimulant-dependent sleep disorder	Excessive sleepiness occurs during abrupt withdrawal of stimulant medications. MSLT demonstrates a decrease in mean sleep latency.

Evaluation of Excessive Sleepiness

Excessive sleepiness can be evaluated using both subjective and objective measures (Table 4–25).

Therapy for Hypersomnia

General Measures

Any underlying medical, neurologic, or psychiatric disorder that can give rise or contribute to sleepiness should be properly treated, if possible. Sleep hygiene, including maintaining a regular sleep-wake schedule and obtaining an adequate amount of sleep each night, is paramount.

Countermeasures for Sleep Deprivation

The effectiveness of behavioral countermeasures, such as increasing levels of activity or external stimulation (eg, loud noises) is limited and unpredictable.

Napping

Sleep is the most effective countermeasure for sleep deprivation. Scheduled naps throughout the day may help alleviate sleepiness. Naps (eg, 45 minutes or longer) scheduled prior to planned prolonged wakefulness and sleep deprivation have beneficial effects on alertness and vigilance.

Table 4–25. Evaluating excessive sleepiness

History	Inquiries into nighttime (sleep latency, duration of nocturnal sleep, and frequency of awakenings) and daytime (overall level of alertness, timing of and activities during periods of sleepiness, decrements in cognitive function and performance, accidents, napping, use of stimulants including caffeine, and other medications) habits and activities are often helpful. Family history, clinical history (sleep, medical, neurologic, and psychiatric) and medication use are also important.
Clinical evaluation	Clinical features suggestive of excessive sleepiness include yawning; head bobbing; ptosis; constricted pupils; and attempts to remain alert by repetitive stretching, standing, or walking.
Sleepiness questionnaires	The Stanford Sleepiness Scale and the Epworth Sleepiness Scale (ESS) can be used to subjectively assess the severity of sleepiness. The Stanford Sleepiness Scale measures sleepiness at a particular moment, and appears to be better at monitoring sleepiness in a specific person over time than for comparing among different individuals. It is sensitive to diurnal changes in sleep propensity and to sleep deprivation. The ESS measures an individual's overall degree of sleepiness. Tendency to fall asleep during eight common real-life situations is graded. Subjectively measured sleepiness by the ESS does not generally correlate with objective severity of sleepiness as determined by the Mean Sleep Latency Test.
Sleep diaries	Sleep and activity patterns over several days or weeks can be charted in a sleep diary, which may help uncover sleep disorders unsuspected from the patient's history such as circadian sleep disorders and insufficient sleep syndrome. Entries can include bedtime; sleep latency; nighttime awakenings (frequency and duration); arising time; number, if any, of naps during the day; mealtimes; exercise times; and the use of medications, alcohol, and caffeine.
Polysomnography	Polysomnography is indicated in the routine evaluation of excessive sleepiness unless the latter is clearly related to insufficient sleep or to a medical, neurologic, or psychiatric disorder, or when sleepiness resolves with appropriate therapy of the underlying condition. Polysomnography should always be performed on the evening preceding an Multiple Sleep Latency Test. It may demonstrate specific sleep disorders, such as obstructive sleep apnea or period limb movements of sleep, which may account for the patient's complaint of excessive sleepiness.
Multiple sleep latency test	MSLT measures the propensity to fall asleep and is the standard test for objectively determining the degree of sleepiness. It is sensitive to the effects of circadian rhythms of sleepiness and wakefulness, and sleep deprivation. A sleep diary is completed for 1 to 2 weeks before the scheduled test. Stimulants and REM sleep suppressants should ideally be discontinued for 2 weeks prior to the MSLT. Four to five nap periods in a dark and quiet room are scheduled after an overnight polysomnography every 2 hours, beginning about 2 hours after awakening from nighttime sleep. Naps opportunities are continued for 20 minutes if no sleep episode is identified or for 15 minutes following the first epoch of sleep unless REM sleep occurs. Sleep is terminated if unequivocal REM sleep occurs. A urine drug abuse screen should be done on the day of the study.

Table 4-25. Evaluating excessive sleepiness—cont'd

	Sleep latency is defined as the time from the start of the study (lights out) to the first recorded sleep epoch (clinical studies), or to the first three consecutive epochs of NREM stage 1 sleep or first epoch of NREM stage 2 sleep (sleep latency is recorded as 20 minutes if no sleep occurs). Mean sleep latency is the average of the sleep latencies across all naps. Mean sleep latency correlates with severity of sleepiness. The presence of sleep onset REM periods is useful in the diagnosis of narcolepsy.
Maintenance of wakefulness test	MWT measures a person's ability to stay awake. It consists of four nap periods each lasting 40 minutes in which the patient is asked to try to stay awake. Most normal persons without excessive sleepiness can remain awake during these naps. MWT is sensitive to sleep deprivation and the effects of circadian sleep-wake rhythms.
Performance vigilance testing	Tests that involve repetitive tasks, such as driving simulators, which measure performance, attention, and alertness, can be used to assess excessive sleepiness.
Actigraphy	A person's periods of rest/sleep and activity can be discerned using wrist actigraphs. These devices produce a signal whenever movement is detected. Because of its portability, it permits extended monitoring over several days to weeks.
Pupillometry	Sleepiness is generally associated with pupillary instability and constriction whereas a large pupil is seen with wakefulness. The diameter and stability of the pupil can be evaluated using pupillometry. Lack of a reference standard limits its clinical application.
Laboratory tests	Drug screening for stimulants, opiates, and benzodiazepines may be considered. Depending on the clinical presentation, laboratory testing for restless legs syndrome (eg, serum ferritin) and hypothyroidism may be indicated as well.

Environmental Manipulation

Provision of bright ambient light during the night augments alertness among night shift workers. Physical activity, changes in posture (such as standing), or environmental stimulation (eg, noise, cold air) does not enhance alertness or vigilance.

Pharmacologic Therapy for Sleepiness

Psychostimulant agents are often required to control pathologic sleepiness. These agents improve alertness, cognitive performance, and mood. Commonly used agents include caffeine, amphetamines (eg, dextroamphetamine), and modafinil. They increase the availability of norepinephrine and dopamine at the synaptic junctions.

General guidelines regarding the use of stimulant agents for the therapy of excessive sleepiness include using the lowest possible effective dose, monitoring clinical response as well as adverse effects (including abuse and dependency), and timing drug administrating to meet specific individual needs. For instance, amphetamines and methylphenidate should be given at least 1 hour prior to the time of desired effectiveness. Shorter acting medications (eg, methylphenidate) may be combined with longer acting agents (eg, modafinil) to achieve rapid onset as well as sustained duration of alertness. It is recommended that all stimulants be used only on an acute basis to maintain effectiveness. They should not be used chronically to replace obtaining sufficient duration of sleep.

Abuse liability of a drug can be defined as the probability of developing dependency, either physiologic (withdrawal symptoms with drug discontinuation), behavioral (drug seeking) or both, with its repeated use. Dependency, in turn, increases the likelihood of drug self-administration. It is one of the adverse effects of stimulants (Box 4–7).

Caffeine

Caffeine is the most frequently ingested stimulant worldwide. It acts by decreasing adenosine transmission from both central nervous system A_1 and A_{2A} receptors. Physiologic changes related to caffeine use include increases in metabolic rate, blood pressure, heart rate, and body temperature. There is enhanced secretion of epinephrine and norepinephrine. In addition, caffeine possesses a significant diuretic effect.

Caffeine increases objective measures of wakefulness (ie, increase in sleep latency during MSLT and MWT), as well as subjective alertness. In sleep-deprived individuals, caffeine ingestion improves alertness, vigilance, short-term memory, reasoning, reaction time, and psychomotor performance, and decreases fatigue. When ingested close to bedtime, caffeine can result in sleep disturbance with an increase in sleep latency, decrease in total sleep time, and decrease in NREM stages 3 and 4 sleep. Adverse effects on sleep, which are dose-dependent, may last up to 8 hours after caffeine ingestion. *The elimination half-life of caffeine, which is usually 3 to 6 hours, is decreased among smokers.*

Habitual use of caffeine can give rise to tolerance and withdrawal symptoms with a decrease in performance. Tolerance to caffeine may develop within a few days in some individuals after repeated ingestion; therefore, administration to habitual caffeine users may not lead to any significant improvement in psychomotor functioning. Tolerance to subjective reports of alertness may develop more rapidly compared to objective measures. Caffeine has a moderate abuse liability, with physical dependency and withdrawal symptoms (eg, fatigue, sleepiness, and headaches) developing

Box 4–7.

Adverse effects of stimulant agents

Abuse liability and dependency

Anorexia

Development of tolerance

Gastrointestinal symptoms

Hallucinations and paranoia

Headaches

Increase in blood pressure

Insomnia

Irritability

Nervousness

Tachycardia/palpitations

Tremors

Withdrawal symptoms following drug discontinuation

in some high-dose habitual caffeine users. Doses under 100 mg daily appear to pose no hazard to health. Overdosage (ie, doses greater than approximately 600 mg) can produce insomnia, anxiety, palpitations, diaphoresis, nervousness, agitation, dizziness, headache, tremors, jitteriness, and nausea/vomiting.

Amphetamine

Amphetamine is a stimulant agent approved for the treatment of excessive sleepiness related to narcolepsy, as well as attention deficit hyperactivity disorder (ADHD). It acts by releasing norepinephrine and dopamine at neuronal terminals.

Dextroamphetamines are the most commonly administered form of amphetamines. Amphetamine use results in dose-related improvements in alertness, vigilance, memory, mood, performance, and reaction time, as well as reductions in sleepiness and fatigue. Sleep disturbance may develop, such as sleep initiation insomnia, frequent awakenings, and decrease in sleep quality.

Amphetamines may decrease sleepiness by increasing the release, and decreasing the reuptake of dopamine at the mesencephalic ventral tegmental area of Tsai and ventral periaqueductal gray area. See Box 4–8 for more information about the effects of amphetamines on sleep. The incidence of physiologic effects (tachycardia, and increases in body temperature and blood pressure) and adverse effects (insomnia, headaches, nervousness, anxiety, depression, paranoia, delusions, tremulousness, restlessness, agitation, paresthesias, nausea, anorexia, dry mouth, stomach cramping, postural hypotension, palpitations and ventricular arrhythmias) are dose-dependent. Euphoria and pupillary dilation are commonly noted. Tolerance develops rapidly.

Dextroamphetamines have a half-life of about 10 to 30 hours. Usual daily dosage ranges from 5 to 60 mg. They have an FDA Schedule II rating, with a high abuse liability and risk of dependency. Withdrawal symptoms are common following drug discontinuation.

Methamphetamine

Following sleep deprivation, administration of methamphetamine (formed by adding a methyl group to the amine of amphetamine) improves alertness, vigilance, reaction time, and task performance, and it decreases fatigue and sleepiness. In addition, its use can give rise to a decrease in subjective sleep duration and quality, insomnia, headaches, dizziness, nervousness, anxiety, confusion, tremulousness, anorexia, nausea, diaphoresis, palpitations, chills and extremity numbness.

Box 4–8. **Polysomnographic features during amphetamine use**	↑ Sleep latency
	↓ Sleep efficiency
	↓ Total sleep time
	↑ Wake time after sleep onset
	↑ Frequency of awakenings
	↑ NREM stage 1 sleep
	↓ NREM stages 2, 3 and 4 sleep
	↑ REM sleep latency
	↓ REM sleep

Increases in blood pressure, heart rate, respiratory rate, and body temperature are described. Changes in sleep architecture include decreases in sleep efficiency, total sleep time and NREM sleep, and an increase in frequency of awakenings.

Methamphetamine has significant neurotoxicity and undesirable effects on the cardiovascular system.

Methylphenidate

Methylphenidate, a piperidine derivative, acts by blocking dopamine reuptake and enhancing the release of dopamine and norepinephrine. This drug has been shown to improve alertness and psychomotor performance. It produces an increase in sleep latency during MSLT and MWT. Methylphenidate is indicated for the treatment of ADHD and excessive sleepiness related to narcolepsy. Physiologic effects of methylphenidate administration include an increase in heart rate and blood pressure. It increases plasma concentrations of epinephrine, growth hormone, and cortisol, and it decreases levels of prolactin. Patients taking methylphenidate may complain of insomnia, anorexia, headaches, palpitations, nervousness, tremulousness and irritability. Sleep disturbance can be minimized if medications are not administered after 4 PM.

Methylphenidate has a FDA Schedule II rating and is available in an immediate-release form (elimination half-life of approximately 2.5 to 3.5 hours), an extended-release form (duration of action of 8 to 12 hours), and combinations of both immediate- and extended-release formulations. Usual daily dosage generally ranges from 10 to 60 mg. It appears to have less abuse liability than amphetamines. Development of tolerance has been described.

Pemoline

Pemoline is an oxazolidine psychostimulant that acts by increasing the release and inhibiting the reuptake of dopamine. Improvements in performance and alertness have been described following its administration. It has an elimination half-life of approximately 12 hours. Because of the risk of hepatotoxicity, it has been withdrawn from the market.

Modafinil

Modafinil is an alerting and wakefulness-promoting agent indicated for the therapy of excessive sleepiness related to narcolepsy and shift work sleep disorder. It is also approved for treating persistent sleepiness despite continuous positive airway pressure therapy for OSA.

Its precise mechanism of action is incompletely understood, but is believed to partly involve dopaminergic systems. It also appears to possess direct α-1 noradrenergic agonist action, activate hypocretin-containing neurons, and reduce GABA.

Modafinil administration results in a dose-dependent improvement in alertness, psychomotor performance, memory, reaction time, and mood when given to sleep-deprived individuals. Efficacy decreases as the duration of prior wakefulness increases. Effects on sleep architecture within 14 hours of drug administration include a decrease in sleep efficiency and total sleep time. Sleep latency measured by MSLT and MWT is increased.

Physiologic effects consist of increases in blood pressure, heart rate, and body temperature, especially at higher doses. Adverse effects such as nervousness, agitation, anxiety, depression, confusion, headaches, palpitations, tremor, insomnia, dry mouth, and nausea are especially prominent at higher doses.

Modafinil is a FDA Schedule IV drug. Compared with amphetamine or methylphenidate, modafinil has less abuse liability and is not associated with significant tolerance or withdrawal symptoms.

Table 4–26. Drug Enforcement Administration (DEA) Classification and Food and Drug Administration (FDA) Labeling

Category II	High abuse potential; severe physical or psychologic dependency with use
Category III	Some abuse potential; low-to-moderate physical dependency or high psychologic dependency with use
Category IV	Low abuse potential; limited physical or psychologic dependency with use
Category V	Low abuse potential; state and local regulation

Because modafinil's elimination half-life is approximately 12 to 14 hours, it can be administered once daily. Its usual starting dose is 100 to 200 mg daily. Maximum dose is 400 mg daily. The drug is metabolized in the liver. Significant drug interactions include diazepam, diphenylhydantoin, and propranolol. It can also interact with, and reduce the efficacy of, birth control pills. Drug discontinuation does not result in rebound of NREM stages 3 and 4, or REM sleep.

Other Medications

Selegiline is a MAO inhibitor with stimulating and anticataplectic actions. Adverse effects include confusion, dizziness, dry mouth, and nausea. As with other MAO inhibitors, a diet low in tyramine is recommended.

See Table 4–26 for Drug Enforcement Administration classification of drugs based on their abuse potential.

References

General References

American Academy of Sleep Medicine. *The International Classification of Sleep Disorders: Diagnostic and Coding Manual.* 2nd ed. Westchester, IL: American Academy of Sleep Medicine, 2005.

Bowman TJ. *Review of Sleep Medicine.* Burlington, MA: Butterworth-Heinemann, 2002.

Berry RB. *Sleep Medicine Pearls.* 2nd ed. Philadelphia, PA: Hanley & Belfus, 2002.

Chokroverty S. *Clinical Companion to Sleep Disorders Medicine.* 2nd ed. Butterworth-Heinemann, 2000.

Lavie P, Pillar G, Malhotra A. *Sleep Disorders Handbook.* New York, NY: Taylor & Francis, 2002.

Lee-Chiong TL, ed. *Sleep: A Comprehensive Handbook.* Hoboken, NJ: John Wiley & Sons, 2006.

Lee-Chiong TL, Sateia M, Carskadon M, eds. *Sleep Medicine.* Philadelphia, PA: Hanley & Belfus (Elsevier), 2002.

Perlis ML, Lichstein KL, eds. *Treating Sleep Disorders: Principles and Practice of Behavioral Sleep Medicine.* Hoboken, NJ: John Wiley & Sons, 2003.

Rechtschaffen A, Kales A. *A Manual of Standardized Terminology, Techniques and Scoring System for Sleep Stages of Human Subjects.* Los Angeles, CA: Brain Information Service/Brain Research Institute, University of California, 1968.

Reite M, Ruddy J, Nagel K. *Concise Guide to Evaluation and Management of Sleep Disorders* (3rd ed.). Arlington, VA: American Psychiatric Publishing, April 2002.

Sleep Deprivation and Stimulant Task Force of the American Academy of Sleep Medicine. The use of stimulants to modify performance during sleep loss: a review. *Sleep.* 2005;28(9).

Sleep Disorders. Medical Clinics of North America. Philadelphia, PA: Elsevier Saunders, 2004.

Sleep Medicine. Primary Care: Clinics in Office Practice. Philadelphia, PA: Elsevier Saunders, 2005.

Wise MS. Narcolepsy and other disorders of excessive sleepiness. *Sleep Disorders.* Medical Clinics of North America. Elsevier Saunders, 2004.

Definition

Lee-Chiong TL. Manifestations and classification of sleep disorders. In: Lee-Chiong TL, Sateia M, Carskadon M, eds. *Sleep Medicine.* Philadelphia, PA: Hanley & Belfus (Elsevier), 2002.

Mysliwiec V, Henderson JH, Strollo PJ. Epidemiology, consequences and evaluation of excessive daytime sleepiness. In: Lee-Chiong TL, Sateia M, Carskadon M, eds. *Sleep Medicine.* Philadelphia, PA: Hanley & Belfus (Elsevier), 2002.Wise MS. Narcolepsy and other disorders of excessive sleepiness. *Sleep Disorders.* Medical Clinics of North America. Elsevier Saunders, 2004.

Demographics

Mysliwiec V, Henderson JH, Strollo PJ. Epidemiology, consequences and evaluation of excessive daytime sleepiness. In: Lee-Chiong TL, Sateia M, Carskadon M, eds. *Sleep Medicine.* Philadelphia, PA: Hanley & Belfus (Elsevier), 2002.

Wise MS. Narcolepsy and other disorders of excessive sleepiness. *Sleep Disorders.* Medical Clinics of North America. Elsevier Saunders, 2004.

Classification of Excessive Sleepiness

American Sleep Disorders Association. *International classification of sleep disorders, revised: diagnostic and coding manual.* Rochester, MN: American Sleep Disorders Association, 1997.

Lee-Chiong TL. Manifestations and classification of sleep disorders. In: Lee-Chiong TL, Sateia M, Carskadon M, eds. *Sleep Medicine.* Philadelphia, PA: Hanley & Belfus (Elsevier), 2002.

Consequences of Excessive Sleepiness

Mysliwiec V, Henderson JH, Strollo PJ. Epidemiology, consequences and evaluation of excessive daytime sleepiness. In: Lee-Chiong TL, Sateia M, Carskadon M, eds. *Sleep Medicine.* Philadelphia, PA: Hanley & Belfus (Elsevier), 2002.

Wise MS. Narcolepsy and other disorders of excessive sleepiness. *Sleep Disorders.* Medical Clinics of North America. Elsevier Saunders, 2004.

Etiology of Excessive Sleepiness

American Sleep Disorders Association. *International classification of sleep disorders, revised: diagnostic and coding manual.* Rochester, MN: American Sleep Disorders Association, 1997.Chimelli L, Scaravilli F. Trypanosomiasis. *Brain Pathology.* 1997;7:599–611.

Lee-Chiong TL. Manifestations and classification of sleep disorders. In: Lee-Chiong TL, Sateia M, Carskadon M, eds. *Sleep Medicine.* Philadelphia, PA: Hanley & Belfus (Elsevier), 2002.

Lins O, Castonguay M, Dunham W, Nevsimalova S, Broughton R. Excessive fragmentary myoclonus: time of night and sleep stage distributions. *Can J Neurol Sci.* 1993;20:142–146.

Wilmer JP, Broughton RJ. Neurogenic sleep related polypnea—a new disorder? *Sleep Res.* 1989;18:322.

Wise MS. Narcolepsy and other disorders of excessive sleepiness. *Sleep Disorders.* Medical Clinics of North America. Elsevier Saunders, 2004.

Narcolepsy

Aldrich MS. Diagnostic aspects of narcolepsy. *Neurology.* 1998;50(2 Suppl 1):S2–S7.

American Sleep Disorders Association. *International classification of sleep disorders, revised: diagnostic and coding manual.* Rochester, MN: American Sleep Disorders Association, 1997.

Bassetti C, Aldrich MS. Narcolepsy. *Neurol Clin.* 1996;14:545–571.

Brooks SN, Mignot E. Narcolepsy and idiopathic hypersomnia. In: Lee-Chiong TL, Sateia M, Carskadon M, eds. *Sleep Medicine.* Philadelphia, PA: Hanley & Belfus (Elsevier), 2002.

Choo KL, Guilleminault C. Narcolepsy and idiopathic hypersomnolence. *Clin Chest Med.* 1998;19:169–181.

Lee-Chiong TL. Manifestations and classification of sleep disorders. In: Lee-Chiong TL, Sateia M, Carskadon M, eds. *Sleep Medicine.* Philadelphia, PA: Hanley & Belfus (Elsevier), 2002.

Littner M et al. Practice parameters for the treatment of narcolepsy: an update for 2000. *Sleep.* 2001; 24(4).

Stores G. Recognition and management of narcolepsy. *Arch Dis Child.* 1999;81:519–524.

Wise MS. Narcolepsy and other disorders of excessive sleepiness. *Sleep Disorders.* Medical Clinics of North America. Elsevier Saunders, 2004.

Idiopathic Hypersomnia

Bassetti C. Aldrich MS. Idiopathic hypersomnia. A series of 42 patients. *Brain.* 1997;120(Pt 8): 1423–1435.

Billiard M, Merle C, Carlander B, Ondze B, Alvarez D, Besset A. Idiopathic hypersomnia. *Psychiatr Clin Neurosci.* 1998;52:125–129.

Brooks SN, Mignot E. Narcolepsy and idiopathic hypersomnia. In: Lee-Chiong TL, Sateia M, Carskadon M, eds. *Sleep Medicine.* Philadelphia, PA: Hanley & Belfus (Elsevier), 2002.

Dyken ME, Yamada T. Narcolepsy and disorders of excessive sleepiness. *Sleep Medicine. Primary Care: Clinics in Office Practice.* Elsevier Saunders, 2005.

Lee-Chiong TL. Manifestations and classification of sleep disorders. In: Lee-Chiong TL, Sateia M, Carskadon M, eds. *Sleep Medicine.* Philadelphia, PA: Hanley & Belfus (Elsevier), 2002.

Wise MS. Narcolepsy and other disorders of excessive sleepiness. *Sleep Disorders.* Medical Clinics of North America. Elsevier Saunders, 2004.

Insufficient Sleep Syndrome

Lee-Chiong TL. Manifestations and classification of sleep disorders. In: Lee-Chiong TL, Sateia M, Carskadon M, eds. *Sleep Medicine.* Philadelphia, PA: Hanley & Belfus (Elsevier), 2002.

Post-traumatic Hypersomnia

D'Ambrosio CM. Miscellaneous syndromes causing excessive daytime sleepiness. In: Lee-Chiong TL, Sateia M, Carskadon M, eds. *Sleep Medicine*. Philadelphia, PA: Hanley & Belfus (Elsevier), 2002.

Guilleminault C, Yuen KM, Gulevich MG, Karadeniz D, Leger D, Philip P. Hypersomnia after head-neck trauma: a medicolegal dilemma. *Neurology*. 2000;54:653–659.

Lee-Chiong TL. Manifestations and classification of sleep disorders. In: Lee-Chiong TL, Sateia M, Carskadon M, eds. *Sleep Medicine*. Philadelphia, PA: Hanley & Belfus (Elsevier), 2002.

Wise MS. Narcolepsy and other disorders of excessive sleepiness. *Sleep Disorders*. Medical Clinics of North America. Elsevier Saunders, 2004.

Recurrent Hypersomnia

American Sleep Disorders Association. *International classification of sleep disorders, revised: diagnostic and coding manual*. Rochester, MN: American Sleep Disorders Association, 1997.

D'Ambrosio CM. Miscellaneous syndromes causing excessive daytime sleepiness. In: Lee-Chiong TL, Sateia M, Carskadon M, eds. *Sleep Medicine*. Philadelphia, PA: Hanley & Belfus (Elsevier), 2002.

Lee-Chiong TL. Manifestations and classification of sleep disorders. In: Lee-Chiong TL, Sateia M, Carskadon M, eds. *Sleep Medicine*. Philadelphia, PA: Hanley & Belfus (Elsevier), 2002.

Manni R, Martinetti M, Ratti MT, Tartara A. Electrophysiological and immunogenetic findings in recurrent monosymptomatic-type hypersomnia: a study of two unrelated Italian cases. *Acta Neurol Scand*. 1993;88:293–295.

Tanabe E, Yara K, Mastuura M, Takahashi S, Sakai T, Kojima T. Prolonged polysomnography in a case with recurrent hypersomnia. *Psychiatr Clin Neurosci*. 1998;52:204–205.

Subwakefulness Syndrome

American Sleep Disorders Association. *International classification of sleep disorders, revised: diagnostic and coding manual*. Rochester, MN: American Sleep Disorders Association, 1997.

D'Ambrosio CM. Miscellaneous syndromes causing excessive daytime sleepiness. In: Lee-Chiong TL, Sateia M, Carskadon M, eds. *Sleep Medicine*. Philadelphia, PA: Hanley & Belfus (Elsevier), 2002.

Hisanaga A, Tsutsumi M, Yasui S, Fukuda H, Tachibana H, Hagino H, et al. A case of subwakefulness syndrome. *Psychiatr Clin Neurosci*. 1998;52:206–207.

Lee-Chiong TL. Manifestations and classification of sleep disorders. In: Lee-Chiong TL, Sateia M, Carskadon M, eds. *Sleep Medicine*. Philadelphia, PA: Hanley & Belfus (Elsevier), 2002.

Miscellaneous Disorders

D'Ambrosio CM. Miscellaneous syndromes causing excessive daytime sleepiness. In: Lee-Chiong TL, Sateia M, Carskadon M, eds. *Sleep Medicine*. Philadelphia, PA: Hanley & Belfus (Elsevier), 2002.

Dyken ME, Yamada T. Narcolepsy and disorders of excessive sleepiness. *Sleep Medicine. Primary Care: Clinics in Office Practice*. Elsevier Saunders. 2005.

Lee-Chiong TL. Manifestations and classification of sleep disorders. In: Lee-Chiong TL, Sateia M, Carskadon M, eds. *Sleep Medicine*. Philadelphia, PA: Hanley & Belfus (Elsevier), 2002.

Differential Diagnosis

D'Ambrosio CM. Miscellaneous syndromes causing excessive daytime sleepiness. In: Lee-Chiong TL, Sateia M, Carskadon M, eds. *Sleep Medicine*. Philadelphia, PA: Hanley & Belfus (Elsevier), 2002.

Lee-Chiong TL. Manifestations and classification of sleep disorders. In: Lee-Chiong TL, Sateia M, Carskadon M, eds. *Sleep Medicine*. Philadelphia, PA: Hanley & Belfus (Elsevier), 2002.

Wise MS. Narcolepsy and other disorders of excessive sleepiness. *Sleep Disorders*. Medical Clinics of North America. Elsevier Saunders, 2004.

Evaluation of Excessive Sleepiness

Benbadis SR, Mascha E, Perry MC, Wolgamuth BR, Smolley LA, Dinner DS. Association between the Epworth Sleepiness Scale and the Multiple Sleep Latency Test in a clinical population. *Ann Intern Med*. 199;130:289–292.

Chervin RD, Aldrich MS. The Epworth Sleepiness Scale may not reflect objective measures of sleepiness or sleep apnea. *Neurology*. 1999;52:125–131.

Johns MW. A new method for measuring daytime sleepiness: the Epworth Sleepiness Scale. *Sleep*. 1991;14:540–545..

Mitler MM, Gujavarty KS, Browman CP. Maintenance of wakefulness test: a polysomnographic technique for evaluating treatment efficacy in patients with excessive somnolence. *Electroencephalogr Clin Neurophysiol*. 1982;53:658–661.

Mysliwiec V, Henderson JH, Strollo PJ. Epidemiology, consequences, and evaluation of excessive daytime sleepiness. v

Newman J, Broughton R. Pupillometric assessment of excessive daytime sleepiness in narcolepsy-cataplexy. *Sleep*. 1991;14:121–129.

Sangal RB, Thomas L, Mitler MM. Maintenance of wakefulness test and multiple sleep latency test. *Chest*. 1992;101:898–902.

Thorpy MJ. The clinical use of the Multiple Sleep Latency Test. The Standards of Practice Committee of the American Sleep Disorders Association. *Sleep*. 1992;15:268–276.

Wise MS. Narcolepsy and other disorders of excessive sleepiness. *Sleep Disorders*. Medical Clinics of North America. Elsevier Saunders, 2004.

Therapy of Hypersomnia

Dyken ME, Yamada T. Narcolepsy and disorders of excessive sleepiness. *Sleep Medicine. Primary Care: Clinics in Office Practice*. Elsevier Saunders, 2005.

Wise MS. Narcolepsy and other disorders of excessive sleepiness. *Sleep Disorders*. Medical Clinics of North America. Elsevier Saunders, 2004.

Sleep-Related Breathing Disorders 5

Several conditions can cause disordered respiration during sleep, including:

1. Obstructive sleep apnea (OSA) syndrome in which inadequate ventilation occurs despite continued efforts to breath due to upper airway obstruction

2. Central sleep apnea (CSA) syndrome resulting from absent or diminished respiratory effort

3. Chronic alveolar hypoventilation syndromes, with hypercapnia (partial pressure of arterial carbon dioxide [$PaCO_2$] > 45 mm Hg)

Some abbreviations frequently used in this chapter are listed in Box 5–1.

Obstructive Sleep Apnea Syndrome

Definition of Terms

Apnea in an adult is defined as the absence of nasal and oral airflow for at least 10 seconds in duration. It is classified as *central* if respiratory efforts are absent, *obstructive* if cessation of airflow is noted despite the persistence of respiratory effort, or *mixed* apnea if it consists of an initial central apnea followed by an ineffectual respiratory effort consistent with obstructive apnea. The definition of hypopnea is less established; a reduction of airflow or amplitude of thoracoabdominal movement by at least 30% from baseline and accompanied by oxyhemoglobin desaturation of 4% or more for at least 10 seconds in duration is commonly used. Apneas and hypopneas share similar mechanisms and adverse physiologic effects, and they are generally considered together when determining disease severity. Definitions of terms used in the discussion of apneas and hypopneas are given in Table 5–1.

Box 5–1. Abbreviations		
	AHI	apnea hypopnea index
	CPAP	continuous positive airway pressure
	CSA	central sleep apnea
	NREM	non–rapid eye movement
	OSA	obstructive sleep apnea
	PaCO$_2$	partial pressure of arterial carbon dioxide
	PaO$_2$	partial pressure of arterial oxygen
	RDI	respiratory disturbance index
	REM	rapid eye movement
	SaO$_2$	oxygen saturation
	UARS	upper airway resistance syndrome
	UPPP	uvulopalatopharyngoplasty

Table 5–1. Definitions of terms related to sleep-related breathing disorders

Term	Definition
Apnea	Cessation of nasal and oral airflow for a duration of at least 10 seconds. There are three types of apnea, namely central, obstructive and mixed.
Hypopnea	Reduction of airflow or amplitude of thoraco-abdominal movement by at least 30% from baseline, for at least 10 seconds in duration, and accompanied by oxyhemoglobin desaturation of 4% or more
Respiratory event related arousal (RERA)	Reduction in airflow that does not meet the criteria for either apnea or hypopnea and is not associated with significant oxygen desaturation
Obstructive event	Cessation or reduction of airflow that occurs despite the persistence of ventilatory efforts
Central event	Cessation or reduction of airflow that occurs in association with the absence of ventilatory efforts
Mixed event	Cessation or reduction of airflow with an initial central component and a terminal obstructive component
Cheyne-Stokes respiration	Crescendo-decrescendo variability in respiratory rate and tidal volume
Apnea index (AI)	Number of apneas per hour of sleep time
Apnea-hypopnea index (AHI)	Number of apneas *plus* hypopneas per hour of sleep time
Respiratory disturbance index (RDI)	Number of apneas *plus* hypopneas plus RERAs per hour of sleep time

Classification

The severity of OSA can be classified based on the apnea index (AI) or the apnea hypopnea index (AHI) (Table 5–2). Several other factors also influence the clinical severity of OSA, namely the degree of daytime sleepiness and functional impairment, nadir of oxygen saturation (SaO_2), extent of sleep fragmentation, presence of nocturnal arrhythmias related to respiratory events, and presence of comorbid disorders (ischemic heart disease, hypertension, or congestive heart failure [CHF]). Severity of daytime sleepiness appears to correlate better with the extent of sleep fragmentation than with AHI, whereas the degree of arterial oxygen desaturation may be related to the subsequent development of pulmonary artery hypertension.

Table 5-2. Severity of obstructive sleep apnea based on the apnea hyopnea index	Severity	Apnea-hypopnea index (events/hour)
	Mild	5–15
	Moderate	16–30
	Severe	> 30

Demographics

OSA is estimated to affect 24% of males aged 30 to 60 years and 9% of similarly aged females if the disorder is defined by the presence of an AHI of 5 or more, or in 4% of men and 2% of women with an AHI ≥ 5 *plus* complaints of daytime sleepiness. OSA is most prevalent between the fifth and seventh decades. It is more common in men than in women with a ratio of 2–10:1. Prevalence in women increases with menopause. Greater prevalence has also been reported among African Americans, Pacific Islanders, and Mexican-Americans compared to Caucasians. Prevalence increases with aging, with OSA possibly affecting up to 30% to 80% of older adults.

Pathophysiology

The upper airway, from the nares to the larynx, is a flexible collapsible tube that performs various functions in respiration, swallowing, and phonation. An obstructive apnea or hypopnea occurs when the forces that maintain upper airway patency such as activation of dilator muscles (genioglossus, tensor palatini, geniohyoid, and sternohyoid) are insufficient to counteract the factors that promote upper airway closure during sleep (eg, negative intraluminal pressure). The upper airways of patients with OSA tend to be narrower (due to altered anatomical structures, fat accumulation in soft tissues, mucosal swelling or muscle hypertrophy) and are more vulnerable to collapse compared to that among persons without this disorder.

OSA can be considered the extreme end of a spectrum of repetitive upper airway obstruction resulting from reduced activity of the upper airway dilating muscles during sleep that includes, in order of severity, intermittent snoring, continuous snoring, upper airway resistance syndrome, and symptomatic hypopnea/apnea. The diminished tone of the muscles maintaining upper airway patency is part of the generalized muscle hypotonia that occurs during sleep.

The critical closing pressure (P_{crit}) is the pressure at which collapse of the upper airway occurs, and it is less negative among patients with OSA compared to normal persons. The most common sites of upper airway obstruction are the airspaces behind the palate (retropalatal) and behind the tongue (retrolingual).

During sleep, episodes of loud snoring alternate with periods of silence due to marked diminution or total absence of airflow. Blood oxygen saturation may drop during this hypopneic-apneic phase. In addition, respiratory efforts against an occluded upper airway can result in a decrease in intrathoracic pressure, which, in turn, can give rise to reductions in blood pressure and cardiac output. Systemic and pulmonary artery blood pressures then rise as apnea progresses, reaching their peak in the immediate postapneic period. Relative bradycardia may develop during airway obstruction followed by tachycardia during termination of apnea.

After a variable period of time, the apneic episode is terminated by an arousal that manifests as gross body movements, loud grunting, gasping or choking. The brief arousal reestablishes airway patency. Oxygen saturation generally returns to its baseline level with resumption of normal respiration. Sleep then resumes and the cycle repeats itself.

Respiratory events occur more frequently during rapid eye movement (REM) sleep than in NREM sleep. In addition, events occurring during REM sleep tend to be longer in duration and are associated with greater falls in oxygen saturation. Factors determining the severity of oxygen desaturation in sleep apnea are listed in Box 5–2.

Box 5–2. **Factors determining increased severity of oxygen desaturation in sleep apnea**	↓ Baseline awake supine SaO_2 ↓ Baseline sleep SaO_2 ↑ Percentage of sleep time with apnea or hypopnea ↑ Duration of apnea or hypopnea ↓ Duration of ventilation between periods of apnea ↓ Functional residual capacity and expiratory reserve volume Presence of comorbid lung disorders (eg, chronic obstructive pulmonary disease) Stage of sleep (more severe during REM than NREM sleep) Type of apnea (more severe with obstructive than central apneas)

Respiratory events typically recur throughout the evening, at times reaching numbers substantial enough to produce sleep fragmentation and subsequent daytime sleepiness. The severity of excessive daytime sleepiness in individuals with OSA varies from person to person and from one day to another. Naps are unrefreshing; this contrasts with narcolepsy.

Risk Factors

Several risk factors might possibly increase the likelihood of developing OSA. These include a positive family history of the disorder, male gender, increasing age, excess body weight, medical and neurologic disorders, smoking, alcohol and medication use, and specific craniofacial and oropharyngeal characteristics (Table 5–3).

Table 5–3. Risk factors for obstructive sleep apnea

Factor	Description
Genetics	Patients with OSA often have a positive family history of the disorder. Risk of developing OSA is greater among offsprings and first-degree relatives of OSA patients.

Continued

Table 5-3.   Risk factors for obstructive sleep apnea—cont'd

Factor	Description
Gender	Male gender is a risk factor for the occurrence of adult OSA. Among women, menopause increases the predisposition for developing OSA. In contrast, there appears to be no gender difference in OSA prevalence among children. There are several factors that could possibly account for the gender differences in the predisposition for developing OSA, including variations in *distribution of body fat* (peripheral obesity in women and central obesity in men), upper airway anatomy (narrower oropharynx in men), *hormones* (female estrogen and progesterone stimulate respiration and upper airway muscle tone; male androgens inhibit them), and *central ventilatory control systems.*
Age	OSA is relatively more common in childhood (ages 3 to 5 years) than during adolescence and early adulthood. Prevalence progressively increases in middle-aged individuals until the sixth and seventh decade of life Although the risk of developing OSA increases with aging, no specific age-related anatomic or functional factors primarily account for this increased risk.
Race	Prevalence may be higher among African -Americans, Mexican -Americans and Pacific Islanders compared with Caucasians.
Anatomic features	Certain craniofacial and cervical anatomic features increase the risk of developing OSA. These include: 1. Increasing neck circumference (> 17 inches in men and > 16 inches in women) is correlated with greater apnea hypopnea indices (however, not independent of body mass index [BMI]) 2. Nasal features (nasal narrowing, deviated septum, polyps, prominent turbinates, or chronic congestion) 3. Lingual features (macroglossia or posteriorly displaced tongue) 4. Palatal features (large broad uvula, low-lying soft palate) 5. Enlarged tonsils and adenoids (especially in children) 6. Restricted oropharyngeal size (generally narrowest at the level of the velopharynx), especially its lateral dimensions 7. Maxillomandibular features (midface hypoplasia, retrognathia, micrognathia, or mandibular hypoplasia) 8. Hereditary syndromes (Down, Pierre-Robin sequence, achondroplasia, Crouzon, Apert, Treacher-Collin, and Cornelia De Lange)
Excess body weight	Excess body weight (overweight defined as a BMI $\geq$ 25 kg/m^2 and obese as BMI $\geq$ 30–40 kg/m^2) is a major risk factor for OSA. The prevalence of OSA increases with greater excess body weight and is especially high among morbidly obese persons. Other factors influencing the risk of OSA include fat skin-fold thickness, intra-abdominal fat, and percentage of body fat. Excess body weight may be particularly important in persons without any apparent craniofacial or oropharyngeal features that would predispose them to developing OSA. Distribution of fat is important because central or nuchal obesity (increased waist-hip ratio and neck circumference) appears to correlate better with OSA severity than obesity in general (ie, body weight). The apnea hypopnea index is correlated with leptin levels. Excess body weight can contribute to the development of OSA either by fatty deposition in the upper airways leading to reduced airway size and decreased muscle tone, or by reducing lung volumes, which, in turn, decreases upper airway size. Aside from obesity, increased fat deposition in the upper airways can be seen in patients with acromegaly or myxedema.

Table 5-3. Risk factors for obstructive sleep apnea—cont'd

Factor	Description
Endocrinologic disorders	Untreated hypothyroidism (myxedema) can precipitate or exacerbate existing OSA, possibly secondary to upper airway narrowing, macroglossia (due to deposits of mucoproteins), upper airway myopathy, or impairment of ventilatory control systems. (Note: Routine screening for hypothyroidism in patients presenting with OSA is not warranted unless other clinical features suggestive of hypothyroidism are present.) Acromegaly is also associated with a greater risk of OSA.
Neurologic disorders	OSA and central sleep apnea (CSA) may develop following strokes. OSA has also been described in association with several neuromuscular conditions, such as Duchene muscular dystrophy, myotonic dystrophy, postpolio syndrome, neuropathies, and myopathies.
Smoking	Smoking can induce edema in the upper airways and increases risk for the development of OSA.
Alcohol use	Ingestion of alcohol close to bedtime can aggravate OSA. Alcohol inhibits the activity of the upper airway muscles and increases airway collapsibility. In addition, it can diminish arousal responses to airway obstruction, prolong apnea duration, and worsen oxygen desaturation.
Medication use	Several medications, including muscle relaxants, sedative -hypnotics (benzodiazepines and barbiturates), narcotics, and anesthetics can induce OSA by reducing upper airway dilator muscle tone. Some studies, but not all, have demonstrated that administration of benzodiazepines is associated with an increase in the frequency and duration of apneas as well as greater nocturnal oxygen desaturation. Morphine, an opioid analgesic, can depress ventilatory drive and give rise to obstructive and central apneas. Neither zolpidem, zaleplon nor eszopiclone, nonbenzodiazepine benzodiazepine receptor agonist hypnotic agents used for the treatment of insomnia, appear to significantly affect the AHI.
Nasal congestion	Nasal congestion, due to allergic or nonallergic chronic rhinitis, can worsen snoring and OSA.
Miscellaneous conditions	Amyloidosis

Upper Airway Anatomic Abnormalities Associated With Obstructive Sleep Apnea

Anatomic abnormalities of the upper airway, from the nose to the vocal cords, may predispose to the development of OSA (Table 5–4). This region becomes more collapsible during sleep due to the relative lack of bony or cartilaginous supporting structures.

Table 5-4. Upper airway anatomic abnormalities that can cause obstructive sleep apnea

Anatomic abnormality	Characteristics
Choanal atresia	Congenital absence of the posterior nasal passages may be unilateral or bilateral. It can present with (1) feeding difficulty at birth (bilateral atresia) or with (2) recurrent sinusitis or rhinorrhea (unilateral atresia). It may be associated with other congenital abnormalities, particularly in patients with bilateral disease. Surgical correction is required in most cases.

Table 5–4.   Upper airway anatomic abnormalities that can cause obstructive sleep apnea—cont'd

Anatomic abnormality	Characteristics
Nasal obstruction	Nasal obstruction increases the likelihood of snoring or obstructive sleep apnea. Causes include adenoid hypertrophy (in young children), nasal septal deviation, nasal polyps, antrochoanal polyps and enlarged turbinates. In addition, oral breathing due to nasal obstruction in children may result in alterations of the craniofacial structures during development. Efficacy of surgery to correct nasal obstruction appears higher among children with OSA than in adults; success rates may be especially limited in adults with craniofacial abnormalities or severe obesity.
Laryngomalacia	In this condition, there is a lack of cartilaginous or muscular support of the larynx; it can be congenital or acquired. Laryngomalacia typically presents with stridor and, if severe, dyspnea, cyanosis, and difficulties with feeding.
Tracheal stenosis	Cases of obstructive and central apneas due to tracheal stenosis have been described.

Genetic Syndromes Associated With Obstructive Sleep Apnea

Craniofacial anomalies (eg, enlarged tongue, or maxillary or mandibular hypoplasia) may compromise upper airway patency and cause OSA in children and adults. Critical upper airway compromise may arise during the newborn period in some infants with craniofacial syndromes,

Several mechanisms may be responsible for the development of OSA. These include (1) abnormal bony structures, (2) overgrowth of soft tissues, or (3) impaired neuromuscular control of the upper airways. More than one mechanism may be responsible for upper airway narrowing in some patients, and there may be more than one specific site of obstruction. Furthermore, the degree of craniofacial disfigurement may not correlate with the severity of OSA.

Maxillary Hypoplasia

The syndromic craniosynostoses (eg, Apert syndrome, Crouzon syndrome, and Pfeiffer syndrome), Stickler syndrome, Antley-Bixler syndrome, and Down syndrome are associated with maxillary (midface) hypoplasia. The syndromic craniosynostoses arise as a result of mutations in fibroblast growth factor receptor (FGFR) genes that inhibit the anterior-posterior growth of the cranium. Individuals typically possess a facial profile that is either flattened or scaphoid in shape. Midfacial hypoplasia displaces the palate posteriorly closer to the posterior wall of the nasopharynx. Syndromes associated with maxillary hypoplasia are described in Table 5–5.

Table 5–5.   Syndromes associated with maxillary hypoplasia

Syndrome	Characteristics
Antley-Bixler syndrome	This disorder is characterized by craniosynostosis, frontal bossing, midfacial hypoplasia, choanal atresia or stenosis, and depression of the nasal bridge. Periods of apnea may occur. Most cases are sporadic but some present as an autosomal recessive disorder.
Apert syndrome (acrocephalosyndactyly type I)	A small nose and large jaw develop secondary to premature fusion of the cranial bones. Upper airway abnormalities can give rise to OSA. Breathing difficulties may develop early in life but resolve by 3 to 4 months with growth of the nasal passages. Most cases appear to arise as fresh mutations but some cases are inherited in an autosomal dominant pattern. Both genders can be affected.

Table 5-5.   Syndromes associated with maxillary hypoplasia—cont'd

Syndrome	Characteristics
Crouzon syndrome	Abnormally early fusion of the cranial bones leads to a small head. Additional features include a small jaw, nasal septal deviation, exophthalmos, short upper lip, and, in some cases, a cleft palate. OSA can develop secondary to upper airway obstruction occurring as a result of choanal stenosis, maxillary hypoplasia, posterior displacement of the tongue, and lengthened soft palate. It can either be inherited as an autosomal dominant disorder or arise as a new mutation. Both genders can be affected.
Down syndrome (trisomy 21)	Characteristic craniofacial features include a small head, maxillary hypoplasia, a small nose, an enlarged tongue, and a short neck, all of which increase the risk of developing OSA. In addition, patients may develop central apneas, hypoventilation and hypoxemia. It is caused in most cases by an extra chromosome at the 21 position. Incidence increases with advanced maternal age. Both genders can be affected.
Pfeiffer syndrome (acrocephalosyndactyly type V)	OSA may develop due to abnormalities of the upper airway, specifically involving the pharyngeal area, or secondary to a tracheal cartilaginous sleeve (a congenital cartilage malformation).
Stickler syndrome	This is an autosomal dominant connective tissue disorder with ophthalmologic and nonophthalmologic features. *Ophthalmologic features* include cataracts, glaucoma, myopia, retinal detachment, and vitreoretinal degeneration. *Nonophthalmologic features* consist of cleft palate, dysplastic bony abnormalities, and midfacial hypoplasia.
Cleft palate repair	A cleft palate is often accompanied by significant narrowing of the anterior-posterior dimension of the pharynx, a lower hyoid position, and a longer uvula. Clinically significant OSA can develop following repair of cleft palates using flap pharyngoplasty, sphincter pharyngoplasty, or velopharyngeal ring ligation procedure. OSA can occur in the immediate postoperative period, and may, in some cases, resolve spontaneously within several months.

Mandibular Hypoplasia

OSA can develop as a result of posterior displacement of the base of the tongue closer to the posterior pharynx. Associated symptoms are described in Table 5–6.

Table 5-6.   Syndromes associated with mandibular hypoplasia

Syndrome	Characteristics
Goldenhar syndrome	This syndrome is characterized by vertebral abnormalities, dermal cysts, and auricular malformations. Abnormalities of the upper airway can lead to upper airway obstruction. It can either be inherited as an autosomal dominant or recessive disorder, or it may occur sporadically. Males are affected more commonly than women.

Continued

Table 5-6. Syndromes associated with mandibular hypoplasia—cont'd

Syndrome	Characteristics
Pierre-Robin syndrome	Features of this syndrome include a small jaw, retropositioned tongue and soft palate, displacement of the larynx, and, in some cases, a cleft palate. Mandibular hypoplasia in utero displaces the tongue posteriorly, which, in turn, impairs the midline closure of the palate. Breathing difficulties that develop in the early days of life improve significantly during the first 2 years, with growth of the lower jaw in relation to the cranial dimensions. Persistent micrognathia can increase the risk of snoring and OSA in later life, and serial polysomnography is recommended.
Treacher Collins syndrome	This syndrome is characterized by an underdeveloped mandible, receding chin, malar hypoplasia and cleft palate. Other features include an antimongoloid palpebral fissure slant, eyelid coloboma, ear deformities, and conductive hearing loss. It is inherited as an autosomal dominant disorder and is caused by mutations in the TCOF1 gene coding for the Treacle protein. Resolution of OSA by mandibular advancement surgery has been described.

Tongue Enlargement

Features of Beckwith-Wiedemann syndrome include unusually large tongues, small noses, umbilical abnormalities (eg, hernia or omphalocele), and renal/adrenal tumors. It can affect both genders. Macroglossia is also present in Hunter syndrome.

Mucopolysaccharidosis

Hurler (mucopolysaccharidosis type I) and Hunter (mucopolysaccharidosis type II) syndromes are characterized by the accumulation of glycosaminoglycans in various tissues and organs of the body. Clinical features of Hurler syndrome, an autosomal recessive disorder, include dwarfism, mental retardation, and increased urinary levels of chondroitin sulfate B and heparin sulfate. Patients with Hunter syndrome, a rare X-linked recessive disorder, can have skeletal abnormalities, hepatosplenomegaly, macroglossia, adenotonsillar hypertrophy, tracheomalacia, and a high arched palate. Both conditions can present with OSA due to glycosaminoglycan deposition in the upper airways.

Evaluation and Management of Upper Airway Anatomic Abnormalities

Routine screening for OSA is recommended for patients with craniofacial syndromes. Periodic reassessment is important because growth-related alterations in craniofacial structures may significantly affect upper airway anatomy and function.

Patients with craniofacial syndromes may require more extensive evaluation. After the presence of OSA has been established by polysomnography, additional studies may be required to assess the anatomic site/s of upper airway obstruction. Imaging studies include lateral cephalometric views, computed tomography, or magnetic resonance imaging to visualize both key skeletal structures and soft tissues such as tonsils and adenoids, and their relationships to each other. Nasendoscopy enables visualization of the site(s) of upper airway obstruction. Interventions may involve staged ortho-dontic and surgical procedures. Continuous positive airway pressure (CPAP) therapy or, in severe cases, tracheostomy may be required prior to, or between specific surgical procedures.

Clinical Features of Obstructive Sleep Apnea

Clinical manifestations that should alert the clinician to the possibility of OSA include complaints of daytime sleepiness, snoring, accounts of witnessed apneas, repeated awakenings with gasping or choking, nighttime diaphoresis, morning headaches, nocturia, and alterations in mood. Daytime sleepiness is the most common complaint; however, the absence of daytime sleepiness does not exclude the presence of this disorder. See Table 5–7 for more information.

Common physical findings include excess body weight, nasal septal deviation or turbinate hypertrophy, enlarged tonsils and adenoids, narrow oropharynx, macroglossia, retro- or micrognathia, and a large neck circumference. Nevertheless, physical examination may be entirely unremarkable.

Table 5–7. Manifestations of obstructive sleep apnea

Clinical features	Associated features	Physical features
Attention deficit (in children)	Cardiac arrhythmias	Crowded posterior pharyngeal space
Awakenings with a sensation of gasping or choking	Congestive heart failure	Dental malocclusion
Behavioral disorders	Ischemic heart disease	Enlarged tonsils and adenoids; prominent tonsillar pillars (especially among children)
Changes in mood (eg, depression) or personality	Nocturnal seizures	High, narrow hard palate
Daytime sleepiness or fatigue	Parasomnias (eg, confusional arousals, sleep-related eating disorder)	Large neck circumference
Decline in performance at work or school	Pulmonary hypertension and cor pulmonale (severe disease)	Large uvula
Dry mouth/throat sensation on awakening	Systemic hypertension	Low-lying soft palate
Excessive body movements during sleep	Type 2 diabetes mellitus	Lower extremity edema
Gastroesophageal reflux		Macroglossia
Hearing impairment		Narrow oropharynx (maxilla and mandible)
Hyperactivity (in children)		Nasal septal deviation
Impaired cognition (memory and concentration)		Nasal turbinate hypertrophy
Impotence or diminished libido		Obesity (body mass index > 25)
Insomnia		Retro- or micrognathia
Morning headaches		
Mouth breathing (in children)		
Nocturia or enuresis		
Nocturnal diaphoresis		Note: Physical examination may be normal.
Nonrestorative or unrefreshing sleep or naps		
"Restless" sleep with frequent movements		
Snoring		
Witnessed apneas, gasping, or choking		

Consequences

OSA has been associated with greater mortality as well as significant adverse cardiovascular, gastrointestinal, genitourinary, endocrine, psychiatric, and social consequences (Table 5–8). OSA, by impairing vigilance and alertness, increases driving and work-related accident rates, and has a negative impact on neurocognitive function and performance.

Table 5–8. Consequences of obstructive sleep apnea

Physiologic effects	Decrease in SaO_2 and PaO_2 Severity of oxygen desaturation is dependent on baseline oxygen saturation prior to the apnea, lung volume, and duration of apnea; thus, oxygen desaturation is more severe with lower baseline oxygen levels, lesser lung volumes and longer apneic episodes. Increase in $PaCO_2$ Increase in systemic and pulmonary artery pressure Decrease in left and right ventricular output Increased vascular resistance secondary to heightened sympathetic nervous system activity
Sleep	Disturbances in sleep continuity, consolidation, and architecture Arousal occurs at the termination of the apneic-hypopneic event
Mortality	Increase in mortality among young and middle-age adults In one retrospective study, increased mortality at 8 years was noted in untreated male patients with AI > 20 compared to those with AI < 20; this normalized with therapy using CPAP or tracheostomy but not with uvulopalatopharyngoplasty.
Cardiovascular	<u>Systemic hypertension (independent of obesity)</u> Increased risk of hypertension associated with greater frequency of apneic episodes and nocturnal oxygen desaturation. In one study, each additional apneic event per hour of sleep increased the odds of hypertension by about 1%, whereas each 10% decrease in nocturnal oxygen saturation increased the odds by 13%. Conversely, prevalence of OSA is increased in patients with hypertension (about 30%). Respirstory disturbance index is a predictor of systolic and diastolic blood pressure after adjustment for gender, age and body mass index. Systemic blood pressure normally falls during NREM sleep ("dipping"). Many patients with OSA may fail to demonstrate this sleep-related fall in blood pressure ("nondipping") Blood pressure increases following termination of apneas or hypopneas possibly secondary to arousals and accompanying increases in sympathetic activity. Other factors that could possibly contribute to hypertension include intermittent hypoxemia and negative intrathoracic pressure swings. Treatment of OSA may result in a decrease in blood pressure and improved hypertension control. <u>Pulmonary hypertension and cor pulmonale</u> These are seen particularly in severe OSA, especially in patients with daytime hypoxemia and hypercapnia due to concurrent chronic obstructive pulmonary disease ("overlap" syndrome) or morbid obesity (obesity-hypoventilation syndrome) OSA, by itself, may not be sufficient for the development of significant pulmonary hypertension. <u>Coronary artery disease (CAD)</u> The increased risk of CAD in patients with OSA may be related to endothelial dysfunction and accelerated atherosclerosis. Nocturnal ischemia in patients with CAD and OSA may be due to increased sympathetic activity, arousal-related tachycardia, and increased left ventricular afterload, and it may improve with therapy for OSA. <u>Congestive heart failure (CHF)</u> The relationship between OSA and CHF appears bidirectional Prevalence of OSA is increased in patients with moderate to severe CHF and asymptomatic left ventricular dysfunction.

Table 5–8. Consequences of obstructive sleep apnea—cont'd

	There are two possible mechanisms by which OSA can give rise to CHF: 1. Increase in left ventricular afterload due to greater peripheral resistance (hypertension) and more negative intrathoracic pressure (inspiration against a closed airway) 2. Sympathetic nervous system activation by hypoxemia and repeated arousals during sleep Cardiac arrhythmias Includes sinus arrhythmia [most common], bradycardia, sinus pauses, sinus arrest, premature ventricular contractions, ventricular tachycardia, and atrioventricular block Higher recurrence rate of atrial fibrillation after successful cardioversion Cerebrovascular disease OSA can increase the risk for strokes and vice versa. Increase in stroke risk is due to several factors, including impaired cerebral vascular autoregulation, decrease in cerebral blood flow, hypertension, endothelial dysfunction, enhanced thrombogenesis, and accelerated atherosclerosis Patients with OSA have higher carotid artery intimamedia thickness values. OSA may adversely affect prognosis and survival following strokes.
Neurocognitive and psychiatric/behavioral	Excessive daytime sleepiness Present in a majority of patients Secondary to sleep fragmentation Poor correlation between apnea indices and objective (Multiple Sleep Latency Test) and subjective (Epworth Sleepiness Scale) measures of sleepiness Sleepiness improves with therapy of OSA. Depression Anxiety "Irritable" mood Changes in personality Diminished quality of life Decreased alertness Impairment of cognitive performance Deterioration of learning and memory Possibly due to chronic sleep deprivation or recurrent nocturnal hypoxemia
Gastrointestinal	Gastroesophageal reflux Secondary to significant negative intrathoracic pressures prior to resumption of breathing at the termination of apnea
Genitourinary	Nocturia Erectile dysfunction Decreased libido Poor sexual function
Endocrine/metabolism	Insulin resistance
Social	Negative impact on academic and occupational performance Social withdrawal Increased risk of accidents (due to decreased alertness and impaired neurocognitive function) Increased marital difficulties

Evaluation

Clinical History

Clinical features that suggest the diagnosis of OSA include obesity, habitual snoring, reports of apneas, hypertension, and a large neck circumference. Questionnaires, such as the Berlin Questionnaire, may be useful in helping identify patients with OSA. For information about the differential diagnosis of OSA, see Table 5–9.

Table 5-9. Differential diagnosis of obstructive sleep apnea

Sleepiness	Nighttime awakenings	Nocturnal oxygen desaturation
Insufficient sleep	Laryngospasm	Chronic obstructive pulmonary
Narcolepsy	Stridor	disease
Idiopathic hypersomnia	Panic disorder	Nocturnal asthma
Periodic limb movement	Parasomnias	Central sleep apnea
disorder	Gastroesophageal reflux	Alveolar hypoventilation syndromes
Medication use or withdrawal	Nocturnal asthma	Congestive heart failure
	Chronic obstructive pulmonary disease	
	Congestive heart failure (paroxysmal nocturnal dyspnea or orthopnea)	

Polysomnography

Because clinical and physical examination features are neither sufficiently sensitive nor specific, a polysomnography (PSG) is required for the diagnosis of OSA. Recordings should ideally include sleep in all sleep stages and in all sleep positions, and should be at least 6 hours in duration. Polysomnographic features of OSA are listed in Box 5–3.

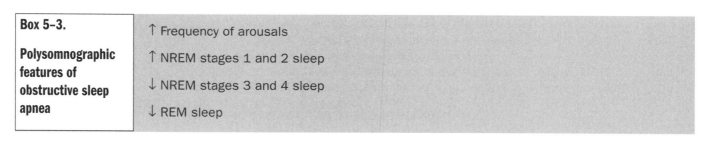

Box 5-3. **Polysomnographic features of obstructive sleep apnea**	↑ Frequency of arousals
	↑ NREM stages 1 and 2 sleep
	↓ NREM stages 3 and 4 sleep
	↓ REM sleep

Respiratory events consist of cessation or reduction of airflow despite ongoing respiratory efforts. These events are accompanied by oxygen desaturation (with the decline in oxygen saturation [SaO_2] starting shortly after the onset of apnea or hypopnea and reaching a nadir about 6 to 8 seconds following the termination of the event, usually when normal respiration resumes), and arrhythmias (bradyarrhythmia or tachyarrhythmia) (Box 5–4). Apneas and hypopneas terminate with a brief electroencephalographic (EEG) arousal (often with a burst of chin electromyographic [EMG] activity). Respiratory events typically are more frequent, last longer, and are associated with more profound oxygen desaturation during REM sleep.

Paradoxical breathing or "out-of-phase" motion of the rib cage and abdomen suggesting the presence of increased upper airway resistance can be observed during apneic episodes. This phenomenon is due to downward displacement of the diaphragm occurring simultaneously with occlusion of the upper airway that (1) creates negative intrapleural pressures causing retraction of the thoracic cage and (2) positive intraabdominal pressure pushing the abdominal wall outward.

Box 5–4.	Brady-tachycardia
Cardiac arrhythmias related to obstructive sleep apnea	Relative bradycardia at the onset of apnea
	Relative tachycardia during arousals following apnea termination
	Heart rate remains between 60 and 100 beats per minute in many patients
	Heart blocks (second– and third–degree)
	Premature ventricular complexes

Esophageal manometry demonstrates large inspiratory and expiratory pressure swings. Using esophageal pressure or nasal pressure monitoring, two patterns of increased respiratory effort have been described, namely *crescendo* (progressive increase), or *persistent* (sustained increase), that occur prior to the reversal that accompanies arousals.

Pulse transit time (PTT) is the time it takes the arterial pulse pressure wave to travel from the aortic valve to the periphery. PTT increases during the OSA-related inspiratory fall in blood pressure and decreases during the arousal-related rise in blood pressure. PTT is useful to distinguish obstructive from central respiratory events.

The current standard of practice in the United States is an attended laboratory PSG with technologist-attended positive airway pressure titration using either a full- or split-night protocol. Split-night studies consist of an initial diagnostic portion and a subsequent CPAP titration on the same night.

Multiple Sleep Latency Test

The Multiple Sleep Latency Test (MSLT) is useful in assessing the presence and degree of sleepiness. It may be indicated in patients with OSA whose sleepiness persists despite optimal CPAP therapy.

Imaging Studies

Imaging studies, including lateral cephalometric views, computed tomography, or magnetic resonance imaging of the upper airways, might be required for patients with craniofacial syndromes or for those in whom surgical therapy is being considered.

Laboratory Tests

Thyroid function tests may be helpful in patients with a clinical history suggestive of hypothyroidism.

Rapid Eye Movement Sleep–Associated Obstructive Sleep Apnea

In some patients, OSA occurs primarily or exclusively during REM sleep. For more information, see Box 5–5. There are no generally accepted guidelines regarding the therapy of patients with REM sleep–associated OSA with normal overall AHI. Some clinicians have opted to treat such patients, especially if they had presented with complaints of excessive sleepiness.

Therapy

The goals of therapy for OSA include improving sleep quality, relieving daytime symptoms such as excessive sleepiness, enhancing quality of life, and preventing long-term neurocognitive and cardiovascular consequences of untreated or partially treated sleep apnea. A variety of therapies for OSA have been described (Table 5–10). These include general measures such as avoidance of alcohol and muscle relaxants, weight reduction for patients who are overweight, positional therapy for those whose apnea occurs exclusively or predominantly during a supine sleep position, oxygen supplementation if concurrent hypoxemia is present and persists despite optimal positive airway pressure therapy, pharmacotherapy, positive airway pressure therapy, oral devices, and upper airway surgery.

Box 5-5. **Effect of rapid eye movement sleep on sleep-related breathing disorders**	Decrease in upper airway dilating muscle activity (especially during phasic REM sleep)
	Decrease in lung volumes (eg, end expiratory lung volume, and functional residual capacity)
	Decrease in hypoxic and hypercapnic ventilatory drive
	Longer duration of apneic and hypopneic events
	More severe oxygen desaturation related to obstructive respiratory events

General Measures

Certain drugs known to either induce or worsen obstructive apneic events are best avoided in patients with OSA. Patients should be advised to refrain from using alcohol, benzodiazepines, narcotic agents, sedatives, and muscle relaxants that might decrease the activity of the upper airway dilating muscles and, thus, worsen sleep-related breathing disorders. Smoking should be avoided.

Sleep deprivation may prolong apnea duration and increase arousal threshold. Issues regarding sleep hygiene (including obtaining an adequate amount of sleep each night and maintaining a regular bedtime and waking time each day) as well as safety, with counseling to not operate motor vehicles or engage in other potentially dangerous activities unless fully alert, should be discussed with the patient. See Box 5–6 for more information.

Table 5-10. Treatment of obstructive sleep apnea

Therapy	Comments
General measures	Avoidance of alcohol, muscle relaxants and sedative agents Correction of precipitating factors (eg, hypothyroidism) Smoking cessation
Weight reduction	Reduction of dietary caloric consumption Increase in physical activity Bariatric surgery for morbid obesity
Positional therapy	Avoidance of a supine sleep position, and promotion of a lateral or upright sleep position
Oxygen therapy	Low-level supplemental oxygen
Pharmacotherapy	Selective serotonin reuptake inhibitors Medroxyprogesterone Nasal decongestants
Positive airway pressure	Continuous positive airway pressure Bi-level positive airway pressure Automated positive airway pressure Noninvasive nighttime ventilation

Table 5-10. Treatment of obstructive sleep apnea—cont'd

Therapy	Comments
Oral devices	Mandibular advancers Tongue retainers
Upper airway surgery	Nasal surgery Uvulopalatopharyngoplasty Genioglossal advancement Maxillomandibular advancement Tracheostomy

Box 5-6. **Sleep hygiene measures for patients with obstructive sleep apnea**	Avoidance of alcohol, sedatives, narcotics, and other central nervous system suppressants that can decrease upper airway muscle tone Cessation of smoking that can cause airway mucosal irritation and congestion Avoidance of sleep deprivation

In certain situations, it is reasonable to report patients with excessive sleepiness due to OSA to appropriate authorities, particularly if there had been prior episodes of vehicular accidents related to excessive sleepiness, if expeditious therapy for OSA cannot be provided, if the patient refuses therapy for his or her OSA, if the patient fails to restrict driving until his or her OSA has been adequately controlled, and if such conditions are considered reportable based on local legislation.

Weight Reduction

Factors related to obesity that enhance the risk of developing OSA include an increase in upper airway collapsibility (less negative pharyngeal critical closing pressure), fatty tissue deposition in the cervical area, dysfunction of the upper airway dilating muscles, and decrease in lung volumes (Box 5–7). All obese patients with OSA should be encouraged to lose weight, either by changes in lifestyle, dietary modifications (eg, low caloric diets) or, in selected individuals with morbid obesity, surgical procedures (eg, gastric stapling or bypass) to aid with weight reduction. Weight loss can be combined with other therapeutic approaches such as avoidance of supine sleep or CPAP therapy.

Weight loss, even of modest proportions (eg, 5% to 10% of baseline weight) can result in improvements in sleep apnea indices (Box 5–8). However, weight loss alone, is often insufficient to reverse sleep-related breathing disorders in patients with OSA related to morbid obesity or an abnormal upper airway anatomy. The magnitude of weight reduction that can improve sleep apnea varies across patients; apparently, a critical level of weight reduction in each individual must be

Box 5-7. **Mechanisms by which obesity may cause obstructive sleep apnea**	Reduction of upper airway caliber due to fat deposition Alteration of upper airway compliance (increase in collapsibility) due to changes in muscle tone Decrease in lung residual volume

<table>
<tr><td>

Box 5–8.

Effects of weight reduction in patients with obstructive sleep apnea

</td><td>

Upper airway and lung parameters

  ↓ Adipose tissue in the upper airways

  ↑ Airway caliber

  ↓ Airway collapsibility (more negative upper airway critical closing pressure)

  ↑ Oxygen saturation

  ↑ Vital capacity, functional residual capacity, and residual volume

  ↓ Respiratory work of breathing

Sleep parameters

  ↑ Sleep quality

  ↑ Sleep efficiency

  ↑ Total sleep time

  ↓ Frequency of arousals

Neurocognitive parameters

  ↓ Subjective daytime sleepiness

  ↑ Measures of mood

  ↑ Quality of life

Sleep-related breathing disorder parameters

  ↓ Apnea-hypopnea index

  ↓ Snoring

  Decrease in level of CPAP required to treat OSA

Cardiovascular parameters

  ↓ Resting systolic and diastolic blood pressures

  Enhanced blood pressure control

</td></tr>
</table>

Long-term benefits remain uncertain.

achieved before a significant reduction in AHI occurs. In one study, a 3% change in AHI was associated with each percent change in weight. However, the amount of weight loss often fails to correlate with the extent of improvement in sleep apnea in an individual. The timing of a repeat PSG should be individualized but is generally recommended following weight loss of about 20 to 50 lbs.

Optimal weight can be difficult to maintain, and many persons regain weight after initially losing it with recurrence or worsening of their OSA. OSA may also recur despite maintenance of weight loss.

Positional Therapy

Positional sleep apnea has been defined as OSA in which the supine sleep-related AHI is at least twice that of sleep in a non-supine (eg, lateral recumbency) position. Patients with positional sleep apnea have a greater likelihood of being less overweight and of having lower AHIs compared with patients whose apnea is present in all sleep positions. In many patients with OSA, the upper airway is most vulnerable to collapse during supine sleep. Due to the effects of gravity, the tongue tends to be displaced closer to the posterior pharynx. There is, thus, greater reduction of the pharyngeal area in a supine than an upright position.

In selected patients in whom respiratory events occur exclusively or predominantly during a supine sleep position and if PSG demonstrates a normal AHI in the lateral posture, elevation of the head or restricting sleep to lateral recumbency might be tried. Techniques available for positional therapy include:

1. Placing three to four tennis balls in a pocket sewn on the back of a well-fitted pajama top

2. Pinning a sock filled with tennis balls to the back of a sleep garment

3. Sleeping with a Styrofoam-filled backpack

4. Using a posture alarm that is triggered whenever a person remains in a supine position

5. Elevating the head and trunk at a 30–60 degree angle.

Sleep position training alone may be sufficient for patients with OSA who's AHI is normal during lateral recumbency sleep. For more information about the effects of this therapy in patients with OSA, see Box 5–9. However, long-term adherence to, and enduring efficacy of, sleep position training are not well established. Patients whose OSA is not position dependent do not generally benefit from this kind of intervention.

Box 5–9. **Effects of sleep-position therapy in patients with obstructive sleep apnea**	Sleep parameters ↑ Sleep quality ↓ Frequency of arousals Neurocognitive parameters ↓ Daytime sleepiness ↑ Neurocognitive performance Sleep-related breathing disorder parameters ↓ Apnea-hypopnea index

Cervical Positional Therapy

The efficacy of head extension using a cervical pillow appears to be limited to patients with mild OSA (respiratory disturbance indices between 5 and 20 per hour).

Oxygen Therapy

The role of oxygen therapy in the treatment of OSA is not clearly established. Although oxygen supplementation can decrease central and mixed apneas, it does not control OSA. Oxygen supplementation can potentially improve nocturnal oxygen saturation but at the risk of possibly increasing apnea duration. Patients with the *overlap syndrome* (OSA plus chronic obstructive pulmonary disease) may develop worsening hypercapnia during oxygen therapy. In addition, because the definition of a hypopnea often includes a measured reduction in oxygen saturation, administration of oxygen during PSG can minimize oxygen desaturation related to respiratory events and thus decrease the frequency of recorded hypopneas.

Oxygen supplementation may be considered for patients with marked nocturnal oxygen desaturation that is not controlled by CPAP therapy alone. However, there is no general consensus regarding the level of nocturnal oxygen desaturation that would benefit from oxygen therapy.

Nasal Dilators

Nasal passage dilators can decrease nasal resistance due to congestion or mechanical obstruction that can produce upper airway obstruction during sleep. Such devices, including external nasal strips and intranasally-applied dilators, can reduce snoring but are generally not sufficiently effective, when used alone, to reverse OSA.

Pharyngeal Muscle Stimulation

Direct hypoglossal nerve or genioglossal muscle electrical stimulation by augmenting muscle tone and lowering upper airway P_{crit} can stabilize the upper airway and decrease upper airway narrowing. However, this approach does not generally eliminate OSA and is still experimental. Possible adverse effects include nerve injury and bradycardia.

Pharmacologic Treatment

Several medications, including acetazolamide, medroxyprogesterone, serotonin-active agents, and modafinil, have been investigated for the therapy of OSA (Table 5–11). Mechanisms whereby these pharmacologic agents might improve sleep-related breathing disorders include enhancement of upper airway muscle tone during sleep, increase in ventilatory drive, reduction of REM sleep during which the frequency and duration of apneas and hypopneas tend to be greater, and alleviation of excessive sleepiness that occurs as a consequence of sleep fragmentation. OSA associated with endocrinologic conditions (eg, hypothyroidism) might improve with resolution of the underlying disorder with hormone replacement therapy.

Published studies commonly include small sample sizes and are often not controlled. To date, no pharmacologic agent is entirely effective in treating OSA. The recommendations of the American Academy of Sleep Medicine (AASM) for the pharmacologic therapy of OSA are listed in Box 5–10.

Table 5–11. Medications that have been used for treating obstructive sleep apnea

Agent	Effect on apnea
Acetazolamide	A carbonic anhydrase inhibitor, which acts by increasing urinary excretion of bicarbonate and sodium, produces metabolic acidosis and a compensatory increase in respiratory drive. It has been suggested that acetazolamide might have a beneficial effect in mild cases of OSA through an augmentation of central ventilatory drive and a stabilizing effect on ventilatory control. Studies have demonstrated that acetazolamide reduces apnea/hypopnea frequency, decreases frequency of oxygen desaturation, improves sleep architecture, and decreases clinical symptoms in patients with OSA.
Almitrine	A respiratory stimulant that acts by sensitizing peripheral chemoreceptors in the carotid body. It also improves gas exchange by enhancing hypoxic pulmonary vasoconstriction. One study reported that almitrine failed to reduce the number of respiratory events in patients with OSA. However, there was a reduction in mean duration of respiratory events during NREM sleep.
Bromocriptine	A direct-acting dopamine agonist, bromocriptine improved sleep apnea in a patient with long-standing acromegaly complicated by OSA. However, in another study, bromocriptine produced no significant beneficial effects on the number and duration of apneas and hypopneas, or oxygen desaturation in patients with OSA.
Caffeine	A stimulant that has been used in the treatment of apneas in premature infants. Caffeine decreased apnea frequency in one infant with Arnold-Chiari malformation and severe apnea.
Cannabinoids	Cannabinoid receptor agonist that can inhibit excitatory effects of serotonin, and, like other serotonin antagonists, might reduce sleep-related breathing disorders. Intraperitoneal injection of delta-9-tetrahydrocannabinol decreases apnea index during NREM and REM sleep in Sprague-Dawley rats.
Chlorimipramine	A tricyclic antidepressant, chlorimipramine has not been shown to be effective in the treatment of patients with OSA.
Cilazapril	A long-acting angiotensin-converting enzyme inhibitor, cilatapril has been shown to decrease apnea and hypopnea indices in patients with OSA and hypertension. Cilazapril lowers respiratory disturbance index and apnea index during NREM sleep but not during REM sleep.
Clonidine	A centrally-acting alpha 2-adrenergic agonist antihypertensive agent with REM-suppressant activity, clonidine decreases or totally suppresses REM sleep and improves nocturnal hypoxemia. It has no effect on the frequency and duration of NREM breathing abnormalities.
Domperidone	A selective dopamine D2-receptor antagonist, domperidone enhances hypercapnic ventilatory response and peripheral chemosensitivity in patients with OSA.
Doxapram	A respiratory stimulant, doxapram improves oxygen saturation during apneic/hypopneic episodes and decreases average apnea length. However it does not decrease the number of disordered breathing events during sleep.

Continued

Table 5–11. Medications that have been used for treating obstructive sleep apnea—cont'd

Agent	Effect on apnea
Fluoxetine	A serotonin-receptor uptake inhibitor, fluoxetine has been shown to decrease percentage of REM sleep time and the number of apneas or hypopneas during NREM sleep.
Imipramine	A tricyclic antidepressant, imipramine decreases total number of apneas and improves symptoms in patients with sleep-related breathing disorders, including central sleep apnea.
L-tryptophan	L-tryptophan improves OSA, especially during NREM sleep.
Medroxyprogesterone	The prevalence of OSA among women before menopause is less compared to men. Risk of snoring and OSA increases among postmenopausal women. It has been suggested that female hormones may exert a protective effect on sleep-related breathing disorders. In some studies, medroxyprogesterone significantly improves apnea frequency and duration as well as daytime sleepiness in postmenopausal women. Possible mechanisms for the beneficial therapeutic effect of medroxyprogesterone include a mild activating action on central nervous system arousal systems, improvement in esophageal pressure nadir, and enhancement of hypercapnic ventilatory responses. It has been suggested that progestins may require concomitant estrogen administration to stimulate breathing during sleep. In men, therapy with medroxyprogesterone fails to abolish OSA.
Naloxone	An opioid antagonist, naloxone fails to produce any significant beneficial effects on the frequency or duration of apneas-hypopneas in patients with OSA, or on respiratory pattern and occurrence of periodic apneas in infants with severe OSA.
Naltrexone	An oral semisynthetic opiate antagonist, administration results in significant improvements in arterial blood gases possibly as a result of a decrease in REM sleep time and an increase in intrasleep awakenings in patients with OSA. In a separate study, apnea index, and the number, duration and intensity of hypoxic events were reduced in patients with OSA.
Nicotine	A central nervous system stimulant, nicotine increases the activity of the upper airway dilator muscles. This action could reduce upper airway obstruction during sleep. Nicotine's effects on sleep architecture include an increase in sleep latency and decrease in total sleep time, sleep efficiency, and % REM sleep. In one study, nicotine reduced apneas during the first 2 hours of sleep in eight patients with OSA. Other studies showed that nicotine failed to significantly improve apnea index, apnea duration, and minimum oxygen saturation in persons with OSA.
Ondansetron	A selective serotonin 5-HT (3)-type receptor antagonist, ondansetron reduces respiratory disturbance index during REM sleep (but not during NREM sleep) in the English Bulldog, an animal model of OSA.
Paroxetine	This serotonin-receptor uptake inhibitor has no effect on apnea-hypopnea indices as reported in a study of eight adult male patients with severe OSA. In another study, paroxetine reduced apnea indices during NREM sleep but not during REM sleep; it did not affect hypopnea indices in 20 male patients with OSA.

Table 5-11. Medications that have been used for treating obstructive sleep apnea—cont'd

Agent	Effect on apnea
Protriptyline	Beneficial effects of protriptyline appear related primarily to a reduction in REM sleep, with a reduction of more severe REM-associated apneas, but it may also decrease the number of apneas/hypopneas during NREM sleep. A study, however, reported no significant effect on symptoms or the frequency of apneas, hypopneas, arousals, and 4% oxygen desaturations in 10 patients with OSA given protriptyline. Patients with mild to moderate OSA may respond more favorably to protriptyline therapy than those with severe disease. The use of protriptyline can be complicated by anticholinergic side effects, including dry mouth, urinary hesitancy, mild constipation, and difficulty in maintaining an erection, which may necessitate cessation of therapy.
Sabeluzole	An agent with antiexcitatory amino acid activity used in the treatment of Alzheimer disease. In one study, administration of sabeluzole reduced oxygen desaturation index during sleep in 13 patients with OSA.
Somatostatin	Patients with untreated acromegaly may develop OSA, and indices of sleep apnea severity, oxygen saturation, and sleep quality may improve, along with normalization of growth hormone levels, during somatostatin or octreotide (a somatostatin analog) therapy. This beneficial effect might be mediated, at least in part, by a reduction in the volume of the upper airway soft tissues and tongue.
Steroids (nasal)	Allergic rhinitis and nasal stuffiness increase both the risk of developing OSA and its severity. Nasal steroids improve apnea hypopnea indices in children with mild OSA.
Theophylline	Some studies have demonstrated a decrease in apnea index and an increase in oxygen saturation during treatment, with this bronchodilator and respiratory stimulant. Nevertheless, although theophylline might reduce apnea frequency, it generally does not normalize the apnea index. Theophylline is less effective than CPAP therapy in improving respiratory variables (apnea-hypopnea index and oxygen desaturation), and in normalizing sleep architecture in patients with OSA. However, some studies have reported no significant beneficial effects on the number or duration of apneas and hypopneas or on oxygen desaturation with theophylline therapy. Theophylline appears to have no effect on snoring. Theophylline may disrupt sleep architecture, decrease sleep efficiency, and increase sleep fragmentation.
Thyroid hormone	Hypothyroidism is associated with an increased prevalence of OSA. Thyroid hormone replacement in hypothyroid patients with OSA can decrease apnea frequency and increase oxygen saturation. However there seems to be no correlation between the severity of OSA and serum levels of thyroid hormones. Angina can develop in patients with ischemic heart disease and untreated OSA during thyroid hormone replacement therapy. Nevertheless, restoration of the euthyroid state does not completely abolish apnea and hypopnea events in every hypothyroid patient with OSA. A repeat polysomnography is recommended after reversal of the hypothyroid state to determine if significant OSA persists.

Continued

Table 5–11. Medications that have been used for treating obstructive sleep apnea—cont'd

Agent	Effect on apnea
Trazodone	In the English bulldog, an animal model of OSA, the combination of serotonergics, trazodone (an antidepressant agent that selectively inhibits serotonin reuptake), and L-tryptophan, reduces respiratory events during NREM and REM sleep and minimizes sleep-related suppression of upper airway dilator activity. Trazodone therapy in a patient with progressive olivopontocerebellar degeneration, excessive daytime sleepiness, and OSA resulted in resolution of daytime sleepiness and improvement of sleep architecture.

Box 5–10.

American Academy of Sleep Medicine (AASM) recommendations regarding medical therapy of obstructive sleep apnea

WEIGHT REDUCTION

Dietary weight reduction may improve the apnea-hypopnea index (AHI) in obese patients with obstructive sleep apnea (OSA) (guideline).

Dietary weight reduction should be used in conjunction with a primary treatment for OSA (option).

In obese patients, bariatric surgery may be considered as an adjunct in the treatment of OSA (option).

PHARMACOLOGIC AGENTS

The following pharmacologic agents are not recommended for the therapy of OSA:

a. Selective serotonin reuptake inhibitors (standard)

b. Protriptyline as primary treatment (guideline)

c. Methylxanthine derivatives, including aminophylline and theophylline (standard)

d. Estrogen therapy with or without progesterone (standard)

e. Short-acting nasal decongestants (option)

Topical nasal corticosteroids may be a useful adjunct to primary therapies for OSA in patients with concurrent rhinitis. (guideline)

Modafinil is recommended for treating residual daytime sleepiness in patients with OSA on effective positive airway pressure (PAP) treatment and with no other known cause for sleepiness (standard).

There was no or insufficient data in the literature to formulate any recommendations regarding androgen blockade, bromocriptine (for acromegaly), medroxyprogesterone (for men with OSA), mirtazapine, nicotine, and thyroid hormone (for hypothyroidism).

SUPPLEMENTAL OXYGEN

Supplemental oxygen is not recommended as a primary therapy for OSA (option).

(continued from page 194)
Box 5-10.

American Academy of Sleep Medicine (AASM) recommendations regarding medical therapy of obstructive sleep apnea

POSITIONAL THERAPY

Methods to permit sleep only in a non-supine position are effective either as secondary therapy or as supplement to primary therapies for OSA in patients with a low AHI in the non-supine versus the supine position (guideline).

Source: Adapted and modified from Morgenthaler T, Kapen S, Lee-Chiong T, et al. Practice parameters for the medical therapy of obstructive sleep apnea. Sleep. 2006;29(8):1031-1035.

AASM Definition of Terms

Standard	Generally accepted practice with a high level of clinical certainly
Guideline	Practice associated with a moderate degree of clinical certainty
Option	Practice of uncertain clinical use

Positive Airway Pressure Therapy

Administration of positive airway pressure therapy is the treatment of choice for most patients with OSA (Table 5–12). CPAP treatment is generally recommended for all patients with an AHI greater than or equal to 15/hour and for symptomatic patients (eg, excessive daytime sleepiness, insomnia, impaired cognition, mood disorder, hypertension, ischemic heart disease, or stroke) with an AHI between 5–30/hour.

Table 5-12.   Treatment modalities for positive airway pressure therapy

Continuous positive airway pressure	Provides a constant pressure throughout the respiratory cycle
Bi-level positive airway pressure	Provides two pressure levels during the respiratory cycle: a higher level during inspiration and a lower pressure during expiration
Autotitrating positive airway pressure	Provides variable pressures using device-specific diagnostic and therapeutic algorithms
Nocturnal noninvasive positive pressure ventilation	Provides two pressure levels at a set rate to assist ventilation

Mechanism of Action

Positive airway pressure, via a fan or turbine generated flow of air, is generally believed to function as a pneumatic splint that maintains the patency of the vulnerable portions of the nasopharyngeal airway. Positive airway pressure increases nasal pressure above P_{crit}.

Determining Optimal Continuous Positive Airway Pressure

With CPAP, the patient sleeps with a single constant pressure throughout the night. A variety of methods have been used to determine a single optimal CPAP level. These include:

1.   In-laboratory attended polysomnographically guided CPAP titration

a. Full-night studies

b. Split-night studies (consists of an initial diagnostic portion and a subsequent CPAP titration on the same night);

2. Unattended laboratory or home titration

3. Use of autotitrating devices

4. Formula-derived pressures from clinical, PSG, and/or anthropometric variables

The current standard of practice involves an attended pressure titration during a laboratory PSG, during which sleep stages and respiratory variables are monitored. The goal is to determine a single fixed pressure that eliminates apneas, hypopneas, snoring, and respiratory effort–related arousals (RERAs); maintains adequate oxygen saturation; and improves sleep architecture and quality in all sleep positions and in all sleep stages. It is generally accepted that higher pressures are required to reverse airway occlusion during REM sleep and during sleep in a supine position.

A split-night study in which an initial diagnostic portion is followed by CPAP titration on the same night is successful in identifying an adequate pressure in about 60% to 80% of patients. Criteria for a split-night study are given in Box 5–11. Because respiratory events tend to be more common during REM sleep, which predominates during the second half of the night, spit-night studies can potentially underestimate the severity of OSA.

Box 5–11. **Criteria for split-night continuous positive airway pressure (CPAP) titration**	At least 2 hours of recorded sleep time during the initial diagnostic portion of the study Apnea-hypopnea indices during the diagnostic portion of the study: AHI > 40 AHI = 20–40 (accompanied by significant oxygen desaturation) At least 3 hours are available for CPAP titration with the presence of REM sleep during a supine sleep position

Central apneas may develop or become more frequent during CPAP titration. In some cases, this may simply be a temporary phenomenon, possibly postarousal, and will disappear once the patient gets used to the positive airway pressure and his or her sleep stabilizes. Persistent central apneas, especially if associated with frequent arousals and significant sleep disruption, may respond to changes in CPAP pressure (either an increase or decrease), the addition of supplemental low-flow oxygen (between 1–2 liters per minute), or changing CPAP to bilevel positive pressure or adaptive servoventilation.

AASM recommendations for CPAP and bilevel positive airway pressure (BPAP) therapy for adult patients with sleep-related breathing disorders are listed in Box 5–12.

Effects of Positive Airway Pressure Therapy

Positive airway pressure therapy has salutary effects on mortality, cardiovascular parameters, daytime alertness, neurocognitive function, mood, sleep quality, and health care utilization. CPAP is effective in symptomatic patients with moderate to severe OSA, and the beneficial effects of CPAP

Box 5-12.

American Academy of Sleep Medicine (AASM) recommendations for CPAP and BPAP therapy for adult patients with sleep-related breathing disorders

1. The presence of obstructive sleep apnea (OSA) based on an acceptable diagnostic method should be established prior to continuous positive airway pressure (CPAP) therapy (standard).

2. Indications for CPAP therapy include:

   a. Moderate to severe OSA (standard)

   b. Mild OSA (option)

   c. Improvement of subjective sleepiness in patients with OSA (standard)

   d. Improvement of quality of life in patients with OSA (option)

   e. As an adjunctive therapy to lower blood pressure in patients with OSA and hypertension (option)

3. The preferred CPAP titration method to determine optimal positive airway pressure is an in-laboratory, full-night, attended polysomnography, but split-night (initial diagnostic and subsequent titration portion) studies are usually adequate (guideline).

4. Objective monitoring of CPAP use is recommended to ensure optimal utilization (standard).

5. Close monitoring of CPAP utilization and any problems that might develop, especially during the first few weeks of use, is important, as is the correction of problems if needed (standard).

6. Addition of heated humidification and a systematic educational program enhance adherence to CPAP use (standard).

7. Patients with OSA treated with CPAP therapy should be followed up yearly or more frequently as needed to correct problems related to its use (option).

8. CPAP and bilevel positive airway pressure (BPAP) therapy are generally safe with minor adverse effects (standard).

9. BPAP can be considered as an optional therapy to CPAP in selected patients who require high pressures, who report difficulty exhaling against a fixed CPAP pressure, or who have coexisting central hypoventilation (guideline).

10. BPAP may also be beneficial in patients with some forms of restrictive lung disease or hypoventilation syndromes with daytime hypercapnia (option).

Source: Adapted and modified from Kushida CA, Littner MR, Hirshkowitz M, et al. Practice parameters for the use of continuous and bilevel positive airway pressure devices to treat adult patients with sleep-related breathing disorders. Sleep. 2006;29(3):375–380.

For the AASM definition of terms, see Box 5-10.

are sustained over time. See Table 5–13 for further information. The extent to which asymptomatic patients with mild OSA and no associated medical or psychiatric disorders benefit from CPAP is less certain. The minimal severity level of OSA at which patients benefit from CPAP treatment is not well characterized. Intermittent use of CPAP should be avoided, because virtually all of the gains in sleep quality and daytime alertness derived from sleeping with CPAP are rapidly reversed with CPAP discontinuation.

Table 5–13. **Beneficial effects of positive airway pressure therapy in obstructive sleep apnea**

Sleep quality	Improvement in sleep quality Decrease in number of arousals
Upper airway anatomy and function	Reduction or elimination of upper airway collapse Reduction or elimination of snoring Decrease in apneahypopnea index (AHI) Increase in arterial oxygen saturation (SaO_2)
Sleepiness and other daytime symptoms	Decrease in sleepiness (subjective and objective) Improvement in quality of life Enhancement of neurocognitive function Improvement in mood Improvement in driving simulator steering performance
Mortality	Reversal of the increase in mortality associated with sleep apnea
Hypertension	Improvement in blood pressure and heart rate profiles in patients with hypertension Decrease in nighttime and daytime mean arterial, systolic and diastolic blood pressures Restoration of normal circadian "dipping" pattern of blood pressure ("dipping" is defined as an average blood pressure reduction ≥ 10 mm Hg systolic and ≥ 5 mm Hg diastolic at night compared to daytime values)
Congestive heart failure	Improvement in cardiac function in patients with OSA and congestive heart failure
Health care utilization	Reduction in physician claims and hospital stay

Adverse Consequences of Positive Airway Pressure Therapy

The use of positive airway pressure therapy can give rise to a number of adverse consequences due to the prescribed pressure or mask. See Box 5–13 for a list of adverse effects.

Adherence to Positive Airway Pressure Therapy

CPAP therapy is only as beneficial as its utilization. Less than optimal CPAP utilization is a significant problem in clinical practice. A large proportion of patients report not being able to tolerate the device.

Self-reports often overestimate actual CPAP use. Therapeutic adherence in the different studies has varied from 46% to 80% of patients who use CPAP for 4 or more hours nightly on at least 70% of monitored nights.

Approximately 50% of patients are consistent CPAP users, and the rest are intermittent users with a wide range of nightly use. Average nightly use is between 4 to 5 hours each night among CPAP users. The percent of days in which CPAP was not used correlated with decreased duration of nightly use. Factors influencing long-term use include snoring history, severity of illness (AHI), perceived benefit from therapy, and self-reported sleepiness (Epworth Sleepiness Scale [ESS]). Patients with mild OSA have a particularly high rate of CPAP discontinuation. Long-term use of CPAP does not appear to be related to the prescribed pressure. Finally, CPAP usage tends to

Box 5–13.	
Adverse consequences of positive airway pressure therapy	Aerophagia and gastric distention
	Arousals
	Barotrauma (eg, pneumothorax, pneumomediastinum, pneumocephalus)
	Chest discomfort and tightness
	Claustrophobia, sensation of suffocation or difficulty with exhalation
	Eye irritation (conjunctivitis)
	Facial skin irritation, rash or abrasion
	Mask and mouth leaks
	Nasal congestion, dryness, epistaxis or rhinorrhea
	Sleep disruption due to noise from the device
	Sinus discomfort or pain

be greater among patients who underwent full-night CPAP titration studies compared to those who had split-night CPAP titration.

Patterns of nightly use are often discernible by the first few days or weeks of initiating treatment. Reasons for non-adherence to positive airway pressure therapy and suggestions for how to correct them are described in Table 5–14.

Adherence to CPAP therapy may be improved with education (eg, additional home visits, participation in group clinics, periodic phone calls to uncover any problems and to encourage use, and even simple written information on the importance of regular CPAP use), airway humidification, proper selection of the CPAP interface, desensitization procedures for CPAP, early follow-up, prompt and aggressive management of adverse effects related to CPAP use, and regular assessment of CPAP adherence. For a summary of these techniques, see Table 5–15.

Table 5–14.   Reasons for non-adherence to positive airway pressure therapy

Reason	Possible corrective measures
Perception of lack of benefit	Patient education
Discomfort with its use (including mask)	Mask refitting (nasal masks, nasal pillows, full-face masks, or oral masks)
Noise from the device	Placing device in another room adjacent to bedroom Use of ear plugs or noise-attenuating devices
Air leaks from the mask or mouth	Mask refitting for mask leaks Use of chin strap or full face mask for mouth leaks Airway humidification Treatment of nasal congestion
Difficulty with exhaling against high expiratory pressures	Trial of CPAP with C-flex technology or bilevel positive airway pressure (BPAP)

Table 5–14. Reasons for non-adherence to positive airway pressure therapy—cont'd

Reason	Possible corrective measures
Excessively high pressures	Trial of automated positive airway pressure or Adjunctive therapy with sleep position treatment or oral devices
Inconvenience related its use	Patient education
Frequent nocturnal awakenings	Reassessment of delivered CPAP pressures Brief trial of hypnotic agents during the acclimatization phase of initial CPAP use
Claustrophobia	Mask refitting (eg, nasal pillows or oral masks) Formal program of CPAP desensitization

Nasal problems
  Dryness
  Rhinorrhea
  Congestion
  Sneezing
  Epistaxis
	Airway humidification (preferably heated)
	Use of nasal lubricants, decongestants (short-term use), anticholinergic agents, or corticosteroids
	Immunotherapy, oral decongestants, or antihistamine agents may also be tried for allergic rhinitis
	Nasal surgery (in selected patients with nasal anatomic abnormalities)

Gastric distention due to aerophagia	BPAP therapy

Table 5–15. Techniques that may increase continuous positive airway pressure utilization

Technique	Description
CPAP education and support	A variety of CPAP support programs, including outpatient group clinics designed to encourage CPAP use, home CPAP education, phone calls, providing written information about OSA and the importance of regular CPAP use, verbal reinforcement, cognitive-behavioral techniques, motivational enhancement to reduce ambivalence regarding treatment, and desensitization, have been shown to improve CPAP utilization.
Humidification	Nasal dryness, rhinorrhea, nasal congestion, sneezing, or epistaxis are common problems in patients using CPAP therapy and can adversely affect optimal CPAP utilization. Humidification can help alleviate these problems. Many individuals using CPAP develop increased nasal resistance. Nasal resistance is affected by mouth leakage and can be attenuated by heated (less commonly by cold) humidification. Factors predicting the need for heated humidification include age older than 60 years, use of drying medications, presence of chronic mucosa disease, and a previous uvulopalatopharyngoplasty.

Table 5–15. Techniques that may increase continuous positive airway pressure utilization—cont'd

Technique	Description
Pressure ramp	A ramp, which is available in many CPAP devices, allows the pressure to be reset to a lower level, which is then gradually increased over time to the prescribed pressure setting. The amount of time and rate of increase is usually adjustable. The pressure ramp has been proposed to enhance patient comfort by allowing the patient sufficient time to fall asleep before higher and more uncomfortable pressures are reached. The ramp mode can also be activated following awakenings during the night. However, having lower pressures at sleep onset may permit obstructive events during subtherapeutic CPAP levels and allow sleep-onset central apnea episodes to occur. Some patients find the ramp feature useful; however, others do not.
Correction of nasal problems	Nasal congestion can be alleviated with the use of nasal corticosteroids or judicious use of topical nasal decongestants.
Nasal vs. full-face masks	Patients who are having difficulty with nasal breathing or who have a large mouth leak may benefit from a full face mask that allows them to breathe through both the nose and mouth. Full face masks have valves that allow entry of room air in case of failure of the CPAP device. Edentulous patients may have greater difficulty obtaining satisfactory mask seal with full face masks.
Sedative-hypnotics	Sedative-hypnotics have been used during the acclimatization phase of initial CPAP use to assist patients reporting difficulty sleeping with CPAP. However, benzodiazepines may increase arousal threshold, prolong apnea duration, and worsen oxyhemoglobin desaturation in patients with OSA.
C-flex	This device allows a reduction in pressure during expiration following delivery of positive airway pressure. It may be beneficial for patients who complain of having difficulty breathing out against the delivered CPAP pressure.
BPAP	BPAP delivers different positive airway pressures during inspiration and expiration. It has been proposed that the lower expiratory pressure may enhance patient comfort, especially in those complaining of having difficulty breathing out against the delivered CPAP pressure, or of gastric distention due to aerophagia. Nevertheless, BPAP has not been noted to consistently alter patient acceptance and CPAP adherence.

Other Modes of Positive Airway Pressure

Autotitrating Positive Airway Pressure   Because the required positive airway pressure can differ considerably with sleeping posture and sleep stages, optimal positive airway pressure may have significant intranight and internight variability. The causes of this variability are listed in Box 5–14. Auto-titrating positive airway pressure (APAP) devices automatically and continuously adjust the delivered pressure, as required, to maintain airway patency. Pressure is increased if apneas, hypopneas, airflow limitation or snoring are present, or is gradually reduced if no respiratory events are detected over a predetermined period. These devices have been used to help identify a fixed single pressure for subsequent treatment with a conventional CPAP device (APAP titration) or in a self-adjusting mode for nightly therapy of OSA (APAP treatment).

Using a fixed single continuous pressure for the entire night based on parameters obtained during REM-supine sleep (when pressure requirements are expected to be greater) may result in using more pressure than is needed for certain portions of sleep. This might possibly increase mask

Box 5-14.	Changes in percentage of REM sleep
Etiology of night-to-night variability of apnea hypopnea index in patients with obstructive sleep apnea	Changes in percentage of different sleep positions (supine vs. nonsupine)
	Changes in nasal resistance (eg, congestion)
	Use of alcohol
	Use of muscle relaxants, sedatives and opioids
	Change in weight

and mouth air leaks as well as pressure intolerance. These, in turn, might reduce CPAP acceptance and therapeutic adherence. Compared to constant CPAP, mean delivered pressure is generally lower during APAP, but peak airway pressure may be higher. APAP use can be limited by the development of significant mask or mouth air leaks or central apneas. Thus, proper mask fitting is crucial prior to unattended APAP use.

Studies have shown no significant differences between conventional in-laboratory CPAP titration and APAP titration in reductions of AHI and arousal indices, changes in sleep architecture, oxygenation, or subsequent CPAP acceptance. In addition, APAP treatment has been demonstrated to be comparable to conventional constant-pressure CPAP therapy.

Nevertheless, clinicians should realize that not all APAP systems are equal in efficacy and that published outcomes regarding one APAP model from a specific manufacturer may not necessarily be applicable to other systems. Different devices may utilize different algorithms for monitoring respiratory events (eg, snoring, airflow limitation, apnea-hypopneas, or impedance) and for altering delivered pressures. Patients who are being offered APAP for titration or therapy rather than conventional sleep laboratory CPAP titration should be informed of these limitations. AASM recommendations for auto-titrating continuous positive airway pressure for obstructive sleep apnea are presented in Box 5–15.

Bilevel Positive Airway Pressure   Patients with OSA who have persistent oxygen desaturation due to hypoventilation despite CPAP therapy may benefit from BPAP. BPAP devices provide two pressure levels during the respiratory cycle, namely a higher level during inspiration (inspiratory positive airway pressure; IPAP) and a lower pressure during expiration (expiratory positive airway pressure; EPAP).

Box 5-15.	**STANDARD**
American Academy of Sleep Medicine (AASM) recommendations for autotitrating continuous positive airway pressure for obstructive sleep apnea	1. The presence of obstructive sleep apnea (OSA) must be diagnosed using an acceptable method.
	2. APAP titration or treatment is not indicated for patients with the following medical conditions:
	• Congestive heart failure
	• Significant respiratory diseases such as chronic obstructive pulmonary disease or daytime hypoxemia and respiratory failure from any cause
	• Nocturnal arterial oxygen desaturation secondary to disorders other than OSA (eg, obesity hypoventilation syndrome)

(continued from page 202)
Box 5–15.

American Academy of Sleep Medicine (AASM) recommendations for autotitrating continuous positive airway pressure for obstructive sleep apnea

3. Nonsnorers should not be titrated with APAP devices using diagnostic algorithms that rely on vibration or sound production.

4. APAP devices are not recommended for split-night CPAP titration.

5. Patients who are being treated with APAP or with fixed CPAP based on APAP titration should be monitored for effectiveness and safety of therapy.

6. If APAP or CPAP therapy is considered ineffective (ie, symptoms fail to resolve), reevaluation and standard attended CPAP titration should be performed.

GUIDELINE

1. Certain APAP devices may be used to determine a single CPAP pressure during attended polysomnography for the therapy of OSA (APAP titration).

2. Certain APAP devices may be used in a self-adjusting mode for the therapy of OSA after an initial successful attended polysomnography-guided CPAP or APAP titration (APAP treatment).

OPTION

1. The use of unattended APAP to determine pressures for fixed CPAP or to treat CPAP-naive patients in a self-adjusting APAP mode has not been established

Source: Adapted and modified from Standards of Practice Committee of the American Academy of Sleep Medicine. Practice Parameters for the Use of Auto-Titrating Continuous Positive Airway Pressure Devices for Titrating Pressures and Treating Adult Patients with Obstructive Sleep Apnea Syndrome. An American Academy of Sleep Medicine Report. Sleep. 2003;25143–147.

For an AASM definition of terms, See Box 5-10.

When used for patients with OSA, levels of EPAP are titrated to eliminate apneas, and IPAP is progressively increased until hypopneas and snoring are controlled. A commonly used titration strategy starts at low IPAP and EPAP pressures (usually IPAP of 5–6 cm H_2O and EPAP of 3–4 cm H_2O). Both pressures are then increased in a stepwise fashion (typically by 2 cm H_2O increments) until apneas are eliminated. IPAP is then increased without changing EPAP until hypopneas and snoring are controlled.

BPAP may also be considered for (1) patients with OSA who are unable to tolerate CPAP and complain of being unable to breathe out against high CPAP expiratory pressures, significant mouth leaks or aerophagia, (2) those with concurrent chronic obstructive pulmonary disease (overlap syndrome), or (3) those in whom hypoventilation (eg, obesity hypoventilation syndrome or neuromuscular weakness) is suspected. If used for patients with hypoventilation syndromes, the difference between IPAP and EPAP is equivalent to the delivered pressure support (ie, a pressure support of 5 cm H_2O is provided by a BPAP setting of 20 (IPAP)/15 (EPAP) cm H_2O [20–15 = 5]).

Studies have not shown consistent advantages of BPAP over CPAP in patient preference and device utilization.

Noninvasive Positive Pressure Ventilation   Noninvasive positive pressure ventilation (NIPPV) may be required in selected patients with persistent sleep-related hypoventilation and

CO_2 retention despite therapy with CPAP and supplemental oxygen. NIPPV, which can be provided using a volume-cycled ventilator, can improve ventilation and arterial blood gas values during both wakefulness and sleep. Some patients on NIPPV are able to resume CPAP therapy at a later time.

Oral Devices

Oral devices worn during sleep may be considered for snorers and individuals with mild to moderate OSA who are intolerant of positive airway pressure therapy or whose OSA persists following upper airway surgery. These devices are designed to reposition the mandible and tongue in an anterior or forward position to enlarge pharyngeal dimensions and to prevent their collapse into the airways during sleep. The goals of treatment include improvement or resolution of snoring and/or obstructive sleep apnea. A conservative degree of advancement is initially applied; this is then increased gradually over several weeks until the desired goals are achieved. The degree of anterior displacement of the tongue is considered the primary factor in influencing the effectiveness of these devices.

Oral devices are fairly well tolerated and many patients may prefer them to CPAP devices. Overall, oral devices appear to be effective in about 80% of patients with snoring or mild to moderate OSA and in about 30% of those with severe OSA. Patients with positional sleep apnea (whose apnea is worse during a supine sleep position) may have higher success rates. Because response rates are unpredictable, a repeat sleep study is recommended once the device has been optimally adjusted to assess its therapeutic efficacy.

Two types of oral devices are currently available for the therapy of OSA, namely tongue-retaining devices and mandibular repositioners (Table 5–16). A third device, palatal lifter, is not generally used at this time.

Table 5–16. Oral devices for obstructive sleep apnea

Device	Characteristics
Mandibular repositioners	They advance the mandible (and tongue) forward, and are the most commonly used oral devices. Contraindicated in patients with inadequate dentition to adequately support the oral device, compromised dentition (ie, loose, broken or diseased teeth), or significant temporomandibular joint dysfunction
Tongue-retaining devices	These devices hold the tongue in an anterior (forward) position by securing the tip of the tongue in a soft bulb located anterior to the teeth. They are preferred for edentulous patients or for those with compromised dentition.

Oral devices should be avoided in patients who are unable to breathe nasally or who have high resistances to nasal airflow, as well as in those whose sleep apnea is primarily central in nature. Complications related to the use of oral devices include a dry mouth sensation related to mouth breathing, excessive salivation (usually resolves by the first week of use), tooth pain, undesirable dental movements associated with mandibular repositioning devices, bite changes (generally occurring in the first half hour following device removal in the morning and tend to resolve spontaneously), and jaw or temporomandibular joint pain or discomfort. Guaranteeing a good lip seal can prevent a dry mouth sensation and excessive salivation. Muscle relaxants and physical therapy may help alleviate temporomandibular joint pain or discomfort.

AASM recommendations for the treatment of snoring and OSA with oral devices (1995) are presented in Box 5–16. More current AASM recommendations for the use of oral devices for OSA are presented in Box 5–17.

Box 5-16.

American Academy of Sleep Medicine (AASM) recommendations for the treatment of snoring and obstructive sleep apnea with oral devices (1995)

1. The diagnosis of obstructive sleep apnea (OSA) must be established before starting therapy using oral appliances.

2. The goals of therapy using oral appliances include:

   - For patients with primary snoring — to reduce snoring to an acceptable level

   - For patients with OSA — to normalize clinical signs and symptoms, apnea-hypopnea index, and oxygen saturation

3. Oral appliances are indicated for patients with:

   - Primary snoring or mild OSA who have failed to respond to or are not candidates for behavioral therapy (eg, weight reduction)

   - Moderate or severe OSA who are intolerant or unwilling to adhere to prescribed continuous positive airway pressure (CPAP) therapy, or are not appropriate candidates for upper airway surgery

4. Qualified personnel should fit oral appliances. They may perform cephalometric evaluation whenever this is considered necessary.

5. A follow-up polysomnography with the oral appliance in place is indicated for patients with moderate or severe OSA to ensure therapeutic efficacy of the device. Follow-up evaluations at regular intervals with the clinician and dentist are recommended to monitor outcomes, compliance, overall oral health, and complications (eg, temporomandibular joint disease, dental misalignment, oral discomfort, and appliance deterioration). A follow-up polysomnography is not indicated for patients with primary snoring or mild OSA unless symptoms worsen or do not resolve.

Source: Adapted and modified from Thorpy M, et al. Practice parameters for the treatment of snoring and obstructive sleep apnea with oral appliances. Sleep. 1995;18:511–513.

Upper Airway Surgery

Upper airway surgery may be considered in patients who are either unwilling or unable to use positive airway pressure therapy. Surgical procedures may be particularly useful for patients with definitive craniofacial or upper airway abnormalities. Easily reversible causes of upper airway obstruction, such as nasal mucosal swelling, enlarged turbinates, nasal polyps, and enlarged tonsils should be addressed.

Box 5-17.

American Academy of Sleep Medicine (AASM) recommendations for use of oral devices for obstructive sleep apnea (2005)

1. The presence and severity of obstructive sleep apnea (OSA) should be determined prior to starting therapy using oral devices (standard).

2. Fitting of oral devices should be performed by qualified dental personnel, and dental management of patients with OSA should be supervised by those with training in sleep medicine (option).

3. Cephalometric evaluation, although not always required, should be performed when indicated (option).

4. The objective of therapy using oral devices for patients with primary snoring (ie, without OSA or upper airway resistance syndrome) is the reduction of snoring to a subjectively acceptable level (standard).

(continued from page 205)
Box 5–17

American Academy of Sleep Medicine (AASM) recommendations for use of oral devices for obstructive sleep apnea (2005)

5. The objectives of therapy using oral devices for patients with OSA include resolution of symptoms, and normalization of apnea-hypopnea indices (AHI) and oxygen saturation (standard).

6. Indications for oral devices for sleep-related breathing disorders include:

   a. Primary snoring that is unresponsive to or inappropriate for behavioral treatment with weight loss or sleep position therapy (guideline).

   b. Mild to moderate OSA in patients who prefer oral devices over CPAP, or are unresponsive to, fail, or are otherwise not appropriate candidates for CPAP or therapy with weight loss or change in sleep position (guideline).

7. An initial trial of continuous positive airway pressure (CPAP) therapy is recommended for patients with severes OSA prior to using oral devices. For patients in whom upper airway surgeries for OSA are predicted to be highly effective, these operations may also be used prior to oral devices (guideline).

8. Follow-up sleep testing is not required for patients using oral devices for primary snoring (guideline).

9. Follow-up sleep testing (polysomnography or attended cardiorespiratory (type 3) sleep study) is indicated for patients using oral devices for OSA after optimal fit has been achieved to determine therapeutic efficacy and benefit (guideline).

10. Follow-up visits with the dental specialist, including every 6 months for the first year once optimal fit is achieved and at least annually thereafter, to monitor adherence to therapy, oral and dental health, integrity of occlusion, device deterioration, and OSA-related signs and symptoms, are recommended (option).

11. Periodic follow-up with the referring clinician, including objective reevaluation of respiration during sleep if manifestations related to OSA recur or worsen, is recommended (option).

Source: Adapted and modified from Kushida CA, Morgenthaler TI, Littner MR, et al. Practice parameters for the treatment of snoring and obstructive sleep apnea with oral appliances: an Update for 2005. Sleep. 2006;29(2):240-243.

For the AASM definition of terms. See Box 5-10.

Pharyngeal narrowing or collapse has been classified based on the region affected into type 1 (retropalatal [region behind the palate]), type 2 (retropalatal and retrolingual [region behind the tongue]) or type 3 (retrolingual). Lateral cephalometry and fiberoptic pharyngoscopy/endoscopy performed while the individual is awake may be used to define the type of pharyngeal narrowing.

Surgical procedures for OSA are designed to increase the dimensions of the retropalatal airspace, retrolingual airway, or both. In rare instances of severe OSA, a tracheostomy, which uses a percutaneous tracheal opening to bypass the area of airway collapse, might be necessary. For information about indications for specific types of surgery, see Table 5–17. For information about individual surgical techniques, see Table 5–18.

Any single type of surgery may not be effective for a particular patient with OSA given the varying location, degree, and complexity of upper airway narrowing or collapse. Surgery may be sequentially staged, with most patients first undergoing uvulopalatopharyngoplasty, and genio-glossal advancement and/or hyoid myotomy and suspension, followed by maxillomandibular oste-otomy and advancement if significant sleep-related breathing disorder persists.

A formal PSG following upper airway surgery is recommended to determine its therapeutic efficacy. Data on long-term surgical effectiveness is limited. Many patients report greater subjective

Table 5-17. Upper airway surgical therapy for obstructive sleep apnea

Indications	Procedures
To increase dimensions of the retropalatal airspace	Radiofrequency palatal submucosal tissue volume reduction Laser-assisted uvulopalatoplasty Uvulopalatopharyngoplasty Transpalatal advancement pharyngoplasty
To increase dimensions of the retrolingual airway	Radiofrequency tongue base ablation Laser midline glossectomy and lingualplasty Tongue base reduction with hyoepiglottoplasty Genioglossal advancement Hyoid myotomy and suspension Mandibular advancement
To increase dimensions of the retrolingual, retropalatal and transpalatal airway	Uvulopalatopharyngoglossoplasty Maxillomandibular advancement
To bypass the upper airway	Tracheostomy — uses a percutaneous tracheal opening to bypass the area of airway collapse

Table 5-18. Surgical techniques proposed for snoring or obstructive sleep apnea

Procedure	Description
Nasal surgeries	Septal reconstruction (septoplasty), polyp removal, and/or turbinectomy Enlarges nasal airway
Tonsillectomy and adenoidectomy	Removal of the tonsils and enlarged adenoids May be particularly effective in children with OSA due to adenotonsillar enlargement
Radiofrequency palatal submucosal tissue volume reduction	Radiofrequency submucosal tissue volume reduction (Somnoplasty®) of the soft palate Repeated treatments may be required Enlarges retropalatal airway
Radiofrequency tongue base ablation	Radiofrequency submucosal tissue volume reduction (Somnoplasty®) of the tongue base Enlarges retrolingual airway
Laser midline glossectomy and lingualplasty	Laser excision of a midline portion of the posterior tongue and lateral portions of the tongue Enlarges retrolingual airway
Tongue base reduction with hyoepiglottoplasty	Excision of tongue base and suspension of the hyoid from the mandible Enlarges retrolingual airway
Uvulopalatopharyngoplasty	Excision of uvula, posterior portion of the soft palate, redundant pharyngeal tissue, and tonsils (if present), and trimming of the tonsillar pillars Enlarges retropalatal airway Less effective than CPAP therapy Successful in reducing AHI by half of the preoperative level in 30% to 50% of patients (some investigators have reported a decrease in frequency of apneas, but an increase in number of hypopneas)

Continued

Table 5-18.   Surgical techniques proposed for snoring or obstructive sleep apnea—cont'd

Procedure	Description
	Subsequent use of nasal CPAP may be compromised by UPPP (increase in mouth leaks).
	Complications include velopharyngeal insufficiency (nasal regurgitation of fluid during swallowing), nasopharyngeal stenosis, changes in voice and taste, globus (a foreign body sensation in the throat) and pain, bleeding, apnea and oxygen desaturation in the postoperative period.
	Later recurrence of snoring or OSA after an initial beneficial response has been described
Uvulopalatopharyngoglossoplasty	UPPP *plus* limited tongue base resection
	Enlarges retropalatal and retrolingual airway
Laser-assisted uvulopalatoplasty	Carbon dioxide laser ablation of the uvula and posterior portion of the soft palate
	Enlarges retropalatal airway
	Used for treatment of snoring
	Performed under local anesthesia in an ambulatory setting and requires no postoperative hospitalization
Transpalatal advancement pharyngoplasty	Resection of the posterior hard palate and anterior advancement of the soft palate
	Enlarges retropalatal airway
Orthognathic surgery	Maxillary expansion in patients with constriction of the maxilla
Genioglossal advancement	Anterior advancement of the genial tubercle of the mandible (where the tongue is attached) by limited parasagittal mandibular osteotomy
	Enlarges retrolingual airway
Hyoid myotomy and suspension	Anterior traction of the tongue, hyoid, and suprahyoid muscle by suspension of the hyoid either from the mandible or from the thyroid cartilage
	Enlarges retrolingual airway
	Complications include anesthesia of the lower teeth (transient).
Mandibular advancement	Anterior displacement of the tongue by sagittal osteotomies of the mandible
	Enlarges retrolingual airway
Maxillomandibular osteotomy and advancement	Advancement of both the maxilla and mandible by Le Fort I maxillary and sagittal-split mandibular osteotomies
	Complications include transient (6 to 12 months) chin and cheek numbness
	Enlarges retrolingual and retropalatal airway
	Reported positive response rates up to 90%
Tracheostomy	Percutaneous tracheal opening distal to the pharynx that bypasses the area of upper airway obstruction
	Indicated in patients with severe life-threatening OSA (severe sleepiness, cardiac arrhythmias, severe hypoxemia, severe hypoventilation, or cor pulmonale) who are intolerant or unresponsive to other types of therapy
	The external end of the tracheostomy can be plugged while the patient is awake
	Complications include formation of granulation tissue at the stoma site, infection, and accidental decannulation

improvements in sleep quality, daytime alertness, and quality of life compared to objective measures of disease severity based on polysomnographic data.

AASM recommendations for the surgical treatment of obstructive sleep apnea in adults are presented in Box 5–18. AASM recommendations for laser-assisted uvulopalatoplasty are presented in Box 5–19.

Management of Residual Sleepiness

Excessive daytime sleepiness may persist despite regular use of CPAP in patients with OSA. This may be due to suboptimal CPAP pressures or coexisting sleep disorders, such as insufficient sleep, narcolepsy, idiopathic hypersomnia, or periodic limb movements of sleep. The use of sedating medications and the presence of depression must be excluded. The differential diagnosis of persistent sleepiness in patients with OSA on positive airway pressure therapy is presented in Box 5–20.

Box 5-18.
 	
American Academy of Sleep Medicine (AASM) recommendations for the surgical treatment of obstructive sleep apnea in adults
	STANDARD
	
	1. The presence and severity of obstructive sleep apnea (OSA) should be determined before starting surgical therapy for OSA.
	
	2. The goals of therapy for OSA include resolution of its associated signs and symptoms, and normalization of sleep quality, apnea hypopnea index (AHI), and oxygen saturation.
	
	3. Patients seeking therapy for OSA should be informed of the effectiveness and complications of the various treatment modalities such as continuous positive airway pressure (CPAP), oral appliances, and upper airway surgery.
	
	GUIDELINE
	
	1. CPAP is the therapy of choice for moderate to severe OSA.
	
	2. Surgery is indicated for patients with an underlying specific surgically correctable abnormality that is responsible for their OSA.
	
	3. Surgery may be indicated for the therapy of OSA when:
	
	  • Other noninvasive treatments are rejected or unsuccessful
	
	  • Surgery is desired
	
	  • Patients are medically stable to undergo surgery
	
	4. Follow-up evaluation, including objective measures of apnea severity and sleep quality, should be performed in patients with preoperatively symptomatic, moderate or severe OSA to determine the presence of any residual OSA.
	
	OPTION
	
	1. *Tracheostomy* is the only surgical procedure that is consistently effective as a sole procedure for OSA and may be considered when other therapeutic options are absent, are refused, or have failed.
	
	2. *Uvulopalatopharyngoplasty* (with or without tonsillectomy) may be appropriate for patients with retropalatal narrowing or collapse.

Box 5-18

American Academy of Sleep Medicine (AASM) recommendations for the surgical treatment of obstructive sleep apnea in adults

(continued from page 209)

3. *Inferior sagittal mandibular osteotomy* and *genioglossal advancement* with or without *hyoid myotomy* and *suspension* appear to be the most promising of the procedures designed to enlarge the retrolingual region.

4. A stepwise surgical approach is acceptable and patients should be informed of the possible need for multiple procedures and the effectiveness of each operation.

5. Long-term follow-up is recommended for patients who had undergone surgical therapy for OSA.

Source: Adapted and modified from Thorpy M, et al. Practice parameters for the rreatment of obstructive sleep apnea in adults: the efficacy of surgical modifications of the upper airway. Sleep. 1996;19:152-155.

For the AASM definition of terms, see Box 5-10.

Box 5-19.

American Academy of Sleep Medicine (AASM) recommendations for laser-assisted uvulopalatoplasty

STANDARD

1. Preoperative evaluation of patients undergoing laser-assisted uvulopalatoplasty (LAUP) to treat snoring should include:

   • Polysomnography or cardiorespiratory study to determine the presence of sleep-disordered breathing

   • Assessment of medications to be used during the perioperative period that might affect respiration

2. The risks and complications of LAUP should be explained to the patient.

3. Patients who had LAUP for snoring should undergo periodic evaluation for possible later development of obstructive sleep apnea.

GUIDELINE

1. LAUP is not recommended for treating sleep-disordered breathing including obstructive sleep apnea.

2. LAUP appears comparable to uvulopalatopharyngoplasty (UPPP) for treating snoring.

Source: Littner et al. Practice parameters for laser-assisted uvulopalatoplasty. Sleep. 2001;24:604.

For the AASM definition of terms, see Box 5-10.

Polysomnography can be repeated with CPAP retitration to determine better treatment parameters. Other sleep disorders, if present, should be appropriately treated.

Modafinil, a wake-promoting agent, may be considered as an adjunct therapy for improving alertness and wakefulness in patients with residual daytime sleepiness despite optimal CPAP therapy for OSA. This agent is a central nervous system stimulant indicated for the therapy of excessive sleepiness. It is used primarily in patients with narcolepsy, idiopathic hypersomnia, or

Box 5-20.	Suboptimal CPAP pressure
Differential diagnosis of persistent sleepiness in patients with obstructive sleep apnea on positive airway pressure therapy	Nonadherence to CPAP therapy Coexisting sleep disorders (insufficient sleep, narcolepsy, periodic limb movements of sleep, and idiopathic hypersomnolence) Use of sedating medications Mood disorders

shift work sleep disorder. Modafinil enhances daytime vigilance and long-term memory without modifying nocturnal sleep or respiratory events. However, not every study has demonstrated improvement in daytime sleepiness with modafinil therapy in patients with OSA receiving effective CPAP therapy. Modafinil does not reverse the negative impact of OSA on cardiovascular morbidity.

Snoring

Definition

Snoring is produced by vibration of upper airway structures, including the soft palate, uvula, and lateral walls of the pharynx, which occurs with airway narrowing during sleep. The site(s) of vibration influences the character and timbre of the audible sound produced.

The term, *primary* or *simple snoring*, refers to isolated snoring unaccompanied by clinical and polysomnographic features suggestive of OSA. Primary snorers do not complain of insomnia, excessive sleepiness, or nighttime sleep disturbance.

Demographics

Snoring can occur in all age groups. Approximately 10% to 12% of children snore. The prevalence of snoring is greater in men than in women and increases with aging. Primary snoring is seen in about 20% to 40% of men and women, and it occurs in up to 40% to 60% of adults over 65 years of age. Women may first develop snoring during pregnancy. A positive family history of snoring can often be elicited. Although data from the Wisconsin Sleep Cohort Study revealed that habitual snorers have a higher prevalence of elevated AHIs, snoring, by itself, lacks sufficient specificity for OSA. It has been estimated that OSA is present in about 25% to 95% of snorers.

Risk Factors

Risk factors for snoring include sleep deprivation; supine sleep position; obesity; nasal obstruction (eg, allergic rhinitis); smoking; and the ingestion of alcohol, muscle relaxants, narcotics, and sedative-hypnotic agents (eg, benzodiazepines). These factors either narrow the upper airway dimensions or decrease upper airway muscle tone. Genetic studies have demonstrated a higher concordance of habitual snoring among monozygotic compared to dizygotic twins.

Consequences

Snorers may complain of a dry or irritated throat and mouth on awakening. Some investigators, but not others, have noted that habitual snorers appear to have an increased risk of developing hypertension, ischemic heart disease, and stroke even after controlling for age and body mass index.

Pathophysiology

Snoring is produced by vibrations of the soft palate, uvula, pharyngeal walls, and faucial pillars related to turbulent airflow when the inspiratory luminal negative pressure exceeds the distending activity of the upper airway muscles. Snoring is often noted during inspiration, but it can occur during exhalation as well. Upper airway collapsibility increases during sleep due to the reduction in upper airway muscle tone. Snoring, hypopneas, or apneas are produced depending on the differences in collapsibility of the upper airway, defined by its P_{crit}. Snoring also stems from, or is made worse by, nasal obstruction.

Evaluation

Snorers may present for evaluation if there is concern that snoring is associated with OSA, or if snoring is causing significant disruption of the bed partner's or roommate's sleep. Inquiries should be made about the duration, frequency and intensity of snoring. Snorers share many of the upper airway physical examination features of patients with OSA (Box 5–21).

Box 5–21. Physical examination findings in snorers	Swollen nasal mucosa
	Enlargement of the tonsils, uvula, and tongue
	Narrowing of lateral pharyngeal dimensions
	Low palate
	Retrognathia or micrognathia

Otorhinolaryngology referral for evaluation and, possibly, fiberoptic pharyngoscopy can provide additional information, especially in patients with incomplete response to medical therapy or for those who are considering surgery for their snoring. However, pharyngoscopic features do not reliably predict responses to surgical interventions for snoring.

Polysomnography

PSG is not routinely indicated in the evaluation of snorers. Nevertheless, it may be helpful in patients contemplating upper airway surgery, especially if other symptoms suggestive of OSA, such as daytime sleepiness, are present. Primary snoring is not associated with arousals, oxygen desaturation, apnea-hypopneas, hypoventilation, or significant cardiac arrhythmias. Snoring is often most frequent and loudest during NREM stages 3 and 4 sleep. Snoring intensity often diminishes during REM sleep. Snoring is identified (1) during PSG by using microphones or sound/vibration sensors placed on the neck or near the oronasal opening or (2) from reports of audible snoring by sleep technologists.

Snoring can produce changes in airflow or oscillations in the nasal pressure or pneumotachograph tracing and greater negative deflections in esophageal pressure recordings. Blood pressure may rise, or fail to decrease, with episodes of snoring.

Differential Diagnosis

Differential diagnosis of snoring includes stridor due to laryngeal narrowing, sleep talking, and expiratory groaning during sleep (catathrenia).. Otorhinolaryngologic and neurologic evaluation is typically normal in patients with catathrenia.

Therapy

Patients with problematic snoring should be advised to avoid smoking and alcohol consumption, as well as to restrict the use of muscle relaxants and sedatives. Weight reduction may benefit those who are overweight. If snoring occurs predominantly or exclusively during a supine sleep position, measures to maintain a nonsupine posture during sleep may be useful. Alternatively, the bed partner can be offered noise-reducing therapies, such as the use of earplugs.

Nasal congestion, if present, should be addressed appropriately. Medical therapies for nasal congestion may include avoidance of allergens, oral antihistamines, and nasal sprays (decongestants, anticholinergics, or corticosteroids). The Clinical Practice Committee of the AASM recently reported that there is currently insufficient information to provide standards of practice recommendations for external nasal dilator strips, internal nasal dilator devices, and oral-nasal lubricants for snoring because of limited data available on the beneficial effect of these therapeutic approaches. Nasal surgery (eg, septoplasty for nasal septal deviation, polypectomy for nasal polyps, and turbinectomy for engorged nasal turbinates) may be indicated for patients with significant nasal narrowing or obstruction.

Although appropriately titrated CPAP therapy eliminates snoring, medical insurers do not universally cover this form of therapy.

Oral devices designed to advance the mandible or tongue anteriorly are effective treatment options for snoring. Clinical guidelines for the use of oral devices in patients with snoring or OSA have been published.

Surgery to reduce or eliminate snoring includes radiofrequency surgery of the soft palate, laser-assisted uvulopalatoplasty (LAUP), uvulopalatopharyngoplasty (UPPP), injection snoreplasty, and palatal implants to reduce palatal flutter.

Upper Airway Resistance Syndrome

Definition

Upper airway resistance syndrome (UARS) is a term that has been proposed to describe a pattern of repetitive sleep-related episodes of increasing resistance in the upper airways with a decrease in inspiratory airflow, increased or constant respiratory effort, and arousals from sleep (referred to as respiratory effort related arousals [RERAs]). The AHI is less than five events per hour, and there is no accompanying oxygen desaturation. Snoring may or may not be present.

It is postulated that patients with UARS have a lower arousal threshold in response to increases in respiratory effort compared to patients with OSA.

Demographics

UARS can affect individuals of all ages. There is no apparent gender difference in prevalence. Compared to patients with OSA, those with UARS are generally younger and leaner.

Consequences

Frequent arousals associated with UARS can result in sleep fragmentation. Affected individuals often complain of excessive sleepiness and fatigue. Patients may also present with less specific somatic complaints, such as sleep-onset insomnia, headaches, myalgias, history of fainting, and irritable bowel syndrome. There appears to be a higher prevalence of systemic hypertension associated with this syndrome. Hypotension can also develop.

Evaluation

UARS should be excluded in patients presenting with unexplained daytime sleepiness or in those with a presumptive diagnosis of idiopathic hypersomnia. Minor and subtle upper airway abnormalities may be appreciated during physical examination. Other possible features include postural hypotension, cold extremities, and orthostasis during tilt table testing. PSG often demonstrates an increase in wake time after sleep onset and decreased duration of NREM stages 3 and 4 sleep. Alpha delta sleep and bruxism may be present.

Accurate identification of UARS is hampered by the lack of standardized diagnostic criteria. Various definitions have been used, including the presence of EEG arousals following one to three breaths with increased inspiratory effort (more negative peak end-inspiratory esophageal pressure [Pes] swings) and decrement in airflow. Pes is an indicator of respiratory effort. This is then followed by less negative Pes excursions as airflow increases during arousals.

Nasal cannula/pressure transducers may demonstrate an inspiratory "plateau" pattern (flattened contour of the tracing) corresponding to the increasingly negative pleural pressure excursions preceding arousals, followed by a rounded contour during arousals. Nasal cannula/pressure transducers are more accurate than thermistors in detecting UARS, but may, nonetheless, still fail to detect all abnormal breathing episodes during sleep. Two types of breathing patterns have been described in patients with UARS, namely a crescendo pattern or a continuously high respiratory effort pattern (Table 5–19). Respiratory events may be accompanied by increases in heart rate and blood pressure and changes in electrocardiographic R-R intervals.

Table 5–19. Types of breathing patterns in upper airway resistance syndrome

Breathing patterns	Sleep stage
Crescendo pattern consisting of a progressively more negative peak end-inspiratory esophageal pressures	NREM stages 1 and 2 sleep
Regular and continuously high respiratory efforts	NREM stages 3 and 4 sleep

Therapy

A variety of therapeutic approaches have been described for patients with UARS, including nasal CPAP, anterior mandibular positioning devices, and upper airway surgery (eg, tonsillectomy and adenoidectomy for pediatric cases, or palatal surgery).

Central Sleep Apnea Syndrome

Central sleep apnea (CSA) is characterized by repetitive apneic episodes lasting at least 10 seconds each occurring during sleep without associated ventilatory efforts. Many patients with CSA also have some obstructive respiratory events.

Demographics

The true incidence of idiopathic CSA is not known but appears to be rare. CSA is estimated to represent about 5% to 10% of patients with sleep-related breathing disorders. CSA also accounts for up to 12% of adult patients with insomnia. Prevalence of CSA is greater among men, and increases in middle-aged and older adults.

CSA can result from a failure of ventilatory drive (idiopathic form) or may be due to secondary causes such as CHF or neurologic disorders. The idiopathic form is less common than secondary causes. Central apneas can also occur during sleep-onset in otherwise healthy individuals and during sleep at high altitude.

Risk Factors

Factors that increase the risk of developing CSA include:

1.   High CO_2 ventilatory drive

2.   Sleep disturbance: Increased frequency of sleep-wake transitions

3.   Gender: Men are more likely to have central apneas due to a higher hypocapnic apneic threshold during NREM sleep

4.   Age: Central apneas are more common in older adults due to the increased prevalence of underlying medical disorders (eg, CHF), neurologic disorders, or greater sleep disturbance and awakenings

5.   Altitude: Central apneas can develop acutely following ascent to high altitudes

6.   Nasal obstruction

Clinical Features

Clinical manifestations are diverse and may include insomnia, daytime hypersomnolence, and repetitive nighttime awakenings. Manifestations of CSA are presented in Table 5–20.

Table 5–20.   Manifestations of central sleep apnea

Clinical features	Associated features	Physical features
Excessive sleepiness	Nocturnal hypoxemia and hypercapnia	Peripheral edema
Sleep disturbance with repeated nocturnal awakenings	Cardiovascular disorders	Cyanosis
Nocturnal sensation of dyspnea	Systemic hypertension	Shallow breathing
Morning headaches	Pulmonary hypertension	
Insomnia	Cor pulmonale	
Note: Patients may be asymptomatic.	Cardiac arrhythmias (sinus arrhythmia [with bradycardia occurring at apnea termination], bradycardia, sinus arrest, premature ventricular contractions, or ventricular tachycardia)	
	Respiratory insufficiency	
	Polycythemia	
	Depression	
	Cognitive impairment	
	Impotence	

Classification of Central Sleep Apnea

Central sleep apnea can be classified based on:

1.   Underlying level of ventilation—hypercapnic or non-hypercapnic; or

2.   Etiology—idiopathic or secondary

In hypercapnic CSA, persons with ventilatory impairment due to neuromuscular diseases affecting the respiratory apparatus or due to diminished chemoresponsiveness can manifest with central apneas or hypopneas. On the other hand, nonhypercapnic CSA consists of idiopathic CSA or central apnea in patients with CHF. For further information, see Table 5–21.

Table 5–21. Classification of central sleep apnea based on ventilatory response

Classification	Characteristics
Hypercapnic	Associated with daytime hypoventilation (high waking $PaCO_2$) Diminished response to hypercapnia Hypoventilation continues during sleep. Includes patients with central alveolar hypoventilation, neuromuscular disorders, or neurologic disorders (affecting the brainstem)
Nonhypercapnic	Not associated with daytime hypoventilation (normal or low waking $PaCO_2$) Increased ventilatory response to hypercapnia $PaCO_2$ levels increase during sleep; brief arousals are accompanied by a hyperventilatory "overshoot" that decreases $PaCO_2$ levels below the apneic threshold and leads to central apneas Includes patients with idiopathic CSA, postarousal CSA, congestive heart failure, sleep at high altitude, or during CPAP titration

CSA can be idiopathic (primary) or secondary to other medical disorders, such as cardiac, renal and neurologic (eg, brainstem lesions) conditions. Finally, central sleep apnea can arise from chronic use of long-acting opioids, including methadone, hydrocodone (time-release preparations), and morphine (time-release preparations). Secondary forms of CSA are more common than the idiopathic form.

Pathophysiology of Central Sleep Apnea

During the waking state, respiration is controlled by two processes, namely the metabolic (automatic) and behavioral (voluntary) systems (Table 5–22). During NREM sleep, the wake-related

Table 5–22.   Respiratory control systems

Control system	Characteristics
Metabolic	Consists of chemoreceptors for hypoxia (carotid body) and hypercapnia (carotid body and medulla) as well as brainstem systems that regulate ventilation to maintain stable levels of pH, PaO_2 and $PaCO_2$
Behavioral	Respiration can be altered by behavior (eg, eating or talking) via input from the forebrain

drive to breathe and behavioral control systems are abolished, and respiration is controlled entirely by the metabolic control system, primarily by the hypercapnic ventilatory drive (ie, ventilation is stimulated by hypercapnia) and to a lesser degree by the hypoxic ventilatory drive (ie, ventilation is stimulated by hypoxia). A $PaCO_2$ above the apneic threshold stimulates ventilation, whereas a $PaCO_2$ below this threshold leads to a central apnea that continues until $PaCO_2$ increases and once again exceeds the apneic threshold.

Etiology

Central sleep apnea has diverse causes, each with its specific pathophysiologic mechanism(s). The causal factors involved in CSA are presented in Box 5–22.

Box 5–22. Etiology of central sleep apnea	Medical disorders
	
	    Congestive heart failure
	
	    Endocrine disorders (eg diabetes mellitus, acromegaly, or myxedema)
	
	    Nasal obstruction
	
	Neurologic disorders
	
	    Autonomic dysfunction (familial dysautonomia, multisystem atrophy, Parkinson disease, Shy-Drager syndrome, or diabetes mellitus)
	
	    Brainstem (medulla) tumors, infarctions, or hemorrhage
	
	    Encephalitis
	
	    Head injury
	
	    Amyotrophic lateral sclerosis
	
	    Neuromuscular diseases (myasthenia gravis, myopathy, muscular dystrophy, or myotonia congenita)
	
	    Poliomyelitis and postpolio syndrome
	
	    Stroke
	
	Miscellaneous
	
	    At sleep onset
	
	    Following therapy of OSA with CPAP or tracheotomy
	
	    After ascent to high altitude
	
	    Medication use (eg, opiates)
	
	    Prematurity

Idiopathic Central Sleep Apnea

The etiology of idiopathic CSA is unknown. In patients with idiopathic CSA, carbon dioxide (CO_2) ventilatory drive is increased. Thus, $PaCO_2$ is low during wakefulness and sleep.

Congestive Heart Failure

Both central and obstructive apneas can develop in persons with CHF, and the predominant type of respiratory event appears to depend on the size and collapsibility of the individual's upper airway. CSA is present in about 50% of patients with CHF. A correlation between CSA and decreased left ventricular function (due to a delay in circulatory time to respiratory control centers) and lower awake $PaCO_2$ is present. CSA is more common in persons with increased hypercapnic chemoresponsiveness during wakefulness than in those with a normal $PaCO_2$.

Types of sleep-related breathing disorders in patients with CHF are listed in Box 5–23.

Box 5–23. **Types of sleep-related breathing disorders in patients with congestive heart failure**	Central sleep apnea Cheyne-Stokes respiration Obstructive sleep apnea

Neurologic Disorders

Several neurologic and neuromuscular disorders can decrease central ventilatory drive and give rise to CSA. Patients are usually hypercapnic.

Sleep-Onset Central Apneas

As sleep states oscillate between sleep and wake-drowsiness at sleep onset, repetitive episodes of central apneas may occur if $PaCO_2$ (higher during sleep and lower during wakefulness) fluctuates above or below the apneic threshold. Sleep-onset central apneas are generally transient, disappearing once stable sleep is attained (ie, when $PaCO_2$ is maintained continuously at higher levels). Frequency of central apneas is normally less than five episodes per hour of sleep. Repetitive sleep-onset central apneas can result in sleep-initiation insomnia.

Central Sleep Apnea Related to Medication Use

Central apneas can develop during administration of opiate drugs. Aside from central apneas, other respiratory pattern abnormalities, such as periodic breathing, Biot respiration, and obstructive hypoventilation, can develop due to μ-receptor-related depression of the hypercapnic ventilatory drive and increase in hypoxic ventilatory drive.

Central Apnea During Positive Airway Pressure Titration

Central sleep apnea may emerge during CPAP titration in patients with OSA. This may be due to unmasking of a previously concurrent central apnea that becomes apparent when the more predominant obstructive events are controlled by CPAP therapy. Alternatively, it may be due to recurrent arousals related to the use of CPAP with central arousals occurring in the postarousal period.

Clinical Course

Prognosis of persons with CSA is variable. When CSA is related to another condition (eg, CHF), the clinical outcome is related to the severity of the underlying disorder. Cheyne-Stokes respiration (CSR) is believed to be a poor prognostic sign for patients with CHF.

Evaluation

Polysomnography is necessary for the diagnosis of CSA. See Box 5–24 for further information. Central apneas tend to occur more frequently at sleep onset and during NREM stages 1 and 2 sleep. Respiratory events are less frequent during NREM stages 3 and 4 sleep, and REM sleep.

Awake $PaCO_2$ is typically normal or low.

Differential Diagnosis

Central sleep apnea has to be differentiated from Cheyne-Stokes respiration, which has a crescendo-decrescendo breathing pattern. A comparison of central and obstructive apneas is given in Table 5–23.

Therapy

The decision to initiate treatment should be individualized, as is the selection of therapeutic modalities (Box 5–25). Intervention is generally not necessary for sleep-onset central apneas that resolve spontaneously as sleep progresses and that do not give rise to sleep-initiation insomnia. Therapy varies depending on whether the patient has (1) idiopathic or secondary CSA or (2) hypercapnic or nonhypercapnic forms of CSA. Response to therapy should be closely monitored. Therapy for sleep-related breathing disorders in patients with CHF may improve cardiac function (left ventricular ejection fraction). Data regarding benefits related to cardiac transplantation rates and survival are conflicting.

Box 5-24. **Polysomnographic features of central apneas**	Pauses in respiration and absent ventilatory effort lasting 10 seconds or longer
	Loss of chest and abdominal movement (strain gauge or respiratory inductance plethysmography)
	No electromyographic (EMG) activity of the respiratory muscles including diaphragm
	No change in intrathoracic pressures (esophageal balloon)
	Central hypopneas have a rounded profile on nasal pressure monitoring
	Associated with oxygen desaturation (generally mild) and, occasionally, arousals
	In patients with obstructive, central and mixed apneas, at least 80% of the respiratory events are central in nature
	At least five central apneas per hour of sleep
	Snoring may occur (less prominent than in obstructive sleep apnea)
	Changes in sleep architecture
	↑ NREM stages 1 and 2 sleep
	↓ NREM stages 3 and 4 sleep

Table 5–23. Comparison between central and obstructive apneas

Characteristic	Central apneas	Obstructive apneas
Oxygen desaturation	Mild	Worse
Hemodynamic changes	Less	Greater
Concurrent respiratory effort	Absent	Present

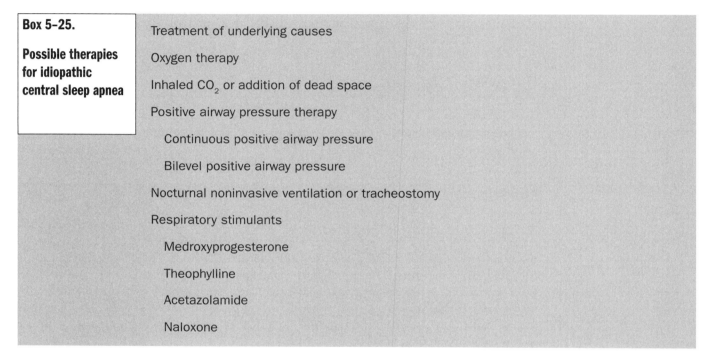

Box 5–25.

Possible therapies for idiopathic central sleep apnea

Treatment of underlying causes

Oxygen therapy

Inhaled CO_2 or addition of dead space

Positive airway pressure therapy

    Continuous positive airway pressure

    Bilevel positive airway pressure

Nocturnal noninvasive ventilation or tracheostomy

Respiratory stimulants

    Medroxyprogesterone

    Theophylline

    Acetazolamide

    Naloxone

Therapy for Underlying Causes of Central Sleep Apnea

Treatment of underlying causes of CSA (eg, CHF) may reduce or eliminate central apneas. Benzodiazepines, narcotics, and other sedatives that may suppress respiratory drive should be avoided in patients with hypercapnic forms of CSA.

Oxygen Therapy

By stabilizing the respiratory control centers, supplemental oxygen therapy may reduce nonhypercapnic CSAs in some but not all patients. It minimizes hypoxemia, and in so doing, reduces the hypocapnia induced by reflex hyperventilation, and increases the level of $PaCO_2$ above the apneic threshold. Hypoxemia can also directly suppress ventilation; this is reversed by oxygen therapy. Close monitoring of arterial blood gas (ABG) parameters is crucial, because oxygen therapy in some patients (particularly those with hypercapnic central sleep apnea) can result in worsening hypercapnia.

Positive Airway Pressure Therapy

Positive airway pressure therapy can improve cardiac function (increase in left ventricular ejection fraction and reduction in left ventricular afterload) in patients with CSA due to CHF, particularly those with elevated pulmonary capillary wedge pressures. Mechanisms by which positive airway pressure therapy improve CSA are listed in Box 5–26.

Box 5–26. **Mechanisms by which positive airway pressure therapy improves central sleep apnea**	Improvement of oxygen saturation Mild increase in PaCO$_2$ (moving it closer to the apneic threshold) Prevention of reflex inhibition of ventilation following upper airway obstruction or narrowing

Nocturnal Noninvasive Ventilation

Patients with severe CSA can be mechanically ventilated during sleep. Ventilation can improve ABG parameters. Titration of positive airways pressures can be aided by PSG accompanied by serial ABG measurements.

Pharmacologic Therapy

Several pharmacologic agents, including acetazolamide, theophylline, and hypnotic agents, have been used to treat CSA.

Acetazolamide, a carbonic anhydrase inhibitor, acts by inducing a mild degree of metabolic acidosis from bicarbonate diuresis, which, in turn, increases respiratory drive. It is effective in improving CSA in some patients (eg, high-altitude periodic respiration).

Theophylline, an adenosine antagonist, is a respiratory stimulant as well as a positive inotropic agent. Its use has been described in CSA or CSR associated with CHF, and in CSA related to immaturity in newborns.

Medroxyprogesterone can stimulate ventilation and has been used in patients with obesity hypoventilation syndrome.

Hypnotic agents can be tried in patients without significant hypoxemia to help consolidate sleep and decrease sleep fragmentation. Hypnotic agents may permit patients to sleep through sleep-onset central apneas and allow them to reach deeper stages of sleep. Patients must be monitored closely for adverse effects because benzodiazepines could inhibit ventilation and worsen hypoventilation and oxygenation in patients with hypercapnic forms of CSA.

Cheyne-Stokes Respiration

Cheyne Stokes respiration CSR is characterized by periodic breathing with recurring periods of crescendo-decrescendo ventilation separate by central apneas or hypopneas.

Etiology

The mechanism is believed to be instability of the control of ventilation related, in part, to a long circulation time, lower daytime and sleep-related PaCO$_2$ levels (< 45 mm Hg), and greater hypercapnic respiratory drive (leading to an "overshoot" of ventilation, as well as a fall in PaCO$_2$ below the apneic threshold) compared with patients with CHF but without CSR. In patients with CHF, hyperventilation can also arise from stimulation of pulmonary vagal receptors by pulmonary congestion.

CSR-related arousals generally occur at the peak of ventilation or a few breaths after ventilation resumes (unlike that of OSA in which arousals occur at the termination of apnea). In addition, the period of hyperpnea is longer, and the waxing and waning of ventilation is less abrupt (typically > 45 seconds in duration) compared with other forms of CSA. Cycle length is related inversely to cardiac output, and directly to circulation time. There is typically also a delay in the nadir of oxygen desaturation following the apneic events. Arousals, if frequent, result in sleep fragmentation, insomnia, or daytime sleepiness. Patients may also report nocturnal episodes of dyspnea.

The development of CSR in patients with CHF is correlated with ejection fraction and is associated with a worse prognosis (ie, increased risk of death and higher frequency of transplantation). In addition to CHF in which CSR can be seen in up to 40% to 50% of patients, CSR can also be caused by neurologic disorders (eg, prevalence of about 10% in strokes), renal failure, or occur in an idiopathic form without any identifiable underlying cause. In patients with CHF, the likelihood of CSR is increased in those with atrial fibrillation, low awake $PaCO_2$, and age > 60 years. Males are affected more commonly than women.

Differential Diagnosis

Differential diagnosis includes OSA, primary CSA, periodic breathing related to high altitude, and sleep-related hypoventilation syndromes.

Evaluation

During PSG, CSR generally occurs during the transition from wakefulness to sleep and during NREM stages 1 and 2 sleep. It attenuates or resolves during NREM stages 3 and 4 sleep and REM sleep. By definition, there are at least 10 episodes of central apneas/hypopneas per hour of sleep. Arousals and modest oxygen desaturation may accompany the respiratory events.

Therapy

Therapy consists of improving cardiac function (via a reduction in both sympathetic tone and afterload), low-flow oxygen supplementation (1 to 4 liters per minute), nasal CPAP, BPAP, or adaptive servoventilation (ASV). With ASV, the pressure support delivered (difference between maximum IPAP and minimum IPAP) increases during periods of hypoventilation and decreases with hyperventilation.

CPAP appears to reduce CSR by increasing $PaCO_2$, enhancing cardiac function, and improving oxygen saturation. CPAP has also been shown to improve survival in patients with CHF in some studies but not in others. Nasal CPAP can be started at an empiric pressure of 10 to 12 cm H20 with follow-up PSG recommended to assess therapeutic efficacy.

Periodic Breathing Secondary to High Altitude

Periodic breathing, or cycles of central apneas and hyperpneas, can occur on ascent to high altitude (usually > 4000 to 7600 meters). Severity of symptoms is influenced by elevation, speed of ascent, and individual predisposition. Persons with increased hypoxic ventilatory chemoresponsiveness appear to have a greater risk for developing high-altitude–related periodic breathing. Rapid ascent and extreme altitudes also increase the risk and severity of high-altitude periodic breathing. Men may be affected more commonly than women.

Hyperventilation due to hypoxia on ascent to altitude gives rise to hypocapnic (low $PaCO_2$) alkalosis that, in turn, results in central apneas during sleep, particularly NREM sleep, on the first few nights at altitude. Ventilation resumes as $PaCO_2$ rises and PaO_2 falls during the apneic episode. Respiration stabilizes during REM sleep, possibly related to the decrease in hypoxic ventilatory response. Symptoms, including frequent awakenings, nocturnal dyspnea, sleepiness, and fatigue, generally improve over time with adaptation unless elevation is extreme.

Polysomnographic features of high-altitude periodic breathing are listed in Box 5–27. Therapy consists of either oxygen therapy or administration of acetazolamide.

Box 5-27.
 	
Polysomnographic features of high-altitude periodic breathing
	Repetitive central apneas 10 seconds or longer in duration occurring about every 12 to 34 seconds primarily during NREM sleep
	
	  Can be associated with oxygen desaturation
	
	  Can result in arousals
	
	Respiration is more regular during REM sleep
	
	Sleep architecture
	
	  No change in total sleep time
	
	  ↑ Frequency of arousals
	
	  ↑ NREM stages 1 and 2 sleep
	
	  ↓ NREM stages 3 and 4 sleep
	
	  No change in REM sleep

Obesity Hypoventilation Syndrome

Definition

The two essential features of obesity hypoventilation syndrome (OHS) are the presence of severe obesity (defined as a body mass index $\geq$ 40 kg/m^2) and hypercapnia ($PaCO_2$ > 45 mmHg) during wakefulness. Hypoventilation is not due to another respiratory or neuromuscular disorder. Many patients with OHS also have OSA.

Clinical Features

Clinical manifestations include excessive sleepiness, insomnia, sleep fragmentation with frequent arousals, decreased attention or concentration, peripheral edema and cyanosis. Chronic hypoxemia can result in polycythemia, pulmonary hypertension, and cor pulmonale.

Pathophysiology

Excess weight is important in the pathogenesis of OHS. Severe obesity can be associated with mild to moderate degrees of restrictive ventilatory impairment. However, OHS is uncommon even among obese persons.

The causes of hypercapnia in OHS are presented in Box 5–28.

Box 5-28.
 	
Etiology of hypercapnia in obesity hypoventilation syndrome
	Increased production of CO_2 due to greater work of breathing
	
	   Decreased chest wall compliance
	
	Decreased ventilation
	
	   Decreased expiratory reserve volume
	
	   Decreased tidal volume
	
	   Increased resistive load
	
	   Increased dead space
	
	Decreased ventilatory response to hypercapnia and hypoxemia

Box 5-29. Causes of hypercapnia in patients with obstructive sleep apnea	OSA and obesity hypoventilation syndrome Overlap syndrome (OSA and chronic obstructive pulmonary disease)

Evaluation and Differential Diagnosis

Evaluation may disclose the presence of periodic respiration, hypoxemia, pulmonary hypertension, and polycythemia. Differential diagnosis includes other causes of chronic hypoventilation (eg, severe chronic obstructive pulmonary disease [FEV_1 < 1 liter or < 40% of predicted], neuromuscular disorders, demyelinating illnesses, brainstem strokes, poliomyelitis, or diaphragmatic paralysis). *Overlap syndrome* consists of both OSA and chronic obstructive pulmonary disease. Idiopathic central alveolar hypoventilation involving nonobese individuals is due to a defect in ventilatory chemoreceptors in the medulla and has also been described. OSA is present in many cases of OHS, but patients may present without OSA. The causes of hypercapnia in OSA are listed in Box 5–29.

Compared with patients with OSA, diurnal ABG measurements are worse and pulmonary artery hypertension is more prevalent in those with OHS.

Therapy

Noninvasive mechanical ventilation (NIMV), including BPAP delivered by a nasal mask, during sleep are effective therapies. The use of NIMV can improve sleepiness, dyspnea, morning headaches, leg edema and ABG parameters. Gastric surgery for morbid obesity may also be beneficial for selected individuals.

No pharmacologic agent has been found to be consistently effective for OHS. Medroxyprogesterone, theophylline, and acetazolamide possess respiratory stimulant properties and can improve hypoxemia and hypercapnia. Acetazolamide is a carbonic anhydrase inhibitor that induces metabolic acidosis, which, in turn, increases ventilation.

For a summary of therapeutic modalities in OHS, see Box 5–30.

Congenital Central Hypoventilation Syndrome

Definition

In patients with congenital central hypoventilation syndrome (Ondine's curse or primary alveolar hypoventilation syndrome; CCHS), hypoventilation and failure of the autonomic respiratory

| Box 5–30.

Therapy for obesity hypoventilation syndrome | Noninvasive mechanical ventilation with or without oxygen therapy

    Continuous positive airway pressure

    Bilevel positive airway pressure

    Volume cycled ventilation

Weight reduction, including bariatric surgery for morbid obesity.

Pharmacologic therapy (limited usefulness)

    Medroxyprogesterone

    Theophylline

    Acetazolamide

Endotracheal intubation or tracheostomy, and mechanical ventilation (required in cases of severe acute respiratory failure) |

control are present from birth. A disorder of central chemoreceptor responsiveness, rather than respiratory or neuromuscular disorders, CCHS gives rise to impaired ventilatory responses to hypoxia and hypercapnia.

Clinical Features

The onset of this rare disorder is typically during the newborn period. Both genders are affected. Clinical manifestations of CCHS vary depending on disease severity and can include shallow breathing, episodic apnea, cyanosis, feeding difficulties, bradycardia-tachycardia, and diaphoresis. Apparent life-threatening events, respiratory arrest, or pulmonary hypertension may develop during infancy. Most patients have normal cognitive function. Its course is chronic, with death usually due to respiratory failure or cor pulmonale. Associated features of CCHS are listed in Box 5–31.

| Box 5–31.

Associated features and consequences of congenital central hypoventilation syndrome | Dysfunction of autonomic nervous system control of the heart with decreased heart rate variability, hypotension and arrhythmias (eg, heart block and sick sinus syndrome)

Esophageal dysmotility and swallowing difficulty

Growth impairment with hypotonia or motor delay

Heat intolerance

Hirschsprung disease

Impaired mental processing

Metabolic alkalosis

Ophthalmologic abnormalities (strabismus)

Polycythemia

Seizures

Syncope

Tumors of neural crest derivatives (ie, ganglioneuromas and neuroblastomas) |

Pathophysiology

The lack of ventilatory or arousal responses in CCHS can give rise to significant hypoventilation (reduction in tidal volume and respiratory rate) during sleep with the development of hypoxemia and hypercapnia. Hypoventilation is typically most severe during NREM sleep. Frank central apneas, snoring, or paradoxical breathing are uncommon.

Because affected patients have no subjective sensation of dyspnea, activity and exercise can result in worsening gas exchange with greater hypoxemia and hypercapnia, and a lesser increase in heart rate. Increasing respiratory frequency rather than an augmentation of tidal volume is responsible for the increase in minute ventilation during exercise in these patients.

Genetics

Heterozygous de novo mutations in the PHOX2B gene (autosomal dominant with incomplete penetrance) have been described in patients with CCHS and associated autonomic dysfunction. Most mutations consist of five to nine alanine expansions within a 20-residue polyalanine tract (exon 3). Repeat mutation length correlates with the severity of the CCHS phenotype. Less commonly, patients may have an EDN3 frameshift point mutation.

Differential Diagnosis

CCHS should be distinguished from other causes of chronic hypoventilation such as cardiopulmonary (obesity hypoventilation syndrome or diaphragmatic paralysis), neuromuscular (muscular dystrophy or hypothalamic abnormalities), and metabolic (Leigh disease) disorders. Other congenital syndromes that are associated with abnormalities in respiratory control (eg, Prader-Willi syndrome, Arnold-Chiari malformation, and familial dysautonomia) should also be excluded. The diagnosis of CCHS is aided by genetic testing for mutations of the polyalanine expansion sequence of the PHOX2b gene.

Therapy

Ventilatory support can be provided at home with positive-pressure ventilation (via a tracheostomy or a nasal/oronasal mask), a BPAP device, negative-pressure ventilation, or diaphragm pacing using phrenic nerve stimulation. Patients require either continuous 24-hour ventilatory support or, if they are able to maintain adequate spontaneous respiration while awake, ventilatory support only during sleep.

Other Causes of Sleep-Related Hypoventilation

Reduction in ventilation during sleep giving rise to hypoxemia and hypercapnia may be due to lower airway obstruction, or pulmonary, chest wall or neuromuscular disorders (Table 5–24). These disorders may predispose to the development of neurocognitive impairment, cardiac arrhythmias, pulmonary artery hypertension, cor pulmonale, or polycythemia due to chronic hypoxemia

Arterial blood gas (ABG) analysis during sleep demonstrates an absolute ($PaCO_2 > 45$ mm Hg) or relative hypercapnia compared with levels during wakefulness, with $SaO_2 < 90\%$ (nadir of $\leq 85\%$) for greater than 5 minutes, and $SaO_2 < 90\%$ present in $> 30\%$ of total sleep time, that are not related to apneas or hypopneas.

Table 5-24. Causes of sleep-related hypoventilation

Disorder	Characteristics
Idiopathic (primary)	Not associated with lower airway, chest wall, diaphragm, pulmonary, other medical or neuromuscular disorders Hypoxemic and hypercapnic chemoresponsiveness are decreased, leading to reduced tidal volume and ventilation Appears to be more common among males compared to females; often presents during adolescence or early adulthood Repetitive arousals, if present, can result in complaints of insomnia or excessive sleepiness. Hypoventilation is more severe during REM sleep compared to NREM sleep.

Lower airway obstruction	Causes:
	  Alpha-1 antitrypsin deficiency
	  Bronchiectasis
	  Chronic obstructive pulmonary disease (chronic bronchitis and emphysema)
	  Cystic fibrosis
	The likelihood of sleep-related hypoventilation is greater in patients with FEV_1/FVC (ratio of forced expiratory volume exhaled in one second/forced vital capacity) < 60%, with daytime hypoxemia or hypercapnia, or with comorbid obstructive sleep apnea
	Polysomnographic features:
	↑ Sleep latency
	↓ Sleep efficiency
	↓ NREM stages 3 and 4, and REM sleep

Pulmonary disorders	Causes:
	  Interstitial lung diseases
	  Pulmonary hypertension
	  Sickle cell anemia
	The likelihood of sleep-related hypoventilation is greater in patients with more severe pulmonary parenchyma and vascular disease, or with daytime hypoxemia or hypercapnia

Chest wall or diaphragm disorders	Causes:
	  Diaphragmatic paresis or paralysis (especially if bilateral)
	  Severe kyphoscoliosis
	  Severe obesity
	The likelihood of sleep-related hypoventilation is greater in patients with daytime hypoxemia and hypercapnia.
	Polysomnographic features:
	↑ Frequency of arousals
	↑ Wake time after sleep onset
	↓ REM sleep

Neuromuscular disorders	Causes:
	  Amyotrophic lateral sclerosis
	  Muscular dystrophies
	  Myasthenia gravis or Eaton-Lambert syndrome
	  Myopathies
	  Myxedema
	  Postpolio syndrome
	  Spinal cord trauma or injury
	The likelihood of sleep-related hypoventilation is greater in patients with daytime hypoxemia and hypercapnia, reduced chemosensitivity, or neurologic disorders with bulbar dysfunction.

References

General References

American Academy of Sleep Medicine. *The International Classification of Sleep Disorders: Diagnostic and Coding Manual.* 2nd ed. Westchester, IL: American Academy of Sleep Medicine, 2005.

Bowman TJ. *Review of Sleep Medicine.* Burlington, MA: Butterworth-Heinemann, 2002.

Berry RB. *Sleep Medicine Pearls.* 2nd ed. Philadelphia, PA: Hanley & Belfus, 2002.

Chokroverty S. *Clinical Companion to Sleep Disorders Medicine.* 2nd ed. Butterworth-Heinemann, 2000.

Lavie P, Pillar G, Malhotra A. *Sleep Disorders Handbook.* New York, NY: Taylor & Francis, 2002.

Lee-Chiong TL, ed. *Sleep: A Comprehensive Handbook.* Hoboken, NJ: John Wiley & Sons, 2006.

Lee-Chiong TL, Sateia M, Carskadon M, eds. *Sleep Medicine.* Philadelphia, PA: Hanley & Belfus (Elsevier), 2002.

Perlis ML, Lichstein KL, eds. *Treating Sleep Disorders: Principles and Practice of Behavioral Sleep Medicine.* Hoboken, NJ: John Wiley & Sons, 2003.

Rechtschaffen A, Kales A. *A Manual of Standardized Terminology, Techniques and Scoring System for Sleep Stages of Human Subjects.* Los Angeles, CA: Brain Information Service/Brain Research Institute, University of California, 1968.

Reite M, Ruddy J, Nagel K. *Concise Guide to Evaluation and Management of Sleep Disorders.* 3rd ed. Arlington, VA: American Psychiatric Publishing, April 2002.

Sleep Research Society. *SRS Basics of Sleep Guide.* Westchester, IL: Sleep Research Society, 2005.

Obstructive Sleep Apnea Syndrome

Guilleminault C, Abad VC. Obstructive sleep apnea syndromes. *Sleep Disorders.* Medical Clinics of North America. Philadelphia, PA: Elsevier Saunders, 2004.

Olson EJ, Park JG, Morgenthaler TI. Obstructive sleep apnea-hypopnea syndrome. *Sleep Medicine.* Primary Care: Clinics in Office Practice. Elsevier Saunders, 2005.

Sanders M, Gilvelber RJ. Overview of obstructive sleep apnea in adults. In: Lee-Chiong TL, ed. *Sleep: A Comprehensive Handbook.* Hoboken, NJ: John Wiley & Sons, 2006.

Definition of Terms

Meoli AL, Casey KR, Clark RW, Coleman JA Jr, Fayle RW, et al; Clinical Practice Review Committee. Hypopnea in sleep-disordered breathing in adults. *Sleep.* 2001(Jun 15);24(4):469–70.

Demographics

Young T, Palta M, Dempsey J, Skatrud J, Weber S, Badr S. The occurrence of sleep-disordered breathing among middle-aged adults. *N Engl J Med.* 1993(Apr 29);328(17):1230–5.

Pathophysiology

Woodson BT. Physiology of sleep disordered breathing. In: Lee-Chiong TL, ed. *Sleep: A Comprehensive Handbook.* Hoboken, NJ: John Wiley & Sons, 2006.

Risk Factors

Ancoli-Israel S, Kripke DF, Zorick F, Roth T. Effects of a single dose of flurazepam on the sleep of healthy volunteers. *Arzneimittel-Forschung.* 1984;34(1):99–100.

Berry RB, Kouchi K, Bower J, Prosise G, Light RW. Triazolam in patients with obstructive sleep apnea. *Am J Respir Crit Care Med.* 1995(Feb);151(2 Pt 1):450–454.

Camacho ME, Morin CM. The effect of temazepam on respiration in elderly insomniacs with mild sleep apnea. *Sleep.* 1995(Oct);18(8):644–645.

Clyburn PA, Rosen M, Vickers MD. Comparison of the respiratory effects of i.v. infusions of morphine and regional analgesia by extradural block. *British Journal of Anaesthesia.* 1990(Apr); 64(4):446–449.

Dolly FR, Block AJ. Effect of flurazepam on sleep-disordered breathing and nocturnal oxygen desaturation in asymptomatic subjects. *Am J Med.* 1982;73(2):239–243.

Hoijer U, Hedner J, Ejnell H, Grunstein R, Odelberg E, Elam M. Nitrazepam in patients with sleep apnoea: a double-blind placebo-controlled study. *Eur Respir J.* 1994 Nov;7(11):2011–2015.

Lofaso F, Goldenberg F, Thebault C, Janus C, Harf A. Effect of zopiclone on sleep, night-time ventilation, and daytime vigilance in upper airway resistance syndrome. *European Respiratory Journal.* 1997;10(11):2573–2577.

Steens RD, Pouliot Z, Millar TW, Kryger MH, George CF. Effects of zolpidem and triazolam on sleep and respiration in mild to moderate chronic obstructive pulmonary disease. *Sleep.* 1993;16(4):318–326.

Genetic Syndromes Associated with Obstructive Sleep Apnea

Abyholm F, D'Antonio L, Davidson Ward SL, Kjoll L, Saeed M,, et al; VPI Surgical Group. Pharyngeal flap and sphincterplasty for velopharyngeal insufficiency have equal outcome at 1 year postoperatively: results of a randomized trial. *Cleft Palate Craniofac J.* 2005(Sep);42(5):501–11.

Aoe T, Kohchi T, Mizuguchi T. Respiratory inductance plethysmography and pulse oximetry in the assessment of upper airway patency in a child with Goldenhar's syndrome. *Can J Anaesth.* 1990(Apr);37(3):369–71.

Bayraktar S, Bayraktar ST, Ataoglu E, Ayaz A, Elevli M. Goldenhar's syndrome associated with multiple congenital abnormalities. *J Trop Pediatr.* 2005;Dec;51(6):377–9. Epub 2005 Sep 26.

Bull MJ, Givan DC, Sadove AM, et al. Improved outcome in Pierre Robin sequence: effect of multidisciplinary evaluation and management. *Pediatrics.* 1990;86:294–301.

Chan D, Li AM, Yam MC, Li CK, Fok TF. Hurler's syndrome with cor pulmonale secondary to obstructive sleep apnoea treated by continuous positive airway pressure. *J Paediatr Child Health.* 2003;39(7):558–9.

Colmenero C, Esteban R, Albarino AR, Colmenero B: Sleep apnea syndrome associated with maxillofacial abnormalities. *J Laryngology Otology.* 1991;105:94–100.

Cooney TP, Thurlbeck WM. Pulmonary hypoplasia in Down's syndrome. *N Engl J Med.* 1982;307:1170–1173.

Deegan PC, McGlone B, McNicholas WT. Treatment of Robin sequence with nasal CPAP. *Journal of Laryngology and Otology.* 1995;109:328–330.

Donaldson JD, Redmond WM. Surgical management of obstructive sleep apnea in children with Down syndrome. *J Otolaryngology.* 1988;17:398–403.

Freed GF, Pearlman MA, Brown AS, Barot LR. Polysomnographic indications for surgical intervention in Pierre Robin sequence: acute airway management and follow-up studies after repair and take down of tongue lip adhesion. *Cleft Palate J.* 1988;25:151–155.

Hassell S, Butler MG. Antley-Bixler syndrome: report of a patient and review of literature. *Clin Genet.* 1994(Nov);46(5):372–6.

Hui S, Wing YK, Kew J, Chan YL, Abdullah V, Fok TF. Obstructive sleep apnea syndrome in a family with Crouzon's syndrome. *Sleep.* 1998(May 1);21(3):298–303.

Johnston C, Taussig LM, Koopmann C, et al. Obstructive sleep apnea in Treacher-Collins syndrome. *Cleft Palate Journal.* 1981;18:39–44.

Jones KL. Smith's recognizable patterns of human malformation. Philadelphia, PA: WB Saunders, 1997. pp. 234–235.

Kaplan LC. Clinical assessment and multi specialty management of Apert syndrome. *Clinics in Plastic Surgery.* 1991;18:217–225.

Kronwith SD, Quinn G, McDonald DM, Cardonick E, Onyx P, LaRossa D, et al. Stickler's syndrome in the cleft palate clinic. *J Pediatr Ophthalmol Strabismus.* 1990(Sep–Oct);27(5):265–7.

Liao YF, Yun C, Huang CS, Chen PK, Chen NH, Hung KF, et al. Longitudinal follow-up of obstructive sleep apnea following Furlow palatoplasty in children with cleft palate: a preliminary report. *Cleft Palate Craniofac J.* 2003(May);40(3):269–73.

Malone BN, Whitley CB, Duvall AJ, et al. Resolution of obstructive sleep apnea in Hurler syndrome after bone marrow transplantation. *Int J Pediatr Otorhinolaryngol.* 1988;15(1):23–31.

Marcus CL, Keens TG, Bautista DB, et al. Obstructive sleep apnea in children with Down syndrome. *Pediatrics.* 1991;88:132–139.

Mixter RC, David DJ, Perloff WH, Green CG, Pauli RM, Popic PM. Obstructive sleep apnea in Apert's and Pfeiffer's syndromes: more than a craniofacial abnormality. *Plast Reconstr Surg.* 1990 Sep;86(3):457–63.

Monroe CW, Ogo K. Treatment of micrognathia in the neonatal period. *Plast Reconstr Surg.* 1972;50:317–325.

Nielsen CE. Stickler's syndrome. *Acta Ophthalmol (Copenh).* 1981(Apr);59(2):286–95.

Noorily MR, Farmer DL, Belenky WM, Philippart AI. Congenital tracheal anomalies in the craniosynostosis syndromes. *J Pediatr Surg.* 1999(Jun);34(6):1036–9.

Orliaguet O, Pepin JL, Veale D, Kelkel E, Pinel N, Levy P. Hunter's syndrome and associated sleep apnoea cured by CPAP and surgery. *Eur Respir J.* 1999;13(5):1195–7.

Orr WC, Levine NS, Buchanan RT. Effect of cleft palate repair and pharyngeal flap surgery on upper airway obstruction during sleep. *Plast Reconstr Surg.* 1987(Aug);80(2):226–32.

Perkins JA, Sie KC, Milczuk H, Richardson MA. Airway management in children with craniofacial anomalies. *Cleft Palate Craniofac J.* 1997(Mar);34(2):135–40.

Rose E, Thissen U, Otten JE, Jonas I. Cephalometric assessment of the posterior airway space in patients with cleft palate after palatoplasty. *Cleft Palate Craniofac J.* 2003(Sep);40(5):498–503.

Saint Raymond C, Bettega G, Deschaux C, Lebeau J, Raphael B, Levy P, et al. Sphincter pharyngoplasty as a treatment of velopharyngeal incompetence in young people: a prospective evaluation of effects on sleep structure and sleep respiratory disturbances. *Chest.* 2004(Mar);125(3):864–71.

Shapiro J, Strome M, Crocker AC. Airway obstruction and sleep apnea in Hurler and Hunter syndromes. *Ann Otol Rhinol Laryngol.* 1985;94(5 Pt 1):458–61.

Strome M. Obstructive sleep apnea in Down syndrome children: a surgical approach. *Laryngoscope.* 1986;96:1340–1342.

Treacher Collins Syndrome Collaborative Group. Positional cloning of a gene involved in the pathogenesis of Treacher Collins syndrome. *Nature Genet.* 1996;12:130–136.

Uemura T, Hayashi T, Satoh K, Mitsukawa N, Yoshikawa A, Jinnnai T, et al. A case of improved obstructive sleep apnea by distraction osteogenesis for midface hypoplasia of an infantile Crouzon's syndrome. *J Craniofac Surg.* 2001(Jan);12(1):73–7.

Wang KT, Wei FC, Zhao HQ, Song L, Wang Y, Chen AW. A serious complication-obstructive sleep apnea hypopnea syndrome after velopharyngeal ring ligation procedure: report of 6 cases. *Shanghai Kou Qiang Yi Xue.* 2005(Ap)r;14(2):123–6.

Wise CA, Chiang LC, Paznekas W A, et al. TCOF 1 gene encodes a putative nuclear phosphoprotein that exhibits mutations in Treacher Collins syndrome throughout its coding region. *Proc Nat Acad Sci.* 1997;94:3110–3115.

Evaluation and Management of Upper Airway Anatomic Abnormalities

Schwab RJ, Kline NS. Radiographic and endoscopic evaluation of the upper airway. In: Lee-Chiong TL, ed. *Sleep: A Comprehensive Handbook.* Hoboken, NJ: John Wiley & Sons, 2006.

Clinical Features of Obstructive Sleep Apnea

Sanders M, Gilvelber RJ. Overview of obstructive sleep apnea in adults. In: Lee-Chiong TL, ed. *Sleep: A Comprehensive Handbook.* Hoboken, NJ: John Wiley & Sons, 2006.

Consequences

He J, Kryger MH, Zorick FJ, Conway W, Roth T. Mortality and apnea index in obstructive sleep apnea. Experience in 385 male patients. *Chest.* 1988(Jul);94(1):9–14.

Lavie P, Herer P, Hoffstein V. Obstructive sleep apnoea syndrome as a risk factor for hypertension: population study. BMJ. 2000(Feb)19;320(7233):479–82.

Partinen M, Jamieson A, Guilleminault C. Long-term outcome for obstructive sleep apnea syndrome patients. Mortality. *Chest.* 1989(Sep);96(3):703–4.

Peppard PE, Young T, Palta M, Skatrud J. Prospective study of the association between sleep-disordered breathing and hypertension. *N Engl J Med.* 2000(May)11;342(19):1378–84.

Punjabi NM, Shahar E, Redline S, Gottlieb DJ, Givelber R, Resnick HE, Sleep Heart Health Study Investigators. Sleep-disordered breathing, glucose intolerance, and insulin resistance: the Sleep Heart Health Study. *Am J Epidemiol.* 2004(Sep 15);160(6):521–30.

Shahar E, Whitney CW, Redline S, Lee ET, Newman AB, Javier Nieto F, et al. Sleep-disordered breathing and cardiovascular disease: cross-sectional results of the Sleep Heart Health Study. *Am J Respir Crit Care Med.* 2001(Jan);163(1):19–25.

Evaluation

Sanders M, Gilvelber RJ. Overview of obstructive sleep apnea in adults. In: Lee-Chiong TL, ed. *Sleep: A Comprehensive Handbook.* Hoboken, NJ: John Wiley & Sons, 2006.

Littner M. Evaluation of sleep disordered breathing 2: Portable sleep monitoring. In: Lee-Chiong TL, ed. *Sleep: A Comprehensive Handbook*. Hoboken, NJ: John Wiley & Sons, 2006.

Mehra R, Strohl KP. Evaluation of sleep disordered breathing: polysomnography. In: Lee-Chiong TL, ed. *Sleep: A Comprehensive Handbook*. Hoboken, NJ: John Wiley & Sons, 2006.

Therapy

Dave NB, Strollo PJ. Indications for treatment of obstructive sleep apnea in adults. In: Lee-Chiong TL, ed. *Sleep: A Comprehensive Handbook*. Hoboken, NJ: John Wiley & Sons, 2006.

Weight Reduction

Browman CP, Sampson MG, Yolles SF, Gujavarty KS, Weiler SJ, Walsleben JA, et al. Obstructive sleep apnea and body weight. *Chest.* 1984;85:435–436.

Charuzi I, Ovnat A, Peiser J, Saltz H, Weitzman S, Lavie P. The effect of surgical weight reduction on sleep quality in obesity-related sleep apnea syndrome. *Surgery.* 1985;97:535–538.

Garner D, Wooley S. Confronting the failure of behavioural and dietary treatment for obesity. *Clin Psych Rev.* 1991;11:729–780.

Harman EM, Wynne JW, Block AJ. The effect of weight loss on sleep disordered breathing and oxygen desaturation in morbidly obese men. *Chest.* 1982;82:291–294.

Horner RL, Mohiaddin RH, Lowell DG, Shea SA, Burman ED, Longmore DB, et al. Sites and sizes of fat deposits around the pharynx in obese patients with obstructive sleep apnoea and weight matched controls. *Eur Respir J.* 1989;2:613–622.

Kansanen M, Vanninen E, Tuunainen A, Pesonen P, Tuononen V, Hartikainen J, et al. The effect of very low-calorie diet-induced weight loss on the severity of obstructive sleep apnoea and autonomic nervous function in obese patients with obstructive sleep apnoea syndrome. *Clin Physiol.* 1998;18:377–385.

Katz I, Stradling J, Slutsky AS, Zamel N, Hoffstein V. Do patients with obstructive sleep apnea have thick necks? *Am Rev Respir Dis.* 1990;141:1228–1231.

Lojander J, Mustajoki P, Ronka S, Mecklin P, Maasilta P. A nurse-managed weight reduction programme for obstructive sleep apnoea syndrome. *J Intern Med.* 1998;244:251–255.

Loube DI, Loube AA, Mitler MM. Weight loss for obstructive sleep apnea: the optimal therapy for obese patients. *J Am Diet Assoc.* 1994;94(11):1291–1295.

NIH Technology Assessment Conference Panel. Methods for voluntary weight loss and control. *Ann Intern Med.* 1993;119:764–770.

Pasquali R, Colella P, Cirignotta F, Mondini S, Gerardi R, Buratti P, et al. Treatment of obese patients with obstructive sleep apnea syndrome(OSAS): effect of weight loss and interference of otorhinolaryngoiatric pathology. *Int J Obes.* 1990;14:207–217.

Peppard PE, Young T, Palta M, Dempsey J, Skatrud J. Longitudinal study of moderate weight change and sleep disordered breathing. *JAMA.* 2000;284:3015–3021.

Pillar G, Peled R, Lavie P. Recurrence of sleep apnea without concomitant weight increase 7.5 years after weight reduction surgery. *Chest.* 1994;106:1702–1704.

Ryan CF, Love LL. Mechanical properties of the velopharynx in obese patients with obstructive sleep apnea. *Am J Respir Crit Care Med.* 1996;154:806–812.

Sampol G, Munoz X, Sagales MT, Marti S, Roca A, Dolors de la Calzada M, et al. Long-term efficacy of dietary weight loss in sleep apnoea/hypopnoea syndrome. *Eur Respir J.* 1998;12:1156–1159.

Scheuller M, Weider D. Bariatric surgery for treatment of sleep apnea syndrome in 15 morbidly obese patients: long-term results. *Otolaryngol Head Neck Surg.* 2001;125:299–302.

Schwab R, Gefter W, Hoffman E, Gupta KB, Pack AI. Dynamic upper airway imaging during awake respiration in normal subjects and patients with sleep disordered breathing. *Am Rev Respir Dis.* 1993;148:1385–1400.

Schwartz AR, Gold AR, Schubert N, Stryzak A, Wise RA, Permutt S, et al. Effect of weight loss on upper airway collapsibility in obstructive sleep apnea. *Am Rev Respir Dis.* 1991;144:494–498.

Smith PL, Gold AR, Meyers DA, Haponik EF, Bleecker ER. Weight loss in mildly to moderately obese patients with obstructive sleep apnea. *Ann Intern Med.* 1983;103;850–855.

Sugerman HJ, Fairman RP, Sood RK, Engle K, Wolfe L, Kellum JM. Long-term effects of gastric surgery for treating respiratory insufficiency of obesity. *Am J Clin Nutr.* 1992;55:597S–601S.

Suratt P, McTier R, Wilhoit SC. Collapsibility of the nasopharyngeal airway in obstructive sleep apnea. Am Rev Respir Dis. 1985;132;967–971.

Suratt P, McTier R, Findley L, Pohl SL, Wilhoit SC. Effect of very-low calorie diets with weight loss on obstructive sleep apnea. *Am J Clin Nutr.* 1992;56:182–184S.

Positional Therapy

Cartwright RD. Effect of sleep position on sleep apnea severity. *Sleep.* 1984;7:110–114.

Fransson AM. Svenson BA. Isacsson G. The effect of posture and a mandibular protruding device on pharyngeal dimensions: a cephalometric study. *Sleep & Breathing.* 2002;6(2):55–68.

George CF, Millar TW, Kryger MH. Sleep apnea and body position during sleep. *Sleep.* 1988;11:90–99.

Jokic R, Klimaszewski A, Crossley M, Sridhar G, Fitzpatrick MF. Positional treatment vs continuous positive airway pressure in patients with positional bstructive sleep apnea syndrome. *Chest.* 1999;115(3):771–781.

Neil A, Ignacio E, Shaharuddin N, Sajkov D. Upper body elevation improves upper airway stability but not indices of severity in obstructive sleep apnea syndrome. *Australian & New Zealand Journal of Medicine.* 1998;1.28: 270.

Cervical Positional Therapy

Kushida CA, Sherrill CM, Hong SC, Palombini L, Hyde P, Dement WC.Cervical positioning for reduction of sleep-disordered breathing in mild-to-moderate OSAS. *Sleep Breath.* 2001(Jun);5(2):71–8.

Oxygen Therapy

Mayos M, Hernandez Plaza L, Farre A, Mota S, Sanchis J. The effect of nocturnal oxygen therapy in patients with sleep apnea syndrome and chronic airflow limitation. *Arch Bronconeumol.* 2001(Feb);37(2):65–68.

Nasal Dilators

Bahammam AS, Tate R. Manfreda J. Kryger MH. Upper airway resistance syndrome: effect of nasal dilation, sleep stage, and sleep position. *Sleep.* 1999;22(5):592–598.

Hoijer U, Ejnell H, Hedner J, Petruson B, Eng LB. The effects of nasal dilation on snoring and obstructive sleep apnea. *Arch Otolaryngol Head Neck Surg.* 1992;118:281–284.

Pharyngeal Muscle Stimulation

Eisele DW, Smith PL, Alam DS, Schwartz AR. Direct hypoglossal nerve stimulation in obstructive sleep apnea. *Arch Otolaryngol Head Neck Surg.* 1997;123:57–61.

Goding GS Jr, Eisele DW, Testerman R, Smith PL, Roertgen K, Schwartz AR. Relief of upper airway obstruction with hypoglossal nerve stimulation in the canine. *Laryngoscope.* 1998;108:162–169.

Guilleminault C, Powell N, Bowman B, Stoohs R. The effect of electrical stimulation on obstructive sleep apnea. *Chest.* 1995;107:67–73.

Pharmacologic Treatment

Bai Y. Primary hypothyroidism with obstructive sleep apnea syndrome. *Zhongguo Yi Xue Ke Xue Yuan Xue Bao.* 1992(Aug);14(4):267–272.

Berry RB, Desa MM, Branum JP, Light RW. Effect of theophylline on sleep and sleep-disordered breathing in patients with chronic obstructive pulmonary disease. *Am Rev Respir Dis.* 1991(Feb);143(2):245–250.

Berry RB, Yamaura EM, Gill K, Reist C. Acute effects of paroxetine on genioglossus activity in obstructive sleep apnea. *Sleep.* 1999(Dec);22(8):1087–1092.

Block AJ, Wynne JW, Boysen PG, Lindsey S, Martin C, Cantor B. Menopause, medroxyprogesterone and breathing during sleep. *American Journal of Medicine.* 1981(Mar);70(3):506–510.

Brouillette RT, Manoukian JJ, Ducharme FM, Oudjhane K, Earle LG, Ladan S, et al. Efficacy of fluticasone nasal spray for pediatric obstructive sleep apnea. *Journal of Pediatrics.* 2001(Jun);138(6):838–844.

Brownell LG, Perez-Padilla R, West P, Kryger MH. The role of protriptyline in obstructive sleep apnea. *Bull Eur Physiopathol Respir.* 1983(Nov–Dec);19(6):621–624.

Brownell LG, West P, Sweatman P, Acres JC, Kryger MH. Protriptyline in obstructive sleep apnea: a double-blind trial. *New England Journal of Medicine.* 1982(Oct); 307(17):1037–1042.

Carley DW, Paviovic S, Janelidze M, Radulovacki M. Functional role for cannabinoids in respiratory stability during sleep. *Sleep.* 2002(Jun 15);25(4):391–398.

Chiang CH, Tang YC, Wang SE, Hwang JC. Changes in phrenic, hypoglossal and recurrent laryngeal nerve activities after intravenous infusions of aminophylline in cats. *Eur Respir J.* 1995(Apr(8(4):632–636.

Cistulli PA, Barnes DJ, Grunstein RR, Sullivan CE. Effect of short-term hormone replacement in the treatment of obstructive sleep apnoea in postmenopausal women. *Thorax.* 1994(Jul);49(7): 699–702.

Conway WA, Zorick F, Piccione P, Roth T. Protriptyline in the treatment of sleep apnoea. *Thorax.* 1982(Jan);37(1):49–53.

Cook WR, Benich JJ, Wooten SA. Indices of severity of obstructive sleep apnea syndrome do not change during medroxyprogesterone acetate therapy. *Chest.* 1989(Aug);96(2):262–266.

Davila DG, Hurt RD, Offord KP, Harris CD, Shepard JW Jr. Acute effects of transdermal nicotine on sleep architecture, snoring, and sleep-disordered breathing in nonsmokers. *Am J Respir Crit Care Med.* 1994(Aug);150(2):469–74.

Davis JM, Zinman R, Aranda JV. Use of caffeine in the treatment of apnea associated with the Arnold-Chiari malformation. *Dev Pharmacol Ther.* 1989;12(2):70–73.

Di Martino E, Saadi R, Emmerling O, Werner E. Drug therapy of sleep apnea syndromes: results of short-term treatment with theophylline. *Laryngorhinootologie.* 1999(Mar);78(3):120–124.

Dolly FR, Block AJ. Medroxyprogesterone acetate and COPD. Effect on breathing and oxygenation in sleeping and awake patients. *Chest.* 1983(Oct);84(4):394–398.

Esnault S, Merceur C, Kerlan V, Tea SH, le Mevel JC, Bercovici JP, et al. Long-term effects of treatment with SMS 201–995 on sleep apnea syndrome associated with acromegaly. *Neurophysiol Clin.* 1989(Nov);19(5):367–372.

Esnault-Lavandier S, Mabin D. The effects of clomipramine on diurnal sleepiness and respiratory parameters in a case of Prader-Willi syndrome. *Neurophysiol Clin.* 1998(Dec);28(6):521–525.

Espinoza H, Antic R, Thornton AT, McEvoy RD. The effects of aminophylline on sleep and sleep-disordered breathing in patients with obstructive sleep apnea syndrome. *Am Rev Respir Dis.* 1987;136(1):80–84.

Ferber C, Duclaux R, Mouret J. Naltrexone improves blood gas patterns in obstructive sleep apnoea syndrome through its influence on sleep. *Journal of Sleep Research.* 1993;2(3):149–155.

Ferber C, Sanchez P, Lemoine P, Mouret J. Efficacy of the treatment of sleep apnea using naltrexone. A clinical, polygraphic and gasometric study. *C R Acad Sci III.* 1988;307(12):695–700.

Gothe B, Strohl KP, Levin S, Cherniack NS. Nicotine: a different approach to treatment of obstructive sleep apnea. *Chest.* 1985(Jan);87(1):11–17.

Grote L, Wutkewicz K, Knaack L, Ploch T, Hedner J, Peter JH. Association between blood pressure reduction with antihypertensive treatment and sleep apnea activity. *American Journal of Hypertension.* 2000;13(12):1280–1287.

Grunstein RR, Ho KK, Sullivan CE. Effect of octreotide, a somatostatin analog, on sleep apnea in patients with acromegaly. *Ann Intern Med.* 1994(Oct);121(7):478–483.

Guilleminault C, Hayes B. Naloxone, theophylline, bromocriptine, and obstructive sleep apnea. Negative results. *Bulletin Europeen de Physiopathologie Respiratoire.* 1983(Nov–Dec);19(6):632–634.

Guilleminault C, Silvestri R, Mondini S, Coburn S. Aging and sleep apnea: action of benzodiazepine, acetazolamide, alcohol, and sleep deprivation in a healthy elderly group. *J Gerontol.* 1984(Nov);39(6):655–661.

Haidmayer R, Kerbl R, Meyer U, Kerschhaggl P, Kurz R, Kenner T. Effects of naloxone on apnoea duration during sleep in infants at risk for SIDS. *Eur J Pediatr.* 1986(Oct);145(5):357–360.

Hanzel DA, Proia NG, Hudgel DW. Response of obstructive sleep apnea to fluoxetine and protriptyline. *Chest.* 1991(Aug);100(2):416–421.

Hedner J, Grunstein R, Eriksson B, Ejnell H. A double-blind, randomized trial of sabeluzole—a putative glutamate antagonistin—in obstructive sleep apnea. *Sleep.* 1996;19(4):287–289.

Hein H, Kirsten D, Jugert C, Magnussen H. Theophylline in therapy of obstructive sleep apnea? *Pneumologie.* 1993(Dec);47 Suppl 4:750–753.

Inoue Y, Takata K, Sakamoto I, Hazama H, Kawahara R. Clinical efficacy and indication of acetazolamide treatment on sleep apnea syndrome. *Psychiatry Clin Neurosci.* 1999(Apr);53(2):321–322.

Ip MS, Tan KC, Peh WC, Lam KS. Effect of Sandostatin LAR on sleep apnoea in acromegaly: correlation with computerized tomographic cephalometry and hormonal activity. *Clin Endocrinol (Oxf).* 2001(Oct);55(4):477–483.

236 *Sleep-Related Breathing Disorders*</cite>

Issa FG. Effect of clonidine in obstructive sleep apnea. *Am Rev Respir Dis.* 1992;145(2 Pt 1):435–439.

Keefe DL, Watson R, Naftolin F. Hormone replacement therapy may alleviate sleep apnea in menopausal women: a pilot study. *Menopause.* 1999;6(3):196–200.

Kempf P, Mossinger B, Muller B, Kirchheiner T, Ruhle KH. Comparative studies on the effect of nasal CPAP, theophylline and oxygen in patients with sleep apnea syndrome. *Pneumologie.* 1991(May);1.45 Suppl 1:279–282.

Kimura H, Tatsumi K, Kunitomo F, Okita S, Tojima H, Kouchiyama S, et al. Progesterone therapy for sleep apnea syndrome evaluated by occlusion pressure responses to exogenous loading. *Am Rev Respir Dis.* 1989(May);139(5):1198–1206.

Kraiczi H, Hedner J, Dahlof P, Ejnell H, Carlson J. Effect of serotonin uptake inhibition on breathing during sleep and daytime symptoms in obstructive sleep apnea. *Sleep.* 1999(Feb);22(1):61–67.

Krieger J, Mangin P, Kurtz D. Sleep apnea synrome: effects of chlorimipramine in subjects with stable body weight. *Rev Electroencephalogr Neurophysiol Clin.* 1979(Jul–Sep);9(3):250–257.

Mangin P, Krieger J, Kurtz D. Effect of oral almitrine on the sleep apnea syndrome. *Rev Fr Mal Respir.* 1983;11(6):899–906.

Marrone O, Milone F, Coppola P, Oddo S, Giannone G, Macaluso C, et al. Effects of almitrine bismesylate on nocturnal hypoxemia in patients with chronic bronchitis and obesity. *European Journal of Respiratory Diseases—Supplement.* 1986;146:641–648.

Mayer J, Peter JH. First experience with cilazapril in the treatment of sleep apnoea-related hypertension. *Drugs.* 1991;41 Suppl 1:37–47.

Meissner P, Dorow P, Thalhofer S, Heinemann S. Theophylline acceptance in long-term therapy of patients with obstructive sleep related respiratory disorder. *Pneumologie.* 1995(Mar);49 Suppl 1:187–189.

Mulloy E, McNicholas WT. Theophylline in obstructive sleep apnea. A double-blind evaluation. *Chest.* 1992(Mar);101(3):753–757.

Oberndorfer S, Saletu B, Gruber G, Anderer P, Saletu M, Mandl M, et al. Theophylline in snoring and sleep-related breathing disorders: sleep laboratory investigations on subjective and objective sleep and awakening quality. *Methods Find Exp Clin Pharmacol.* 2000(May);22(4):237–245.

Ohshima H. Medroxyprogesterone acetate and sleep apnea. *Jpn J Psychiatry Neurol.* 1987(Dec);41(4):645–650.

Osanai S, Akiba Y, Fujiuchi S, Nakano H, Matsumoto H, Ohsaki Y, et al. Depression of peripheral chemosensitivity by a dopaminergic mechanism in patients with obstructive sleep apnoea syndrome. *Eur Respir J.* 1999(Feb);13(2):418–423.

Peter JH, Gassel W, Mayer J, Herrer-Mayer B, Penzel T, Schneider H, et al. Effect of cilazapril on hypertension, sleep, and apnea. *American Journal of Medicine.* 1989;87(6 B):72S-78S.

Pickett CK, Regensteiner JG, Woodard WD, Hagerman DD, Weil JV, Moore LG. Progestin and estrogen reduce sleep-disordered breathing in postmenopausal women. *Journal of Applied Physiology.* 1989(Apr);66(4):1656–1661.

Rajagopal KR, Abbrecht PH, Jabbari B. Effects of medroxyprogesterone acetate in obstructive sleep apnea. *Chest.* 1986(Dec);90(6):815–821.

Rubin AH, Alroy GG, Peled R, Lavie P. Preliminary clinical experience with imipramine HCl in the treatment of sleep apnea syndrome. *Eur Neurol.* 1986;25(2):81–85.

Saaresranta T, Polo-Kantola P, Rauhala E, Polo O. Medroxyprogesterone in postmenopausal females with partial upper airway obstruction during sleep. European Respiratory Journal. 2001 Dec;18(6):989–995.

Sakamoto T, Nakazawa Y, Hashizume Y, Tsutsumi Y, Mizuma H, Hirano T, et al. Effects of acetazolamide on the sleep apnea syndrome and its therapeutic mechanism. *Psychiatry Clin Neurosci.* 1995(Mar);49(1):59–64.

Salazar-Grueso EF, Rosenberg RS, Roos RP. Sleep apnea in olivopontocerebellar degeneration: treatment with trazodone. *Ann Neurol.* 1988(Apr);23(4):399–401.

Schafer HH, Grieger E, Heitmann J, Koehler U, Peter JH, Ploch T, et al. Long-term theophylline therapy in sleep apnea—follow-up over a period of 12 months. *Pneumologie.* 1993(Dec);47 Suppl 4:741–746.

Schmidt HS. L-tryptophan in the treatment of impaired respiration in sleep. *Bull Eur Physiopathol Respir.* 1983(Nov–Dec);19(6):625–629.

Smith PL, Haponik EF, Allen RP, Bleecker ER. The effects of protriptyline in sleep-disordered breathing. *Am Rev Respir Dis.* 1983(Jan);127(1):8–13.

Strohl KP, Hensley MJ, Saunders NA, Scharf SM, Brown R, Ingram RH Jr. Progesterone administration and progressive sleep apneas. *JAMA.* 1981(Mar 27);245(12):1230–1232.

Sunderram J. Parisi RA. Strobel RJ. Serotonergic stimulation of the genioglossus and the response to nasal continuous positive airway pressure. *Am J Respir Crit Care Med.* 2000(Sep);162(3 Pt 1):925–929.

Suratt PM, Wilhoit SC, Brown ED, Findley LJ. Effect of doxapram on obstructive sleep apnea. *Bulletin Europeen de Physiopathologie Respiratoire.* 1986;22(2):127–131.

Teramoto S, Ohga E, Katayama H, Matsui H, Tomita T, Matsuse T, et al. Effects of thyroid hormone replacement therapy on nocturnal apnea in elderly patients with hypothyroidism. *Nihon Kokyuki Gakkai Zasshi.* 1998(Jul);36(7):590–594.

Tojima H, Kunitomo F, Kimura H, Tatsumi K, Kuriyama T, Honda Y. Effects of acetazolamide in patients with the sleep apnoea syndrome. *Thorax.* 1988(Feb);43(2):113–119.

Tschida U, Winkler A. Efficiency of continuous positive airway pressure versus theophylline therapy in sleep apnea: comparative sleep laboratory studies on objective and subjective sleep and awakening quality. *Neuropsychobiology.* 1999;39(3):151–159.

Veasey SC, Chachkes J, Fenik P, Hendricks JC. The effects of ondansetron on sleep-disordered breathing in the English bulldog. *Sleep.* 2001(Mar)15;24(2):155–160.

Veasey SC, Fenik P, Panckeri K, Pack AI, Hendricks JC. The effects of trazodone with L-tryptophan on sleep-disordered breathing in the English bulldog. *Am J Respir Crit Care Med.* 1999(Nov);160(5 Pt 1):1659–1667.

Whyte KF, Gould GA, Airlie MA, Shapiro CM, Douglas NJ. Role of protriptyline and acetazolamide in the sleep apnea/hypopnea syndrome. *Sleep.* 1988(Oct);11(5):463–472.

Wirth JA. Organic psychosyndrome and sleep apnea. Transdermal nicotine—a new therapy concept? *Pneumologie.* 1995(Mar);49 Suppl 1:183–184.

Ziemer DC, Dunlap DB. Relief of sleep apnea in acromegaly by bromocriptine. *Am J Med Sci.* 1988(Jan);295(1):49–51.

Positive Airway Pressure Therapy

Hirshkowitz M, Lee-Chiong T. Positive airway pressure therapy for obstructive sleep apnea. In: Lee-Chiong TL, ed. *Sleep: A Comprehensive Handbook.* Hoboken, NJ: John Wiley & Sons, 2006.

Mechanism of Action

Hoffstein V, Zamel N, Phillipson EA. Lung volume dependence of pharyngeal cross-sectional area in patients with obstructive sleep apnea. *Am Rev Respir Dis.* 1984(Aug);130(2):175–8.

Smith PL, Wise RA, Gold AR, Schwartz AR, Permutt S. Upper airway pressure-flow relationships in obstructive sleep apnea. *J Appl Physiol.* 1988(Feb);64(2):789–95.

Van de Graaff WB. Thoracic influence on upper airway patency. *J Appl Physiol.* 1988(Nov);65(5): 2124–31.

Van de Graaff WB. Thoracic traction on the trachea: mechanisms and magnitude. *J Appl Physiol.* 1991(Mar);70(3):1328–36.

Determining Optimal Continuous Positive Airway Pressure

Hirshkowitz M, Lee-Chiong T. Positive airway pressure therapy for obstructive sleep apnea. In: Lee-Chiong TL, ed. *Sleep: A Comprehensive Handbook.* Hoboken, NJ: John Wiley & Sons, 2006.

Effects of Positive Airway Pressure Therapy

Akashiba T, Minemura H, Yamamoto H, Kosaka N, Saito O, Horie T. Nasal continuous positive airway pressure changes blood pressure "non-dippers" to "dippers" in patients with obstructive sleep apnea. *Sleep.* 1999(Nov)1;22(7):849–53.

Bahammam A, Delaive K, Ronald J, Manfreda J, Roos L, Kryger MH. Health care utilization in males with obstructive sleep apnea syndrome two years after diagnosis and treatment. Sleep. *1999(Sep 15);22(6):740–7.*

Ballester E, Badia JR, Hernandez L, Carrasco E, de Pablo J, Fornas C, Rodriguez-Roisin R, Montserrat JM. Evidence of the effectiveness of continuous positive airway pressure in the treatment of sleep apnea/hypopnea syndrome. *Am J Respir Crit Care Med.* 1999(Feb);159(2):495–501.

Barnes M, Houston D, Worsnop CJ, Neill AM, Mykytyn IJ, Kay A, et al. A randomized controlled trial of continuous positive airway pressure in mild obstructive sleep apnea. *Am J Respir Crit Care Med.* 2002(Mar 15);165(6):773–80.

Dimsdale JE, Loredo JS, Profant J. Effect of continuous positive airway pressure on blood pressure: a placebo trial. Hypertension. 2000(Jan);35(1 Pt 1):144–7.

Engleman HM, Martin SE, Deary IJ, Douglas NJ. Effect of CPAP therapy on daytime function in patients with mild sleep apnoea/hypopnoea syndrome. *Thorax.* 1997(Feb);52(2):114–9.

Engleman HM, Kingshott RN, Wraith PK, Mackay TW, Deary IJ, Douglas NJ. Randomized placebo-controlled crossover trial of continuous positive airway pressure for mild sleep apnea/hypopnea syndrome. *Am J Respir Crit Care Med.* 1999(Feb);159(2):461–7.

Faccenda JF, Mackay TW, Boon NA, Douglas NJ. Randomized placebo-controlled trial of continuous positive airway pressure on blood pressure in the sleep apnea-hypopnea syndrome. Am J Respir Crit Care Med. *2001(Feb);163(2):344–8.*

Hack M, Davies RJ, Mullins R, Choi SJ, Ramdassingh-Dow S, Jenkinson C, Stradling JR. Randomised prospective parallel trial of therapeutic versus subtherapeutic nasal continuous positive airway pressure on simulated steering performance in patients with obstructive sleep apnoea. *Thorax.* 2000(Mar);55(3):224–31.

He J, Kryger MH, Zorick FJ, Conway W, Roth T. Mortality and apnea index in obstructive sleep apnea. Experience in 385 male patients. *Chest.* 1988(Jul);94(1):9–14.

Jenkinson C, Davies RJ, Mullins R, Stradling JR. Comparison of therapeutic and subtherapeutic nasal continuous positive airway pressure for obstructive sleep apnoea: a randomised prospective parallel trial. *Lancet.* 1999(Jun)19;353(9170):2100–5.

Jenkinson C, Davies RJ, Mullins R, Stradling JR. Long-term benefits in self-reported health status of nasal continuous positive airway pressure therapy for obstructive sleep apnoea. *QJM.* 2001(Feb);94(2):95–9.

Kingshott RN, Vennelle M, Hoy CJ, Engleman HM, Deary IJ, Douglas NJ. Predictors of improvements in daytime function outcomes with CPAP therapy. *Am J Respir Crit Care Med.* 2000(Mar);161(3 Pt 1):866–71.

Lavie P, Herer P, Hoffstein V. Obstructive sleep apnoea syndrome as a risk factor for hypertension: population study. BMJ. *2000(Feb 19);320(7233):479–82.*

Loredo JS, Ancoli-Israel S, Dimsdale JE. Effect of continuous positive airway pressure vs placebo continuous positive airway pressure on sleep quality in obstructive sleep apnea. *Chest.* 1999(Dec);116(6):1545–9.

Mayer J, Becker H, Brandenburg U, Penzel T, Peter JH, von Wichert P. Blood pressure and sleep apnea: results of long-term nasal continuous positive airway pressure therapy. *Cardiology.* 1991;79(2):84–92.

Naughton MT, Bradley TD. Sleep apnea in congestive heart failure. *Clin Chest Med.* 1998(Mar);19(1):99–113.

Rauscher H, Formanek D, Popp W, Zwick H. Nasal CPAP and weight loss in hypertensive patients with obstructive sleep apnoea. *Thorax.* 1993(May);48(5):529–33.

Redline S, Adams N, Strauss ME, Roebuck T, Winters M, Rosenberg C. Improvement of mild sleep-disordered breathing with CPAP compared with conservative therapy. *Am J Respir Crit Care Med.* 1998(Mar);157(3 Pt 1):858–65.

Suzuki M, Otsuka K, Guilleminault C. Long-term nasal continuous positive airway pressure administration can normalize hypertension in obstructive sleep apnea patients. Sleep. *1993(Sep);16(6):545–9.*

Wright J, Johns R, Watt I, Melville A, Sheldon T. Health effects of obstructive sleep apnoea and the effectiveness of continuous positive airways pressure: a systematic review of the research evidence. *BMJ.* 1997(Mar)22;314(7084):851–60.

Adverse Consequences of Positive Airway Pressure Therapy

Hirshkowitz M, Lee-Chiong T. Positive airway pressure therapy for obstructive sleep apnea. In: Lee-Chiong TL, ed. *Sleep: A Comprehensive Handbook.* Hoboken, NJ: John Wiley & Sons, 2006.

Adherence to Positive Airway Pressure Therapy

Berry RB, Kouchi K, Bower J, Prosise G, Light RW. Triazolam in patients with obstructive sleep apnea. *Am J Respir Crit Care Med.* 1995(Feb);151(2 Pt 1):450–4.

Brown LK. Back to basics: if it's dry, wet it: the case for humidification of nasal continuous positive airway pressure air. *Chest.* 2000(Mar);117(3):617–9.

Chervin RD, Theut S, Bassetti C, Aldrich MS. Compliance with nasal CPAP can be improved by simple interventions. *Sleep.* 1997(Apr);20(4):284–9.

Fleury B, Rakotonanahary D, Hausser-Hauw C, Lebeau B, Guilleminault C. Objective patient compliance in long-term use of nCPAP. *Eur Respir J.* 1996(Nov);9(11):2356–9.

Hoffstein V, Viner S, Mateika S, Conway J. Treatment of obstructive sleep apnea with nasal continuous positive airway pressure. Patient compliance, perception of benefits, and side effects. *Am Rev Respir Dis.* 1992(Apr);145(4 Pt 1):841–5.

Hoy CJ, Vennelle M, Kingshott RN, Engleman HM, Douglas NJ. Can intensive support improve continuous positive airway pressure use in patients with the sleep apnea/hypopnea syndrome? *Am J Respir Crit Care Med.* 1999(Apr);159(4 Pt 1):1096–100.

Hui DS, Chan JK, Choy DK, Ko FW, Li TS, Leung RC, Lai CK. Effects of augmented continuous positive airway pressure education and support on compliance and outcome in a Chinese population. *Chest.* 2000(May);117(5):1410–6.

Kribbs NB, Pack AI, Kline LR, Getsy JE, Schuett JS, Henry JN, et al. Effects of one night without nasal CPAP treatment on sleep and sleepiness in patients with obstructive sleep apnea. *Am Rev Respir Dis.* 1993(May);147(5):1162–8.

Kribbs NB, Pack AI, Kline LR, Smith PL, Schwartz AR, Schubert NM, et al. Objective measurement of patterns of nasal CPAP use by patients with obstructive sleep apnea. *Am Rev Respir Dis.* 1993(Apr);147(4):887–95.

Likar LL, Panciera TM, Erickson AD, Rounds S. Group education sessions and compliance with nasal CPAP therapy. *Chest.* 1997(May);111(5):1273–7.

Martins De Araujo MT, Vieira SB, Vasquez EC, Fleury B. Heated humidification or face mask to prevent upper airway dryness during continuous positive airway pressure therapy. *Chest.* 2000(Jan);117(1):142–7.

Massie CA, Hart RW, Peralez K, Richards GN. Effects of humidification on nasal symptoms and compliance in sleep apnea patients using continuous positive airway pressure. *Chest.* 1999(Aug);116(2):403–8.

McArdle N, Devereux G, Heidarnejad H, Engleman HM, Mackay TW, Douglas NJ. Long-term use of CPAP therapy for sleep apnea/hypopnea syndrome. *Am J Respir Crit Care Med.* 1999(Apr);159(4 Pt 1):1108–14.

Mortimore IL, Whittle AT, Douglas NJ. Comparison of nose and face mask CPAP therapy for sleep apnoea. *Thorax.* 1998(Apr);53(4):290–2.

Pepin JL, Krieger J, Rodenstein D, Cornette A, Sforza E, Delguste P, et al. Effective compliance during the first 3 months of continuous positive airway pressure. A European prospective study of 121 patients. *Am J Respir Crit Care Med.* 1999(Oct);160(4):1124–9.

Pressman MR, Peterson DD, Meyer TJ, Harkins JP, Gurijala L. Ramp abuse. A novel form of patient noncompliance to administration of nasal continuous positive airway pressure for treatment of obstructive sleep apnea. *Am J Respir Crit Care Med.* 1995(May);151(5):1632–4.

Rakotonanahary D, Pelletier-Fleury N, Gagnadoux F, Fleury B. Predictive factors for the need for additional humidification during nasal continuous positive airway pressure therapy. *Chest.* 2001(Feb);119(2):460–5.

Reeves-Hoche MK, Hudgel DW, Meck R, Witteman R, Ross A, Zwillich CW. Continuous versus bilevel positive airway pressure for obstructive sleep apnea. *Am J Respir Crit Care Med.* 1995(Feb);151(2 Pt 1):443–9.

Richards GN, Cistulli PA, Ungar RG, Berthon-Jones M, Sullivan CE. Mouth leak with nasal continuous positive airway pressure increases nasal airway resistance. *Am J Respir Crit Care Med.* 1996(Jul);154(1):182–6.

Rosenthal L, Gerhardstein R, Lumley A, Guido P, Day R, Syron ML, et al. CPAP therapy in patients with mild OSA: implementation and treatment outcome. *Sleep Med.* 2000(Jul 1);1(3):215–220.

Strollo PJ Jr, Sanders MH, Costantino JP, Walsh SK, Stiller RA, Atwood CW Jr. Split-night studies for the diagnosis and treatment of sleep-disordered breathing. *Sleep*. 1996(Dec);19(10 Suppl): S255–9.

Weaver TE, Kribbs NB, Pack AI, Kline LR, Chugh DK, Maislin G, et al. Night-to-night variability in CPAP use over the first three months of treatment. *Sleep*. 1997(Apr);20(4):278–83.

Wiest GH, Lehnert G, Bruck WM, Meyer M, Hahn EG, Ficker JH. A heated humidifier reduces upper airway dryness during continuous positive airway pressure therapy. *Respir Med*. 1999(Jan);93(1):21–6.

Autotitrating Positive Airway Pressure

Berry RB, Parish JM, Hartse KM. The use of auto-titrating continuous positive airway pressure for treatment of adult obstructive sleep apnea. An American Academy of Sleep Medicine review. *Sleep*. 2002(Mar 15);25(2):148–73.

d'Ortho MP, Grillier-Lanoir V, Levy P, Goldenberg F, Corriger E, Harf A, et al. Constant vs. automatic continuous positive airway pressure therapy: home evaluation. *Chest*. 2000(Oct);118(4):1010–7.

Littner M, Hirshkowitz M, Davila D, Anderson WM, Kushida CA, et al; Standards of Practice Committee of the American Academy of Sleep Medicine. Practice parameters for the use of auto-titrating continuous positive airway pressure devices for titrating pressures and treating adult patients with obstructive sleep apnea syndrome. An American Academy of Sleep Medicine report. *Sleep*. 2002(Mar 15);25(2):143–7.

Meurice JC, Marc I, Series F. Efficacy of auto-CPAP in the treatment of obstructive sleep apnea/hypopnea syndrome. *Am J Respir Crit Care Med*. 1996(Feb);153(2):794–8.

Sharma S, Wali S, Pouliot Z, Peters M, Neufeld H, Kryger M. Treatment of obstructive sleep apnea with a self-titrating continuous positive airway pressure (CPAP) system. *Sleep*. 1996(Jul);19(6):497–501.

Standards of Practice Committee of the American Academy of Sleep Medicine. Practice Parameters for the Use of Auto-Titrating Continuous Positive Airway Pressure Devices for Titrating Pressures and Treating Adult Patients with Obstructive Sleep Apnea Syndrome. An American Academy of Sleep Medicine Report. *Sleep*. 2002;25(2):143–147.

Stradling JR, Barbour C, Pitson DJ, Davies RJ. Automatic nasal continuous positive airway pressure titration in the laboratory: patient outcomes. *Thorax*. 1997(Jan);52(1):72–5.

Bilevel Positive Airway Pressure

Schafer H, Ewig S, Hasper E, Luderitz B. Failure of CPAP therapy in obstructive sleep apnoea syndrome: predictive factors and treatment with bilevel-positive airway pressure. *Respir Med*. 1998(Feb);92(2):208–15.

Noninvasive Ventilation Positive Pressure Ventilation

Piper AJ, Sullivan CE. Effects of short-term NIPPV in the treatment of patients with severe obstructive sleep apnea and hypercapnia. *Chest*. 1994(Feb);105(2):434–40.

Oral Devices

Bailey DR. Dental therapy for obstructive sleep apnea. *Semin Respir Crit Care Med*. 2005(Feb);26(1):89–95.

Millaman R, Rosenberg C, Carlisle C, Kramer N, Kahn D, Bonitati A. The efficacy of oral appliances in the treatment of persistent sleep apnea after uvulopalatopharyngoplasty. *Chest*. 1998;113:992–996.

Schmidt-Nowara W, Lowe A, Wiegand L, Cartwright R, Perez-Guerra F, Menn S. Oral appliances for the treatment of snoring and obstructive sleep apnea: a review. *Sleep*. 1995;18:501–510.

Thorpy M, et al. Practice parameters for the treatment of snoring and obstructive sleep apnea with oral appliances. *Sleep*. 1995;18:511–513.

Wilhelmsson B, Teglberg A, Walker-Engstrom M, et al. A prospective randomized study of a dental appliance compared with uvulopalatopharyngoplasty in the treatment of obstructive sleep apnea. *Acta Otolaryngol*. 1999;119:503–509.

Upper Airway Surgery

Fujita S. Midline laser glossectomy with lingualplasty: A treatment of sleep apnea syndrome. *Op Tech Otolaryngol HNS*. 1991;2:127–131.

Sher AE. Obstructive sleep apnea syndrome: a complex disorder of the upper airway. *Otolaryngol Clin North Am*. 1990;92:593–608.

Sher AE. Upper airway surgery for obstructive sleep apnea. *Sleep Medicine Reviews*. 2002;6: 195–212.

Sher AE. Upper airway surgery for obstructive sleep apnea. In: Lee-Chiong TL, ed. *Sleep: A Comprehensive Handbook*. Hoboken, NJ: John Wiley & Sons, 2006.

Sher AE. Schechtman KB, Piccirillo JF. The efficacy of surgical modifications of the upper airway in adults with obstructive sleep apnea syndrome. *Sleep*. 1996;19:156–177.

Management of Residual Sleepiness

Arnulf I, Homeyer P, Garma L, Whitelaw WA, Derenne JP. Modafinil in obstructive sleep apnea-hypopnea syndrome: a pilot study in 6 patients. *Respiration*. 1997;64(2):159–161.

Black JE, Hirshkowitz M. Modafinil for treatment of residual excessive sleepiness in nasal continuous positive airway pressure-treated obstructive sleep apnea/hypopnea syndrome. *Sleep*. 2005(Apr 1);28(4):464–71.

Kingshott RN, Vennelle M, Coleman EL, Engleman HM, Mackay TW, Douglas NJ. Randomized, double-blind, placebo-controlled crossover trial of modafinil in the treatment of residual excessive daytime sleepiness in the sleep apnea/hypopnea syndrome. *Am J Respir Crit Care Med*. 2001(Mar);163(4):918–923.

Pack AI, Black JE, Schwartz JR, Matheson JK. Modafinil as adjunct therapy for daytime sleepiness in obstructive sleep apnea. *Am J Respir Crit Care Med*. 2001(Nov);64(9):1675–1681.

Snoring

Ayappa I, Rapoport DM. The upper airway in sleep: physiology of the pharynx. *Sleep Med Rev*. 2003(Feb);7(1):9–33.

Ferguson KA. The role of oral appliance therapy in the treatment of obstructive sleep apnea. In: Lee-Chiong T, Mohsenin V. *Clinics in Chest Medicine*. Philadelphia, PA: WB Saunders, 2003. pp. 355–364.

Gleadhill IC, Schwartz AR, Schubert N, Wise RA, Permutt S, Smith PL. Upper airway collapsibility in snorers and in patients with obstructive hypopnea and apnea. *Am Rev Respir Dis.* 1991(Jun);143(6):1300–3.

Littner M, Kushida CA, Hartse K, Anderson WM, Davila D, Johnson SF, et al. Practice parameters for the use of laser-assisted uvuloplasty: an update for 2000. *Sleep.* 2001;24(5):603–619.

Maurer JT, Hein G, Verse T, Hormann K, Stuck BA. Long-term results of palatal implants for primary snoring. *Otolaryngol Head Neck Surg.* 2005(Oct);133(4):573–8.

Meoli AL, Rosen CL, Kristo D, Kohrman M, Gooneratne N, Aguillard RN, et al; Clinical Practice Review Committee, American Academy of Sleep Medicine. Nonprescription treatments of snoring or obstructive sleep apnea: an evaluation of products with limited scientific evidence. *Sleep.* 2003(Aug);26(5):619–24.

American Sleep Disorders Association. Practice parameters for the treatment of snoring and obstructive sleep apnea with oral appliances. American Sleep Disorders Association. *Sleep.* 1995(Jul);18(6):511–3.

Rappai M, Collop N, Kemp S, deShazo R. The nose and sleep-disordered breathing: what we know and what we do not know. *Chest.* 2003(Dec);124(6):2309–23.

Stuck BA, Sauter A, Hormann K, Verse T, Maurer JT. Radiofrequency surgery of the soft palate in the treatment of snoring. A placebo-controlled trial. *Sleep.* 2005(Jul 1);28(7):847–50.

Vetrugno R, Provini F, Plazzi G, Vignatelli L, Lugaresi E, Montagna P. Catathrenia (nocturnal groaning): a new type of parasomnia. *Neurology.* 2001(Mar 13);56(5):681–3.

Wetter DW, Young TB, Bidwell TR, Badr MS, Palta M. Smoking as a risk factor for sleep-disordered breathing. *Arch Intern Med.* 1994(Oct 10);154(19):2219–24.

Young T, Palta M, Dempsey J, Skatrud J, Weber S, Badr S. The occurrence of sleep-disordered breathing among middle-aged adults. *N Engl J Med.* 1993(Apr 29);328(17):1230–5.

Upper Airway Resistance Syndrome

Ayappa I, Norman RG, Krieger AC, Rosen A, O'Malley RL, Rapoport DM. Non-Invasive detection of respiratory effort-related arousals (REras) by a nasal cannula/pressure transducer system. *Sleep.* 2000(Sep 15);23(6):763–71.

Bao G, Guilleminault C. Upper airway resistance syndrome—one decade later. *Curr Opin Pulm Med.* 2004(Nov);10(6):461–7.

Gold AR, Dipalo F, Gold MS, O'Hearn D. The symptoms and signs of upper airway resistance syndrome: a link to the functional somatic syndromes. *Chest.* 2003(Jan);123(1):87–95.

Guilleminault C, Stoohs R, Duncan S. Snoring (I). Daytime sleepiness in regular heavy snorers. *Chest.* 1991(Jan);99(1):40–8.

Guilleminault C, Stoohs R, Clerk A, Cetel M, Maistros P. A cause of excessive daytime sleepiness. The upper airway resistance syndrome. *Chest.* 1993(Sep);104(3):781–7.

Guilleminault C, Stoohs R, Clerk A, Simmons J, Labanowski M. From obstructive sleep apnea syndrome to upper airway syndrome: consistency of daytime sleepiness. *Sleep.* 1992;15 (6 Suppl):S13–6.

Guilleminault C, Poyares D, Palombini L, Koester U, Pelin Z, Black J. Variability of respiratory effort in relation to sleep stages in normal controls and upper airway resistance syndrome patients. *Sleep Med.* 2001(Sep);2(5):397–405.

Lofaso F, Goldenberg F, d'Ortho MP, Coste A, Harf A. Arterial blood pressure response to transient arousals from NREM sleep in nonapneic snorers with sleep fragmentation. Chest. 1998(Apr);113(4):985–91.

Lofaso F, Coste A, Gilain L, Harf A, Guilleminault C, Goldenberg F. Sleep fragmentation as a risk factor for hypertension in middle-aged nonapneic snorers. *Chest.* 1996(Apr);109(4):896–900.

Yoshida K. Oral device therapy for the upper airway resistance syndrome patient. *J Prosthet Dent.* 2002(Apr);87(4):427–30.

Central Sleep Apnea Syndrome

Badr MS. Central sleep apnea. *Sleep Medicine. Primary Care: Clinics in Office Practice.* Elsevier Saunders, 2005.

Bradley T, Holloway RM, McLaughlin PR, Ross BL, Walters J, Liu PP. Cardiac output response to continuous positive airway pressure in congestive heart failure. *Am Rev Respir Dis.* 1992;145:377–82.

Bradley T, Phillipson EA. Central sleep apnea. *Clin Chest Med.* 1992;13:493–505.

DeBacker W, Verbaecken J, Willemen M, Wittesaelle W, DeCock W, Van deHeyning P. Central apnea index decreases after prolonged treatment with acetazolamide. *Am J Respir Crit Care Med.* 1995;151:87–91.

Franklin KA, Eriksson P, Sahlin C, Lundgren R. Reversal of central apnea with oxygen. *Chest.* 1997;111:163–169.

Grunstein RR, Ho KY, Berthon-Jones M, et al. Central sleep apnea is associated with increased ventilatory response to carbon dioxide and hypersecretion of growth hormone in patients with acromegaly. *Am J Respir Crit Care Med.* 1994;150:496.

Hanly PJ, Millar TW, Steljes DG, Baert R, et al. The effect of oxygen on respiration and sleep in patients with congestive heart failure. *Ann Intern Med.* 1989;111:777–782.

Javaheri S, Parker TJ, Wexler L, et al. Occult sleep-disordered breathing in stable congestive heart failure. *Ann Intern Med.* 1995;122:487–92.

Javaheri S. A mechanism of central sleep apnea in patients with heart failure. *N Engl J Med.* 1999;341:949–954.

Levin B, Margolis G. Acute failure of autonomic respirations secondary to unilateral brainstem infarct. *Ann Neurol.* 1977;1:583–586.

McNicholas W, Carter JL, Rutherford R, Zamet N, Phillipson EA. Beneficial effect of oxygen in primary alveolar hypoventilation with central sleep apnea. *Am Rev Respir Dis.* 1982;125:773–5.

Naughton MBD, Rutherford R, Bradley TD. Effect of continuous positive airway pressure on central sleep apnea and nocturnal PCO_2 in heart failure. *Am J Respir Crit Care Med.* 1994;150: 1598–604.

White D, Zwillich C, Pickett C, et al. Central sleep apnea: improvement with acetazolamide therapy. *Arch Intern Med.* 1982;142:1816–1819.

Cheyne-Stokes Respiration

Hanly P, Zuberi N, Gray R. Pathogenesis of Cheyne-Stokes respiration in patients with congestive heart failure. *Chest.* 1993;104:1079–84.

Periodic Breathing Secondary to High Altitude

Chatila W, Krachman S. Sleep at high altitudes. In: Lee-Chiong TL, ed. *Sleep: A Comprehensive Handbook*. Hoboken, NJ: John Wiley & Sons, 2006.

Obesity Hypoventilation Syndrome

Kessler R, Chaouat A, Schinkewitch P, Faller M, Casel S, Krieger J, et al. The obesity-hypoventilation syndrome revisited: a prospective study of 34 consecutive cases. *Chest*. 2001(Aug);120(2):369–76.

Masa JF, Celli BR, Riesco JA, Hernandez M, Sanchez De Cos J, Disdier C. The obesity hypoventilation syndrome can be treated with noninvasive mechanical ventilation. *Chest*. 2001(Apr);119(4):1102–7.

Nowbar S, Burkart KM, Gonzales R, Fedorowicz A, Gozansky WS, Gaudio JC, et al. Obesity-associated hypoventilation in hospitalized patients: prevalence, effects, and outcome. *Am J Med*. 2004 (Jan 1);116(1):1–7.

Sugerman HJ, Fairman RP, Sood RK, Engle K, Wolfe L, Kellum JM. Long-term effects of gastric surgery for treating respiratory insufficiency of obesity. *Am J Clin Nutr*. 1992(Feb);55(2 Suppl):597S–601S.

Sullivan CE, Berthon-Jones M, Issa FG. Remission of severe obesity-hypoventilation syndrome after short-term treatment during sleep with nasal continuous positive airway pressure. *Am Rev Respir Dis*. 1983(Jul);128(1):177–81.

Congenital Central Hypoventilation Syndrome

Amiel J, Laudier B, Attie-Bitach T, Trang H, de Pontual L, Gener B, et a;. Polyalanine expansion and frameshift mutations of the paired-like homeobox gene PHOX2B in congenital central hypoventilation syndrome. *Nat Genet*. 2003(Apr);33(4):459–61. Epub 2003 Mar 17.

Gozal D. Congenital central hypoventilation syndrome: an update. *Pediatr Pulmonol*. 1998(Oct);26(4):273–82.

Paton JY, Swaminathan S, Sargent CW, Keens TG. Hypoxic and hypercapnic ventilatory responses in awake children with congenital central hypoventilation syndrome. *Am Rev Respir Dis*. 1989(Aug);140(2):368–72.

Paton JY, Swaminathan S, Sargent CW, Hawksworth A, Keens TG. Ventilatory response to exercise in children with congenital central hypoventilation syndrome. *Am Rev Respir Dis*. 1993(May);147(5):1185–91.

Silvestri JM, Weese-Mayer DE, Flanagan EA. Congenital central hypoventilation syndrome: cardio-respiratory responses to moderate exercise, simulating daily activity. *Pediatr Pulmonol*. 1995(Aug);20(2):89–93.

Weese-Meyer DE, Shannon DC, Keens TG, Silvestri JM. 1999. American Thoracic Society Consensus Statement. Idiopathic congenital central hypoventilation syndrome. diagnosis and management. *Am J Respir Crit Care Med*. 160:368–373.

Weese-Mayer DE, Silvestri JM, Menzies LJ, Morrow-Kenny AS, Hunt CE, Hauptman SA. Congenital central hypoventilation syndrome: diagnosis, management, and long-term outcome in thirty-two children. *J Pediatr*. 1992(Mar);120(3):381–7.

Weese-Mayer DE, Berry-Kravis EM, Zhou L, Maher BS, Silvestri JM, Curran ME, et al. Idiopathic congenital central hypoventilation syndrome: analysis of genes pertinent to early autonomic nervous system embryologic development and identification of mutations in PHOX2b. *Am J Med Genet A*. 2003(Dec 15);123(3):267–78.

Woo MS, Woo MA, Gozal D, Jansen MT, Keens TG, Harper RM. Heart rate variability in congenital central hypoventilation syndrome. *Pediatr Res.* 1992(Mar);31(3):291–6.

Other Causes of Sleep-Related Hypoventilation

American Academy of Sleep Medicine. *The International Classification of Sleep Disorders: Diagnostic and Coding Manual.* 2nd ed. American Academy of Sleep Medicine, 2005.

Circadian Rhythm Disorders 6

Definition of Chronobiologic Terms

Rhythmicity in biological processes is a fundamental characteristic of life. There is simply insufficient cellular energy for organisms to perform all their functions at the same constant rate (steady state) and all at the same time. Biological rhythms are ubiquitous, being found in prokaryotic and eukaryotic microbes; plants; insects; and animals, including humans. Endogenous rhythm generators or pacemakers as well as environmental factors, such as cycles of light and darkness, control these biologic rhythms.

Rhythms are characterized by specific frequency, period length, amplitude, and phase. See Table 6–1 for more information.

Table 6-1. Definitions		
Frequency	Number of oscillations per unit time	
	Ultradian–one oscillation lasting less than 24 hours	
	Circadian–one oscillation approximately every 24 hours	
	Infradian–one oscillation lasting greater than 24 hours	
	Circaseptan–one oscillation every 7 days	
	Circannual–one oscillation per year	
Period length	Time interval between two consecutive events (eg, between two peaks)	
Amplitude	Maximal excursion from peak to trough	
	Acrophase–peak	
	Mesor–mean	
	Nadir–trough	
Phase	Temporal position in relation to an external cue (eg, light-dark cycle)	
	Phase advance–shift of an episode to an earlier time in the 24-hour cycle	
	Phase delay–shift of an episode to a later time in the 24-hour cycle	
Chronobiology	Study of the influence of circadian rhythms on biological processes	
Chronotherapy	Treatment approach utilizing manipulation of circadian rhythms	

Circadian Rhythms in Biologic Processes

The term "circadian" is derived from the Latin words *circa*, which means "about," and *dien*, which means "day." There are specific, genetically determined circadian fluctuations in most biochemical and physiologic variables, with each oscillating at its own frequency, period length, amplitude, peak, trough, and phase. Different variables attain peak levels of activity at different points in time throughout a circadian period—some peak during the sleep phase, some peak in the awake phase, and others peak during the transition between sleep and wakefulness (Table 6–2).

Basic Principles of Chronobiology

Free-Running

Circadian rhythms *free-run* at their genetically determined frequency in the absence of synchronizing environmental time cues. Most free-running intrinsic human circadian rhythms have been

Table 6–2. Circadian rhythms of physiologic variables

Peak activity	Physiologic variables	Associated disease events
During the sleep phase	Adrenocorticotropic hormone Cortisol Follicle-stimulating hormone Luteinizing hormone Lymphocyte and eosinophil counts Melatonin Prolactin Thyroid-stimulating hormone	Angina (Prinzmetal's) Gastric ulcer Nocturnal asthma Strokes (late night)
During the transition from sleep to wakefulness	Catecholamine surges	Blood pressure surges
During the active phase	Blood chemistry Acid phosphatase Cholesterol Triglycerides Uric acid Body temperature Forced expiratory volume Blood viscosity Hemoglobin concentration Platelet adhesiveness Red blood cell count Insulin levels	Angina Myocardial infarction (early morning)
During the transition from activity to sleep	Gastric acid secretion White blood cell count	

shown to not be exactly 24 hours, having a frequency ranging from slightly under or, more frequently, over 24 hours (most commonly about 24.2 hours). This endogenous circadian period is referred to as "*tau.*"

Entrainment

Entrainment is the process by which external time cues adjust the phase of the endogenous circadian rhythms. Entrainment synchronizes the intrinsic circadian cycle, which is generally not equivalent to 24 hours, to the environmental 24-hour period. For instance, the phase of the sleep-wake cycle can be reset forward or backward with light presented at dusk or dawn, respectively.

Zeitgebers

Zeitgebers (from the German word "time-giver") are environmental cues that are capable of entraining endogenous circadian rhythms. These external stimuli can either be photic or nonphotic (eg, meals or social interactions). Interactions of inputs from these environmental sources are complex with varying degrees of inhibition or synergy. Environmental light is the dominant synchronizer for the circadian sleep-wake pacemaker. Light exposure can induce phase shifts, the direction and extent of which depends on the intensity and duration of light exposure, and its timing in relation to the circadian rhythm. Changing the circadian phase of the sleep-wake cycle requires high intensity light (> 2000 lux). Indoor room lighting, which is typically less than 100 lux, possess less significant phase-changing effects.

Several nonphotic synchronizers are also capable of entraining circadian sleep-wake rhythms. These include meals, activities, social cues, and ambient temperature. Physical exercise in the evening can phase delay rhythms, whereas physical exercise in the morning can give rise to phase advance of rhythms. Phase delay can also result from passive body heating in the evening. These nonphotic stimuli have a weaker influence on the sleep-wake cycle compared to environmental light.

Phase Shifting

A phase shift is a forward or backward displacement of intrinsic circadian rhythms in response to entrainment by a zeitgeber. For instance, a phase delay is produced when light is presented near the start of the subjective night (ie, before the core body temperature nadir [CTmin]), whereas a phase advance follows light exposure near the end of the subjective night (ie, after the CTmin). Greatest phase shifting is seen when light exposure occurs closest to the CTmin. Exposure to light during the subjective day generates either no phase shifts (dead zone) or much lesser amounts of phase shifts compared with exposure during the subjective night.

The phase response curve is a graphical depiction of the process of entrainment that plots the timing of presentation of zeitgebers (eg, light) and the magnitude of the shift in phase of the circadian rhythms.

Constant Routine

A constant routine is a testing protocol of the endogenous circadian rhythms that involves placing a subject under a constant routine of activity, mealtime, and light exposure. This is performed to minimize the effects of zeitgebers on the rhythms being evaluated.

Biological Markers of Circadian Rhythms

Two biological markers have been utilized to estimate the timing of circadian rhythms, namely *dim light melatonin onset (DLMO)*, and *minimum of the core body temperature rhythm [CTmin]*). DLMO, defined as the time when melatonin levels start to rise (> 3 and 10 pg/ml for salivary and plasma melatonin, respectively), generally occurs 2 to 3 hours before bedtime in normally entrained persons. CTmin occurs 2 to 4 hours prior to the end of the sleep period.

Circadian Timing Systems

Circadian rhythms (eg, sleep-wake, core body temperature or hormonal levels) persist even under constant environmental conditions (ie, they are endogenous). In mammals, the suprachiasmatic nuclei (SCN) in the anterior hypothalamus, located dorsal to the optic chiasm, serve as the master neural generator of circadian rhythms. The SCN exert a pervasive influence on the timing of various physiologic and neurobehavioral variables both in relation to the exogenous environment and to each other. Other anatomical sites may also harbor endogenous clocks.

Suprachiasmatic Nuclei

Circadian rhythms in mammals are generated by a circadian pacemaker located in the SCN in the anterior hypothalamus. The SCN can be divided into two components, namely a core and a shell region (Table 6–3). The SCN oscillate independently of the environment, firing more frequently during the daytime compared to nighttime, and during wake and rapid eye movement (REM) sleep compared with non–rapid eye movement (NREM) sleep.

Table 6–3. Regions of the suprachiasmatic nuclei

Region	Location	Neurotransmitter	Size of neurons	Function
Core	Ventrolateral	Vasoactive intestinal peptide	Small (30 μm²)	Resetting of endogenous circadian rhythms
Shell	Dorsomedial	Arginine vasopressin	Large (45 μm²)	Control of endogenous circadian rhythms

The actions of the SCN include promoting wakefulness during the day and enhancing sleep consolidation during the night. Experimental bilateral ablation of the SCN leads to loss of the circadian rhythm of the sleep-wake cycle, with sleep being distributed randomly throughout the day and night. In some cases, it can result in a reduction in the duration of waking periods.

Several neurotransmitters are involved with the circadian timing system, such as gamma-aminobutyric acid (GABA), glutamate, histamine, neuropeptide γ, serotonin, vasoactive intestinal peptide, and vasopressin.

The SCN receive inputs from several sources, including:

1. Afferent pathways from *photic* stimuli

   • Photosensitive retina ganglion cells containing the photopigment, melanopsin, via the retinohypothalamic tract, using glutamate and pituitary adenylate cyclase–activating polypeptide as its neurotransmitters (main afferent connection). Retinal photoreceptors involved with circadian processes are most sensitive to visible light of shorter wavelengths (from 450 nm [blue] to 500 nm [blue-green])

   • Thalamic intergeniculate leaflet of the lateral geniculate nuclei via the geniculohypothalamic tract using neuropeptide γ and GABA as its neurotransmitters (alternate afferent connection)

   • Tuberomammillary complex neurons in the posterior basal hypothalamus via histaminergic pathways

   • Basal forebrain (eg, septum, diagonal band of Broca and substantia innominata) and brainstem (eg, pedunculopontine tegmentum and parabigeminal nucleus) neurons via cholinergic pathways

2. Afferent pathways from nonphotic stimuli, including midbrain medial raphe nuclei via serotonergic pathways

Although disruption of the retinohypothalamic tract results in loss of light entrainment, the latter appears to be unaffected by interruption of the alternate geniculohypothalamic tract.

Details about the afferent SCN pathways are provided in Table 6–4.

Table 6–4. Afferent suprachiasmatic nuclei pathways

Afferent inputs	Pathway	Neurotransmitter
Glutamatergic	From the eyes via retinohypothalamic tract	Glutamate
Alternate afferent connection	From the eye via the geniculohypothalamic tract	Neuropeptide γ, GABA
Histaminergic	Hypothalamus	Histamine
Cholinergic	From the basal forebrain and brainstem	Acetylcholine
Serotonergic	From the midbrain	Serotonin

The SCN has efferent projections to several areas of the central nervous system (CNS), including the:

1. Hypothalamus (subparaventricular zone, dorsal medial area, medial preoptic area, ventral tuberal area)

2. Locus ceruleus

3. Ventrolateral preoptic nucleus

4. Basal forebrain

5. Hypocretin neurons

6. Pineal gland (the pineal gland, in turn, influences the SCN via its production of melatonin [see below])

7. Thalamus (paraventricular nucleus, intergeniculate leaflet)

The pathway from the SCN to the pineal gland is shown in Figure 6–1. Transforming growth factor-α and prokineticin 2 are among the efferent SCN neurotransmitters.

Genetics

Circadian rhythms are under genetic control. Circadian rhythmicity appears to be related to auto-regulated cyclic oscillations in clock-related proteins.

Research into clock genes has been carried out in cyanobacteria, *Neurospora*, *Drosophila*, and mice. Mutations in clock genes are associated with faster or slower cycles than normal clocks and cause phase-advanced or phase-delayed sleep-wake rhythms. At least six genes related to the

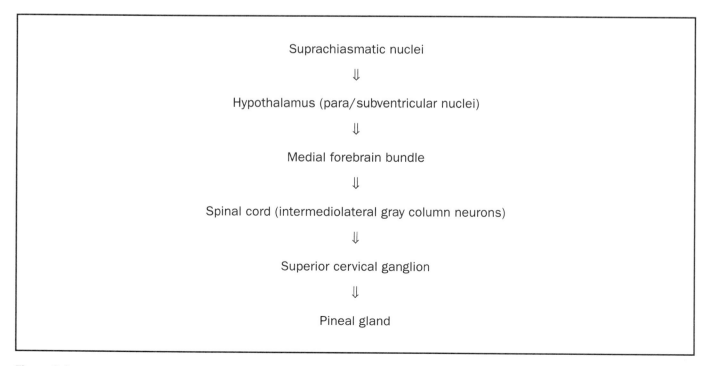

Figure 6-1
Neural pathway from the suprachiasmatic nuclei to the pineal gland

timing of circadian rhythms have been identified in the *Drosophila melanogaster*. These include *Casein kinase 1 (CK1), Clock (clk), Cryptochrome (cry), Cycle (cyc), Period (per)*, and *Timeless (tim)*. There is a high degree of similarity in sequence between *Drosophila* and mice genes. Corresponding mammalian circadian genes consist of *B-ma11, Casein kinase 1 (CK1), Clock (clk), Cryptochrome (Cry1* and *Cry2), Period (per1, per2* and *per3)*, and *Timeless (tim)*. It is likely that other genes may be involved. Variations in the *Clock gene* are responsible, in part, for the Horne-Ostberg "evening-ness" or "morningness" chronotypes.

Circadian rhythms are controlled by transcription-translation positive and negative feedback loops involving the clock genes and regulatory factors (eg, casein kinase I epsilon [CKIε]). Circadian gene feedback loops are shown in Figure 6–2. *Period* and *Timeless* transcription starts in the early morning to midday, with peak protein levels of *Period* and *Timeless* by mid-evening. Levels then decrease due to phosphorylation. Downregulation of *Period* and *Timeless* transcription occurs due to interactions with *Clock* and *Cycle*. *Cryptochrome* is required for light-related degradation of *Timeless*.

Transcription of *Clock* and *Bmal1* genes into mRNA

⇓

Translation of *Clock* and *Bmal1* mRNA into proteins

⇓

Translocation of *Clock* and *Bmal1* proteins into the nucleus

⇓

Activation of transcription and translation of *Period, Cryptochrome*, and *Timeless* that are then translocated into the nucleus

⇓

Inhibition of *Clock* and *Bmal1*

Figure 6-2 Circadian gene feedback loop

Melatonin

Melatonin is synthesized and released by the pineal gland in a rhythmic fashion with greatest secretion at night and suppression of secretion in the daytime. Production and secretion of melatonin is regulated by light stimuli via the SCN. In the pineal gland, the amino acid tryptophan is enzymatically converted into serotonin (5-hydroxytryptamine), which is, in turn, converted into melatonin (N-acetyl-5-methoxytryptamine). Production of melatonin decreases with aging. Exposure to light inhibits melatonin secretion. The liver metabolizes melatonin.

Melatonin, in turn, influences the SCN and alters the phase of circadian rhythms. Appropriately timed administration of melatonin can phase shift the circadian sleep-wake rhythms (ie, phase delay when taken in the morning, and phase advance when given in the afternoon or early evening). Melatonin is less effective in phase shifting the circadian rhythm compared to light exposure. Melatonin also possesses a mild hypnotic effect that helps promote sleep onset.

Circadian Rhythm Sleep Disorders

Proper alignment between the desired sleep-wake schedule and the circadian rhythm-related propensity for sleep and wakefulness is necessary for optimal sleep and wakefulness to occur. Circadian rhythm sleep disorders are caused by a recurrent or persistent mismatch between the sleep-wake schedules of the environmental day and endogenous circadian rhythms. They can give rise to insomnia or excessive sleepiness (or both), distress, and functional impairment.

There are six basic disorders of the circadian cycle. These can be classified as either *primary* (eg, delayed sleep phase syndrome, advanced sleep phase syndrome, irregular sleep-wake rhythm, free-running or nonentrained type), which results from a possible alteration of the endogenous circadian pacemakers, or *secondary* (eg, jet lag and shift work disorder), which is produced by an inability to adjust promptly to a change in environmental time. A list of circadian rhythm sleep disorders is presented in Box 6–1.

Delayed Sleep Phase Syndrome

Delayed sleep phase syndrome (DSPS) is characterized by a chronic or recurrent inability to sleep during desired hours, with a delayed habitual bedtime coupled with an equally delayed arising time (ie, the major nocturnal sleep period occurs later than the conventional or socially acceptable bedtime). Individuals complain of being unable to fall asleep until the early morning hours (eg, 1:00 to 6:00 AM) as well as difficulty arising until late morning or early afternoon (eg, 10:00 AM to 2:00 PM). Patients often report feeling most alert late in the evening and most sleepy in the morning. If they attempt to sleep and arise at times closer to socially accepted norms, both sleep-onset insomnia and morning sleepiness occur. Occasionally, marked difficulty awakening in the morning may be associated with confusion.

If untreated, DSPS tends to be persistent, but the severity may lessen with increasing age. Although individuals with DSPS are unable to voluntarily advance their sleep time, they typically have no difficulty remaining asleep following the onset of sleep, with normal (or prolonged) sleep duration and quality for age during their preferred sleep schedules, if sleep is allowed to continue *ad libitum* until spontaneous awakening.

Box 6–1. **Classification of circadian rhythm sleep disorders**	Delayed sleep phase syndrome
	Advanced sleep phase syndrome
	Irregular sleep-wake rhythm
	Free-running or nonentrained type (non–24–hour sleep-wake disorder)
	Jet lag
	Shift work sleep disorder
	Secondary to a medical condition
	Secondary to drug or substance Use

Source: Adapted from American Academy of Sleep Medicine. The International Classification of Sleep Disorders: Diagnostic and Coding Manual. 2nd ed. American Academy of Sleep Medicine, 2005.

Demographics

Excluding shift work sleep disorder and jet lag, DSPS is the most common of the circadian sleep disorders. It has a prevalence in the general population of about 0.1% to 0.2%. DSPS accounts for an estimated 5% to 10% of chronic insomnia cases seen in sleep clinics. Prevalence appears to be highest among adolescents and young adults. Mean age of onset is about 20 years. Both genders are affected equally.

Genetics

A significant number of individuals with DSPS report a positive family history. However, the genetic basis for DSPS remains incompletely understood. An autosomal dominant inheritance pattern has been described in a single family with DSPS. Associations between DSPS, human leukocyte antigen DR1 (HLA-DR1); and certain human Period 3 (hPer3), casein kinase I epsilon (CKIε), and arylalkylamine N-acetyltransferase gene polymorphisms have been described.

Associated Disorders

Associations between DSPS and affective disorders (eg, depression) and personality disorders have been described. DSPS has also been observed following traumatic brain injury.

Consequences

Consequences of DSPS include sleep deprivation if earlier wake times are enforced. Habitual absence or tardiness for early work or school schedules could negatively impact job performance or academic advancement. Attempts to fall asleep at earlier times may lead to prolonged periods of time awake in bed; this, in turn, can give rise to secondary conditioned insomnia.

Pathophysiology

DSPS results from both a phase delay of the circadian pacemaker in relation to conventional sleep-wake schedules and an inability to advance the phase in order to correct the disturbance. Postulated pathogenetic mechanisms include an altered endogenous phase relative to the environmental light-dark cycle, a markedly prolonged intrinsic period, changes affecting the entrainment of the endogenous clock to synchronizing agents, decreased sensitivity to morning light exposure or hypersensitivity to nocturnal light exposure, impaired ability to phase advance, or disturbance in homeostatic regulation of sleep.

Social and behavioral factors may contribute to the genesis and maintenance of DSPS. Many individuals habitually choose to voluntarily delay bedtimes by engaging in social, academic, occupational, and recreational activities until the late evening or early morning hours. In addition, they may then nap in the afternoon to compensate for their shortened nocturnal sleep, thereby delaying sleep onset on subsequent evenings. Finally, exposure to environmental light in the evening while awake and decreased light exposure in the morning when patients are still asleep can further delay the circadian phase.

Evaluation

Diagnosis relies mainly on history, often aided by well-kept sleep diaries. Actigraphy or sleep logs monitored for at least 7 days reveal a stable delay of the habitual sleep period. Individuals typically score as evening types on the Horne-Ostberg "eveningness or morningness" chronotype scale.

Polysomnography

Polysomnography (PSG) is not routinely indicated for the diagnosis of DSPS. Polysomnographic findings depend on the timing of the study in relation to the habitual or desired sleep times. PSG commonly demonstrates an increase in sleep latency and decrease in total sleep time when performed during desired conventional sleep-wake times. In contrast, sleep architecture is normal for age when PSG is recorded at the habitual delayed sleep periods. Corresponding delays in the timing of the temperature rhythm nadir and DLMO are also present.

Differential Diagnosis

Differential diagnosis includes disorders that may also present with sleep-onset insomnia such as psychophysiologic insomnia, idiopathic insomnia, psychiatric conditions (eg, mood and anxiety disorders), restless legs syndrome, and other circadian rhythm sleep disorders (eg, irregular sleep-wake rhythm, free-running sleep-wake disorder, and shift work sleep disorder). Distinction has to be made between the altered sleep-wake patterns due to an acquired lifestyle or poor sleep hygiene and DSPS that they may resemble.

Therapy

Therapy for DSPS includes chronotherapy, phototherapy, and pharmacotherapy. Although hypnotic medications may improve sleep latency, this benefit is often partial and temporary, and these agents generally are not effective for long-term use. See Table 6–5 for more information about the treatment of DSPS. See Box 6–2 for the recommendations of the American Academy of Sleep Medicine for the use of light therapy in circadian rhythm sleep disorders.

Table 6–5. Therapy for delayed sleep phase syndrome

Therapy	Description
Chronotherapy	Both progressive phase delay and progressive phase advancement of the major sleep episode have been described for the therapy of DSPS.
	With the progressive phase delay approach, bedtime and wake times are delayed usually by about 2 to 3 hours each day on successive days. The major sleep episode is, therefore, allowed to "march" around the clock until the desired or conventional bedtime is reached. Napping should be avoided. Physical activities, meal times and light exposure should be timed to coincide with the progressive delay in wake times. This method relies on the individual's tendency to phase delay. However, this approach requires several days to complete, and many patients might find this approach cumbersome. School and work schedules are affected during those days when the individual is sleeping during the daytime.
	Progressive phase advance is achieved by gradually advancing bedtimes (usually by 30 to 60 minutes) and the time of awakening over several days until more conventional sleep-wake schedules are attained.
	Free-running or nonentrained type (non–24-hour sleep-wake disorder) has developed following chronotherapy in patients with DSPS.
	Alternatively, a schedule shift technique, consisting of six consecutive nights on the usual sleep schedule followed by a night of sleep deprivation, then six subsequent days with a 90-minute advance in sleep schedule can be tried. This protocol is repeated until the desired bedtime is attained.

Table 6–5. Therapy for delayed sleep phase syndrome—cont'd

Therapy	Description
Phototherapy	Phototherapy, or light treatment, utilizes timed early morning exposure and evening avoidance of bright light to produce a phase advance in the sleep-wake circadian cycle. The intensity and duration of light exposure should be individualized, with adjustments made as necessary depending on the person's response to the therapy. Suggested schedules have included 2 hours of morning light exposure at 2500 lux, or shorter durations of exposure at greater light intensities (eg, 10,000 lux for 30 to 40 minutes).
	The optimal timing of light exposure is equally important. Exposure *might* be of greatest benefit if timed close after the temperature nadir (CTmin). In theory, the closer such exposure is to the temperature nadir (on the dawn side), the more robust the phase advance should be. However, light administered prior to the temperature nadir could further phase delay circadian rhythms. The body temperature nadir is often about 1 to 2 hours after the habitual midsleep time.
	Because measuring temperature nadir is difficult and impractical for most patients, many clinicians simply initiate bright light therapy at the patient's habitual awakening time. If no significant phase advancement is achieved, bright lights can be applied at successively earlier times (e.g., 30 minutes to 1 hour earlier) until phase advancement is noted.
	Neither optimum nor minimum length of therapy has been standardized and, again, should be individualized. Maintenance dosing may be useful to help prevent relapse.
	Commercial bright light boxes generate light at 5,000 to 10,000 lux and generally filter out harmful ultraviolet rays.
	Phototherapy should not be used in patients with retinopathy, photosensitivity, mania, and possibly migraines. An ophthalmologic examination is recommended in patients with significant retinal and ocular disorders prior to initiating bright light therapy.
	Adverse effects of light therapy include headaches, eye irritation, nausea, dryness of the eyes and skin, skin erythema, and precipitation of a hypomanic state in patients with bipolar disorder.
Melatonin	Trials of melatonin for DSPS have utilized various response measures and melatonin dosage and duration. Generally, melatonin given in the evening is effective in inducing a phase advance of the sleep period with a decrease in sleep latency. Its phase shifting effect is less potent than that of bright light. Relapse to pretreatment sleep patterns has been reported to be high in patients on long-term melatonin therapy for DSPS.
	Melatonin also has a mild hypnotic effect when ingested in supraphysiologic (> 0.5-mg) doses. Patients taking melatonin should be cautioned against driving or engaging in potentially dangerous activities for several hours after ingesting melatonin.
	The FDA does not approve melatonin as a therapy for circadian sleep disorders. Melatonin may worsen asthma symptoms. Its use should be avoided in pregnant or breastfeeding women.
Other pharmacologic treatments	Vitamin B_{12} and sedative-hypnotic agents have been described for the therapy of DSPS but few systematic investigations regarding their efficacy have been performed. Vitamin B_{12} is believed to augment the entraining effect of light on the SCN.
Behavioral interventions	Once a desired sleep-wake schedule has been established, efforts shift to the maintenance of the new sleep pattern because the risk of relapse may be high. Because subsequent delays in bedtime and arising times could initiate a new cycle of sleep phase delay, patients should be instructed to maintain a regular sleep schedule throughout the week. Careful attention to sleep hygiene is essential. Patients with a previous history of repeated relapses may benefit from ongoing maintenance therapy with periodic timed bright light exposure or melatonin administration.

Box 6–2.

American Academy of Sleep Medicine (AASM) recommendations for the use of light therapy for circadian rhythm sleep disorders

1. A physician planning to use light therapy should know recommended dosages and intensity limits, and adverse effects of this form of treatment (standard).

2. When used within recommended guidelines regarding intensity and duration of exposure, light therapy used for some circadian rhythm disorders is generally safe (guideline).

3. Light therapy appears to have potential utility for the treatment of the following circadian rhythm disorders:

   • Delayed sleep phase syndrome (guideline)

   • Advanced sleep phase syndrome (guideline)

   • Some blind patients with Non-24-hour sleep-wake syndrome (option)

4. Neither the minimum nor optimal duration of light therapy is known for the following circadian rhythm disorders:

   • Delayed sleep phase syndrome (option)

   • Advanced sleep phase syndrome (option)

   • Non-24-hour sleep-wake syndrome (Option)

5. For jet lag, light therapy at destination appears potentially useful for individuals traveling across multiple time zones (option).

6. For shift workers:

   • Light exposure *before* the core body temperature minimum may be helpful for a *day to evening to night* rotating work schedule (option)

   • Light exposure *after* the core body temperature minimum may be helpful for a *night to evening to day* schedule (option)

7. No recommendations are provided regarding the use of light therapy for patients with dementia, or other causes of insomnia among the healthy elderly.

Source: Adapted and modified from Chesson, et al. Practice parameters for the use of light therapy in the treatment of sleep disorders. Sleep, 1999;22:5.

AASM Definition of Terms

Standard	Generally accepted practice with a level of clinical certainly
Guideline	Practice associated with a moderate degree of clinical certainty
Option	Practice of uncertain clinical use

Advanced Sleep Phase Syndrome

Advanced sleep phase syndrome (ASPS) involves a stable shift of the major sleep period to an earlier time relative to desired or conventional bedtimes. This results in a marked inability to delay sleep time and a spontaneous morning awakening that is several hours earlier than desired. Patients generally report being most alert in the morning. Sleep typically occurs between 6:00 and 9:00 PM and wake time occurs between 2:00 and 5:00 AM. Sleep, itself, is normal for age and undisturbed.

Clinical Features

Typical complaints include excessive sleepiness in the late afternoon or early evening and an inability to remain asleep until the desired morning awakening time. Affected individuals may voluntarily restrict nighttime activities to permit earlier bedtimes. Psychophysiologic or conditioned insomnia may develop if maladaptive responses to the early morning awakenings occur. In addition, sleep deprivation may ensue due to the persistence of early morning awakenings if the person stays up later than is customary due to job or social responsibilities.

Demographics

ASPS is estimated to affect approximately 1% of middle-aged adults and is less common than DSPS. Onset is typically during middle age. Prevalence increases with age, and the elderly are at greater risk of developing ASPS due to their tendency for mild sleep phase advancement. Cases not involving middle age and elderly adults are rare. Both genders are affected equally. Individuals with ASPS are commonly rated as "morning types" on the Horne-Ostberg questionnaire, which assesses an individual's "eveningness" or "morningness."

Genetics

Familial cases of ASPS have been described. The gene of familial ASPS, an autosomal dominant variant, has been localized near the telomere of chromosome 2q. A serine to glycine mutation within the casein kinase I epsilon (CKIε) binding region of *hPer2* (human Period 2) causes hypophosphorylation of *hPer2* protein by CKIε in vitro. This, in turn, results in a shortening of the cycle duration of the transcription-translation feedback loop. Other cases of familial ASPS involve a mutation of the casein kinase I delta (CKI_δ) gene.

Pathophysiology

The precise pathogenetic mechanism of ASPS remains unknown. It is possible that affected individuals may have a deficiency in their ability to phase delay, an overly dominant phase-advance capability, a naturally faster circadian rhythm, or a very short endogenous period length. There is also an earlier phase in the timing of melatonin onset (DLMO) and temperature rhythm (CTmin). Finally, consistent early awakenings can lead to greater morning light exposure and earlier bedtimes limit evening light exposure, both of which can contribute to phase advances.

Evaluation

Diagnosis relies on sleep logs or actigraphy performed over several days. If PSG is performed over the usual advanced sleep schedule, sleep latency, duration, and quality are normal. In contrast, a short sleep latency and decrease in total sleep time are observed if PSG is recorded during conventional sleep-wake times. There can be a decrease in REM sleep latency.

Occasionally, a psychiatric evaluation may be required to exclude major mood disorders because depression may also present with early morning awakenings. Depression is often associated with a decrease in REM sleep latency as well as frequent awakenings, whereas sleep quality prior to the final awakening is normal in ASPS.

Therapy

Bright light therapy for 30 to 45 minutes or longer during the early evening (7:00 to 9:00 PM) prior to the body temperature nadir in order to phase delay the circadian sleep-wake timing rhythm may be useful in persons with ASPS. Light exposure in the early morning should be minimized. Chronotherapy involves gradually shifting the usual sleep time until the desired bedtime is achieved.

Administration of melatonin during the early morning has been proposed but, given its hypnotic properties, can lead to unwanted daytime sleepiness.

Irregular Sleep-Wake Pattern

In the irregular sleep-wake pattern (ISWP) syndrome, stable circadian sleep-wake rhythms are absent. Sleep and wake times are disorganized, with three or more short "naps" comprising the fragmentary remnants of the major sleep episode. There is temporal variability in sleep and wake activity from one day to the next, with inconsistent, unpredictable sleep onset and wake times throughout the day. Nonetheless, the aggregate sleep time over a 24-hour period is typically near normal or normal for age.

Affected individuals may complain of insomnia, daytime sleepiness, and/or cognitive impairment.

Demographics

ISWP may arise from abnormalities of the circadian clock or severely disrupted entrainment by environmental synchronizing factors. The disorder is rare in the general population and is most frequently encountered in persons with severe brain dysfunction (eg, mental retardation, dementia, head injury or recovery from coma). However, ISWP may be observed in normal cognitively intact individuals who repetitively ignore environmental and social time cues with indiscriminate daytime napping or spending disproportionately excessive time in bed (voluntary irregular sleep schedule). Onset can occur at any age. It appears to affect both genders equally and has no identified familial pattern.

Evaluation

In addition to a comprehensive history, diagnosis often requires sleep logs and wrist actigraphic monitoring over several days, none of which demonstrates any apparent regular sleep-wake circadian pattern. Poor sleep hygiene must be excluded.

The loss of the normal pattern of sleep and wakefulness is clearly evident during a 24-hour PSG, and if recordings are continued for several days, the sleep and wake schedules will be observed to be variable and disorganized. Other chronobiologic rhythms, including body temperature and hormones, may demonstrate flattened profiles with loss of periodic fluctuations.

Therapy

Therapy for ISWP needs to be individualized. Successful outcomes with both properly timed bright light therapy and evening melatonin administration have been reported. The use of vitamin B_{12} or hypnotics has also been described. Behavioral modifications, including maintaining regular schedules of sleep and wakefulness, limiting the aggregate daily time spent in bed, and having structured daytime activities, including mealtimes and social activities, can be of benefit. Chronic use of hypnotic agents should be avoided.

Free-Running or Nonentrained Type (Non–24-Hour Sleep-Wake Disorder)

Definition

In free-running or nonentrained type (non–24-hour sleep-wake disorder or hypernychthemeral syndrome), there is abnormal synchronization between the endogenous sleep-wake circadian rhythm and the 24-hour environmental light-dark cycle. Sleep-wake patterns seem to rely solely on intrinsic biologic rhythms. Freed of exogenous entraining influences such as light and social activities, the free-running internal rhythms behave with a periodicity of slightly over 24 hours.

Clinical Features

Sleep onset and wake times are delayed by about 1 hour or more each day. Less commonly, longer cycles may be observed resulting in greater daily delays. The major sleep period therefore progressively "marches" throughout the day, into the afternoon and on to the evening. The relationship between the external 24-hour world and the internal 25-hour clock then tends to vary from one extreme of total asynchrony to the other extreme of complete conformity. The severity of symptoms shares this cyclic variability and range from considerable sleep and daytime disturbances to the complete, albeit brief, disappearance of symptoms. Despite the progressive delay in sleep schedules, sleep duration and daytime performance may be normal if patients are allowed to sleep *ad libitum*.

As sleep onset and offset are progressively delayed, affected individuals complain of periodically recurring problems of insomnia or excessive daytime sleepiness. They are often incapable of maintaining the tightly scheduled lifestyle required for schooling and employment.

Demographics

This syndrome is rarely encountered in the general population, and most reported cases involved totally blind individuals who lack photic entrainment, many of whom also have psychiatric or behavioral disorders. About 70% of blind individuals complain of chronic sleep-wake disturbances and 40% have chronic, recurring and cyclical insomnia.

Light stimuli to the SCN are absent in most blind individuals. However, some blind persons are able to partially entrain to the environment using nonphotic factors (social schedules) or photic cues via an intact retinohypothalamic pathway (ie, they demonstrate melatonin suppression with light exposure). Unlike totally blind persons with absent retinas who are incapable of entraining to environmental light, blind persons with intact functioning retinohypothalamic tracts are able to synchronize to external photic zeitgebers and are, thus, less likely to develop progressive phase delays in their circadian sleep-wake rhythms.

Less commonly, this condition can affect sighted individuals with severely schizoid or avoidant personality disorders, mental retardation, or dementia. Cases associated with hypothalamic tumors or brain injuries have also been described.

There are no known gender differences or familial patterns. Onset can occur at any age. If left untreated, its course tends to be chronic and unrelenting.

Pathophysiology

Several mechanisms have been postulated to account for the lack of stable entrainment to the 24-hour environment, including a weakness of zeitgebers or environmental entraining influences, a decreased sensitivity to zeitgebers, or a circadian system period that is markedly longer than 24- hours. The melatonin rhythm may be dampened, deficient, or delayed, with low nighttime levels of plasma melatonin. In addition, there may be internal desynchronization among the various endogenous circadian rhythms, such as body temperature. In sighted individuals, the non–24-hour sleep-wake syndrome may arise from a reduced sensitivity to the phase-altering effects of light, voluntary disregard of entraining environmental or social cues, or an extremely lengthy endogenous circadian period that is beyond the range for external 24-hour entrainment.

Environmental influences may modify the expression of sleep-wake rhythm disorders. A report described two female siblings with non–24-hour sleep-wake rhythm at home who developed DSPS immediately following admission to a hospital.

Evaluation

The non–24-hour sleep-wake syndrome should be considered in any blind individual who presents with complaints of periodic and recurring episodes of insomnia and excessive daytime somnolence.

Diagnosis is made by sleep logs or actigraphy performed over several days or weeks that demonstrate a progressive delay of the circadian sleep-wake timing that is present for at least 1 to 2 months. PSG and continuous 24-hour body temperature monitoring seldom provide additional useful diagnostic information not obtainable from carefully kept sleep-wake logs or actigraphy. Despite variations in sleep onset and offset times, sleep efficiency is usually normal. If PSG is recorded at a fixed time over several days, sleep latency becomes progressively longer, and total sleep time becomes commensurately shorter. Twenty-four-hour core body temperature monitoring and measurements of DLMO demonstrate a progressive delay of the temperature and melatonin rhythms.

A thorough neurologic evaluation is recommended for sighted persons to exclude any occult CNS pathology.

Differential Diagnosis

Differential diagnosis includes a delayed sleep phase syndrome that might occasionally occur with a progressive delay in bedtime. Other causes of altered circadian rhythms, such as medical, neurologic, psychiatric, or behavioral disorders, as well as medication use or abuse, should be excluded.

Therapy

Melatonin administered in the evening or at bedtime to entrain the circadian rhythm is the initial treatment of choice. Light therapy may be an option in sighted persons or blind persons with light perception. Nonphotic entrainment by strict regulation of the timing of bedtime, arising times, activities, and meals, or the use of hypnotic agents and stimulants, are less effective. Although its mechanism of action is unknown, oral vitamin B_{12} has been tried with some success in persons with this syndrome.

Time Zone Change (Jet Lag) Syndrome

Clinical Features

Rapid eastward or westward air travel across multiple time zones can precipitate both transient insomnia and hypersomnolence. In time zone change syndrome or jet lag, the person's intrinsic circadian rhythm remains temporarily aligned to the home time zone and has not yet synchronized to the external cues in the new local time zone. Individuals traveling westward are phase-advanced relative to the new clock time and those traveling eastward are phase-delayed.

Common complaints include nighttime insomnia, disturbed sleep, frequent arousals, excessive daytime sleepiness, and diminished daytime alertness and performance developing within a day or two of transmeridian air travel. A westward flight is associated with early evening sleepiness as well as increased wakefulness during the early morning hours. Conversely, eastward flights result in both difficulty falling asleep and difficulty awakening the next day. Individuals may also present with nonspecific gastrointestinal disturbances, malaise, fatigue, and decreased mood.

There are individual differences in susceptibility, and not every traveler develops jet lag. Symptoms tend to increase in severity with greater amounts and rates of time zone transitions as well as with increasing age. The direction of travel (symptoms may be more pronounced with eastward travel that entails a phase advance) and factors associated with travel itself, such as prior sleep deprivation, psychologic stress, and prolonged inactivity during flights, may also influence symptom severity. North-south travel does not lead to jet lag symptoms.

Depending on the direction of jet travel, PSG performed at the new sleep schedule demonstrates prolonged sleep latency or early morning awakenings, and diminished sleep efficiency.

Jet lag is self-limited, and symptoms typically remit spontaneously within a few days (approximately a day for every time zone change). Adjustment is characteristically more difficult following eastward travel, which requires advancing the circadian phase, compared with westward travel. Resynchronization may be delayed among the elderly and by inappropriate timing of light exposure. Nonetheless, another diagnosis, such as psychophysiologic insomnia, should be considered if sleep disturbance persists for longer than 2 weeks.

Therapy

Sleep-wake schedules should be immediately changed to accommodate to the new destination time on the day of arrival. Individuals may choose to begin the shift in sleep-wake schedule even prior to travel. Appropriately timed exposure to bright lights (ie, morning exposure after westward travel and evening exposure after eastward travel) may hasten synchronization to the new time zone. Administration of melatonin several hours prior to bedtime starting a few days prior to eastward travel and continuing for several days at the new destination has been reported. Short-acting hypnotic agents taken at the new bedtime can also help alleviate complaints of insomnia. Caffeine may be tried to minimize excessive daytime sleepiness.

Shift Work Sleep Disorder

Shift work may take several forms, including permanent night or early morning hours, rotating schedules or random work assignments. Workers who have rotating shifts or have regular nighttime or early morning shift schedules but revert back to a traditional daytime routine on nonworking days (eg, weekends and vacations) may experience a disparity in the timing between the requirements of work and the demands for sleep. In addition, the conventional time cues of sunlight and social activities are frequently out of phase with the altered sleep time.

Complaints of insomnia and sleep disruption are common. When working the night shift, sleep begun the following morning may have a prolonged latency. Conversely, persons who have to arise shortly after midnight to start an early morning work schedule (eg, between 3:00 and 7:00 AM) may complain of difficulty falling asleep in the early evening hours and difficulty waking up. Sleep is often described as nonrestorative or unsatisfying. Other presenting features include excessive sleepiness, chronic fatigue, malaise, mood disorder, and nonspecific gastrointestinal (eg, dyspepsia), cardiovascular (eg, ischemic heart disease), and endocrine (eg, decreased glucose tolerance) disturbances. Shift workers may be at greater risk for alcohol and substance dependency.

Not every shift worker develops the disorder; some workers can adapt more readily to nonconventional work and sleep hours than others. Factors that may influence a person's ability to tolerate shift work schedules include age, diurnal preference ("eveningness" versus "morningness"), comorbid sleep disorders, and extent of daytime activities. Shift work sleep disorder can affect workers of all ages. Both genders are affected equally. Its course parallels the schedule of the shift work period and remits with termination of shift work.

Shift work sleep disorder poses a significant hazard in the work environment. Serious physical injuries and faulty decision-making may arise due to diminished vigilance secondary to sleep deprivation and circadian changes in levels of alertness. Shift work sleep disorder also has a negative impact on work performance and family life.

Evaluation

Sleep logs or actigraphy recorded over several days may reveal a reduction in total sleep time in addition to the circadian misalignment in sleep-wake times. PSG is rarely required to diagnose shift work sleep disorder. However, if PSG is indicated to exclude other sleep disorders, it is preferable to perform the recording during the usual shift work schedule. Common polysomnographic features include an increase in sleep latency, decrease in total sleep time, and decrease in sleep efficiency with frequent arousals and awakenings. Reductions in NREM stage 2 sleep and REM sleep are also seen. Polysomnographic features of this disorder are listed in Box 6–3.

Box 6-3. **Polysomnographic features of shift work sleep disorder**	↑ Sleep latency ↓ Total sleep time ↓ Sleep efficiency ↑ Frequency of arousals ↓ NREM stage 2 sleep ↓ REM sleep

Therapy

Maintaining a regular and comparable sleep-wake schedule during both work and nonwork days is important. Intermittent use of hypnotics can alleviate insomnia, as can minimizing environmental factors (eg, light or noise) in the bedroom that might disrupt sleep. Light exposure should also be minimized during the morning trip home from work (eg, using dark sunglasses).

Intermittent exposure to bright lights in the workplace, administration of psychostimulants (eg, caffeine or modafinil) during evening work hours, and scheduled napping can enhance alertness and reduce sleepiness. Other causes of excessive sleepiness, such as inadequate sleep hygiene, obstructive sleep apnea or narcolepsy, must be addressed and managed.

Family counseling may be useful if significant disruptions of social and family life arising from the worker's shift schedules are present. Organizations can help alleviate sleep disturbances and enhance alertness during nighttime work among their shift workers by scheduling phase delays in shifts (ie, evening to night to day), rather than phase advances. In addition, random work schedules or rapidly rotating shifts should be avoided.

Secondary to a Medical Condition

Disturbances of circadian sleep rhythms may be secondary to a medical (eg, encephalopathy from liver cirrhosis) or neurologic disorder (eg, dementia). Individuals may present with complaints of insomnia, poor sleep quality, or daytime sleepiness. A misalignment between the endogenous sleep-wake cycle and external circadian synchronizing agents can be discernible on sleep logs or actigraphy recorded over several days.

Secondary to Drug or Substance Use

In this disorder, disturbances of circadian sleep-wake rhythms are secondary to the use of specific drugs or substances and not to other circadian rhythm sleep disorders.

References

General References

American Academy of Sleep Medicine. *The International Classification of Sleep Disorders: Diagnostic and Coding Manual*. 2nd ed. Westchester, IL: American Academy of Sleep Medicine, 2005.

Bowman TJ. *Review of Sleep Medicine*. Burlington, MA: Butterworth-Heinemann, 2002.

Berry RB. *Sleep Medicine Pearls*. 2nd ed. Philadelphia, PA: Hanley & Belfus, 2002.

Chokroverty S. *Clinical Companion to Sleep Disorders Medicine*. 2nd ed. Burlington, MA: Butterworth-Heinemann, 2000.

Lavie P, Pillar G, Malhotra A. *Sleep Disorders Handbook*. New York, NY: Taylor & Francis, 2002.

Lee-Chiong TL, ed. *Sleep: A Comprehensive Handbook*. Hoboken, NJ: John Wiley & Sons, 2006.

Lee-Chiong TL, Sateia M, Carskadon M, eds. *Sleep Medicine*. Philadelphia, PA: Hanley & Belfus (Elsevier), 2002.

Perlis ML, Lichstein KL, eds. *Treating Sleep Disorders: Principles and Practice of Behavioral Sleep Medicine*. Hoboken, NJ: John Wiley & Sons, 2003.

Rechtschaffen A, Kales A. *A Manual of Standardized Terminology, Techniques and Scoring System for Sleep Stages of Human Subjects*. Los Angeles, CA: Brain Information Service/Brain Research Institute, University of California, 1968.

Reid KJ, Burgess HJ. Circadian rhythm sleep disorders. *Sleep Medicine. Primary Care: Clinics in Office Practice*. Elsevier Saunders, 2005.

Reid KJ, Chang AM, Zee PC. Circadian rhythm sleep disorders. *Sleep Disorders*. Medical Clinics of North America. Philadelphia, PA: Elsevier Saunders, 2004.

Reite M, Ruddy J, Nagel K. *Concise Guide to Evaluation and Management of Sleep Disorders* (3rd ed.). Arlington, VA: American Psychiatric Publishing, April 2002.

Sleep Deprivation and Stimulant Task Force of the American Academy of Sleep Medicine. The use of stimulants to modify performance during sleep loss: a review. *Sleep*. 2005;28(9).

Sleep Disorders. Medical Clinics of North America. Elsevier Saunders, 2004.

Sleep Medicine. Primary Care: Clinics in Office Practice. Elsevier Saunders, 2005.

Sleep Research Society. *SRS Basics of Sleep Guide*. Sleep Research Society, 2005.

Definition of Chronobiologic Terms

Lee-Chiong TL, ed. *Sleep: A Comprehensive Handbook*. Hoboken, NJ: John Wiley & Sons, 2006.

Lee-Chiong TL, Sateia M, Carskadon M, eds. *Sleep Medicine*. Philadelphia, PA: Hanley & Belfus (Elsevier), 2002.

Sleep Research Society. *SRS Basics of Sleep Guide*. Sleep Research Society, 2005.

Circadian Rhythms in Biologic Processes

Lee-Chiong TL, ed. *Sleep: A Comprehensive Handbook*. Hoboken, NJ: John Wiley & Sons, 2006.

Lee-Chiong TL, Sateia M, Carskadon M, eds. *Sleep Medicine.* Philadelphia, PA: Hanley & Belfus (Elsevier), 2002.

Sleep Research Society. *SRS Basics of Sleep Guide.* Sleep Research Society, 2005.

Basic Principles of Chronobiology

Hastings M, Maywood ES. Circadian clocks in the mammalian brain. *BioEssays.* 2000;22:23–31.

Vitaterna MH, King DP, Chang AM, Kornhauser JM, Lowrey PL, McDonald JP, et al. Mutagenesis and mapping of a mouse gene, Clock, essential for circadian behavior. *Science.* 1994;264: 719–725.

Circadian Timing Systems

Lee-Chiong TL, ed. *Sleep: A Comprehensive Handbook.* Hoboken, NJ: John Wiley & Sons, 2006.

Lee-Chiong TL, Sateia M, Carskadon M, eds. *Sleep Medicine.* Philadelphia, PA: Hanley & Belfus (Elsevier), 2002.

Sleep Research Society. *SRS Basics of Sleep Guide.* Sleep Research Society, 2005.

Suprachiasmatic Nuclei

Lee-Chiong TL, ed. *Sleep: A Comprehensive Handbook.* Hoboken, NJ: John Wiley & Sons, 2006.

Lee-Chiong TL, Sateia M, Carskadon M, eds. *Sleep Medicine.* Philadelphia, PA: Hanley & Belfus (Elsevier), 2002.

Sleep Research Society. *SRS Basics of Sleep Guide.* Sleep Research Society, 2005.

Genetics

Lee-Chiong TL, ed. *Sleep: A Comprehensive Handbook.* Hoboken, NJ: John Wiley & Sons, 2006.

Lee-Chiong TL, Sateia M, Carskadon M, eds. *Sleep Medicine.* Philadelphia, PA: Hanley & Belfus (Elsevier), 2002.

Melatonin

Lee-Chiong TL, ed. *Sleep: A Comprehensive Handbook.* Hoboken, NJ: John Wiley & Sons, 2006.

Lee-Chiong TL, Sateia M, Carskadon M, eds. *Sleep Medicine.* Philadelphia, PA: Hanley & Belfus (Elsevier), 2002.

Sleep Research Society. *SRS Basics of Sleep Guide.* Westchester, IL: Sleep Research Society, 2005.

Delayed Sleep Phase Syndrome

Czeisler CA, Richardson GS, Zimmerman JC, Moore-Ede MC, Weitzman ED. Entrainment of human circadian rhythms by light-dark cycles: a reassessment. *Photochem Photobiol.* 1981;34(2):239–47.

Czeisler CA, Richardson GS, Coleman RM, Zimmerman JC, Moore-Ede MC, Dement WC, et al. Chronotherapy: resetting the circadian clocks of patients with delayed sleep phase insomnia. *Sleep.* 1981;4:1–21.

Dagan Y, Eisenstein M. Circadian rhythm sleep disorders: toward a more precise definition and diagnosis. *Chronobiol Int.* 1999;16:213–22.

Dagan Y, Stein D, Steinbock M, Yovel I, Hallis D. Frequency of delayed sleep phase syndrome among hospitalized adolescent psychiatric patients. *J Psychosom Res.* 1998;45:15–20.

Dagan Y, Yovel I, Hallis D, Eisenstein M, Raichik I. Evaluating the role of melatonin in the long-term treatment of delayed sleep phase syndrome (DSPS). *Chronobiol Int.* 1998;15(2):181–90.

Ebisawa T, Uchiyama M, Kajimura N, Mishima K, Kamei Y, Katoh M, et al. Association of structural polymorphisms in the human period3 gene with delayed sleep phase syndrome. *EMBO Rep.* 2001;2:342–346.

Hoelscher TJ, Bond T, Ware JC. Treatment of delayed sleep phase syndrome with sleep schedule manipulation. *Sleep Res.* 1992;1: 211.

Hohjoh H, Takahashi Y, Hatta Y, Tanaka H, Akaza T, Tokunaga K, et al. Possible association of human leucocyte antigen DR1 with delayed sleep phase syndrome. *Psychiatry Clin Neurosci.* 1999;53:527–529.

Kamei Y, Hayakawa T, Urata J, Uchiyama M, Shibui K, Kim K, et al. Melatonin treatment for circadian rhythm sleep disorders. *Psychiatry Clin Neurosci.* 2000;54:381–382.

Kamei Y, Urata J, Uchiyaya M, Hayakawa T, Ozaki S, Shibui K, et al. Clinical characteristics of circadian rhythm sleep disorders. *Psychiatry Clin Neurosci.* 1998;52:234–235.

Okawa M, Uchiyama M, Ozaki S, Shibui K, Kamei Y, Hayakawa T, et al. Melatonin treatment for circadian rhythm sleep disorders. *Psychiatry Clin Neurosci.* 1998;52:259–260.

Pelayo RT, Govinski P. Prevalence of delayed sleep phase syndrome among adolescents. *Sleep Res.* 1988;17:392.

Quinto C, Gellido C, Chokroverty S, Masdeu J. Posttraumatic delayed sleep phase syndrome. *Neurology.* 2000;54:250–252.

Regestein QR, Monk TH. Delayed sleep phase syndrome: a review of its clinical aspects. *Am J Psychiatry.* 1995;152:602–608.

Reme CE, Rol P, Grothmann K, Kaase H, Terman M. Bright light therapy in focus: lamp emission spectra and ocular safety. *Technol Health Care.* 1996;4(4):403–13.

Rosenthal NE, Joseph-Vanderpool JR, Levendosky AA, Johnson SH, Allen R, Kelly KA, Souetre E, Schultz PM, Starz KE. Phase-shifting effects of bright morning light as treatment for delayed sleep phase syndrome. *Sleep.* 1990;13:354–361.

Schrader H, Bovim G, Sand T. The prevalence of delayed and advanced sleep phase syndromes. *J Sleep Res.* 1993;2(1):51–55.

Ulrich V, Olesen J, Gervil M, Russell MB. Possible risk factors and precipitants for migraine with aura in discordant twin-pairs: a population-based study. *Cephalalgia.* 2000;20(9):821–5.

Weitzman E, Czeisler CA, Coleman RM. Delayed sleep phase syndrome: a biological rhythm sleep disorder. *Sleep Res.* 1979;8:221.

Weitzman ED, Czeisler CA, Coleman RM, Spielman AJ, Zimmerman JC, Dement W, et al. Delayed sleep phase syndrome. A chronobiological disorder with sleep-onset insomnia. *Arch Gen Psychiatry,* 1981;38:737–746.

Yamadera H, Takahashi K, Okawa M. A multicenter study of sleep-wake rhythm disorders: therapeutic effects of vitamin B$_{12}$, bright light therapy, chronotherapy and hypnotics. *Psychiatry Clin Neurosci.* 1996;50:203–209.

Advanced Sleep Phase Syndrome

Ando K, Kripke DP, Ancoli-lsrael S. Estimated prevalence of delayed and advanced sleep phase syndromes. *Sleep Research.* 1995;24:509.

Chesson AL Jr, Littner M, Davila D, Anderson WM, Grigg-Damberger M, Hartse K, et al. Practice parameters for the use of light therapy in the treatment of sleep disorders. Standards of Practice Committee, American Academy of Sleep Medicine. *Sleep.* 1999;22:641–660.

Toh KL, Jones CR, He Y, Eide EJ, Hinz WA, Virshup DM, et al. An hPer2 phosphorylation site mutation in familial advanced sleep phase syndrome. *Science.* 2001;291:1040–1043.

Wagner DR. Disorders of the circadian sleep-wake cycle. *Neurol Clin.* 1996;14:651–670.

Irregular Sleep-Wake Pattern

Wagner DR. Disorders of the circadian sleep-wake cycle. *Neurol Clin.* 1996;14:651–670.

Free-Running or Nonentrained Type (Non–24-Hour Sleep-Wake Disorder)

Chesson AL Jr, Littner M, Davila D, Anderson WM, Grigg-Damberger M, Hartse K, et al. Practice parameters for the use of light therapy in the treatment of sleep disorders. Standards of Practice Committee, American Academy of Sleep Medicine. *Sleep.* 1999;22:641–660.

Hayashi E. Effect of melatonin on sleep-wake rhythm: the sleep diary of an autistic male. *Psychiatry Clin Neurosci.* 2000;54:383–384.

Kamei Y, Hayakawa T, Urata J, Uchiyama M, Shibui K, Kim K, et al. Melatonin treatment for circadian rhythm sleep disorders. *Psychiatry Clin Neurosci.* 2000;54:381–382.

Kamgar-Parsi B, Wehr TA, Gillin JC. Successful treatment of human non-24-hour sleep-wake syndrome. *Sleep.* 1983;6:257–264.

Kohsaka M. Non-24-hour sleep-wake syndrome. *Nippon Rinsho.* 1998;56:410–415.

Martens H, Endlich H, Hildebrandt G, et al. Sleep/wake distribution in blind subjects with and without sleep complaints. *Sleep Research.* 1990;9:398.

McArthur AJ, Lewy AJ, Sack RL. Non-24-hour sleep-wake syndrome in a sighted man: circadian rhythm studies and efficacy of melatonin treatment. *Sleep.* 1996;19:544–553.

Miles LE, Wilson MA. High incidence of cyclic sleep-wake disorders in the blind. *Sleep Research.* 1977;6:192.

Mukai M, Uchimura N, Takeuchi N, Waseda Y, Takaishi J, Sakamoto T, et al. Therapeutic progress of two sibling cases exhibiting sleep-wake rhythm disorder. *Psychiatry Clin Neurosci.* 2000;54: 354–355.

Nakamura K, Hashimoto S, Honma S, Honma K, Tagawa Y. A sighted man with non-24-hour sleep-wake syndrome shows damped plasma melatonin rhythm. *Psychiatry Clin Neurosci.* 1997;51:115–119.

Palm L, Blennow G, Wetterberg L. Long-term melatonin treatment in blind children and young adults with circadian sleep-wake disturbances. *Dev Med Child Neurol.* 1997;39:319–325.

Uchiyama M, Okawa M, Shibui K, Kim K, Tagaya H, Kudo Y, et al. Altered phase relation between sleep timing and core body temperature rhythm in delayed sleep phase syndrome and non-24-hour sleep-wake syndrome in humans. *Neurosci Lett.* 2000;294:101–114.

Wagner DR. Disorders of the circadian sleep-wake cycle. *Neurol Clin.* 1996;14:651–670.

Yamadera H, Takahashi K, Okawa M. A multicenter study of sleep-wake rhythm disorders: therapeutic effects of vitamin B$_{12}$, bright light therapy, chronotherapy and hypnotics. *Psychiatry Clin Neurosci.* 1996;50:203–209.

Time Zone Change (Jet Lag) Syndrome

Lee-Chiong TL, ed. *Sleep: A Comprehensive Handbook.* Hoboken, NJ: John Wiley & Sons, 2006.

Lee-Chiong TL, Sateia M, Carskadon M, eds. *Sleep Medicine.* Philadelphia, PA: Hanley & Belfus (Elsevier), 2002.

Parasomnias and Abnormal Sleep-Related Movements

7

Parasomnias

Parasomnias are undesirable physical phenomena or behavior that develop during the sleep period. These abnormal events or experiences are not principally abnormalities of the states of sleep and wakefulness, and they are not generally associated with major complaints of excessive sleepiness or insomnia. Parasomnias can manifest as activation of skeletal muscles or the autonomic nervous system during sleep. They usually occur intermittently or episodically either within sleep or during its transition to and from wakefulness. Occasionally, parasomnias may give rise to violent and potentially injurious behavior.

Classification

Parasomnias can be classified into three groups based on the American Academy of Sleep Medicine International Classification of Sleep Disorders (ICSD; second edition; see References) (Box 7–1).

1. Disorders of arousal from non–rapid eye movement (NREM) sleep, including confusional arousals, sleepwalking, and sleep terrors

2. Parasomnias usually associated with rapid eye movement (REM) sleep, including REM sleep behavior disorder (including parasomnia overlap disorder and status dissociatus), recurrent isolated sleep paralysis, and nightmare disorder

3. Other parasomnias, including sleep-related dissociative disorder, sleep enuresis, sleep-related groaning (catathrenia), exploding head syndrome, sleep-related hallucinations, and sleep-related eating disorder.

Parasomnias may also be categorized either as primary (ie, disorders of the sleep states per se, such as disorders of arousal or REM sleep behavior disorder), or secondary (ie, disorders of other systems that emerge during sleep, such as nocturnal seizures).

Box 7–1.

Parasomnias

Disorders of arousal (from NREM sleep)

    Confusional arousals

    Sleepwalking

    Sleep terrors

Parasomnias usually associated with REM sleep

    REM sleep behavior disorder

        Parasomnia overlap disorder

        Status dissociatus

    Recurrent isolated sleep paralysis

    Nightmare disorder

Other parasomnias

    Sleep-related dissociative disorders

    Sleep enuresis

(continued from page 272)
Box 7-1.

Parasomnias

Sleep-related groaning (catathrenia)

Exploding head syndrome

Sleep-related hallucinations

Sleep-related eating disorder

Unspecified

Due to drug or substance

Due to medical condition

Source: Adapted from the American Academy of Sleep Medicine. The International Classification of Sleep Disorders, second edition: Diagnostic and Coding Manual. American Academy of Sleep Medicine, 2005.

Disorders of Arousal

The disorders of arousal are believed to result from abnormal arousal processes (during which motor activity is restored without an accompanying full consciousness) and consist of confusional arousals, sleepwalking, and sleep terrors. They occur out of NREM sleep, particularly stages 3 and 4 sleep, during the first third of the night. These disorders are most commonly encountered during childhood, and their frequency diminishes with increasing age as NREM stages 3 and 4 decline. There is often a strong familial pattern.

Predisposing factors for these disorders include febrile illness, alcohol, prior sleep deprivation, irregular sleep-wake schedules, emotional stress, and pregnancy or menstruation. Partial arousals can be precipitated by forced arousals from sleep, obstructive sleep apnea (OSA), periodic limb movements of sleep, nocturnal seizures, or endogenous factors such as a distended bladder. Events have also been described following alcohol ingestion and during administration of several medications, including sedative-hypnotics, neuroleptics, minor tranquilizers, stimulants, and antihistamines.

Differential diagnosis includes nightmares (occur during REM sleep, with full alertness and recall of the preceding dream on awakening), and REM sleep behavior disorder (occur during REM sleep with apparent "acting out" of dreams).

Pathogenesis

Pathogenetic mechanisms underlying most of the parasomnias remain incompletely understood. Interactions between the sleep environment and genetically determined predisposition are likely to be present for some parasomnias. Simultaneous occurrence of, or rapid oscillation between, the various state-determining variables of wakefulness, NREM sleep, and REM sleep can result in intrusion of elements of one state into another. Parasomnias are especially likely to emerge during the transition periods of one state to another. Thus, combinations of wakefulness and NREM sleep give rise to confusional arousals, and the persistence of REM sleep into wakefulness produces REM sleep behavior disorder.

Genetics

A high degree of concordance (monozygotic versus dizygotic) is present in twin studies of sleepwalking, sleep terrors and idiopathic sleep paralysis. An increase in prevalence of arousal disorders has been described among family members of affected individuals. Finally, an association between REM sleep behavior disorder and the human leukocyte antigen (HLA)-DQl has been reported.

Clinical Features

Some parasomnias occur predominantly during NREM sleep (eg, disorders of arousal and bruxism) or during REM sleep (eg, REM sleep behavior disorder). Others, such as enuresis or the parasomnia overlap syndrome, can manifest during both NREM and REM sleep.

Evaluation

Diagnosis for most parasomnias is based on its clinical presentation and, except for REM sleep behavior disorder, seldom requires polysomnographic documentation. A formal polysomnographic study is recommended for possible parasomnias associated with very frequent episodes, complaints of excessive sleepiness, unusual presentation or significant sleep disturbance, significant disruption of the bed partner, or those that have resulted in injury to the individual or bed partner. Polysomnography is also indicated if an underlying seizure activity is suspected, or in cases that have medicolegal implications. A single normal polysomnogram (PSG) does not exclude the presence of parasomnias. Multiple studies, preferably with time-synchronized video recording (ie, simultaneous video and sleep monitoring), performed over several nights may be required. Additional electroencephalographic (EEG) electrodes are required for patients in whom a seizure disorder is being excluded. Evaluation of patients presenting with violent behavior duringsleep should be more comprehensive, and it may include an extensive neurologic and psychiatric assessment.

Differential Diagnosis

Differential diagnosis of parasomnias includes seizure activity (tends to occur more frequently during NREM sleep than REM sleep), panic attacks (most frequently seen during NREM sleep), and the sleep-related movement disorders.

1. Seizures should be considered in the differential of any parasomnia-like behavior that is accompanied by atypical features or stereotypic activities. Seizures can occur at any time during sleep but appear to start more frequently during NREM sleep. Seizures of frontal and temporal lobe origins may be associated with complex activities or behavior. This disorder should be highly suspected in patients who report urinary incontinence or tongue biting accompanying abnormal sleep-related behaviors.

2. Nocturnal wandering secondary to dementia ("sundowning")

3. Panic attacks and post-traumatic stress disorder

4. Status dissociatus is a disorder characterized by the presence of complex behavior and activities due to a complete dissolution of sleep state boundaries with polysomnographic features of wakefulness, NREM sleep and REM sleep occurring simultaneously. Status dissociatus can be encountered in fatal familial insomnia, alcohol withdrawal, and in some patients with narcolepsy.

5. "Sleep drunkenness" (state of sleep inertia with partial awakening).

6. Dissociative state is a psychogenic condition in which abnormal behavior, although appearing to occur during sleep at night, actually develops during wakefulness.

7. Münchhausen syndrome and malingering both consist of false symptoms that masquerade as actual clinical conditions.

Therapy

Unless injurious or associated with significant distress, sleep disturbance, or daytime impairment, a majority of parasomnias require no specific therapy. Known risk or precipitating factors should be avoided or eliminated. Instructions regarding proper sleep hygiene and safety issues are important.

Sleep-Related Movement Disorders

Unlike parasomnias that consist of relatively complex, apparently purposeful, behavior or movements, these disorders are characterized by simple, often stereotypical, movements that give rise to sleep disturbance. A list of sleep-related movement disorders is given in Box 7–2.

Box 7–2. Sleep-related movement disorders	Restless legs syndrome
	Periodic limb movement disorder
	Sleep-related leg cramps
	Sleep-related bruxism
	Sleep-related rhythmic movement disorder

Source: Adapted from American Academy of Sleep Medicine. The International Classification of Sleep Disorders, second edition: Diagnostic and Coding Manual. American Academy of Sleep Medicine, 2005.

Confusional Arousals

Confusional arousals are characterized by episodes of confusion following spontaneous or forced arousals from sleep, typically from NREM stages 3 and 4 sleep. They usually occur in the first third of the night. Disorientation, confusion, inappropriate behavior (moving around in bed, thrashing, crying, or sleep talking), amnesia for the event, and inconsolability are common. Other features include diminished vigilance and blunted response to questions or external stimuli. Behavior may, at times, become violent. However, signs of fear or autonomic hyperactivity are minimal or absent. Episodes may last from several minutes to hours, with most cases spontaneously resolving within 5 to 15 minutes.

The ICSD has described two clinical variants of confusional arousals: (1) severe morning sleep inertia (sleep drunkenness), which occurs during morning awakenings from sleep, and (2) sleep-related abnormal sexual behaviors (eg, sexual vocalizations, sexual assaults or masturbation). Sleep-related abnormal sexual behaviors or "sleep sex" can also occur during episodes of sleepwalking.

Confusional arousals may be precipitated by sleep deprivation, irregular sleep-wake schedules (e.g., shift work), use of central nervous system (CNS)–active agents or alcohol, neurologic disorders, OSA, periodic limb movement disorder, or forced awakenings from deep sleep.

These conditions are most prevalent in children, especially those with frequent sleep terrors and sleepwalking. The prevalence rate in children 3 to 13 years of age is estimated to be 17%. Childhood cases of confusional arousals typically diminish in frequency as children get older. Confusional arousals are less common among adults in whom the prevalence is approximately 4%. There is no gender difference. Genetic factors play an important role, and there is a strong familial pattern in cases of idiopathic confusional arousals seen in families of deep sleepers. During an episode of confusional arousal, polysomnographic recordings may demonstrate an alpha rhythm, repetitive microsleeps, or NREM sleep stage 1 activity. A single normal PSG does not exclude the diagnosis of confusional arousals, and multiple studies, preferably with time-synchronized video recording, over several nights may be required.

Off-label use of tricyclic antidepressants and benzodiazepines or nonpharmacologic therapy (psychotherapy, progressive relaxation or hypnosis) have been suggested for disorders of arousal that are potentially injurious or disruptive to household members. With scheduled awakenings, parents are instructed to awaken the child about 15 minutes before their usual time of arousal and then allow the child to return to sleep. Specific behavioral treatments of disorders of arousals are listed in Box 7–3.

Box 7–3. **Behavioral treatment of disorders of arousal**	Avoidance of sleep deprivation Trial of sleep extension Maintenance of a regular sleep-wake schedule Scheduled awakenings Psychotherapy (if marked psychologic distress is present)

Enuresis

Sleep enuresis is described as recurrent involuntary bed-wetting occurring during sleep after 5 years of age. It can arise throughout the night and during any stage of sleep, although most tend to occur early during sleep in the first third of the evening. Children with enuresis may report embarrassment or guilt about their problem.

Pathophysiology involves a variety of factors, including failure to arouse in response to a sensation of bladder fullness, impaired ability to transiently delay bladder contraction when a need to void develops, greater urine production during sleep in relation to age-related nocturnal bladder capacity, or a maturational delay in bladder development resulting in a smaller bladder capacity. By 18 months to 3 years of age, children develop the ability to postpone voiding in response to a full bladder, initially during wakefulness and eventually during sleep as well.

Sleep enuresis is classified as primary if recurrent sleep-related micturition occurring at least twice a week persists in children older than 5 years of age who have not been consistently dry during sleep or secondary if bed-wetting recurs at least twice a week for at least 3 months after the child or adult has maintained dryness for at least six consecutive months. Information about the classification of enuresis is presented in Table 7–1. Sleep enuresis is more common among boys than girls in children at all ages. The demographics of primary enuresis are presented in Table 7–2. Secondary sleep enuresis accounts for approximately 5% to 10% of cases, and can occur at any age. Both primary and secondary enuresis can result from organic or functional causes. An organic etiology should be suspected if urgency or an abnormality in urinary flow is present, or involuntary voiding occurs during wakefulness as well. Secondary sleep enuresis may be associated with increased production of urine due to the use of diuretics, ingestion of caffeine, or impairment in the ability to concentrate urine (eg, diabetes mellitus or diabetes insipidus); urinary tract infection; pelvic abnormalities (eg, urinary bladder outlet obstruction or anomalies of the bladder, urethra, and ureters); psychosocial stressors (eg, birth of a sibling); depression; OSA; congestive heart failure; dementia; seizures; and chronic constipation.

Table 7–1. Classification of enuresis

Primary enuresis	Secondary enuresis
Most childhood cases of enuresis are primary. Primary enuresis commonly results from an impaired arousal response secondary to very deep sleep or high nighttime urine volume due to impaired release of vasopressin during sleep. Other contributory factors include inappropriate or inadequate toilet training, and residence in disorganized families. The prevalence of primary enuresis is greater among children with attention deficit/ hyperactivity disorder.	Bedwetting incidents can be precipitated by neglect, recent stressful events, or physical or sexual abuse. Coexisting chronic constipation and fecal soiling are not uncommon.

Table 7–2. Demographics of primary enuresis

Age (years)	Prevalence
4	30%
5	12% (males: 7%–15%; females: 3%–10%)
6	10%
7	7%
10	5% (males: 3%–5%; females: 2%)
12	3%
15	1%–2%

Genetics appear to have an important role in the development of enuresis. Children with primary enuresis often have a positive family history among their siblings or parents.

Differential diagnosis includes nocturia secondary to diuretic therapy, diabetes mellitus, diabetes insipidus, or prostate hypertrophy. In contrast to enuresis, nocturia involves frequent awakenings from sleep to urinate in the bathroom.

Evaluation includes an extensive medical, neurologic, psychiatric, and sleep history. A diary consisting of the frequency of nighttime enuretic incidents and daytime urination is often helpful. Physical examination and laboratory evaluations (eg, urinalysis, urine culture, and measurements of voiding and urinary flow) are indicated to exclude organic causes of enuresis such as neurologic and urologic abnormalities. Although sleep architecture is generally normal, polysomnography or EEG may be required, in the appropriate clinical setting, to rule out the presence of OSA or seizure disorder, respectively.

The spontaneous cure rate in children with primary sleep enuresis is estimated at 15% annually. Treatment consists of pharmacotherapy or behavioral therapy. A secondary cause of enuresis, if identified, should be addressed and corrected.

Medications useful for enuresis include desmopressin and the tricyclic antidepressants (eg, imipramine). Desmopressin is an analog of vasopressin (antidiuretic hormone) that decreases urine production by enhancing renal water reabsorption. It is administered intranasally using a nasal spray. Tricyclic antidepressants work via their anticholinergic action. Pharmacotherapy is indicated primarily for specific situations that require acute control (eg, sleepovers or camping trips). Recurrence of enuresis is common following discontinuation of pharmacologic therapy.

Behavioral therapy starts with patient and parental education about the pathophysiology, clinical course, and consequences of enuresis. Proper sleep hygiene is important, including restricting fluid intake after dinner and voiding prior to going to bed. Older children may be asked to launder their own soiled clothes and bed sheets. Rewards for dry nights are preferable to punishing or humiliating the child for bedwetting.

In addition, behavioral therapy may involve an enuresis alarm system that consists of an alarm attached to a pad placed in the underwear of the sleeping child, who is then awakened when moisture is detected. This then prompts the child to get up and go to the bathroom. It often takes several weeks of regular use to work, but it provides effective long-term control. Other behavior approaches to the therapy of enuresis include bladder training exercises wherein the child is made to consume a large amount of liquid and asked to hold the urine as long as possible before voiding. This exercise is believed to provide the child with a sense of being able to control urination, strengthen the urinary sphincter, and possibly increase functional bladder capacity.

Exploding Head Syndrome

Persons with exploding head syndrome describe a sensation of an "explosion" or a "sudden loud noise" in their head as they are falling asleep or upon awakening. A flash of light, a myoclonic jerk, or a sense of fear or concern may accompany the experience. There are commonly no complaints of significant pain. The syndrome is likely a variant of sleep starts with a typically benign course, although frequent attacks can give rise to complaints of insomnia.

The frequency of attacks varies significantly among individuals, may increase with stress or fatigue, and tends to diminish over time. The syndrome appears to be more common among women than in men. A seizure disorder should be considered in its differential diagnosis.

Polysomnographic features consist of sudden arousals during the sleep-wake transition with EEG demonstrating alpha and theta activity.

Impaired Sleep-Related Penile Erections

The ability to achieve penile erection during sleep of sufficient rigidity and duration necessary for sexual intercourse can be used to differentiate organic from other causes of male impotence. Impaired or absent sleep-related penile tumescence supports an organic basis for impotence. Organic impotence can be related to an underlying medical illness (eg, hypertension, diabetes mellitus, cardiac disease, renal failure, and alcoholism), pelvic/urogenital injury or surgery (eg, prostatectomy), or spinal cord disorder. A reduction in penile tumescence during sleep is also observed with aging.

Nightmares

Nightmares are unpleasant and frightening dreams, often involving threats to life or security, that occur during REM sleep and that commonly abruptly awaken the sleeper from sleep. Episodes typically occur in the latter half of the night. Once awakened, the person is fully alert and profoundly fearful and anxious, can recall vividly the preceding dream, and has difficulty returning to sleep. Some minor autonomic activation, such as tachycardia and tachypnea, is evident. Nightmares may also occur during NREM sleep, particularly in persons who have experienced a traumatic event (eg, acute stress disorder or post-traumatic stress disorder). Nightmares can cause distress or functional impairment. Recurring nightmares can result in insomnia, sleep avoidance due to fear of falling asleep, excessive daytime sleepiness, and anxiety.

Nightmares can be precipitated by illness, traumatic experiences, acute alcohol ingestion, and medications. Risk factors for frequent post-traumatic nightmares include severity of the traumatic event, any underlying psychopathology, low levels of education, low socioeconomic status and female gender. Post-traumatic nightmares can persist throughout life. Pharmacologic agents that affect the neurotransmitters norepinephrine, serotonin, and dopamine (eg, antidepressants, antihypertensives, particularly beta-blockers, or dopamine agonists) can induce nightmares. Additionally, a possible association exists between the occurrence of nightmares and some anesthetics, antipsychotics, and antiepileptic agents as well as medications affecting the neurotransmitters acetylcholine, gamma-aminobutyric acid or/and histamine. Nightmares have been observed during withdrawal of REM-sleep suppressive agents (eg, tricyclic antidepressants [TCAs] or selective serotonin reuptake inhibitors [SSRIs]), benzodiazepines, and barbiturates.

Occasional nightmares are not uncommon. An estimated 10% to 50% of children report recurrent nightmares. Onset of nightmares is usually at 3 to 6 years of age and the prevalence peaks at 6 to 10 years of age. Nightmares generally become less frequent during adulthood. Chronic nightmares in adults can be encountered in persons with cardiac diseases or post-traumatic stress disorder and after severe burns. There is no difference in nightmare prevalence in children based on gender. Among adults, nightmares appear to be more common in women than in men. Most nightmare sufferers have no underlying psychiatric disorder.

Nightmares should be distinguished from both sleep terrors, which occur shortly after sleep onset and consist only of vague dream images, as well as REM sleep behavior disorder with its seemingly purposeful and potentially violent acts (Table 7–3). Nocturnal panic attacks occur following awakenings from NREM sleep.

Polysomnography demonstrates abrupt awakenings from REM sleep. REM sleep abnormalities (eg, decrease in REM sleep latency, increased REM density [number of eye movements per minute of REM sleep], and increase in percent REM sleep) can be seen in some patients.

Generally, no specific therapy aside from reassurance that the condition is benign is necessary. In cases in which treatment may be desired because of the frequency of events or extremely disturbing nature of the dream content, behavioral treatment (eg, imagery) or psychotherapy may be considered. Any underlying post-traumatic stress disorder should be addressed. Medications known to trigger nightmares may need to be changed. The use of REM sleep suppressant agents (TCAs or SSRIs) to reduce the occurrence of nightmares has been described.

Table 7–3. Differences between nightmares and sleep terrors

Characteristics	Nightmares	Sleep terrors
Time of night	Latter half of the night	First half of the night
Sleep stage	Emerges during REM sleep	Emerges during NREM stages 3 and 4 sleep
Level of consciousness	Awake and alert	Confused and disoriented
Memory of episode	Full recall	Partial or complete amnesia
Subsequent return to sleep	Delayed	Rapid

Nocturnal Eating (Drinking) Syndrome

This syndrome consists of repetitive arousals from sleep with involuntary eating or drinking. Affected individuals are unaware or only partly conscious of the abnormal behavior. Characteristic features include partial recall or total amnesia for the episodes and consumption of high-caloric foodstuffs or inappropriate substances. Alcohol is not typically ingested. There is typically no associated daytime abnormal eating behavior, such as binge eating, anorexia, bulimia, or purging. These episodes, if frequent, can give rise to weight gain and obesity. Other potential consequences include insomnia, excessive sleepiness due to sleep fragmentation, injuries, dyspepsia, and abdominal distention.

Onset can either be insidious or abrupt. Episodes often occur nightly, and the course is generally chronic. Episodes can be observed any time during sleep, often many times each night. Nocturnal eating (drinking) syndrome is a rare condition in the general population, but appears to be more common among individuals with an underlying eating disorder. Women are affected more frequently than men. Onset is typically during early adulthood.

Some cases are idiopathic, whereas others can be related to another sleep disorder (eg, sleepwalking, OSA, restless legs syndrome, periodic limb movement disorder, or narcolepsy). Additional factors that can precipitate episodes of nocturnal eating or drinking include acute stress, mood disorder, poor sleep hygiene, variable sleep schedules, cessation of alcohol, substance or tobacco use, medications (eg, anticholinergic agents, lithium, triazolam or zolpidem), encephalitis, and dieting during the daytime. In many instances, the awakenings appear to be triggered by learned behavior and not by real hunger or thirst.

Differential diagnosis involves gastrointestinal conditions that can be relieved with food intake (eg, peptic ulcer disease), nocturnal eating syndrome, Kleine-Levin syndrome (recurrent episodes of excessive sleepiness associated with hypersexuality and increased food consumption), Klüver-Bucy syndrome (a rare disorder in which individuals may place objects in their mouths and engage in inappropriate sexual behavior), and hypoglycemia. With nocturnal eating syndrome, compulsive eating occurs at night while awake.

Polysomnography may reveal the presence of a primary sleep disorder, primarily sleepwalking. Common features consist of multiple arousals typically from NREM stages 3 and 4 sleep, but occasionally from REM sleep as well.

Several treatment approaches have been recommended for patients with this disorder. Suggested pharmacotherapy has consisted of benzodiazepines (eg, clonazepam), antidepressants (eg, SSRIs), or dopaminergic agonists (eg, carbidopa/levodopa). Any underlying mood disorder as well as alcohol or substance use should be addressed.

Nocturnal Leg Cramps

Persons with nocturnal leg cramps or "charley horse" are awakened by painful spasms or tightening of the muscles of the calves or feet. Sleep is reestablished only after the painful sensation is relieved by forcible stretching of the affected muscle group or by local massage. Residual muscle discomfort may persist for several minutes to hours thereby delaying the return to sleep. Nocturnal leg cramping is an almost universal experience, and most individuals complain of having had these symptoms during their lifetime.

Onset peaks during adulthood. Its prevalence may be increased among the elderly; in women during pregnancy; with use of oral contraceptives; with dehydration; after vigorous exercise; and in persons with diabetes mellitus and other endocrine disorders, fluid and electrolyte imbalances (eg, hypocalcemia), peripheral vascular disease, neuromuscular disorders, Parkinson disease, and musculoskeletal disorders. A significant number of cases are idiopathic.

The differential diagnosis is extensive and includes cramps related to heat, hemodialysis and electrolyte disturbances, muscular contractures secondary to metabolic myopathies and thyroid disease, tetany, and dystonias resulting from antipsychotic medications. Diagnosis is usually made by history alone. Polysomnography, if performed, demonstrates an awakening coinciding with nonperiodic bursts of high-frequency gastrocnemius electromyographic (EMG) activity.

Evaluation should consist of neurologic, musculoskeletal, and vascular examinations. Laboratory investigation includes assessment of thyroid function, platelet counts, and serum levels of electrolytes, calcium, and magnesium.

If they occur frequently, nocturnal legs cramps can give rise to insomnia or daytime sleepiness due to sleep disruption. Quinine is reported to be effective in decreasing the frequency of nocturnal leg cramps but not their severity or duration. Potentially fatal immunologically-mediated hypersensitivity reactions and thrombocytopenia can occur with the use of quinine. Quinine use should be monitored closely by physicians, and avoided during pregnancy and in persons with hepatic failure. Lower starting doses should be considered for older adults and patients with impaired renal function. Muscle relaxants (eg, baclofen) have also been tried. Finally, local massage or hot baths may be considered.

Nocturnal Paroxysmal Dystonia

Nocturnal paroxysmal dystonia (NPD) is characterized by abrupt complex behavior, with dystonic-dyskinetic, choreoathetoid, ballistic posturing, or semipurposeful activity, arising repeatedly from NREM sleep. Events may occur several times nightly, often in clusters, and can be either short (lasting 15 to 60 seconds) or more prolonged (duration of 2 minutes to under an hour). Automatisms and vocalization can be present. Return to sleep is rapid following each episode. Affected individuals may report partial recall of the events.

NPD was initially considered a specific movement disorder, and the 1997 International Classification of Sleep Disorders (ICSD) included it within the category of parasomnias. Recently, it has been suggested that NPD, particularly the short attack type, might, instead, be epileptic in nature. In one report, attacks of NPD in a child originated from the right orbitofrontal cortex, and surgical ablation of a cortical dysplastic lesion resulted in full control of the disorder. NPD is clinically similar to frontal lobe seizures that arise mesially or in depth. Additionally, generalized tonic-clonic seizures can follow an episode of NPD.

NPD is also classified as a nocturnal frontal lobe epilepsy (NFLE) along with two other disorders, paroxysmal arousals and episodic nocturnal wanderings. These three conditions often coexist. Paroxysmal arousals are brief, sudden awakenings during NREM sleep associated with transient stereotyped dystonic-dyskinetic posturing. Episodic nocturnal wanderings consist of prolonged episodes of agitated ambulation, with unintelligible speech, screaming, and complex motor behavior and dystonic postures involving the head, trunk, and limbs.

NFLE is more common among males and usually begins during adolescence. It affects individuals of all ages and, if left untreated, tends to have a chronic course. Most cases are sporadic. An autosomal dominant mode of inheritance has been documented in a minority of cases.

Neurologic evaluation, including EEG, computed tomography and magnetic resonance imaging (MRI), is typically normal in NPD. Polysomnography may reveal repeated arousals at the start of each attack.

Carbamazepine controls, or significantly reduces, seizures in most patients with the short-duration attack type. Therapy using barbiturates and phenytoin has been described. The prolonged-duration attack type is less responsive to therapy.

Rapid Eye Movement Sleep Behavior Disorder

Definition

In REM sleep behavior disorder (RBD), abnormal behaviors develop during REM sleep and are accompanied by loss of REM-related muscle atonia or hypotonia. These dream-enacting behaviors can result in sleep disruption or injury to the sleeper or bed partner. There is often no history of violent or aggressive behavior during the day while awake.

Clinical Features

Abnormal behaviors occurring during REM sleep range from simple motions to highly elaborate activities (eg, screaming, punching, kicking, jumping, or running). Affected individuals appear to be "acting out their dreams." Dream content can be altered or unpleasant, often involving defense of the sleeper against attack. The eyes are usually closed, in contrast to the sleepwalker, whose eyes are open during the episode. Episodes end with a rapid awakening and full alertness. Associated features include good dream recall on awakening.

Episodes are more common during the second half of the night (eg, early morning hours) when REM sleep percentage is greatest.

Demographics

The prevalence of RBD is unknown, but it appears to affect less than 1% of the general population. RBD is predominantly seen in males and in elderly adults (50 years of age and older). Cases of idiopathic RBD involving women and children are less common.

Classification

Most forms of RBD are idiopathic (approximately 60% of cases). RBD can also be associated with various neurologic and medical disorders, including Parkinson disease, dementia with Lewy bodies, and multiple system atrophy. Various medications (eg, tricyclic antidepressants) can induce or aggravate RBD. The disorder can also occur during withdrawal from alcohol or REM sleep suppressants.

Clinical Subtypes

There are three clinical subtypes of RBD, namely subclinical RBD, parasomnia overlap syndrome, and status dissociatus (Table 7–4).

Table 7–4. Clinical subtypes of rapid eye movement sleep behavior disorder

Subtype	Characteristics
Subclinical RBD	Polysomnographic features consistent with RBD without clinical manifestations of the disorder. Clinical RBD may develop subsequently in some cases.
Parasomnia overlap syndrome	Elements of disorders of arousal (confusional arousals, sleep terrors, and sleepwalking) and RBD are present. It can affect all age groups, and onset is generally during childhood or adolescence.
Status dissociatus	Admixture of the different states of wakefulness, NREM sleep, and REM sleep. Abnormal sleep and dream-related behaviors closely resembling RBD in the absence of identifiable sleep stages during polysomnography. Cases are typically associated with an underlying medical disorder, including alcohol withdrawal, dementia, familial fatal insomnia, HIV infection, multiple system atrophy, narcolepsy, or Parkinson disease.

Predisposing Factors

Male gender, aging, and an underlying neurologic condition (Parkinson disease or multiple system atrophy) are important predisposing factors for RBD. RBD may be quite prevalent in Parkinson disease and parkinsonian disorders. Indeed, a substantial number of RBD cases considered to be idiopathic may merely be an early manifestation of a parkinsonian disorder.

Associated Sleep Disorders

Comorbid sleep disorders include the disorders of arousal, narcolepsy and periodic limb movements of sleep. The parasomnia overlap syndrome is a variant of RBD that consists of clinical and polysomnographic features of both RBD and NREM disorders of arousal. In combined RBD-narcolepsy, RBD develops either in tandem with narcolepsy or early in the clinical course of narcolepsy.

Clinical Course

Onset, which is generally during middle age or late adulthood (between 50 to 60 years of age), can either be rapid or gradual. The clinical course is generally chronic and progressive.

Consequences

RBD can lead to injuries to the patient or bed partner. These behaviors may result in repetitive arousals from sleep and sleep fragmentation. Neurodegenerative disorders and Parkinson disease can emerge several years after the onset of RBD in some patients.

Pathophysiology

Muscle atonia is a characteristic feature of REM sleep. In RBD, the REM sleep-related muscular inactivity is intermittently disinhibited, with periods of enhanced muscle tone. The increase in muscle tone during REM sleep is most likely due to a disruption of multisynaptic pathways in the brainstem responsible for suppression of muscle tone during sleep.

REM-related muscle atonia is generated by activation of the medullary reticular formation by the perilocus ceruleus of the pontine tegmentum via the lateral tegmentoreticular tract. This gives rise to inhibition of spinal motor neurons. In animal models, bilateral lesions of the perilocus ceruleus in the dorsal pons result in a syndrome resembling RBD with loss of REM sleep-related muscle atonia-hypotonia and emergence of abnormal motor behavior during sleep.

It is believed that RBD arises from a primary dysfunction of the pedunculopontine nucleus or other key brainstem structures associated with basal ganglia pathology or, alternatively, from abnormal afferent signals in the basal ganglia, leading to dysfunction in the midbrain extrapyramidal area/pedunculopontine nucleus region.

Impaired cortical activation during both wakefulness and REM sleep has been reported in patients with idiopathic RBD. Quantitative analysis of sleep EEG has shown lower beta power in the occipital region during REM sleep in RBD.

Differential Diagnosis

Differential diagnosis includes other parasomnias (eg, sleepwalking, sleep terrors, nightmares, nocturnal paroxysmal dystonia, or rhythmic movement disorder), OSA, periodic limb movements of sleep, nocturnal seizures, nocturnal psychogenic dissociative syndromes, panic attacks, post-traumatic stress disorder, and malingering. RBD may be misdiagnosed as a psychiatric disorder because of the presence of disturbed dreaming and bizarre dream enactment.

Agrypnia excitata is a clinical syndrome that consists of oneirism (REM sleep-related dream enactment), enhanced motor activity, autonomic sympathetic discharge, and sleep disturbances (eg, sleeplessness and loss of NREM stages 3 and 4 sleep). It can be seen in individuals with familial fatal insomnia, delirium tremens, or Morvan fibrillary chorea.

Evaluation

A comprehensive neurologic evaluation, including a thorough examination, EEG, and brain MRI is recommended. Additionally, patients with RBD should be monitored closely for several years for the delayed emergence of Parkinson disease or other neurologic disorders.

Polysomnography

Polysomnography is routinely performed to establish the diagnosis of RBD. Time-synchronized video recording is recommended, and more than a single study may be required. Additional EMG monitoring of the upper extremities (flexor digitorum) may be useful.

Polysomnographic features include persistent augmentation of chin EMG tone, or excessive chin or limb phasic EMG activity during REM sleep associated with abnormal behavior. Limb EMG activity may also be increased during NREM sleep.

REM density can be increased. Occasionally, NREM stages 3 and 4 sleep are increased as well. Otherwise, sleep architecture is normal. No seizure activity is evident on EEG monitoring. Many patients with RBD have periodic limb movements of sleep.

Multiple sleep latency test commonly demonstrates normal sleep latency.

Other Tests

MRI and single photon emission computed tomography (SPECT) of the brain have demonstrated decreased blood flow in the upper portion of both sides of the frontal lobes and pons; however, the decreased blood flow in the frontal lobes shows no correlation with the extent of frontal lobe atrophy. There is also decreased nigrostriatal presynaptic dopamine transporter binding. Nonetheless, neuroimaging is generally not clinically useful in the diagnosis of RBD and is unlikely to reveal any underlying disorder that is not suspected clinically.

Therapy

RBD is treatable. In one series, clonazepam treatment of RBD was completely or partially successful in 87% of patients. However, clonazepam therapy appears to produce minimal changes in polysomnographic parameters. Successful therapy with bupropion, carbamazepine, clonidine, desipramine, doxepin, gabapentin, imipramine, levodopa, and melatonin has also been described. Environmental precautions are essential.

Rapid Eye Movement Sleep-Related Sinus Arrest

This apparently rare cardiac rhythm disorder is characterized by sinus arrest developing during REM sleep. Episodes often occur in clusters, with periods of asystole lasting up to 9 seconds in duration that usually recur frequently. It affects apparently healthy young adults without any identifiable cardiac pathology.

Episodes of nocturnal sinus arrest are not accompanied by arousals, OSA or sleep disruption. Most patients are asymptomatic, although palpitations or vague chest discomfort may occasionally be reported. Its clinical course is not well understood. Daytime electrocardiography (EKG) and angiography are usually unremarkable.

It has been suggested that the underlying pathophysiology involves an autonomic dysfunction. Power spectral analysis of heart rate variability in one case demonstrated abnormal vagal activity, particularly during REM sleep, which was presumably responsible for the bradycardia.

Although treatment is not usually indicated, prophylactic intervention with a cardiac pacemaker, set at a low rate, may be considered in certain patients.

Rhythmic Movement Disorder

Rhythmic movement disorder defines a syndrome consisting of repetitive, rhythmic and stereotypic motions of the head, trunk, or extremities, which usually occurs during drowsiness, in the transition from wakefulness to sleep, or during sustained sleep. Some patients display rhythmic movements during REM sleep as well. This condition is referred to as head banging (jactatio capitis nocturna) if it involves forceful anterior-posterior motions of the head and neck (ie, repeatedly lifting and banging the head back onto the bed). In addition, individuals may display head rolling (lateral movements of the head), body rolling (side-to-side motions of the body), body rocking (entire body is rocked while positioned on hands and knees), leg rolling or banging, and rhythmic vocalizations or humming.

Many infants display rhythmic activity during sleep or quiet wakefulness. This is considered a form of relaxing and soothing self-stimulation. These rhythmic activities become clinically relevant if they are associated with disturbances of sleep and impairment of daytime performance. Other possible complications of head banging, in addition to sleep-onset insomnia, include eye and cranial injuries, such as fractures or soft tissue trauma.

Rhythmic movement disorder most often affects normal infants younger than 18 months of age. Age of onset is typically before the first year of age (mean age of onset of 6 months for body rocking, 9 months for head banging, and 10 months for head rolling). Both genders appear to be affected equally. The condition is typically self-limited; spontaneous resolution before 4 years of age is characteristic. Childhood and adolescent cases are infrequent; in this age group, it may be seen in association with mental retardation, autism, CNS trauma, or other neuropsychiatric disorders. Adult cases are rare.

Differential diagnosis includes self-injurious waking behaviors, periodic limb movement disorder, benign neonatal myoclonus, and seizures. Diagnosis can be greatly enhanced by time-synchronized video recording during polysomnography. During polysomnography, rhythmic movements are demonstrated most frequently during NREM stage 2 sleep.

Therapy includes maintenance of proper sleep hygiene and ensuring a safe sleep environment (eg, padding bed railings and headboard).

Sleep Bruxism

Definition

Sleep bruxism is characterized by repetitive grinding or clenching of the teeth, caused by contractions of the masticatory muscles (eg, masseter and temporalis) during sleep. It is considered a parasomnia in sleep medicine and a parafunction in dentistry. Bruxism during sleep can give rise to arousals.

Bruxism is classified as either *primary* (without an identifiable etiology) or *secondary* (related to medical disorders or medication use).

Demographics

The prevalence of sleep bruxism is difficult to estimate because its frequency and severity can vary considerably between nights. In one study, chronic bruxism was present in 8% of adults. Sleep bruxism commonly begins in the first or second decade of life and affects males and females equally. Prevalence is higher among children with cerebral palsy or mental retardation. The prevalence of tooth grinding decreases with age.

Genetic determinants appear to play a significant role. It is estimated that between 21% and 50% of bruxers have a direct family member who ground his or her teeth during childhood.

The pathophysiology of bruxism is not well understood. Sleep bruxism has been considered an exaggerated form of oromotor masticatory muscle activity that occurs during sleep in most normal individuals. Because of motor suppression during sleep, tooth contact during episodes of bruxism is most likely related to arousals from sleep. It has been postulated that sleep bruxism represents a powerful microarousal event that is associated with central nervous system and autonomic nervous system activity.

Jaw contractions that occur during sleep can either be isolated and sustained, or repetitive (rhythmic masticatory muscle activity [RMMA]). The latter is characterized by jaw muscle contractions (three bursts or more) occurring at a frequency of 1 Hz. It is observed in a majority of normal sleepers in the absence of grinding sounds. Spontaneous RMMA during sleep is noted more frequently following spontaneous transient microarousals. RMMA is more frequent and greater in amplitude among bruxers compared to nonbruxers.

A variety of risk factors for sleep bruxism have been proposed. A history of childhood bruxism appears to predict its presence in adulthood. The risk of developing bruxism is increased among smokers compared to nonsmokers, as well as in persons with restless legs syndrome. Some cases may be related to anxiety, stress, dental disease such as malocclusion or mandibular malformation, caffeine ingestion, alcohol consumption, primary sleep disorders (eg, OSA or REM sleep behavior disorder), neurologic conditions (eg, mental retardation, cerebral palsy, coma, tremors, dystonia or dyskinesia), personality subtypes (eg, vigilant and highly motivated), and medication use (eg, levodopa or SSRIs).

Aside from generating unpleasant noises that might disrupt the bed partner's sleep or causing abnormal dental wear and damage, sleep bruxism can occasionally produce brief arousals, and less commonly full awakenings, from sleep and insomnia. Other consequences include periodontal tissue injury (eg, tooth pain or gum bleeding); dental damage (eg, abnormal tooth wear or destruction of dental restorations); oral, jaw, and facial pain secondary to involvement of the temporomandibular apparatus; headaches; hypertrophy of the masseter muscles; and limitation of mandibular movement.

Diagnosis relies on a current history of witnessed teeth grinding or jaw clenching during sleep and examination of the teeth and periodontal tissue. There is often significant night-to-night variability in the frequency, intensity, and duration of episodes of bruxism. The presence of tooth wear alone is not predictive of ongoing bruxism.

Examination of the teeth may reveal evidence of wear affecting the enamel, most notably on the incisal surfaces of the maxillary canines. With more severe bruxism, the dentin can be affected as well.

During polysomnography, episodes of bruxism are identified as increases in chin and masseter EMG tone that occur rhythmically about every second, with a duration of 0.5 to 15 seconds or longer. These EMG activities may appear as artifacts on the EEG or electro-oculogram channels that are referenced to the masseter or ear electrodes. Rhythmic grinding sounds, which are synchronous with EMG activity, can be detected by audio recording. The ICSD-3 defines sleep-related bruxism as the presence of:

1. ≥ 4 episodes per hour of sleep, or

2. ≥ 25 individual muscle bursts per hour of sleep, and

3. ≥ 2 audible bruxism episodes per polysomnography, and

4. No abnormal EEG activity, such as seizures

Bruxism episodes can occur during all sleep stages, but are especially prominent during NREM stages 1 and 2 sleep; in a particular patient, however, a majority of episodes may occur in one specific sleep stage or another. Although episodes are not typically associated with arousals, shifts of sleep stages can be seen prior to or following episodes of bruxism. Overall, sleep architecture is unremarkable.

Differential Diagnosis

Differential diagnosis of sleep-related bruxism includes rhythmic movement disorder, nocturnal seizures, and facial-mandibular myoclonus.

Therapy

Management goals include protection of the teeth and reduction of the grinding sounds. Therapy involves dental devices, pharmacotherapy, and behavioral therapy.

Evaluation by a dentist can be helpful. A variety of intraoral splints are available. In one report, both occlusal splints and palatal devices significantly reduced the number of bruxism episodes, attenuated episodes with grinding noise, and reduced muscle activity associated with bruxism. Nevertheless, although a dental appliance can protect the teeth from further damage and significantly decrease the noise produced from grinding, rarely does it entirely eliminate bruxism from occurring. Correction of dental malocclusion, if present, is recommended.

Pharmacotherapy (eg, benzodiazepines or muscle relaxants) might be helpful short-term, particularly when bruxism is accompanied by secondary pain. Amitriptyline has not been found to be useful in the management of sleep bruxism. Local administration of botulinum toxin in the masseter muscles has been use to treat severe bruxism, especially for those that have been refractory to conventional therapy or are associated with movement disorders.

In certain patients, behavioral therapy, including stress management, muscle relaxation exercises, hypnosis, biofeedback, and lifestyle modification, may be beneficial, as is observing good sleep hygiene.

Dental wear and masseter hypertrophy are not specific for sleep bruxism. Therefore, it is important to exclude other sleep disorders, such as OSA, that might mimic or precipitate nocturnal bruxism events. When sleep bruxism is related to apnea and hypopneas, successful treatment of sleep-related breathing disorders may eliminate bruxism during sleep.

Sleep Paralysis

In this disorder, there is a generalized transient inability to move the head, body, and extremities, with sparing of the ocular and respiratory muscles. Individuals are unable to speak during these episodes. Skeletal muscle atonia is accompanied by areflexia. It can occur either at sleep onset (hypnagogic) or upon awakening (hypnopompic).

Fright, profound anxiety, and hallucinations (visual, auditory, or tactile) may accompany these attacks, but consciousness and recall are typically unaffected. Paralysis spontaneously resolves after several seconds to several minutes; resolution can be hastened by external stimulation such as a touch or sound. The frequency of episodes ranges from once in a lifetime to almost nightly.

Onset is often during adolescence. Both genders are affected equally. Predisposing and precipitating factors include sleep deprivation, irregular sleep patterns (eg, shift work), a supine sleep position, use of anxiolytic agents, and possibly stress.

Most cases are identified in an isolated form; others occur in a familial form (autosomal dominant in some cases) or in persons with narcolepsy. Isolated sleep paralysis occurs at least once in a lifetime in 40% to 50% of normal individuals. The Hong Kong Chinese "ghost oppression phenomenon" is descriptively identical to sleep paralysis and was reported by 18% of Chinese older than 70 years of age in Hong Kong. It presents much less commonly as a chronic frequently recurring isolated complaint.

PSG recordings are characterized by a REM-wake stage dissociated state with abundant alpha EEG activity and persistence of muscle atonia during wakefulness. Most episodes occur during a sleep-onset REM period.

Differential diagnosis consists of periodic paralysis syndromes (eg, hypokalemic or hyperkalemic periodic paralysis), seizures, conversion disorders, and malingering.

Isolated sleep paralysis is generally a benign condition with no known complications. In the absence of other symptoms of narcolepsy such as excessive sleepiness or cataplexy, further evaluation is unwarranted. Therapy involves addressing known precipitating factors. Sleep deprivation must be avoided, and a regular sleep-wake schedule should be maintained. The use of REM suppressant agents, such as SSRIs or TCAs, for the treatment of sleep paralysis has been described.

Sleep-Related Dissociative Disorders

Dissociative disorders can occur during the daytime, during sleep, or both. Nighttime episodes of violent or sexualized behavior, self-mutilation, screaming, running, eating, or driving a car may last several minutes or hours, and can recur several times nightly. There is generally amnesia for the event.

Demographics

Prevalence is unknown. Onset can occur during childhood or adulthood. Women are affected more commonly than men. Many patients have a history of psychiatric disorders (mood, anxiety or post-traumatic stress disorders), suicide attempts or self-mutilation, or abuse (ie, sexual, physical, or emotional), and demonstrate daytime dissociative behaviors.

Clinical Course

Onset is highly variable and can be either sudden or gradual. The course tends to be chronic.

Consequences

Dissociative disorders can result in injury to the patient or bed partner.

Differential Diagnosis

Sleep-related dissociative disorders should be differentiated from REM sleep behavior disorder, disorders of arousal (confusional arousals, sleep terrors, and sleepwalking), and medical disorders (alcohol or toxic metabolic states).

Polysomnography

Sustained EEG wakefulness is present during these episodes. Abnormal behaviors tend to begin several seconds after an arousal, unlike disorders of arousals wherein activity starts immediately with the arousal from sleep. They can occur during sleep-wake transitions (eg, on falling asleep, or after awakenings from NREM stages 1 and 2 sleep or REM sleep).

Sleep-Related Groaning (Catathrenia)

Catathrenia is a recently described parasomnia that consists of expiratory groaning during sleep. Episodes occur predominantly or exclusively during REM sleep during the second half of the night. This appears to be a rare condition that is more common among males. The individual is asymptomatic with no evident distress and is unaware of the events.

Onset is typically insidious. The course of the condition tends to be chronic with nightly occurrence of groaning.

Differential diagnosis includes sleep talking, seizure activity, and stridor.

Physical examination is generally normal. Polysomnography may demonstrate episodes of bradypnea associated with loud expiratory groaning sounds that occur in clusters recurring several times throughout the night mainly during REM sleep. Although arousals may be observed with these events, unusual movements or cardiac arrhythmias are typically absent. Sleep architecture and oxygen saturation remain normal.

Sleep-Related Hallucinations

Hallucinations can occur during sleep-wake transitions, either at sleep onset (hypnagogic hallucinations) or during awakening (hypnopompic hallucinations). These hallucinatory experiences can take a variety of forms, including visual, auditory, or tactile phenomena, and can last from several seconds to minutes. Sleep paralysis may accompany the hallucinations.

Sleep-related hallucinations can be encountered in patients with narcolepsy or in an isolated form in otherwise healthy individuals in whom they occur more commonly during adolescence or early adulthood. Prevalence decreases with aging. Women are affected more frequently than men.

These hallucinations have also been reported during administration of β-adrenergic blocking agents and in patients with mood disorders, Parkinson disease, Lewy body dementia, or blindness. Other predisposing factors include substance or alcohol use and sleep deprivation.

Polysomnography demonstrates events occurring predominantly during sleep-onset REM periods, but episodes can also arise during NREM sleep.

Sleep-Related Impaired Penile Erections

Sleep-related penile erections (tumescence) can normally be observed during REM sleep among males starting at 3 to 6 months of age. Identifying penile tumescence during sleep and measuring penile rigidity have been used to distinguish between organic (absence of penile erection) and psychogenic (penile erection present) causes of impotence.

The inability to achieve and maintain penile erections during sleep usually indicates the presence of an organic pathology (eg, diabetes mellitus, testosterone deficiency, hyperprolactinemia, depression, peripheral vascular insufficiency, neuropathy, or Peyronie disease). The use of REM sleep suppressing medications, adrenergic blockers, and psychotropic agents can also give rise to impaired tumescence.

Sleep-Related Painful Erections

Painful penile erections occurring during REM sleep can give rise to repetitive awakenings, and, in some cases, insomnia and/or excessive daytime sleepiness. This is a rare condition that often begins after the fourth decade of life and progressively worsens with advancing age. It is not associated with any physical abnormality, or any penile disorder or pain during sexual erections while awake. Sexual function while awake is generally normal. There are no clear predisposing factors or familial patterns.

Differential diagnosis includes Peyronie disease and phimosis.

A PSG may demonstrate a decrease in sleep efficiency, an increase in wake time after sleep onset and a reduced percentage of REM sleep. Impaired nocturnal penile tumescence may also be evident.

Treatment is often not required. If therapy is indicated, several medications, including propranolol, paroxetine, and clozapine, have been reported to be effective in treating this disorder.

Sleep Terrors

Sleep terrors (pavor nocturnus) consist of abrupt awakenings with profound fear usually from NREM stages 3 and 4 sleep, often in the first part of the night. Sleep terrors can cause distress and functional impairment. Individuals may suddenly bolt upright from their beds with a loud yell, cry, or scream, and in rare instances, sleepwalking or running may follow. Associated clinical features include inconsolability, misperception of the environment, confusion, amnesia for the episode, autonomic and behavioral manifestations of intense fear (tachycardia, elevated blood pressure, tachypnea, dilated pupils, and profuse sweating), vocalizations, or urinary incontinence. Affected individuals are usually unresponsive to external stimuli and are difficult to arouse. Although usually benign, these behaviors can become violent and potentially dangerous, and injuries can be sustained during the event. Persons with sleep terrors then spontaneously calm down and return rapidly to sleep.

Sleep terrors are mostly encountered in children between 4 and 12 years of age. They tend to spontaneously abate by adolescence. They appear to affect both genders equally. Persistence or onset during adolescence may be related to psychological factors. Adolescents with sleep terrors and sleepwalking may have an increased prevalence of other sleep disorders (eg, enuresis) and psychiatric disorders (eg, anxiety disorder, panic disorder, or simple phobia).

Sleep terrors are rare in adults; the prevalence is between 1% and 3% in this age group. Many adults with sleep terrors also sleepwalk, and vice versa. A minority of adult patients with sleepwalking or night terrors may have a history of major psychological trauma or psychiatric illness (eg, mood or anxiety disorder). Sleep terrors in adults can begin in NREM stage 2 sleep or during the second half of the night.

Family history is important. A positive family history of sleep terrors is present in a majority of first- to third-degree relatives. Sleep terrors are reported twice as frequently in children in whom one or both parents have a history of sleepwalking compared to children without sleepwalking parents. Episodes of sleep terrors can be triggered by febrile illness, sleep deprivation, stress, excessive ingestion of caffeine, or the use of CNS depressant agents. By inducing arousals from NREM stages 3 and 4 sleep, other sleep disorders such as OSA or periodic limb movement disorder, may increase the risk of developing sleep terrors.

Differential diagnosis includes nocturnal panic attacks, post-traumatic stress disorder, nightmares, seizures, REM sleep behavior disorder, parasomnia overlap disorder, and malingering. As with the other parasomnias, diagnosis is typically arrived at by clinical history alone. Interview of witnesses of the nocturnal event is essential because of the patient's impaired recall of the episode.

Polysomnography

Polysomnographic evaluation is rarely indicated unless the episodes are violent or potentially injurious. Studies should include time-synchronized video recording. Polysomnographic features consist of a decrease in sleep efficiency, more frequent arousals, and greater wake time after sleep onset. There is often a decrease in NREM stage 2 sleep and an increase in NREM stages 3 and 4 sleep. Greater slow wave EEG activity can precede sleep terrors, which usually appear as sudden arousals from NREM stages 3 and 4 sleep.

Therapy

Infrequent episodes of noninjurious sleep terrors require no specific intervention aside from instructions to avoid possible precipitating factors and to maintain a safe bedroom environment. Environmental precautions are similar to those described for sleepwalking (discussed below). Low-dose benzodiazepines, SSRIs, and tricyclic antidepressants can be tried if pharmacologic therapy is indicated.

Sleepwalking

Sleepwalking, or somnambulism, refers to ambulation that occurs during sleep. It is considered a disorder of arousal. Sleepwalking is associated with an altered state of consciousness, diminished arousability, impaired judgment and inappropriate behavior (eg, shouting or climbing out of a window). The behavior can either be calm or agitated and violent. Autonomic activation is generally minimal. The duration of each episode varies widely from several minutes to over an hour. The sleepwalker's eyes are usually open (described as a blank stare), but attempts to communicate with the sleepwalker are generally unsuccessful. Some activities are highly elaborate, such as driving a car. The individual is typically confused when awakened from the episode, with partial or complete amnesia for the event. Sleepwalking can cause distress and functional impairment. Complications consist of physical injuries to the sleepwalker or others (sleep-related violence), social embarrassment, and disturbance of the bed partner's sleep.

Sleepwalking is most commonly seen during the first third or first half of the night and typically originates from NREM stages 3 and 4 sleep. It can, however, occur throughout the entire sleep period in adults, and can begin in NREM stage 2 sleep in this age group.

Sleepwalking is observed in up to 17% to 40% of children. Prevalence peaks between 11 and 12 years of age and decreases significantly with aging, usually disappearing by adolescence. Persistent somnambulism beyond childhood is unrelated to other sleep disturbances, psychopathology, or any known environmental factors.

Children who sleepwalk commonly also present with sleep terrors or sleep talking. It has been hypothesized that sleepwalking and night terrors share a common genetic predisposition, with sleepwalking being a more common but less severe manifestation of the same mechanism responsible for night terrors.

Sleepwalking is less common in adults, with a prevalence of about 0.5% to 4%. A positive history of sleepwalking during childhood is present in most adult sleepwalkers. Furthermore, adult sleepwalking is infrequent among those who had never walked in their sleep during childhood. In rare instances, sleepwalking can begin during adulthood. Like children, most adults who sleepwalk tend to have sleep terrors as well, and vice versa. Whereas both genders are affected equally in childhood sleepwalking, there is a male predominance in adult cases of violent sleepwalking.

Frequency of sleepwalking is increased by any factor that enhances NREM stages 3 and 4 sleep. It may be precipitated or exacerbated by sleep deprivation (most important factor), OSA, febrile illness, stress, and the use of alcohol and certain psychotropic medications (eg, lithium, phenothiazines, tricyclic antidepressants, chloral hydrate, and anticholinergic agents). Additional risk factors for sleepwalking include medical disorders (eg, hyperthyroidism), neurologic illnesses (eg, encephalitis, head injury, migraine headaches, or stroke), environmental disturbances (eg, loud noises), or internal stimuli such as bladder distention. There appears to be no significant association between psychopathology and either childhood or adult sleepwalking.

Familial occurrence is common. Sleepwalking increases from 22% in children without sleepwalking parents to 45% and 60% if one or both parents sleepwalked, respectively. An affected first-degree relative is more than ten times more common than in the general population. Concordance rates vary greatly between monozygotic twins (55%) and dizygotic twins (35%). Finally, specific DQB1 genes have been implicated; DQB1*0501 was present in 35% of sleepwalkers compared to 13% of controls.

Differential diagnosis of sleepwalking includes sleep terrors, REM sleep behavior disorder, parasomnia overlap disorder, seizures, dissociative states, malingering, and "sleep drunkenness" that may occur following arousals related to OSA. Diagnosis is commonly made by history alone. PSG is not routinely indicated in the diagnosis of sleepwalking, and a normal study does not exclude its diagnosis. Nonetheless, PSG may be considered in cases with atypical presentation, forensic implications, or poor response to therapy. If performed, time-synchronized video recording is helpful. Features may include arousals typically occurring from NREM stages 3 and 4 sleep and, occasionally, from stage 2, as well as an increase in NREM stages 3 and 4 sleep. Sleepwalkers have more disturbed sleep during the first NREM-REM sleep cycle with a greater number of disordered arousals and an increase in delta (0.75–2 Hz) activity just prior to arousals. EEG patterns following arousals from NREM stages 3 and 4 sleep in adults with injurious sleepwalking and sleep terrors include (1) diffuse, rhythmic delta activity; (2) diffuse delta and theta activity; and (3) prominent alpha and beta activity. Abrupt heart rate acceleration may be noted postarousal. PSG may also demonstrate the presence of other sleep disorders that could either trigger sleepwalking (eg, OSA), or could be mistaken for it (eg, REM sleep behavior disorder or seizures).

SPECT during sleepwalking has demonstrated activation of thalamocingulate pathways and persistent deactivation of other thalamocortical arousal systems.

No specific treatment is necessary for most cases of sleepwalking. Medications that can potentially trigger sleepwalking episodes should be discontinued, if possible. Therapy, if indicated because of high frequency of events or injurious behavior, includes proper sleep hygiene as well as avoidance of sleep deprivation and other precipitating factors. Environmental safety precautions, such as sleeping on the first floor, removing hazardous objects in the bedroom, locking doors and windows, and covering the windows with heavy drapery, are important.

Scheduled awakenings (ie, having parents awaken their child several hours after the child goes to sleep and just before the typical time of the sleepwalking episode) have been reported to be effective in eliminating sleepwalking with beneficial effects maintained at 3 and 6 months posttreatment. Pharmacologic agents that have been used with some success include low-dose benzodiazepines, SSRIs, tricyclic antidepressants, and trazodone. Nonpharmacologic interventions, including relaxation techniques and hypnosis, can be tried as well.

Parasomnias Secondary to Other Sleep Disorders

Obstructive sleep apnea may be associated with repetitive apnea- or hypopnea-induced arousals from NREM and REM sleep. Behavior during these arousals can be difficult to distinguish from primary REM sleep behavior disorder, disorders of arousal, sleep-related eating disorder, nocturnal seizures, or violent parasomnias.

Parasomnias Secondary to Medications

Disorders of arousal, sleep-related hallucinations, and REM sleep behavior disorder can be precipitated by certain medications (Table 7–5). Sleep-related hallucinations following the administration of β-adrenergic receptor-blocking agents have been described. Medications and substances known to trigger REM sleep behavior disorder include bisoprolol, caffeine, mirtazapine,

Table 7–5. Predisposing factors for rapid eye movement sleep behavior disorder

Conditions	Medications
Aging	Alcohol
Autism	Amphetamines
Cerebrovascular disease (ischemic or hemorrhagic stroke, subarachnoid hemorrhage)	Anticholinergics
	Antidepressants (except bupropion)
Dementia (eg, Alzheimer disease or Lewy body disease)	Mirtazapine
Guillain-Barre syndrome	Monoamine oxidase inhibitors
Hereditary quivering chin syndrome	Selective serotonin reuptake inhibitors (eg, fluoxetine)
Machado-Joseph disease (SCA-3)	Tricyclic antidepressants
Mitochondrial encephalomyopathy	Venlafaxine
Mobius syndrome	Biperiden
Multiple sclerosis	Cocaine
Multiple system atrophy	Sedative-hypnotics
Narcolepsy	Selegiline
Neoplasms (brainstem)	Withdrawal from alcohol, hypnotic agents, and REM sleep suppressants
Normal pressure hydrocephalus	
Olivopontocerebellar degeneration	
Parkinson disease	
Post-traumatic stress disorder	
Shy-Drager syndrome	
Spinocerebellar ataxia	
Striatonigral degeneration	
Tourette syndrome	

monoamine oxidase inhibitors, SSRIs, selegiline, tricyclic antidepressants, and venlafaxine. In addition, withdrawal from alcohol, amphetamines, barbiturates, cocaine, and meprobamate can also give rise to acute REM sleep behavior disorder.

Sleep-Related Violence

Injurious behavior can occur during sleep. Sleep-related violence generally lasts only a few minutes, occurs without apparent purpose or premeditation, may or may not be associated with dreaming, and tends not to be repetitive. There is often complete or partial amnesia for the preceding event. On awakening, individuals generally display genuine horror and remorse for their actions and do not, as a rule, escape the scene of the violence or try to cover up any evidence. Events are classified as "automatisms" because of the absence of conscious awareness or sound judgment; as such, these individuals cannot be held accountable for their actions.

There is a greater prevalence of sleep-related violence among men compared to women. The etiology of sleep-related violence is presented in Box 7–4.

Therapy

Factors known to precipitate sleep-related violence, such as sleep deprivation or alcohol intake, should be avoided. Appropriate use of medications can significantly reduce the frequency of some parasomnias. The patient should be instructed on measures to prevent injury to himself or herself and others.

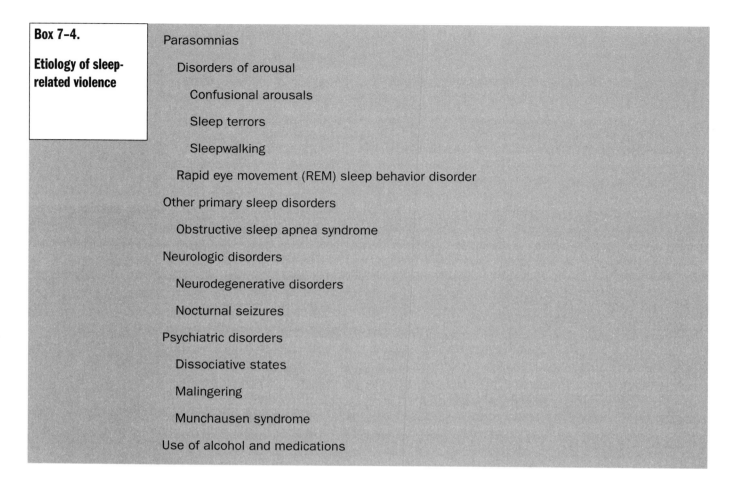

Box 7–4.

Etiology of sleep-related violence

Parasomnias

    Disorders of arousal

        Confusional arousals

        Sleep terrors

        Sleepwalking

    Rapid eye movement (REM) sleep behavior disorder

Other primary sleep disorders

    Obstructive sleep apnea syndrome

Neurologic disorders

    Neurodegenerative disorders

    Nocturnal seizures

Psychiatric disorders

    Dissociative states

    Malingering

    Munchausen syndrome

Use of alcohol and medications

Summary

Parasomnias are common clinical complaints. An extensive history, including medical, neurologic, and psychiatric conditions; sleep disorders; a review of medication, alcohol, or illicit drug use; and a family history of parasomnias, may provide useful clues. A formal sleep evaluation, including polysomnography, is indicated for parasomnias that are violent and potentially injurious; disruptive to the bed partner or other household members; accompanied by excessive daytime sleepiness; or associated with medical, psychiatric, or neurologic symptoms or findings. Distinguishing between a parasomnia and a seizure may be difficult because both can present as recurrent, stereotypical behaviors. Evaluation may be aided by an expanded EEG montage during overnight PSG studies.

Multiple sleep latency testing should be considered for patients with complaints of excessive daytime sleepiness.

References

General References

American Academy of Sleep Medicine. *The International Classification of Sleep Disorders: Diagnostic and Coding Manual.* 2nd ed. Westchester, IL: American Academy of Sleep Medicine, 2005.

Bowman TJ. *Review of Sleep Medicine.* Burlington, MA: Butterworth-Heinemann, 2002.

Berry RB. *Sleep Medicine Pearls.* 2nd ed. Philadelphia, PA: Hanley & Belfus, 2002.

Chokroverty S. *Clinical Companion to Sleep Disorders Medicine.* 2nd ed. Butterworth-Heinemann, 2000.

Lavie P, Pillar G, Malhotra A. *Sleep Disorders Handbook.* New York, NY: Taylor & Francis, 2002.

Lee-Chiong T. Parasomnias and other sleep-related movement disorders. *Sleep Medicine.* Primary Care: Clinics in Office Practice. Elsevier Saunders, 2005.

Lee-Chiong TL, ed. *Sleep: A Comprehensive Handbook.* Hoboken, NJ: John Wiley & Sons, 2006.

Lee-Chiong TL, Sateia M, Carskadon M, eds. *Sleep Medicine.* Philadelphia, PA: Hanley & Belfus (Elsevier), 2002.

Mahowald MW. Arousal and sleep-wake transition parasomnias. In: Lee-Chiong TL, Sateia MJ, Carskadon MA. *Sleep Medicine.* Philadelphia, PA: Elsevier, 2002;207–213.

Mahowald MW. Parasomnias. *Med Clin North Am.* 2004(May);88(3):669–78.

Perlis ML, Lichstein KL, eds. *Treating Sleep Disorders: Principles and Practice of Behavioral Sleep Medicine.* Hoboken, NJ: John Wiley & Sons, 2003.

Rechtschaffen A, Kales A. *A Manual of Standardized Terminology, Techniques and Scoring System for Sleep Stages of Human Subjects.* Los Angeles, CA: Brain Information Service/Brain Research Institute, University of California, 1968.

Reite M, Ruddy J, Nagel K. *Concise Guide to Evaluation and Management of Sleep Disorders.* 3rd ed. Arlington, VA: American Psychiatric Publishing, April 2002.

Sleep Disorders. Medical Clinics of North America. Philadelphia, PA: Elsevier Saunders, 2004.

Sleep Medicine. Primary Care: Clinics in Office Practice. Philadelphia, PA: Elsevier Saunders, 2005.

Sleep Research Society. *SRS Basics of Sleep Guide.* Westchester, IL: Sleep Research Society, 2005.

Confusional Arousals

American Academy of Sleep Medicine. *The International Classification of Sleep Disorders: Diagnostic and Coding Manual.* 2nd ed. American Academy of Sleep Medicine, 2005.

Hublin C, Kaprio J. Genetic aspects and genetic epidemiology of parasomnias. *Sleep Medicine Reviews.* 2003;7(5):413–421.

Mahowald MW. Arousal and sleep-wake transition parasomnias. In: Lee-Chiong TL, Sateia MJ, Carskadon MA. *Sleep Medicine.* Philadelphia, PA: Elsevier, 2002;207–213.

Ohayon MM, Guilleminault C, Priest RG. Night terrors, sleepwalking, and confusional arousals in the general population: their frequency and relationship to other sleep and mental disorders. *J Clin Psychiatry.* 1999;60:268–276.

Enuresis

Brown WD. Other parasomnias. In: Lee-Chiong TL, Sateia M, Carskadon M, eds. *Sleep Medicine.* Philadelphia, PA: Hanley & Belfus (Elsevier), 2002.

Challamel Mj, Cochat P. Nocturnal enuresis in children. In: Lee-Chiong TL, ed. *Sleep: A Comprehensive Handbook.* Hoboken, NJ: John Wiley & Sons, 2006.

Exploding Head Syndrome

American Academy of Sleep Medicine. The International Classification of Sleep Disorders: Diagnostic and Coding Manual. 2nd ed. American Academy of Sleep Medicine, 2005.

Impaired Sleep-Related Penile Erections

Lee-Chiong TL. Manifestations and classification of sleep disorders. In: Lee-Chiong TL, Sateia M, Carskadon M, eds. *Sleep Medicine*. Philadelphia, PA: Hanley & Belfus (Elsevier), 2002.

Nightmares

American Academy of Sleep Medicine. *The International Classification of Sleep Disorders: Diagnostic and Coding Manual*. 2nd ed. American Academy of Sleep Medicine, 2005.

Asplund R. Nightmares, sleep and cardiac symptoms in the elderly. *Neth J Med*. 2003(Jul);61(7): 257–61.

Low JF, Dyster-Aas J, Willebrand M, Kildal M, Gerdin B, Ekselius L. Chronic nightmares after severe burns: risk factors and implications for treatment. *J Burn Care Rehabil*. 2003 (Jul–Aug);24(4):260–7.

Pagel JF, Helfter P. Drug induced nightmares—an etiology based review. *Hum Psychopharmacol*. 2003(Jan);18(1):59–67.

Nocturnal Eating (Drinking) Syndrome

Auger RR, Morgenthaler TI. Sleep-related eating disorders. In: Lee-Chiong TL, ed. *Sleep: A Comprehensive Handbook*. Hoboken, NJ: John Wiley & Sons, 2006.

Lee-Chiong TL. Manifestations and classification of sleep disorders. In: Lee-Chiong TL, Sateia M, Carskadon M, eds. *Sleep Medicine*. Philadelphia, PA: Hanley & Belfus (Elsevier), 2002.

Nocturnal Leg Cramps

Brasic JR. Should people with nocturnal leg cramps drink tonic water and bitter lemon? *Psychol Rep*. 1999(Apr);84(2):355–67.

Leclerc KM, Landry FJ. Benign nocturnal leg cramps. Current controversies over use of quinine. *Postgrad Med*. 1996(Feb);99(2):177–8, 181–4.

Riley JD, Antony SJ. Leg cramps: differential diagnosis and management. *Am Fam Physician*. 1995(Nov 1);52(6):1794–8.

Nocturnal Paroxysmal Dystonia

American Sleep Disorders Association. *International Classification Of Sleep Disorders: Diagnostic and Coding Manual*. Revised. Rochester, MN: American Sleep Disorders Association, 1997.

Hirsch E, Sellal F, Maton B, Rumbach L, Marescaux C. Nocturnal paroxysmal dystonia: a clinical form of focal epilepsy. *Neurophysiol Clin*. 1994(Jun);24(3):207–17.

Lombroso CT. Nocturnal paroxysmal dystonia due to a subfrontal cortical dysplasia. *Epileptic Disord*. 2000(Mar);2(1):15–20.

Montagna P. Nocturnal paroxysmal dystonia and nocturnal wandering. *Neurology*. 1992(Jul); 42(7 Suppl 6):61–7.

Pardal Fernandez JM, Lopez-Agreda JM, Carrillo-Yague R. Nocturnal paroxysmal dystonia, movement disorder and epilepsy. *Rev Neurol*. 2002(May)16–31;34(10):940–4.

Provini F, Plazzi G, Lugaresi E. From nocturnal paroxysmal dystonia to nocturnal frontal lobe epilepsy. *Clin Neurophysiol*. 2000(Sep);111(Suppl 2):S2–8.

Rapid Eye Movement Sleep Behavior Disorder

Abad VC, Guilleminault C. Review of rapid eye movement behavior sleep disorders. *Curr Neurol Neurosci Rep*. 2004(Mar);4(2):157–63.

Boeve BF, Silber MH, Parisi JE, Dickson DW, Ferman TJ, Benarroch EE, et al. Synucleinopathy pathology and REM sleep behavior disorder plus dementia or parkinsonism. *Neurology*. 2003 (Jul 8);61(1):40–5.

Eisensehr I, Linke R, Tatsch K, Kharraz B, Gildehaus JF, Wetter CTet al. Increased muscle activity during rapid eye movement sleep correlates with decrease of striatal presynaptic dopamine transporters. IPT and IBZM SPECT imaging in subclinical and clinically manifest idiopathic REM sleep behavior disorder, Parkinson's disease, and controls. *Sleep*. 2003(Aug 1);26(5):507–12.

Fantini ML, Gagnon JF, Petit D, Rompre S, Decary A, Carrier J, et al. Slowing of electroencephalogram in rapid eye movement sleep behavior disorder. *Ann Neurol*. 2003(Jun);53(6):774–80.

Ferini-Strambi L, Zucconi M. REM sleep behavior disorder. *Clin Neurophysiol*. 2000(Sep);111(Suppl 2): S136–40.

Friedman JH, Fernandez HH, Sudarsky LR. REM behavior disorder and excessive daytime somnolence in Machado-Joseph disease (SCA-3). *Mov Disord*. 2003(Dec);18(12):1520–2.

Fukutake T, Shinotoh H, Nishino H, Ichikawa Y, Goto J, Kanazawa I, et al. Homozygous Machado-Joseph disease presenting as REM sleep behaviour disorder and prominent psychiatric symptoms. *Eur J Neurol*. 2002(Jan);9(1):97–100.

Gilman S, Koeppe RA, Chervin RD, Consens FB, Little R, An H, et al. REM sleep behavior disorder is related to striatal monoaminergic deficit in MSA. *Neurology*. 2003(Jul 8);61(1):29–34.

Olson EJ, Boeve BF, Silber MH. Rapid eye movement sleep behaviour disorder: demographic, clinical and laboratory findings in 93 cases. *Brain*. 2000(Feb);123(Pt 2):331–9.

Onofrj M, Thomas A, D'Andreamatteo G, Iacono D, Luciano AL, Di Rollo A, et al. Incidence of RBD and hallucination in patients affected by Parkinson's disease: 8-year follow-up. *Neurol Sci*. 2002(Sep);23 Suppl 2:S91–4.

Schenck CH, Boyd JL, Mahowald MW. A parasomnia overlap disorder involving sleepwalking, sleep terrors, and REM sleep behavior disorder in 33 polysomnographically confirmed cases. *Sleep*. 1997(Nov);20(11):972–81.

Schenck CH, Mahowald MW: Motor dyscontrol in narcolepsy: rapid-eye-movement (REM) sleep without atonia and REM sleep behavior disorder. *Ann Neurol*. 1992;32:3–10.

Schenck CH. REM-sleep-associated parasomnias. In: Lee-Chiong TL, Sateia MJ, Carskadon MA. Sleep Medicine. Philadelphia, PA: Elsevier, 2002;215–223.

Shirakawa S, Takeuchi N, Uchimura N, Ohyama T, Maeda H, Abe T, et al. Study of image findings in rapid eye movement sleep behavioural disorder. *Psychiatry Clin Neurosci*. 2002(Jun);56(3): 291–2.

Wetter TC, Trenkwalder C, Gershanik O, Hogl B. Polysomnographic measures in Parkinson's disease: a comparison between patients with and without REM sleep disturbances. *Wien Klin Wochenschr*. 2001(Apr 17);113(7–8):249–53.

Rapid Eye Movement Sleep-Related Sinus Arrest

Coccagna G, Capucci A, Pierpaoli S. A case of sinus arrest and vagal overactivity during REM sleep. *Clin Auton Res*. 1999(Jun);9(3):135–8.

Lee-Chiong TL. Manifestations and classification of sleep disorders. In: Lee-Chiong TL, Sateia MJ, Carskadon MA. Sleep Medicine. Philadelphia, PA: Elsevier, 2002.

Schenck CH. REM-sleep-associated parasomnias. In: Lee-Chiong TL, Sateia MJ, Carskadon MA. Sleep Medicine. Philadelphia, PA: Elsevier, 2002:215–223.

Rhythmic Movement Disorder

American Academy of Sleep Medicine. *The International Classification of Sleep Disorders: Diagnostic and Coding Manual*. 2nd ed. American Academy of Sleep Medicine, 2005.

Lee-Chiong TL. Manifestations and classification of sleep disorders. In: Lee-Chiong TL, Sateia MJ, Carskadon MA. Sleep Medicine. Philadelphia, PA: Elsevier, 2002.

Sleep Bruxism

Bader G, Lavigne G. Sleep bruxism; an overview of an oromandibular sleep movement disorder. *Sleep Med Rev*. 2000(Feb);4(1):27–43.

Bader GG, Kampe T, Tagdae T, Karlsson S, Nlomqvist M. Descriptive physiological data on a sleep bruxism population. *Sleep*. 1997;20(11):982–990.

Brown WD. Other parasomnias. In: Lee-Chiong TL, Sateia MJ, Carskadon MA. Sleep Medicine. Philadelphia, PA: Elsevier, 2002:237–244.

Carlsson GE, Egermark I, Magnusson T. Predictors of bruxism, other oral parafunctions, and tooth wear over a 20-year follow-up period. *J Orofac Pain*. 2003(Winter);17(1):50–7.

Dube C, Rompre PH, Manzini C, Guitard F, de Grandmont P, Lavigne GJ. Quantitative polygraphic controlled study on efficacy and safety of oral splint devices in tooth-grinding subjects. *J Dent Res*. 2004(May);83(5):398–403.

Kato T, Thie NM, Montplaisir JY, Lavigne GJ. Bruxism and orofacial movements during sleep. *Dent Clin North Am*. 2001(Oct);45(4):657–84.

Kato T, Rompre P, Montplaisir JY, Sessle BJ, Lavigne GJ. Sleep bruxism: an oromotor activity secondary to micro-arousal. J Dent Res. 2001(Oc)t;80(10):1940–4.

Kato T, Montplaisir JY, Guitard F, Sessle BJ, Lund JP, Lavigne GJ. Evidence that experimentally induced sleep bruxism is a consequence of transient arousal. *J Dent Res*. 2003(Apr);82(4):284–8.

Lavigne GJ, Manzini C. Bruxism. In: Kryger MH, Roth T, Dement WC, eds. *Principles and Practice in Sleep Medicine*. Philadelphia, PA: WB Saunders 2000:773–785.

Lavigne GJ, Montplaisir JY. Restless legs syndrome and sleep bruxism: prevalence and association among Canadians. Sleep. 1994;17(8);739–743.

Lavigne GJ, Kato T, Kolta A, Sessle BJ. Neurobiological mechanisms involved in sleep bruxism. *Crit Rev Oral Biol Med*. 2003;14(1):30–46.

Lavigne GJ, Lobbezoo F, Rompre PH, Nielsen TA, Montplaisir J. Cigarette smoking as a risk factor or an exacerbating factor for Restless Legs Syndrome and Sleep Bruxism. *Sleep.* 1997;20(4): 290–293.

Miyawaki S, Lavigne GJ, Pierre M, Guitard F, Montplaisir JY, Kato T. Association between sleep bruxism, swallowing-related laryngeal movement, and sleep positions. *Sleep.* 2003(); 26(4):461–5.

Oksenberg A, Arons E. Sleep bruxism related to obstructive sleep apnea: the effect of continuous positive airway pressure. *Sleep Med.* 2002(Nov);3(6):513–5.

Raigrodski AJ, Christensen LV, Mohamed SE, Gardiner DM. The effect of four-week administration of amitriptyline on sleep bruxism. A double-blind crossover clinical study. *Cranio.* 2001(Jan);19(1):21–5.

Tan EK, Jankovic J. Treating severe bruxism with botulinum toxin. *J Am Dent Assoc.* 2000(Feb);131(2):211–6.

Tosun T, Karabuda C, Cuhadaroglu C. Evaluation of sleep bruxism by polysomnographic analysis in patients with dental implants. *Int J Oral Maxillofac Implants.* 2003(Mar–Apr);18(2):286–92.

Sleep Paralysis

Buzzi G, Cirignotta F. Isolated sleep paralysis: a web survey. *Sleep Res Online.* 2000;3(2):61–6.

Takeuchi T, Miyasita A, Sasaki Y, Inugami M, Fukuda K. Isolated sleep paralysis elicited by sleep interruption. *Sleep.* 1992(Jun);15(3):217–25.

Wing YK, Chiu H, Leung T, Ng J. Sleep paralysis in the elderly. *J Sleep Res.* 1999(Jun);8(2): 151–5.

Sleep-Related Dissociative Disorders

American Academy of Sleep Medicine. *The International Classification of Sleep Disorders: Diagnostic and Coding Manual.* 2nd ed. American Academy of Sleep Medicine, 2005.

Sleep-Related Groaning (Catathrenia)

American Academy of Sleep Medicine. *The International Classification of Sleep Disorders: Diagnostic and Coding Manual.* 2nd ed. American Academy of Sleep Medicine, 2005.

Sleep-Related Hallucinations

American Academy of Sleep Medicine. *The International Classification of Sleep Disorders: Diagnostic and Coding Manual.* 2nd ed. American Academy of Sleep Medicine, 2005.

Lee-Chiong TL. Manifestations and classification of sleep disorders. In: Lee-Chiong TL, Sateia M, Carskadon M, eds. *Sleep Medicine.* Philadelphia, PA: Hanley & Belfus (Elsevier), 2002.

Sleep-Related Impaired Penile Erections

Lee-Chiong TL. Manifestations and classification of sleep disorders. In: Lee-Chiong TL, Sateia M, Carskadon M, eds. *Sleep Medicine.* Philadelphia, PA: Hanley & Belfus (Elsevier), 2002.

Sleep-Related Painful Erections

Ferini-Strambi L, Oldani A, Zucconi M, Castronovo V, Montorsi F, Rigatti P, et al. Sleep-related painful erections: clinical and polysomnographic features. *J Sleep Res*. 1996(Sep);5(3):195–7.

Steiger A, Benkert O. Examination and treatment of sleep-related painful erections—a case report. *Arch Sex Behav*. 1989(Jun);18(3):263–7.

Sleep Terrors

Abe K, Amatomi M, Oda N. Sleepwalking and recurrent sleeptalking in children of childhood sleepwalkers. *Am J Psychiatry*. 1984;141:800–801.

Espa F, Ondze B, Deglise P, Billiard M, Besset A. Sleep architecture, slow wave activity, and sleep spindles in adult patients with sleepwalking and sleep terrors. *Clin Neurophysiol*. 2000(May);111(5):929–39.

Gau SF, Soong WT. Psychiatric comorbidity of adolescents with sleep terrors or sleepwalking: a case-control study. *Aust N Z J Psychiatry*. 1999(Oct);33(5):734–9.

Guilleminault C, Palombini L, Pelayo R, Chervin RD. Sleepwalking and sleep terrors in prepubertal children: what triggers them? *Pediatrics*. 2003(Jan);111(1):e17–25.

Hartman D, Crisp AH, Sedgwick P, Borrow S. Is there a dissociative process in sleepwalking and night terrors? *Postgrad Med J*. 2001(Apr);77(906):244–9.

Hublin C, Kaprio J, Partinen M, Koskenvuo M. Limits of self-report in assessing sleep terrors in a population survey. *Sleep*. 1999(Feb 1);22(1):89–93.

Kales A, Soldatos CR, Bixler EO, Ladda RL, Charney DS, Weber G, et al. Hereditary factors in sleepwalking and night terrors. *Br J Psychiatry*. 1980;137:111–118.

Sleepwalking

Bassetti C, Vella S, Donati F, Wielepp P, Weder B. SPECT during sleepwalking. *Lancet*. 2000 (Aug 5);356(9228):484–5.

Frank NC, Spirito A, Stark L, Owens-Stively J. The use of scheduled awakenings to eliminate childhood sleepwalking. *J Pediatr Psychol*. 1997(Jun);22(3):345–53.

Gaudreau H, Joncas S, Zadra A, Montplaisir J. Dynamics of slow-wave activity during the NREM sleep of sleepwalkers and control subjects. *Sleep*. 2000(Sep)15;23(6):755–60.

Guilleminault C, Poyares D, Aftab FA, Palombini L, Abat F. Sleep and wakefulness in somnambulism: a spectral analysis study. *J Psychosom Res*. 2001(Aug);51(2):411–6.

Hublin C, Kaprio J, Partinen M, Heikkila K, Koskenvuo M. Prevalence and genetics of sleepwalking: a population-based twin study. *Neurology*. 1997(Jan);48(1):177–81.

Kales A, Soldatos CR, Bixler EO, Ladda RL, Charney DS, Weber G, et al. Hereditary factors in sleepwalking and night terrors. *Br J Psychiatry*. 1980;137:111–118.

Klackenberg G. Somnambulism in childhood—prevalence, course and behavioral correlations. A prospective longitudinal study (6–16 years). *Acta Paediatr Scand*. 1982(May);71(3):495–9.

Lecendreux M, Bassetti C, Dauvilliers Y, Mayer G, Neidhart E, Tafti M. HLA and genetic susceptibility to sleepwalking. *Mol Psychiatry*. 2003(Jan);8(1):114–7.

Ohayon MM, Guilleminault C, Priest RG. Night terrors, sleepwalking, and confusional arousals in the general population: their frequency and relationship to other sleep and mental disorders. *J Clin Psychiatry*. 1999;60:268–276.

Restless Legs Syndrome and Periodic Limb Movement Disorder

Restless Legs Syndrome

Restless legs syndrome (RLS) or Ekbom syndrome is characterized by abnormal and unpleasant sensations (paresthesias or dysesthesias) involving the lower extremities that become apparent or worsen at rest, especially in the evening at bedtime, and are relieved, at least transiently, with movement. Sensations often involve both legs but can be unilateral or may alternate between lower extremities.

Clinical Features

Common complaints include a sensation of creeping, crawling, tingling, wormy, throbbing, pulling, burning, or increased "tension" located deep within the legs (rather than affecting the skin superficially) when sitting or lying down. Some patients are simply unable to describe adequately the sensation they feel. Although symptoms are typically not described as painful, a complaint of pain does not exclude the diagnosis. These uncomfortable sensations extend from the feet and ankle proximally to the legs and, occasionally, thighs. Similar sensations have also been described in the arms. Symptoms tend to occur at night, although unpleasant sensations may emerge during the daytime during prolonged periods of immobility (eg, airplane flights).

There is often an accompanying irresistible urge to move the limbs (motor restlessness) to relieve the uncomfortable sensation. Less frequently, an isolated urge to move is present without any accompanying unpleasant sensations.

Movements or walking result in temporary relief of symptoms. Relief of the unpleasant sensations is typically immediate but can be either partial or complete. With advanced disease, movements may be associated with minimal improvement. Symptoms tend to recur following cessation of leg motion. Improvement in symptoms with local massage or warm soaks has also been reported.

Demographics

Restless legs syndrome can be seen in approximately 1% to 15% of normal individuals. Prevalence is increased with pregnancy, uremia, anemia, and rheumatoid arthritis. Prevalence may be lower among Asians (eg, Singapore and Japan) compared to northern and western Europeans. Women are affected more commonly than men.

Onset can occur at any age. Prevalence increases with aging and is most frequent among middle-aged and elderly adults. Course is chronic, but spontaneous remissions can occur. Significant variability in severity of restless legs is not uncommon.

Concurrent periodic limb movements of sleep (PLMS) occur in a majority of individuals with RLS. About 70% to 90% of patients with RLS have PLMS; conversely, about a third of patients with PLMS have RLS.

Genetics

Genetics appear to have an important role in the development of RLS. A positive family history can be elicited in up to 92% of persons with idiopathic RLS and in about 13% of persons with secondary RLS. An estimated one-third of cases of RLS are associated with an autosomal dominant mode of transmission. There is a high concordance rate of RLS symptoms between twins, and RLS is more frequent in first- and second-degree relatives of individuals with RLS. At least three susceptibility loci (chromosomes 9p, 12q, and 14q) for RLS have been identified.

Classification

RLS can be either idiopathic (ie, primary) or secondary (associated with iron, folate or cobalamin deficiency, uremia, pregnancy, peripheral neuropathy, Parkinson disease, multiple sclerosis, amyotrophic lateral sclerosis, poliomyelitis, vascular insufficiency, diabetes mellitus, rheumatoid arthritis, alcohol use, caffeine ingestion or medication use) (Box 8–1). Primary RLS, in turn, can be classified into two subtypes: early onset (before the age of 35 to 45 years) and late onset. An earlier onset and more gradual progression of symptoms, as well as a greater family history of RLS, characterize the early onset type. The cause of primary RLS is unknown but may involve abnormalities in dopaminergic neurotransmitter systems.

Box 8–1. **Causes of restless legs syndrome**	Idiopathic
	Secondary
	Alcohol use
	Amyotrophic lateral sclerosis
	Attention deficit hyperactivity disorder
	Caffeine ingestion
	Congestive heart failure
	Diabetes mellitus
	Fibromyalgia/fibrositis
	Iron, folate or cobalamin deficiency
	Huntington disease
	Leukemia
	Multiple sclerosis
	Myelopathies
	Parkinson disease
	Poliomyelitis
	Peripheral neuropathy
	Pregnancy
	Radiculopathy
	Rheumatoid arthritis
	Sjogren syndrome

(continued from page 303)
Box 8-1.

Causes of restless legs syndrome

Renal failure or uremia

Vascular insufficiency

Medication use

    Calcium channel blockers

    Dopamine antagonists (eg, metoclopramide)

    Lithium

    Neuroleptics

    Sedating antihistamines

    Selective serotonin reuptake inhibitors

    Tricyclic antidepressants

Withdrawal from narcotics and sedative agents

Drugs that can potentially precipitate or worsen RLS include selective serotonin reuptake inhibitors, tricyclic antidepressants, sedating antihistamines, neuroleptics, lithium, dopamine antagonists (eg, prochlorperazine or metoclopramide), and calcium channel blockers. Bupropion, unlike other antidepressants, increases dopamine and does not cause or aggravate RLS. Finally, RLS can worsen during withdrawal from narcotics and sedative agents.

Severity of RLS can be classified using the International RLS rating scale.

Consequences

The degree of sleep disturbance varies depending on the severity of RLS symptoms. When these sensations occur prior to the desired sleep time, persons may experience difficulty falling asleep (ie, sleep-onset insomnia). Difficulty returning to sleep following awakenings may also be present. Sleep fragmentation, if significant, can result in excessive daytime sleepiness.

Complications also include the development of secondary mood disorders.

Evaluation

The diagnosis of RLS is based on clinical history. For more diagnostic information, see Box 8–2. Among children between the ages of 2 to 12 years, diagnostic criteria, in addition to the adult criteria, include *either*

1.   A description consistent with leg discomfort *or*

2.   No description consistent with leg discomfort but with at least two of the following: a complaint of sleep disturbance, a parent or sibling with RLS, or a periodic limb movement index of at least five per hour of sleep during polysomnography.

Neurologic examination is typically normal in persons with primary RLS. Occasionally, involuntary myoclonic and dystonic movements may be appreciated. Electromyography (EMG) and nerve conduction studies may be needed to exclude the presence of neuropathies.

| **Box 8-2.**

International Restless Legs Syndrome Study Group diagnostic criteria for restless legs syndrome in adults | 1. An urge to move the legs, usually accompanied or caused by uncomfortable and unpleasant sensations (paresthesias or dysesthesias) in the limbs. The arms or other body parts may be involved as well. Occasionally, the urge to move is unaccompanied by uncomfortable sensations and

2. The urge to move or unpleasant sensations:

 • Begin or worsen during periods of rest or inactivity (eg, lying or sitting)

 • Are partially or totally relieved by movement (eg, walking or stretching), at least during the time of the activity

 • Are worse in the evening or night than during the day or only occur in the evening or night

Source: Allen RP, et al. Sleep Med. 2003;4:101-9. |

Polysomnography

If polysomnography is performed, sleep latency is commonly prolonged, and leg movements may be noted during wakefulness prior to sleep onset. A prolonged sleep latency also complicates awakenings that occur during the night.

An increase in frequency of periodic limb movements during wakefulness (PLMW) can be present and, in the appropriate clinical setting, a PLMW index greater than 15 per hour during the entire recording supports the diagnosis of RLS. PLMS can be evident in up to 70% to 90% of cases, some of which can be associated with arousals.

Suggested Immobilization Test

The Suggested Immobilization Test is performed with the patient sitting upright in bed with legs outstretched. Polysomnography is recorded for 1 hour in the evening prior to the habitual bedtime while the patient is awake. The diagnosis of RLS is suggested by the presence of PLMW of more than 40 events per hour.

Differential Diagnosis

Differential diagnosis of RLS includes:

1. *Akathisia* (motor restlessness usually related to the use of neuroleptic agents or dopamine receptor antagonists, and not improved by movement)

2. *Nocturnal leg cramps*

3. *Claudication* (characteristically painful sensations due to peripheral vascular insufficiency aggravated by walking and relieved by rest)

4. *Peripheral neuropathy* (abnormal, unpleasant, or decreased sensations not improved by movement)

5. *Painful toes-moving legs syndrome* (painful sensation not relieved by movement secondary to lumbosacral radiculopathy and accompanied by persistent toe movements)

6. *Arthritic or muscular pain*

7. *Myoclonus*

8. *Sleep starts* or *hypnic jerks*

9. *"Vesper's curse"* (transient lumbar stenosis due to supine-related venous plexus engorgement, giving rise to lower extremity paresthesias and lumbosacral pain)

Periodic Limb Movements of Sleep

PLMS or nocturnal myoclonus consists of stereotypical, intermittent, and repetitive movements of the limbs that occur during sleep.

Clinical Features

Periodic limb movements may also occur while sitting or lying during restful wakefulness (periodic limb movements during wakefulness). The condition usually involves the lower extremities but can affect the arms as well. The characteristic movement consists of partial flexion of the ankle, knee, and hip with extension of the big toe and fanning of the small toes. Involvement of the upper extremity consists of flexion at the elbow.

Demographics

The prevalence of PLMS is difficult to determine because many individuals are asymptomatic. It has been suggested that PLMS affects up to 5% of the general population. It is relatively uncommon during childhood but can be present in children with attention deficit hyperactivity disorder. Prevalence increases with aging and can occur in up to a third of adults 60 years of age or older. This condition is most prevalent among middle-aged and elderly adults. Both genders are affected equally. In some cases, familial aggregation has been described.

Etiology

Many of the conditions that are involved in the genesis of RLS could also trigger or aggravate PLMS. These include low iron levels; peripheral neuropathy; renal failure; Parkinson disease; and medications such as selective serotonin reuptake inhibitors, tricyclic antidepressants, monoamine oxidase inhibitors, phenothiazines, lithium, and dopamine antagonists. Excessive caffeine ingestion and alcohol use can worsen PLMS as can withdrawal of sedative-hypnotics, barbiturates and anticonvulsants. Bupropion is not associated with antidepressant-induced PLMS..

In addition to RLS, other disorders commonly associated with PLMS include primary sleep disorders (eg, narcolepsy, rapid eye movement [REM] sleep behavior disorder, and obstructive sleep apnea), neurologic disorders (eg, Parkinson disease, spinal cord injury, multiple system atrophy, multiple sclerosis, amyotrophic lateral sclerosis, Huntington disease, and neuropathy), medical disorders (eg, diabetes mellitus and fibromyalgia), and psychiatric disorders (eg, post-traumatic stress disorder and attention deficit hyperactivity disorder). In REM sleep behavior disorder, PLMS can be evident during both non–rapid eye movement (NREM) and REM sleep. Conditions associated with PLMS are listed in Box 8–3.

PLMS can emerge during nasal continuous positive airway pressure (CPAP) therapy in persons with obstructive sleep apnea. The mechanism responsible for this is unknown. In many patients, PLMS are transitory phenomena and require no treatment. However, if complaints of sleep disturbance or excessive sleepiness should persist despite optimal therapy of obstructive sleep apnea by CPAP, specific intervention for PLMS may be indicated.

Box 8-3.

Factors related to periodic limb movements during sleep

Sleep disorders

    Narcolepsy

    Obstructive sleep apnea

    REM sleep behavior disorder

    Restless legs syndrome

Neurologic disorders

    Amyotrophic lateral sclerosis

    Huntington disease

    Multiple sclerosis

    Multiple system atrophy

    Neuropathies, radiculopathies and myelopathies

    Parkinson disease

    Seizure disorders

    Spinal cord injury

    Stiff-man syndrome

Medical disorders

    Chronic fatigue syndrome

    Chronic obstructive pulmonary disease

    Congestive heart failure

    Diabetes mellitus

    Fibromyalgia

    Leukemia

Psychiatric disorders

    Attention deficit hyperactivity disorder

    Post-traumatic stress disorder

Medications and substances

    Alcohol use

    Selective serotonin reuptake inhibitors

    Tricyclic antidepressants

Polysomnography

Polysomnography is required for the diagnosis of PLMS. Limb movements are detected using surface EMG recordings over the anterior tibialis muscles. (ie, anterolateral calves). Movements are counted if they occur during sleep, have a duration of 0.5 to 5 seconds, and occur in a series of four or more consecutive contractions with intervals between movements of 5 to 90 seconds from the *onset* of one limb movement to the *onset* of the next. The amplitude of the EMG is at least 25% greater than that of baseline during biocalibrations.

Muscle contractions can be observed in either one or both legs. Contractions occurring simultaneously in both legs are counted as one movement. Arousals can occur before, during or after limb movements (usually within 3 seconds of the leg movements). PLMS can also be accompanied by awakenings. Leg movements occurring during arousals related to sleep-disordered breathing events are not counted. Movements that are observed during wakefulness are scored separately as PLMW.

The periodic limb movement index (PLMI) is defined as the total number of PLMS divided by the total sleep time in hours. The PLMS arousal index is the total number of PLMS associated with arousals per hour of total sleep time. A PLMI is considered abnormal if it is greater than 5 movements per hour of sleep in children, and over 15 movements per hour of sleep among adults. Normative values for the PLMS arousal index are not established.

There is considerable night-to-night variability in the frequency of PLMS. PLMS are more frequent during the first part of the evening. Sleep quality often improves during the latter part of sleep. PLMS also tend to occur more commonly during NREM sleep, particularly stage 2 sleep, and are typically rare or absent during REM sleep.

Periodic Limb Movement Disorder

PLMS can be asymptomatic with the individual unaware of the limb movements, or may be accompanied by arousals, awakenings, sleep fragmentation and complaints of nonrestorative sleep, insomnia, or excessive sleepiness. Periodic limb movement disorder (PLMD) is a clinical syndrome that consists of sleep disturbance related to an abnormal PLMI. The diagnosis of PLMD can also be inferred by a significant improvement in clinical symptoms during a therapeutic trial of a dopaminergic agent.

Although PLMS may be common in the general population, particularly among older adults, the clinical syndrome of PLMD appears to be a less frequent cause of insomnia or excessive sleepiness. Neither the PLMI or PLMS arousal index correlate with the degree of sleep disturbance or subjective sleepiness.

The true significance of PLMD as a clinical entity continues to evolve. Needless to say, asymptomatic PLMS most likely does not need any treatment. Some investigators have proposed that PLMS, rather than a cause of arousals, is instead simply an observable expression of a periodically recurring central neural arousal mechanism.

Differential Diagnosis

Differential diagnosis of PLMS includes:

1.   *Nocturnal seizures*

2.   *Sleep starts* (brief contractions of the extremities or body occurring at sleep onset that can be accompanied by a sensation of falling)

3. *Rhythmic movement disorder* (repetitive, stereotypic, rhythmic movements such as head banging, head or body rolling, or body rocking that continue transiently from sleep onset into early light sleep)

4. *REM sleep behavior disorder* (simple body movements to elaborate enactment of dreams occurring with loss of REM sleep-related muscle atonia)

5. *Movements during phasic REM sleep*

6. *Fragmentary myoclonus* (an isolated brief EMG phenomenon with no observable muscle contraction)

7. *Myoclonic-like activity* related to central nervous system degenerative disorders

8. *Leg movements related to arousals due to obstructive sleep apnea*

Pathophysiology of Restless Legs Syndrome and Periodic Limb Movements of Sleep

The exact mechanisms responsible for both RLS and PLMS remain incompletely understood. Involvement of several areas of the brain (eg, cerebellum, thalamus, red nucleus, brainstem reticular area, pons, and diencephalon) has been associated with clinical symptoms of RLS and PLMS. It has been postulated that dysregulation of the dopaminergic system (eg, decreased receptor binding or dopaminergic hypofunction) may be central to the genesis of these disorders. RLS symptoms and PLMS are diminished by dopaminergic agents and aggravated by dopamine antagonists. Iron plays a key role in dopamine function. Iron is required for tyrosine hydroxylation, a rate-limiting step in dopamine synthesis. Decreased concentrations of brain iron (ie, substantia nigra and putamen) and low levels of serum ferritin (< 50 mg/l) are associated with RLS and PLMS, and are thought to be secondary to abnormal iron uptake or impaired iron transport across the blood-brain barrier (eg, reduced transferrin receptor expression). Reduced cerebrospinal fluid (CSF) ferritin levels and increased CSF transferrin have been reported. In addition, increasing iron stores by oral or parenteral supplementation has been shown to reduce symptoms in those with low serum ferritin levels.

Altered hypocretin or opioid systems might also be present. Evening CSF levels of hypocretin-1 are increased in patients with RLS. Other theories regarding the pathogenesis of RLS and PLMS include neuropathic, vascular, circadian (ie, symptoms are more prominent with fall in core body temperature), and toxic processes.

Therapy for Restless Legs Syndrome and Periodic Limb Movements of Sleep

Therapy of underlying causes of secondary RLS and PLMS can lead to resolution of symptoms. Correction of secondary causes, including iron, folate and cobalamin deficiency or uremia, may be all that is required for some persons. Laboratory evaluation should include complete blood count, serum iron, ferritin, folate, vitamin B12, electrolytes, thyroid function tests, fasting glucose, and renal panel. Resolution of RLS secondary to renal failure has been noted following renal transplantation. Symptoms related to pregnancy typically disappear or significantly diminish with delivery.

Patients should be instructed about proper sleep hygiene, including maintaining regular bedtimes and wake times, and obtaining sufficient duration of nighttime sleep. Patient education should also incorporate avoidance of exacerbating factors, including stress, strenuous physical activity close to bedtime; alcohol; caffeine; medications (antidepressant medications [fluoxetine, mirtazapine, paroxetine, sertraline], beta-blockers, lithium, neuroleptics [olanzapine, risperidone], phenytoin, and sedating antihistamines) (Box 8–4). Local massage, stretching, moderate exercise, or warm baths might be beneficial for some patients.

The American Academy of Sleep Medicine (AASM) recommendations for the treatment of RLS and PLMD are given in Box 8–5.

Box 8-4. **Behavioral treatment of restless legs syndrome and periodic limb movements during sleep**	Avoidance of sleep deprivation Proper sleep hygiene Avoidance of alcohol and caffeine Regular exercise (during the daytime with cessation of activity prior to bedtime)

Box 8-5.
 	
American Academy of Sleep Medicine (AASM) recommendations for the treatment of restless legs syndrome and periodic limb movement disorder
	1. Only patients who meet diagnostic criteria for RLS and/or PLMD should receive pharmacologic therapy for the latter (standard).
	
	2. Physicians evaluating and treating patients with RLS and/or PLMD should be knowledgeable about the following features of RLS and/or PLMD (standard):
	
	  • Idiopathic and secondary forms
	
	  • Risk factors
	
	  • Comorbid conditions
	
	  • Need to monitor adverse effects, augmentation, and tolerance of pharmacologic therapy
	
	2. The following medications are effective in the treatment of RLS and PLMD:
	
	  • Levodopa with decarboxylase inhibitor (guideline)
	
	  • Pergolide (guideline)
	
	  • Oxycodone (guideline)
	
	  • Propoxyphene (guideline)
	
	3. The following medications are effective in the treatment of RLS:
	
	  • Carbamazepine (guideline)
	
	  • Clonidine (option)
	
	  • Gabapentin (option)
	
	  • Iron supplementation in patients with iron deficiency (option).
	
	4. Clonazepam is effective in the treatment of PLMD and possibly RLS (option)
	
	5. No recommendations were provided regarding therapy for RLS or PLMD among children or pregnant women.

Source: Modified and adapted Chesson, et al. Practice parameters for the treatment of restless legs syndrome and periodic limb movement disorder. Sleep. 1999.

AASM definition of terms

Standard	Generally accepted practice with a high level of clinical certainly
Guideline	Practice associated with a moderate degree of clinical certainty
Option	Practice of uncertain clinical use

Pharmacologic Therapy for Restless Legs Syndrome and Periodic Limb Movements of Sleep

Symptoms of RLS and PLMD often respond to the same medications (Box 8–6).

Box 8–6.
 	
Pharmacologic therapy of restless legs syndrome and periodic limb movement disorder
	Adrenergic agonists
	   Clonidine
	Anticonvulsant drugs
	   Carbamazepine
	   Gabapentin
	Benzodiazepines
	   Alprazolam
	   Clonazepam
	   Temazepam
	   Triazolam
	Carbidopa/levodopa (Sinemet)
	Ergotamine dopamine agonists
	   Bromocriptine (Parlodel)
	   Cabergoline
	   Pergolide (Permax)
	Nonergotamine dopamine agonists
	   Pramipexole (Mirapex)
	   Ropinirole (Requip)
	Iron therapy
	N-Methyl-D-Aspartate (NMDA) antagonists
	   Amantadine
	Opioids
	   Codeine
	   Methadone
	   Oxycodone

(continued from page 311)
Box 8-6.

Pharmacologic therapy of restless legs syndrome and periodic limb movement disorder

Propoxyphene

Other medications

    Bupropion

    Entacapone

    Folate

    Selegiline

    Tramadol

Dopaminergic Agents

Dopaminergic medications are considered the first-line therapy for both RLS and PLMD (Box 8–7). These agents decrease the frequency of PLMS, diminish RLS symptoms, and improve sleep quality. They include dopamine precursors (eg, carbidopa/levodopa) and dopamine agonists (eg, pergolide, pramipexole, or ropinirole). Sudden episodes of severe sleepiness can complicate therapy with dopaminergic agents.

Box 8–7.

American Academy of Sleep Medicine (AASM) recommendations for the dopaminergic treatment of restless legs syndrome and periodic limb movement disorder

1. The following medications are effective in the treatment of RLS and PLMD:

   • Levodopa with decarboxylase inhibitor (standard)

   • Pergolide, a dopamine agonist (standard)

   • Pramipexole, a dopamine agonist (guideline)

   • Ropinirole, a dopamine agonist (option)

2. The following dopamine agonists/dopaminergic agents may be effective in the treatment of RLS or PLMD but their level of effectiveness has not been determined (option):

   • Alpha-dihydroergocryptine

   • Amantadine

   • Cabergoline

   • Piribedil

   • Selegiline

   • Talipexole

3. No recommendations were provided regarding the use of dopaminergic agents for RLS or PLMD among children or pregnant women.

Source: Modified and adapted from Standards of Practice Committee of the American Academy of Sleep Medicine. Practice parameters for the dopaminergic treatment of restless legs syndrome and periodic limb movement disorder. Sleep. 2004;27(3):557–9.

Carbidopa/Levodopa Levodopa is a dopamine precursor that is converted to dopamine in the brain. Carbidopa is a decarboxylase inhibitor that is combined with levodopa to diminish the peripheral conversion of levodopa to dopamine and, thereby, increase the availability of levodopa in the central nervous system and decrease its peripheral adverse effects. Levodopa has also been combined with benserazide for this purpose. Compared to the dopamine agonists, carbidopa/levodopa has a more rapid onset of action. It is helpful for cases that are mild or intermittent.

Carbidopa/levodopa is taken at bedtime. Because of its short duration of action, repeated dosing may be required if symptoms recur later in the night or if morning (end-of-dose) rebound of symptoms occur. Alternatively, controlled-release formulations can be used. Entacapone increases the duration of action of carbidopa/levodopa. The typical starting dose for carbidopa/levodopa is 25/100 mg at bedtime.

Chronic administration of levodopa (especially at doses greater than 200 to 300 mg) may give rise to augmentation (ie, RLS symptoms develop earlier in the evening or afternoon, are more severe compared to baseline prior to levodopa therapy, or affect other body parts including the upper extremities). Changing to a dopamine agonist might ameliorate augmentation. Rebound (ie, symptoms recurring late in the night or early morning) can also develop.

Dopamine Agonists Dopamine agonists are classified as either ergotamine compounds (eg, bromocriptine, cabergoline and pergolide) or nonergotamine agents (eg, pramipexole and ropinirole). Ropinirole and pramipexole have a longer duration of action than regular formulations of carbidopa/levodopa and are less likely to cause augmentation than carbidopa/levodopa. Augmentation resulting from dopamine agonists also tends to be less severe than that due to carbidopa/levodopa. Adverse effects of dopamine agonists include nausea, daytime sleepiness and orthostatic hypotension.

Associated with improvements in severity of RLS and frequency of PLMS, ropinirole increases sleep efficiency and total sleep time. The usual starting dose is 0.25 mg 1 to 3 hours before bedtime or before symptom onset. Doses can be increased gradually until symptoms resolve or to a maximum daily dose of 4 mg. Side effects of ropinirole include nausea, sedation, sudden sleep episodes, syncope and postural hypotension. Compulsive behaviors and malignant melanoma have been described.

The initial dose pramipexole is 0.125 mg taken 2 to 3 hours before bedtime or before the onset of symptoms. An earlier dosing can be tried if augmentation develops while on pramipexole. Doses should be reduced in persons with renal insufficiency. Side effects of pramipexole include nausea, sedation, sudden sleep episodes, syncope, orthostatic hypotension, and compulsive behaviors.

Development of pleuropulmonary and cardiac valve fibrosis has been described with pergolide and the medication has been withdrawn from the U.S. market. Side effects of bromocriptine include hypotension. Cabergoline is a long-acting dopamine agonist.

Benzodiazepines

Benzodiazepines (eg, clonazepam, triazolam, alprazolam, or temazepam) can decrease PLMS-related complaints of insomnia and arousals but does not reduce the frequency of leg movements. It can improve sleep quality in RLS. Side effects of benzodiazepines include sedation, development of tolerance, risk of dependency, and possibly increased risk of falls among the elderly.

Iron Therapy

RLS related to iron deficiency may improve with iron supplementation in some patients. Ferritin levels greater than 50 μg/1 are associated with fewer RLS symptoms. It is recommended to monitor ferritin levels 3 months after initiation of iron supplementation therapy and every 6 months thereafter until serum ferritin levels reach 50 μg/1 or greater, during which time iron therapy can be discontinued. Oral iron treatment may cause abdominal discomfort or constipation.

Opioids

Opioids, including codeine, oxycodone, propoxyphene or methadone, can reduce RLS sensations and decrease frequency of PLMS. They are primarily indicated for patients with severe symptoms unresponsive to dopaminergic agonists and benzodiazepines. Side effects of opioids include sedation, constipation, risk of dependency, and worsening of any underlying obstructive sleep apnea. Although development of tolerance and a high abuse liability are major concerns with chronic use of these drugs, many patients with RLS are managed successfully for many years on stable doses of these medications.

Anticonvulsant Drugs

Antiepileptic medications are less effective than dopaminergic agents in treating RLS and PLMD.

Carbamazepine can reduce RLS symptoms but does not alter the frequency of PLMS. Side effects of carbamazepine include nausea, agranulocytosis, and aplastic anemia. Caution should be exercised when using carbamazepine in patients with renal insufficiency or hepatic impairment.

Gabapentin can reduce RLS sensations and decrease frequency of PLMS. It may be considered for patients with mild RLS or those with complaints of pain associated with RLS. Side effects of gabapentin include daytime sleepiness, fatigue, ataxia, and dizziness.

Alpha-2 Adrenergic Agonists

Clonidine can reduce RLS symptoms but does not alter the frequency of PLMS.

Other Medications

Amantadine, baclofen, folic acid, magnesium, propranolol, selegiline, and tramadol have all been tried for patients with RLS and/or PLMD. Baclofen may reduce arousals related to periodic limb movements. Tramadol, a nonnarcotic agent, acts via the mu receptor.

References

General References

American Academy of Sleep Medicine. *The International Classification of Sleep Disorders: Diagnostic and Coding Manual.* 2nd ed. American Academy of Sleep Medicine, 2005.

Bowman TJ. *Review of Sleep Medicine.* Burlington, MA: Butterworth-Heinemann, 2002.

Berry RB. *Sleep Medicine Pearls.* 2nd ed. Philadelphia, PA: Hanley & Belfus, 2002.

Chokroverty S. *Clinical Companion to Sleep Disorders Medicine.* 2nd ed. Butterworth-Heinemann, 2000.

Hoyt BD. Sleep in patients with neurologic and psychiatric disorders. *Sleep Medicine.* Primary Care: Clinics in Office Practice. Elsevier Saunders, 2005.

Itin I, Comella CL. Restless leg syndrome. *Sleep Medicine.* Primary Care: Clinics in Office Practice. Philadelphia, PA: Elsevier Saunders, 2005.

Lavie P, Pillar G, Malhotra A. *Sleep Disorders Handbook.* New York, NY: Taylor & Francis, 2002.

Lee-Chiong TL, ed. *Sleep: A Comprehensive Handbook.* Hoboken, NJ: John Wiley & Sons, 2006.

Lee-Chiong TL, Sateia M, Carskadon M, eds. *Sleep Medicine.* Philadelphia, PA: Hanley & Belfus (Elsevier), 2002.

Perlis ML, Lichstein KL, eds. *Treating Sleep Disorders: Principles and Practice of Behavioral Sleep Medicine.* Hoboken, NJ: John Wiley & Sons, 2003.

Rama AN, Kushida CA. Restless legs syndrome and periodic limb movement disorder. *Sleep Disorders.* Medical Clinics of North America. Philadelphia, PA: Elsevier Saunders, 2004.

Rechtschaffen A, Kales A. *A Manual of Standardized Terminology, Techniques and Scoring System for Sleep Stages of Human Subjects.* Los Angeles, CA: Brain Information Service/Brain Research Institute, University of California, 1968.

Reite M, Ruddy J, Nagel K. *Concise Guide to Evaluation and Management of Sleep Disorders.* 3rd ed. Arlington, VA: American Psychiatric Publishing, April 2002.

Sleep Disorders. Medical Clinics of North America. Elsevier Saunders, 2004.

Sleep Medicine. Primary Care: Clinics in Office Practice. Elsevier Saunders, 2005.

Sleep Research Society. *SRS Basics of Sleep Guide.* Westchester, IL: Sleep Research Society, 2005.

Restless Legs Syndrome

Allen RP, Hening WA, Montplaisir J, et al. Restless legs syndrome: diagnostic criteria, special considerations, and epidemiology: A report from The RLS Diagnosis and Epidemiology workshop at the National Institute of Health. *Sleep Med.* 2003;4(2):101–119.

Diagnostic Classification Steering Committee of the American Sleep Disorders Association. *The International Classification of Sleep Disorders: Diagnostic and Coding Manual.* Rochester, MN: American Sleep Disorders Association, 1997.

Kageyama T, Kabuto M, Nitta H, et al. Prevalences of periodic limb movement-like and restless legs-like symptoms among Japanese adults. *Psychiatry Clin Neurosci.* 2000;54(3):296–8.

Michaud M, Poirier G, Lavigne G, Montplaisir J. Restless legs syndrome: scoring criteria for leg movements recorded during the suggested immobilization test. *Sleep Med.* 2001;2(4):317–321.

Michaud M, Lavigne G, Desautels A, Poirier G, Montplaisir J. Effects of immobility on sensory and motor symptoms of restless legs syndrome. *Mov Disord.* 2002;17(1):112–115.

Michaud M, Paquet J, Lavigne G, Desautels A, Montplaisir J. Sleep laboratory diagnosis of restless legs syndrome. *Eur Neurol.* 2002;48(2):108–113.

Montplaisir J, Boucher S, Poirier G, Lavigne G, Lapierre O, Lesperance P. Clinical, polysomnographic, and genetic characteristics of restless legs syndrome: a study of 133 patients diagnosed with new standard criteria. *Mov Disord.* 1997;12(1):61–65.

Phillips B, Young T, Finn L, Asher K, Hening WA, Purvis C. Epidemiology of restless legs symptoms in adults. *Archives of Internal Medicine.* 2000;160(14):2137–141.

Rothdach AJ, Trenkwalder C, Haberstock J, Keil U, Berger K. Prevalence and risk factors of RLS in an elderly population: the MEMO study. Memory and morbidity in Augsburg elderly. *Neurology.* 2000;54(5):1064–8.

Tan EK, Seah A, See SJ, Lim E, Wong MC, Koh KK. Restless legs syndrome in an Asian population: A study in Singapore. *Movement Disorders.* 2001;16(3):729–32.

The Atlas Task Force. Recording and scoring leg movements. *Sleep.* 1993;16(8):748–759.

The International Restless Legs Syndrome Study Group. The International Restless Legs Syndrome Study Group rating scale for Restless Legs Syndrome. *Sleep Medicine.* 2002;4(2):121–132.

Ulfberg J, Nystrom B, Carter N, Edling C. Prevalence of restless legs syndrome among men aged 18 to 64 years: an association with somatic disease and neuropsychiatric symptoms. *Movement Disorders.* 2001;16(6):1159–63.

Ulfberg J, Nystrom B, Carter N, Edling C. Restless legs syndrome among working aged women. *European Neurology.* 2001;46(1):17–9.

Periodic Limb Movements of Sleep

Chervin RD, Archbold KH, Dillon JE, Pituch KJ, Panahi P, Dahl RE, et al. Associations between symptoms of inattention, hyperactivity, restless legs, and periodic leg movements. *Sleep.* 2002;25(2):213–218.

Exar EN, Collop NA. The association of upper airway resistance with periodic limb movements. *Sleep.* 2001;24(2):188–192.

Gehrman P, Stepnowsky C, Cohen-Zion M, Marler M, Kripke DF, Ancoli- Israel S. Long-term follow-up of periodic limb movements in sleep in older adults. *Sleep.* 2002;25(3):340–343.

Karadeniz D, Ondze B, Besset A, Billiard M. Are periodic leg movements during sleep (PLMS) responsible for sleep disruption in insomnia patients? *European Journal of Neurology.* 2000;7(3):331–6.

Nicolas A, Lesperance P, Montplaisir J. Is excessive daytime sleepiness with periodic leg movements during sleep a specific diagnostic category? *European Neurology.* 1998;40(1):22–6.

Picchietti DL, Walters AS. Moderate to severe periodic limb movement disorder in childhood and adolescence. *Sleep.* 1999;22(3):297–300.

Pathophysiology of Restless Legs Syndrome and Periodic Limb Movements During Sleep

Allen RP, Barker PB, Wehrl F, Song HK, Earley CJ. MRI measurement of brain iron in patients with restless legs syndrome. *Neurology.* 2001;56(2):263–65.

Ancoli-Israel S, Martin J, Jones DW, et al. Sleep-disordered breathing and periodic limb movements in sleep in older patients with schizophrenia. *Biol Psychiatry.* 1999;45(11).

Bucher SF, Seelos KC, Oertel WH, Reiser M, Trenkwalder C. Cerebral generators involved in the pathogenesis of the restless legs syndrome. *Annals of Neurology.* 1997;41(5):639–645.

Connor JR, Boyer PJ, Menzies SL, et al. Neuropathological examination suggests impaired brain iron acquisition in restless legs syndrome. *Neurology.* 2003;61(3):304–9.

Earley CJ, Hyland K, Allen RP. CSF dopamine, serotonin, and biopterin metabolites in patients with restless legs syndrome. *Movement Disorders.* 2001;16(1):44–9.

Earley CJ, Allen RP, Beard JL, Connor JR. Insight into the pathophysiology of restless legs syndrome. *J Neurosci Res.* 2000;62(5):623–8.

Earley CJ, Connor JR, Beard JL, Malecki EA, Epstein DK, Allen RP. Abnormalities in CSF concentrations of ferritin and transferrin in restless legs syndrome. *Neurology.* 2000;54(8):1698–700.

Eisensehr I, Wetter TC, Linke R, et al. Normal IPT and IBZM SPECT in drug-naive and levodopa-treated idiopathic restless legs syndrome. *Neurology*. 2001;57(7):1307–9.

Entezari-Taher M, Singleton JR, Jones CR, Meekins G, Petajan JH, Smith AG. Changes in excitability of motor cortical circuitry in primary restless legs syndrome. *Neurology*. 1999;53(6):1201–1205.

Lindvall O, Bjèorklund A, Skagerberg G. Dopamine-containing neurons in the spinal cord: anatomy and some functional aspects. *Annals of Neurology*. 1983;14(3):255–260.

Mendelson WB. Are periodic leg movements associated with clinical sleep disturbance? *Sleep*. 1996;19(3):219–23.

Montplaisir J, Michaud M, Denesle R, Gosselin A. Periodic leg movements are not more prevalent in insomnia or hypersomnia but are specifically associated with sleep disorders involving a dopaminergic impairment. *Sleep Medicine*. 2000;1(2):163–167.

Nicolas A, Lesperance P, Montplaisir J. Is excessive daytime sleepiness with periodic leg movements during sleep a specific diagnostic category? *European Neurology*. 1998;40(1):22–6.

O'Keeffe ST, Gavin K, Lavan JN. Iron status and restless legs syndrome in the elderly. *Age and Ageing*. 1994;23(3):200–203.

Ruottinen HM, Partinen M, Hublin C, et al. An FDOPA PET study in patients with periodic limb movement disorder and restless legs syndrome. *Neurology*. 2000;54(2):502–4.

Sun ER, Chen CA, Ho G, Earley CJ, Allen RP. Iron and the restless legs syndrome. *Sleep*. 1998;21(4):371–7.

Turjanski N, Lees AJ, Brooks DJ. Striatal dopaminergic function in restless legs syndrome: 18F-dopa and 11C-raclopride PET studies. *Neurology*. 1999;52(5):932–7.

Therapy for Restless Legs Syndrome and Periodic Limb Movements During Sleep

Akpinar S. Treatment of restless legs syndrome with levodopa plus benserazide. *Archives of Neurology*. 1982;39(11):739.

Allen R, Becker PM, Bogan R, et al. Ropinirole decreases periodic leg movements and improves sleep parameters in patients with restless legs syndrome. *Sleep*. 2004;27(5):907–914.

Allen RP, Earley CJ. Augmentation of the restless legs syndrome with carbidopa/levodopa. *Sleep*. 1996(Apr); 19(3): 205–13.

Allen RP, Picchietti D, Hening WA, Trenkwalder C, Walters AS, Montplaisi J. Restless legs syndrome: diagnostic criteria, special considerations, and epidemiology. A report from the restless legs syndrome diagnosis and epidemiology workshop at the National Institutes of Health. *Sleep Medicine*. 2003;4(2):101–119.

Benes H, Kurella B, Kummer J, Kazenwadel J, Selzer R, Kohnen R. Rapid onset of action of levodopa in restless legs syndrome: a double-blind, randomized, multicenter, crossover trial. *Sleep*. 1999;22(8):1073–1081.

Boghen D, Lamothe L, Elie R, Godbout R, Montplaisir J. The treatment of the restless legs syndrome with clonazepam: a prospective controlled study. *Can J Neurol Sci*. 1986;13(3):245–247.

Danoff SK, Grasso ME, Terry PB, Flynn JA, Pleuropulmonary disease due to pergolide use for restless legs syndrome. *Chest*. 2001(Jul);120(1):313–316.

Dressler D, Thompson PD, Gledhill RF, Marsden CD. The syndrome of painful legs and moving toes. *Movement Disorders*. 1994;9(1):13–21.

Earley CJ, Yaffee JB, Allen RP. Randomized, double-blind, placebo-controlled trial of pergolide in restless legs syndrome. *Neurology.* 1998;51(6):1599–602.

Evidente VG, Adler CH, Caviness JN, Hentz JG, Gwinn-Hardy K. Amantadine is beneficial in restless legs syndrome. *Movement Disorders.* 2000;15(2):324–7.

Evidente VG. Piribedil for restless legs syndrome: a pilot study. *Movement Disorders.* 2001;16(3):579–581.

Exar EN, Collop NA. The association of upper airway resistance with periodic limb movements. *Sleep.* 2001;24(2):188–192.

Frucht, S, Rogers JD, Greene, PE, Gordon, MF, Fahn S. Falling asleep at the wheel: motor vehicle mishaps in persons taking pramipexole and ropinirole. *Neurology.* 1999;52(9):1908–10.

Garcia-Borreguero D, Larrosa O, de la Llave Y, Verger K, Masramon X, Hernandez G. Treatment of restless legs syndrome with gabapentin: a double-blind, cross-over study. *Neurology.* 2002;59(10):1573–1579.

Grewal M, Hawa R, Shapiro C. Treatment of periodic limb movements in sleep with selegiline HCL. *Movement Disorders.* 2002;17(2):398–401.

Hening W, Allen R, Earley C, Kushida C, Picchietti D, Silber M. The treatment of restless legs syndrome and periodic limb movement disorder. An American Academy of Sleep Medicine Review. *Sleep.* 1999;22(7):970–999.

Hening WA, Walters AS, Wagner M, et al. Circadian rhythm of motor restlessness and sensory symptoms in the idiopathic restless legs syndrome. *Sleep.* 1999;22(7):901–912.

Jakobsson B, Ruuth K. Successful treatment of restless legs syndrome with an implanted pump for intrathecal drug delivery. *Acta Anaesthesiol Scand.* 2002;46(1):114–7.

LaBan MM, Viola SL, Femminineo AF, Taylor RS. Restless legs syndrome associated with diminished cardiopulmonary compliance and lumbar spinal stenosis—a motor concomitant of "Vesper's curse." *Archives of Physical Medicine and Rehabilitation.* 1990;71(6):384–388.

Mller M. Dopaminergic therapy in children with restless legs/periodic limb movements in sleep and ADHD. Dopaminergic Therapy Study Group. *Pediatric Neurology.* 2000;22(3):182–86.

Montplaisir J, Denesle R, Petit D. Pramipexole in the treatment of restless legs syndrome: a follow-up study. *Eur J Neurol.* 2000;7 (Suppl 1):127–31.

Montplaisir J, Nicolas A, Denesle R, Gomez-Mancilla B. Restless legs syndrome improved by pramipexole: a double-blind randomized trial. *Neurology.* 1999;52(5):938–43.

Montplaisir J, Boucher S, Poirier G, Lavigne G, Lapierre O, Lespâerance P. Clinical, polysomnographic, and genetic characteristics of restless legs syndrome: a study of 133 patients diagnosed with new standard criteria. *Movement Disorders.* 1997;12(1):61–65.

Ondo W. Ropinirole for restless legs syndrome. *Movement Disorders.* 1999;14(1):138–40.

Ondo WG, Vuong KD, Wang Q. Restless legs syndrome in monozygotic twins: clinical correlates. *Neurology.* 2000;55(9):1404–1406.

Picchietti DL, Underwood DJ, Farris WA, et al. Further studies on periodic limb movement disorder and restless legs syndrome in children with attention-deficit hyperactivity disorder. *Movement Disorders.* 1999;14(6):1000–1007.

Pieta J, Millar T, Zacharias J, Fine A, Kryger M. Effect of pergolide on restless legs and leg movements in sleep in uremic patients. *Sleep.* 1998;21(6):617–22.

Pritchett AM, Morrison JF, Edwards WD. Valvular heart disease in patients taking pergolide. *Mayo Clinic Proceedings.* 2002;77(12):1280–1286.

Reuter I, Ellis CM, Ray Chaudhuri K. Nocturnal subcutaneous apomorphine infusion in Parkinson's disease and restless legs syndrome. *Acta Neurologica Scandinavica.* 1999;100(3):163–7.

Saletu M, Anderer P, Saletu-Zyhlarz G, et al. Restless legs syndrome (RLS) and periodic limb movement disorder (PLMD): acute placebo-controlled sleep laboratory studies with clonazepam. *Eur Neuropsychopharmacol.* 2001(Apr);11(2):153–161.

Saletu B, Gruber G, Saletu M, et al. Sleep laboratory studies in restless legs syndrome patients as compared with normals and acute effects of ropinirole. 1. Findings on objective and subjective sleep and awakening quality. *Neuropsychobiology.* 2000;41(4):181–9.

Saletu M, Anderer P, Saletu B, et al. Sleep laboratory studies in restless legs syndrome patients as compared with normals and acute effects of ropinirole. 2. Findings on periodic leg movements, arousals and respiratory variables. *Neuropsychobiology.* 2000;41(4):190–9.

Silber MH, Ehrenberg BL, Allen RP, et al. An algorithm for the management of restless legs syndrome. *Mayo Clinic Proceedings.* 2004;79(7):916–922.

Silber MH, Girish M, Izurieta R. Pramipexole in the management of restless legs syndrome: an extended study. *Sleep.* 2003;26(7):819–821.

Silber MH, Shepard JW, Wisbey HA. Pergolide in the management of restless legs syndrome: an extended study. *Sleep.* 1997;20(10):878–82.

Stiasny K, Moller JC, Oertel WH. Safety of pramipexole in patients with restless legs syndrome. Neurology. 2000;55(10):1589–90.

Stiasny K, Robbecke J, Schuler P, Oertel WH. Treatment of idiopathic restless legs syndrome (RLS) with the D2-agonist cabergoline—an open clinical trial. Sleep. 2000;23(3):349–54.

Stiasny K, Wetter TC, Winkelmann J, et al. Long-term effects of pergolide in the treatment of restless legs syndrome. *Neurology.* 2001;56(10):1399–402.

Trenkwalder C, Brandenburg U, Hundemer HP, Lledo A, Quail D. A randomized longterm placebo controlled multicenter trial of pergolide in the treatment of RLS—The Pearls study. *Neurology.* 2001;56(Suppl 3):A 5.

Trenkwalder C, Walters AS, Hening W. Periodic limb movements and restless legs syndrome. *Neurologic Clinics.* 1996;14(3):629–650.

Van Camp G, Flamez A, Cosyns B, et al. Treatment of Parkinson's disease with pergolide and relation to restrictive valvular heart disease. *Lancet.* 2004;363(9416):1179–1183.

Walters AS, Hening W, Rubinstein M, Chokroverty S. A clinical and polysomnographic comparison of neuroleptic-induced akathisia and the idiopathic restless legs syndrome. *Sleep.* 1991;14(4):339–345.

Walters AS, Mandelbaum DE, Lewin DS, Kugler S, England SJ, Wetter TC, et al. A randomized controlled study of pergolide in patients with restless legs syndrome. *Neurology.* 1999;52(5):944–50.

Walters AS, Wagner ML, Hening WA, et al. Successful treatment of the idiopathic restless legs syndrome in a randomized double-blind trial of oxycodone versus placebo. *Sleep.* 1993;16(4):327–332.

Winkelman JW, Johnston L. Augmentation and tolerance with long-term pramipexole treatment of restless legs syndrome (RLS). *Sleep Medicine.* 2004;5(1):9–14.

Winkelmann J, Muller-Myhsok B, Wittchen HU, et al. Complex segregation analysis of restless legs syndrome provides evidence for an autosomal dominant mode of inheritance in early age at onset families. *Annals of Neurology.* 2002;52(3):297–302.

Zucconi M, Oldani A, Castronovo C, Ferini-Strambi L. Cabergoline is an effective single-drug treatment for restless legs syndrome: clinical and actigraphic evaluation. *Sleep.* 2003;26(7):815–818.

Sleep in the Medical Disorders

321

Many medical disorders can give rise to disturbances of sleep and alter sleep architecture. Sleep can be impaired by the medical conditions themselves or by the medications used to treat them. Several symptoms associated with medical disorders, such as pain, dyspnea, nocturia, and pruritus can potentially disturb sleep, with the severity of sleep complaints waxing and waning in relation to the course of the medical illness. More than one sleep pathology may be present in a particular patient. The sleep disturbance causes distress and functional impairment, and requires independent clinical management. Conversely, sleep impairment can alter the presentation and adversely affect the symptoms of a variety of medical conditions, including respiratory, cardiac, gastrointestinal, renal, rheumatologic and infectious disorders.

Respiratory Disorders

Asthma

Asthma is a disease characterized by episodic dyspnea and wheezing, reversible episodes of bronchoconstriction, and airway hyperreactivity to a variety of specific and nonspecific stimuli.

Sleep Disturbance

Sleep disturbance in patients with asthma can result in complaints of insomnia (including early morning awakenings) or excessive sleepiness. In one study, three of every four asthmatics reported nocturnal awakenings occurring at least once weekly, whereas two-thirds had nocturnal awakenings at least three times a week. Sleep in patients with nocturnal asthma is characterized by poor sleep quality with frequent arousals. They may awaken repeatedly due to coughing, dyspnea, wheezing, and chest discomfort. Complaints of insomnia and/or excessive daytime sleepiness are not infrequent. Some effects of asthma on sleep are listed in Box 9–1.

Box 9-1. **Asthma and sleep**	Insomnia or excessive sleepiness
	Frequent awakenings and arousals
	Nocturnal bronchoconstriction
	Sleep-related hypoxemia
	Polysomnographic features
	$\downarrow$ Sleep efficiency
	$\downarrow$ Total sleep time
	$\uparrow$ Wake time after sleep onset
	$\uparrow$ Frequency of awakenings
	$\downarrow$ NREM stages 3 and 4 sleep

Pathophysiology of Nocturnal Asthma

A number of mechanisms have been postulated to account for the overnight bronchoconstriction noted in nocturnal asthma. There is a circadian variability in airflow, which is greatest in the late afternoon and lowest in the early morning. Sleep, itself, is also a major determinant of the variation in peak expiratory flow rate. In addition, decreases in functional residual capacity, minute ventilation, and tidal volume occur during sleep; these changes may be exaggerated in individuals with nocturnal asthma. Other possible mechanisms for nocturnal bronchoconstriction include increased airway responsiveness, increased airway secretions, as well as circadian changes in vagal (cholinergic) tone, body temperature, cortisol, epinephrine, and inflammatory mediators. A cellular inflammatory response has been described, with an increase in total leukocyte count, neutrophils and eosinophils in bronchoalveolar lavage fluid of subjects with nocturnal asthma.

Evaluation

Diagnosis of nocturnal asthma is aided by monitoring morning and evening peak expiratory flow rates over several days to weeks. There is often a significant fall in airflow rates at night compared to daytime values.

Polysomnographic Features

Polysomnography may demonstrate a decrease in sleep efficiency and total sleep time as well as an increase in both wake time after sleep onset (WASO) and frequency of awakenings. Non–rapid eye movement (NREM) stages 3 and 4 sleep may be reduced (Box 9–1). Hypoxemia can be evident during sleep.

Therapy

Therapy of nocturnal asthma includes the use of inhaled corticosteroids and long-acting bronchodilators (eg, salmeterol or theophylline). Anticholinergic agents (eg, ipratropium bromide) can be tried as well. Corticosteroid administration can diminish the circadian variability in airway tone. Nocturnal symptoms reverse rapidly following administration of bronchodilators. Unfortunately, the medications used to treat acute asthma such as short-acting beta-agonists (eg, albuterol) may, themselves, increase nighttime awakenings.

Both snoring and upper airway obstruction can increase the frequency of nocturnal asthma attacks in individuals with coexisting asthma and obstructive sleep apnea (OSA). In these patients, optimal continuous positive airway pressure (CPAP) therapy for sleep apnea can improve asthma control and increase airway flow rates.

Chronic Obstructive Pulmonary Disease

Chronic obstructive pulmonary disease (COPD) is a disorder characterized by airflow limitation that is usually progressive and is not fully reversible. It is associated with an abnormal inflammatory response of the lungs to noxious particles or gases that results in injury to the small airways and alveoli. Alveolar destruction is predominant in emphysema, whereas airway narrowing and excessive mucus production are more prominent in chronic bronchitis. Dyspnea and/or chronic cough are the chief complaints of patients with COPD. In advanced cases, hypoxemia and hypercapnia can occur during both wakefulness and sleep.

Sleep Disturbance

COPD is associated with poor sleep quality. Nocturnal cough, dyspnea or respiratory distress in persons with COPD may lead to sleep disruption with insomnia, frequent nighttime awakenings, nonrestorative sleep, and excessive sleepiness. Features of COPD and sleep are listed in Box 9–2.

Box 9-2.	Insomnia or excessive sleepiness
Chronic obstructive pulmonary disease and sleep	Frequent nighttime awakenings and non-restorative sleep
	Nocturnal coughing or dyspnea
	Nocturnal hypoxemia and hypercapnia
	"Overlap" syndrome–presence of both COPD and obstructive sleep apnea
	Polysomnographic features
	↑ Sleep latency
	↓ Sleep efficiency
	↓ Total sleep time
	↑ Sleep stage changes
	↑ Frequency of arousals and awakenings
	↓ NREM stages 3 and 4 sleep
	↓ REM sleep

In addition to nocturnal coughing or dyspnea, factors responsible for sleep disturbance in patients with COPD include changes in arterial blood gases (hypoxemia and hypercapnia), and medications for the condition itself (eg, methylxanthines, beta-adrenergic agonists).

Nocturnal Oxygen Desaturation

In patients with moderate to severe COPD, significant oxygen desaturation may develop during sleep. Nocturnal oxygen saturation decreases during NREM sleep compared with levels during wakefulness and decreases further during rapid eye movement (REM) sleep. Episodes of oxygen desaturation are more frequent, of greater duration, and more severe during REM sleep compared to NREM sleep.

The occurrence and severity of arterial oxygen desaturation during sleep are influenced by baseline lung function, and awake PaO_2 and $PaCO_2$ (significant oxygen desaturation is more likely with lower PaO_2 or SaO_2 and higher $PaCO_2$).

Oxygen desaturation occurs during periods of hypoventilation, which is worse during REM sleep. An increase in ventilation-perfusion mismatching and a decrease in lung volumes also contribute to hypoxemia during sleep. Sleep-related hypoxemic episodes appear to be more common among "blue bloaters" than in "pink puffers." Blue bloaters have lower baseline SaO_2, larger falls in SaO_2, more episodes of oxygen desaturation, and longer duration of oxygen desaturation during sleep.

Polysomnographic Features

Polysomnography may demonstrate changes in sleep architecture such as an increase in sleep latency, decrease in sleep efficiency, decrease in total sleep time, and increase in frequency of arousals, awakenings and sleep stage shifts (Box 9–2). Arousals appear to be unrelated to hypoxemia. In one study, reversal of hypoxemia with supplemental oxygen did not diminish arousal frequency. NREM stages 3 and 4 sleep, and REM sleep may be reduced.

Oxygen saturation monitoring demonstrates episodes of sustained desaturation coinciding with periods of REM sleep.

Therapy

Patients with significant nocturnal exacerbations of COPD symptoms may benefit from sustained-action theophylline preparations, long-acting beta-agonists (eg, salmeterol), or long-acting anticholinergic agents (eg, tiotropium). Treatment with low-flow oxygen is the mainstay for oxygen desaturation in patients with COPD. However, there is no consensus regarding the criteria for supplemental oxygen administration in patients with isolated nocturnal hypoxemia. It may be prudent to provide nocturnal oxygen supplementation for patients with cor pulmonale, significant cardiac arrhythmias coinciding with periods of oxygen desaturation, and marked oxygen desaturation ($SaO_2 < 80\%-85\%$). Low-flow oxygen therapy seldom leads to a significant increase in nocturnal $PaCO_2$; nonetheless, caution and close monitoring is indicated in patients with concurrent OSA, in whom apnea duration may lengthen and nocturnal hypercapnia may worsen with oxygen therapy.

Chronic Obstructive Pulmonary Disease and Obstructive Sleep Apnea

An "overlap syndrome" is defined by the presence of both COPD and OSA. Sleep-disordered breathing may have a more severe course in individuals with coexisting COPD. Also, the overlap syndrome is associated with lower PaO_2, higher $PaCO_2$ and higher mean pulmonary artery pressures.

The overlap syndrome should be suspected in patients with mild COPD presenting with daytime hypercapnia. Daytime hypercapnia is unusual in patients with mild COPD. Differential diagnosis for daytime hypercapnia in patients with COPD includes (1) severe COPD ($FEV_1 < 1$ L), (2) overlap syndrome, and (3) obesity hypoventilation syndrome.

Sleep studies are indicated for patients with COPD when there is a possibility of concurrent OSA or obesity-hypoventilation syndrome. Coexisting COPD and OSA can produce a characteristic "saw-tooth" arterial oxygen saturation (SaO_2) tracing.

CPAP therapy is beneficial for patients with the overlap syndrome. Certain patients may respond better to bilevel positive airway pressure therapy.

Cystic Fibrosis

Cystic fibrosis is a multisystemic disease characterized by abnormal transport of sodium and chloride across the epithelium in exocrine tissues. This gives rise to an increased concentration of salt in sweat as well as thick viscous secretions in the lungs, pancreas, intestine, liver, and reproductive tract. It is an autosomal recessive disorder. Patients with cystic fibrosis can present with bronchiectasis and bronchiolectasis, exocrine pancreatic insufficiency, intestinal dysfunction, abnormal sweat gland function, and urogenital dysfunction.

Sleep Disturbance

Patients with cystic fibrosis often report poor sleep quality and sleep fragmentation. Nocturnal episodes of coughing and oxygen desaturation can also occur. The likelihood of sleep-related hypoxemia is greater in patients with a low FEV_1 and a low awake SaO_2. Sleep disturbance in cystic fibrosis is outlined in Box 9–3.

Box 9–3.
 	
Cystic fibrosis and sleep
	Poor sleep quality; can worsen during disease exacerbations
	
	Sleep fragmentation
	
	Nocturnal coughing
	
	Nocturnal oxygen desaturation
	
	Polysomnographic features
	    Normal sleep latency
	    Normal sleep efficiency

Sleep quality is correlated with physiologic variables of disease severity and can worsen significantly during disease exacerbations. Despite poor subjective sleep quality, sleep latency and sleep efficiency are usually normal.

Restrictive Pulmonary Diseases

Reduced lung volumes and diffusion capacity secondary to either pathology involving the lung parenchyma or alterations of the chest wall, pleura, or neuromuscular apparatus characterize restrictive lung diseases. Patient may be totally asymptomatic during the early stages of their illness but, with disease progression, they can develop dyspnea, initially only with exertion but eventually occurring also at rest.

Restrictive lung diseases, including obesity, kyphoscoliosis, interstitial lung disease, and pregnancy, are commonly associated with sleep-related breathing disorders and hypoxemia during sleep (Table 9–1). Patients may complain of disturbed sleep, frequent awakenings, unrefreshing sleep, and excessive daytime sleepiness (Box 9–4).

Table 9–1. Restrictive pulmonary diseases

Interstitial lung disease	Patients with interstitial lung diseases often demonstrate transient or sustained oxygen desaturation during REM sleep. Polysomnographic features can include a decrease in sleep quality and an increase in the number of arousals. An increase in NREM stage 1 sleep and a decrease in REM sleep may be present.
Kyphoscoliosis	A variety of sleep-related breathing syndromes can develop in patients with kyphoscoliosis ranging from obstructive apneas and hypopneas to severe episodes of prolonged central apnea.
Obesity	Obstructive sleep apnea can be identified in more than 50% and nocturnal hypoventilation in over 29% of severely obese individuals. Although sleep latency and REM latency may remain normal, sleep efficiency and percentage of REM sleep are decreased in obese individuals.
Pregnancy	Deterioration of sleep quality can develop during pregnancy. Polysomnography performed during pregnancy can demonstrate a decrease in sleep efficiency and increased frequency of awakenings. There is often an increase in NREM stage 1 sleep and a decrease in REM sleep. Although new onset of snoring may be noted, significant obstructive sleep apnea is relatively uncommon unless it was already present prior to pregnancy.

Box 9–4. **Restrictive pulmonary diseases and sleep**	Sleep disturbance and non–restorative sleep Frequent awakenings Excessive sleepiness Sleep-related breathing disorders Nocturnal oxygen desaturation

TYPES OF DISEASE

Interstitial lung disease

   Nocturnal oxygen desaturation (particularly during REM sleep)

   Polysomnographic features

      ↓ Sleep quality

      ↑ Frequency of arousals

      ↑ NREM stage 1 sleep

      ↓ REM sleep

Kyphoscoliosis

   Obstructive sleep apnea

   Central sleep apnea

Obesity

   Obstructive sleep apnea

   Nocturnal hypoventilation

   Polysomnographic features

      Normal sleep latency

      ↓ Sleep efficiency

      Normal REM sleep latency

      ↓ REM sleep

Pregnancy

   Polysomnographic features

      ↓ Sleep efficiency

      ↑ Frequency of awakenings

      ↑ NREM stage 1 sleep

      ↓ REM sleep

Neuromuscular Disorders

Ventilatory compromise can complicate the course of neuromuscular disorders. The disorders most commonly associated with sleep-related breathing disorders include muscular dystrophy, myotonic dystrophy, amyotrophic lateral sclerosis (ALS), poliomyelitis, and myasthenia gravis (Box 9–5). Nocturnal respiratory impairment, including alveolar hypoventilation, can precede abnormalities during wakefulness by months to years. Individuals with neuromuscular disorders can present with complaints of insomnia, sleep disturbance, excessive sleepiness, fatigue, morning headaches, and nighttime symptoms of dyspnea and intermittent snoring. The likelihood of sleep-related oxygen desaturation is greater in patients with maximal inspiratory pressures less than 60 cm H_2O and forced vital capacity less than 50% of predicted.

Duchenne Muscular Dystrophy

Patients with Duchenne muscular dystrophy can present with both central and obstructive apneas. Polysomnography may reveal an increase in the frequency of arousals and a decrease in REM sleep.

Myotonic Dystrophy

Patients with myotonic dystrophy can have disrupted sleep, apneas or hypopneas, and hypoventilation-induced oxygen desaturation during REM sleep.

Amyotrophic Lateral Sclerosis

Obstructive apneic and hypopneic events in patients with ALS are seen predominantly during REM sleep. The overall apnea-hypopnea index is often only mildly elevated. The development of diaphragmatic dysfunction in patients with ALS can adversely affect survival, and significant nocturnal desaturation secondary to hypoventilation can occur. Compared to those with preserved diaphragm function, these patients can have reduced REM sleep.

Poliomyelitis

Poliomyelitis is a lower motor neuron disease that can involve the respiratory motor nuclei. It can give rise to dysfunction of respiratory muscles including the diaphragm. Sleep-disordered breathing (eg, nocturnal hypoventilation and obstructive apneic and hypopneic events) can develop. Hypersomnolence is a common complaint.

Polysomnographic features consist of a decrease in sleep efficiency and increase in frequency of arousals. There is often an increase in NREM stage 1 sleep and a decrease in REM sleep.

Myasthenia Gravis

Myasthenia gravis is an autoimmune disease characterized by the presence of antibodies directed against acetylcholine receptors that result in impairment of transmission at the neuromuscular junction. There is a higher incidence of both central and obstructive apneas and hypopneas in patients with myasthenia gravis. Significant oxygen desaturation can develop and is seen predominantly during REM sleep.

Box 9–5. **Neuromuscular disorders and sleep**	Insomnia or excessive sleepiness Sleep disturbance Sleep-related breathing disorders Nocturnal dyspnea

TYPES OF DISORDERS

Duchenne muscular dystrophy

  Central and obstructive apneas

  Polysomnographic features

      ↑ Frequency of arousals

      ↓ REM sleep

Myotonic dystrophy

  Disrupted sleep

  Sleep-related breathing disorders

  Hypoventilation (especially during REM sleep)

Amyotrophic lateral sclerosis

  Sleep-related breathing disorders (predominantly during REM sleep)

  Nocturnal hypoventilation

  Polysomnographic features

      ↓ REM sleep

Poliomyelitis

  Excessive sleepiness

  Sleep-related breathing disorders

  Nocturnal hypoventilation

  Polysomnographic features

      ↓ Sleep efficiency

      ↑ Frequency of arousals

      ↑ NREM stage 1 sleep

      ↓ REM sleep

Myasthenia gravis

  Central and obstructive apneas and hypopneas

  Nocturnal oxygen desaturation (predominantly during REM sleep)

Diaphragm Paralysis

Unilateral diaphragmatic paralysis may lead to significant nocturnal hypoxemia but, in the absence of systemic lung disease, it does not generally result in chronic respiratory failure or cor pulmonale. Bilateral diaphragmatic paralysis can give rise to the development of sleep apnea. Unilateral paralysis of the diaphragm is much more common than is bilateral paralysis, the most frequent cause of which is nerve invasion from malignancy (usually a bronchogenic carcinoma). The most common causes of bilateral diaphragmatic paralysis are high spinal cord injury, thoracic trauma, multiple sclerosis, anterior horn disease, and muscular dystrophy.

Polysomnography in patients with diaphragmatic paralysis can demonstrate decreases in NREM stages 3 and 4 sleep and REM sleep (Box 9–6).

Box 9-6.
 	
Diaphragm paralysis and sleep
	Nocturnal hypoxemia
	
	Sleep-related breathing disorders
	
	Polysomnographic features
	
	  ↓ NREM stages 3 and 4 sleep
	
	  ↓ REM sleep

Cardiac Disorders

Hypertension

Sleep-related breathing disorder is a risk factor for hypertension independent of other known confounding factors. In the Sleep Heart Health Study, mean systolic and diastolic blood pressures and the prevalence of hypertension increase significantly with increasing measures of sleep-related breathing disorder (eg, apnea hypopnea index [AHI] and percent sleep time with oxygen saturation below 90%). The odds of developing hypertension were observed to increase by about 1% for each additional apneic event per hour of sleep and to increase by 13% for each 10% decrease in nocturnal oxygen saturation. In the Wisconsin Sleep Cohort Study, over 4 years of follow-up, subjects with an AHI of at least 15 events per hour had an odds ratio of 2.89 for the presence of hypertension compared with those with an AHI of 0 events per hour.

A nocturnal fall in blood pressure can usually be observed in hypertensive patients without OSA ("dippers"). Some patients with obstructive sleep apnea fail to demonstrate this sleep-related nighttime fall in blood pressure ("nondippers"). The risk of cardiovascular disease may be greater among "nondippers" compared to "dippers." In one study, 48% of patients with OSA were found to be systolic nondippers, and 22% were diastolic nondippers. The respiratory disturbance index was the only significant variable related to blood pressure "nondipping."

A reduction in blood pressure was observed during administration of therapeutic CPAP but not subtherapeutic CPAP in patients with coexisting OSA. The benefit was larger in patients with more severe OSA and in those taking drug treatment for blood pressure. Reversal of OSA by CPAP was also noted to reduce nocturnal blood pressure in patients with refractory hypertension. However, some investigators have reported no significant beneficial effect of CPAP on blood pressure in patients with OSA and hypertension.

Hypertension and sleep

Sleep-related breathing disorder is a risk factor for hypertension

Sleep-related Coronary Artery Ischemia

Sleep-related coronary artery ischemia shares many features in common with its daytime counter-part—left-sided or retrosternal chest pressure, pain radiation to the jaw or left upper extremity, dyspnea, diaphoresis, nausea, and palpitations—and can potentially lead to similar complications, including myocardial infarction, congestive heart failure, cardiac arrhythmias, and sudden cardiac death. Chest pain can awaken the patient from sleep (Box 9–7).

Box 9–7. **Coronary artery disease and sleep**	Nocturnal chest pain, dyspnea, or palpitations Frequent arousals and awakenings

Pathogenetic mechanisms responsible for cardiac ischemia developing during sleep include marked sleep-related hypotension as well as sympathetic surges with increase in blood pressure and heart rate during arousals or awakenings from sleep. Hypotension may be particularly prominent during NREM stages 3 and 4 sleep. REM sleep can be associated with instability of heart rate and blood pressure. The risk of sleep-related cardiac events is increased in patients with OSA due, in part, to the hypoxemia that develops during apneic episodes and the postarousal increase in blood pressure and heart rate.

Electrocardiographic (EKG) monitoring during polysomnography may reveal features consistent with myocardial ischemia such as depression or elevation of the ST segment, T wave changes, or atrial or ventricular arrhythmias.

Cardiovascular Disease and Obstructive Sleep Apnea

The risk of developing cardiovascular disease is increased in middle-aged patients with OSA. This elevated risk is independent of age, body mass index, blood pressure, and smoking. The increased risk of cardiovascular disease, including myocardial infarction, angina, coronary revascularization procedure, heart failure, and stroke, is present even in patients with OSA whose AHIs are considered only mildly elevated. Risk is reduced by optimal therapy of OSA.

Several possible mechanisms are responsible for the increased risk of cardiovascular events in patients with OSA.

1. Increase in sympathetic activity during sleep. Reductions in heart rate, blood pressure, and cardiac output occur during normal sleep. However, in patients with OSA, sympathetic activity that is elevated during wakefulness increases further during sleep. CPAP therapy attenuates the sympathetic activation seen in patients with OSA.

2. Inflammation. Proinflammatory cytokines (eg, tumor necrosis factor-α [TNF-α], interleukin-6 [IL-6], and IL-8) and adhesion molecules (intercellular adhesion molecule-1 and vascular cell adhesion molecule-1) are increased in patients with OSA. In addition, elevation of levels of plasma C-reactive protein, a marker of inflammation and of cardiovascular risk, is related to the severity of OSA.

3. Hypercoagulability. Elevated plasma fibrinogen levels, increased platelet activity, and reduced fibrinolytic capacity are present in patients with OSA. Thus, the increased prevalence of cardiovascular disease in OSA may also be related to a hypercoagulable state. CPAP therapy may decrease platelet activity, levels of plasma fibrinogen, and activity of clotting factor VII.

4. Endothelial dysfunction. Endothelial dysfunction has been described in patients with moderate to severe OSA. CPAP therapy can reverse this dysfunction.

5. Oxidative stress. OSA is associated with an increased state of oxidative stress. Biomarkers of oxidative stress are higher in patients with OSA compared with control subjects. Furthermore, these biomarkers correlate positively with the respiratory disturbance index and are decreased during CPAP therapy.

6. Insulin resistance. The AHI and minimum oxygen saturation are independent determinants of insulin resistance, a risk factor for atherosclerosis.

Congestive Heart Failure

OSA, central sleep apnea (CSA), or both can develop in patients with congestive heart failure (CHF). Furthermore, both OSA and CSA are highly prevalent in patients with left ventricular dysfunction but no clinically apparent history of heart failure. Left ventricular systolic dysfunction is an independent risk factor for sleep apnea in patients with CHF. Moreover, untreated severe sleep-related breathing disorders may further impair left ventricular function. The effects of CHF on sleep are summarized in Box 9–8.

Box 9–8. **Congestive heart failure and sleep**	Sleep disruption Obstructive and central sleep apnea Cheyne-Stokes respiration (periodic crescendo/decrescendo breathing with apnea or hypopnea) occurs predominantly during NREM stages 1 and 2 sleep

Why CSA develops in certain patients with CHF and not in others remains incompletely understood. Several possible mechanisms are responsible for the occurrence of CSA in patients with CHF.

1. Pulmonary congestion. Pulmonary congestion with elevated pulmonary capillary wedge pressure is associated with the development of CSA in patients with CHF.

2. Alteration in end-tidal carbon dioxide pressure ($PetCO_2$). Whereas $PetCO_2$ typically increases from wakefulness to sleep, no sleep-related rise in $PetCO_2$ is observed in many patients with stable CHF and CSA.

3. Circulation time. A decrease in circulation time with a delay in response to changes in blood gas concentrations has been proposed as a pathogenetic mechanism for CSA. However, in one study, there were no significant differences in lung-to-ear circulation time, an estimate of circulatory delay, or in left ventricular ejection fraction in patients with CHF with and without Cheyne-Stokes respiration.

Cheyne-Stokes Respiration

Cheyne-Stokes respiration (CSR) is characterized by periodic crescendo/decrescendo breathing with apneas or hypopneas. It can be encountered in patients with CHF. Sleep disruption secondary to arousals associated with the hypercapnic phase of CSR or hypoxemia can develop. CSR occurs predominantly during NREM stages 1 and 2 sleep, and less frequently during NREM stages 3 and 4 sleep and REM sleep.

Mortality may be greater in patients with CHF who also develop CSR during sleep compared to those without CSR. In patients with CHF and CSR, an increased AHI is an independent predictor of poor prognosis.

Therapy of Central Sleep Apnea

Therapy of CSR-CSA in patients with CHF begins with optimization of medical treatment for heart failure. In one study, CPAP therapy improved cardiac function (ie, left ventricular ejection fraction).

Oxygen therapy also reduces CSA with or without CSR and appears to be as effective as CPAP therapy in this regard in patients with CHF and OSA. However, oxygen therapy alone may not significantly improve sleep quality, cardiac function and quality of life.

In patients with CHF, coexisting OSA can contribute to progression of cardiac dysfunction. CPAP therapy in patients with CHF and OSA improves left ventricular systolic function and quality of life, and it may improve prognosis.

Cardiac Arrhythmias

The risk of ventricular arrhythmias appears to be increased during arousals from sleep due to the associated surge in sympathetic activity. In contrast, the frequency of premature ventricular beats may diminish during sleep because of a greater parasympathetic tone.

In OSA, heart rate typically slows at the onset of the apneic episode and increases after the termination of the event. Other rhythm disturbances have been described in patients with OSA and include ventricular tachycardia or fibrillation, complex ventricular ectopy, supraventricular tachycardia, sinus pauses, and second- or third-degree heart blocks. The severity of arrhythmias appears to be correlated with the degree of severity of OSA. The effects of cardiac arrhythmias on sleep are presented in Box 9–9.

Gastrointestinal Diseases

The effects of selected gastrointestinal diseases on sleep are featured in Box 9–10.

Peptic Ulcer Disease

Gastric acid secretion during sleep is greater in patients with peptic ulcer disease compared to normal individuals. Persons may present with repeated arousals and awakenings from their sleep

Box 9–9. **Cardiac arrhythmias and sleep**	Risk of ventricular arrhythmias appears to be increased during arousals from sleep
	Frequency of premature ventricular beats may diminish during sleep
	In OSA, heart rate may slow at the onset of the apneic episode and may increase after the termination of the event
	Other rhythm disturbances in OSA:
	Heart block (second- or third-degree)
	Sinus pauses
	Supraventricular tachycardia
	Ventricular ectopy
	Ventricular tachycardia or fibrillation

Box 9–10. **Gastrointestinal diseases and sleep**	Peptic Ulcer Disease
	Repeated arousals and awakenings
	Nocturnal abdominal pain
	Gastroesophageal reflux
	Insomnia
	Sleep fragmentation
	Recurrent awakenings
	Nocturnal heartburn
	Nocturnal dyspnea, coughing and choking
	"Sleep-related laryngospasm"
	Polysomnographic features
	↑ Frequency of arousals followed by swallowing
	↓ NREM stages 3 and 4 sleep
	Functional bowel disorders
	Poor sleep quality
	Recurrent nighttime awakenings
	Nocturnal abdominal discomfort

due to peptic ulcer disease. The abdominal pain is commonly described as dull, steady, or intermittent and is localized to the epigastric area. Onset of abdominal pain is commonly within the first four hours of sleep.

Gastroesophageal Reflux

Gastroesophageal reflux (GER) is caused by backflow of gastric acid and other gastric contents into the esophagus due to incompetent barriers at the gastroesophageal junction. This leads to irritation and damage to the esophageal mucosa, producing heartburn, pain, or discomfort in the retrosternal area and a sour or bitter taste.

In a nationwide telephone survey conducted in the United States, 79% of respondents reported having heartburn symptoms at night; 75% stated that their sleep was affected by heartburn, and 63% noted that heartburn had an impact on their ability to sleep well. Prevalence increase with aging, and its course is generally chronic.

The primary mechanism for GER is transient relaxation of the lower esophageal sphincter, the main deterrent against GER. The pressure of the upper esophageal sphincter, which acts as a further barrier to nocturnal regurgitation, also diminishes during sleep. Other factors contributing to the pathogenesis of GER include hiatal hernia, poor esophageal clearance, delayed gastric emptying, and impaired mucosal defense factors.

Most episodes of GER occur during wakefulness. They are observed less frequently during sleep. They may also occur during brief periods of arousal from the various sleep stages.

GER during sleep is associated with more prolonged acid contact time. Sleep prolongs esophageal acid clearance times. Furthermore, production of saliva, which helps neutralize acid refluxate, ceases during sleep. Patients with nocturnal GER may complain of recurrent awakenings with a sensation of substernal burning or discomfort, indigestion, sour or bitter taste, or water brash. Dyspnea, coughing, and choking may be reported. Insomnia or sleep fragmentation due to frequent arousals may develop.

Complications of repeated nocturnal GER include esophageal mucosal damage, asthma exacerbation, and sleep disruption. Reflux into the pharynx, larynx, and tracheobronchial tree can cause chronic cough, bronchoconstriction, pharyngitis, laryngitis, bronchitis, or pneumonia. Morning hoarseness may be noted. Recurrent pulmonary aspiration related to GER can cause aspiration pneumonia and pulmonary fibrosis. Esophageal complications include esophagitis, esophageal strictures, and Barrett esophagus, a precancerous condition.

GER may be related to "sleep-related laryngospasm." This condition is characterized by a sudden awakening with a sensation of suffocation and apnea lasting from 5 to 45 seconds, followed by stridor. Breathing generally normalizes within minutes.

Nocturnal GER appears to be common in patients with OSA. In one study, about 50% of episodes of GER occurring in patients with OSA was related to apneas or hypopneas. In some studies, erosive reflux disease appears to be more frequent in patients with severe OSA. However, not all investigators have noted a positive correlation between the severity of GER and OSA.

Diagnosis may require continuous esophageal pH testing with placement of pH probes in the distal esophagus above the lower esophageal sphincter and, in some instances, at the proximal esophagus or pharynx as well. Arousals can accompany falls in distal esophageal pH during episodes of reflux. Esophageal manometry is abnormal with a decrease in lower esophageal sphincter pressure, greater transient lower esophageal sphincter relaxations, and reduced amplitude of peristalsis.

Polysomnographic findings in patients with GER include repeated arousals followed by swallowing (represented as an increase in chin EMG activity). Aside from an increased arousal index, a decrease in duration spent in the deeper stages of sleep has been described.

Therapy may involve elevating the head of the bed, pharmacotherapy (eg, histamine-2 antagonists or proton pump inhibitors) or antireflux surgery. CPAP therapy decreases the frequency of nocturnal GER symptoms, not only in patients with OSA, but also in those without sleep-related breathing disorders. This antireflux activity may be due to elevation of intraesophageal pressure as well as to constriction of the lower esophageal sphincter. Higher CPAP pressures produced greater improvements in GER.

Functional Bowel Disorders

Functional bowel disorders are characterized by chronic gastrointestinal tract symptoms without significant anatomical, metabolic, or infectious abnormalities. These disorders include functional dyspepsia and irritable bowel syndrome (IBS). Patients with functional bowel disorders can have abnormalities of autonomic functioning, and measurements of autonomic functioning during sleep can differentiate these patients from normal controls.

Sleep disturbances, including recurrent nighttime awakenings, poor sleep quality, nonrestorative sleep, and increased daytime fatigue, are common in patients with functional bowel disorders. In one study of patients with sleep disturbances, there was a prevalence of 33% for IBS and 21% for functional dyspepsia. Nighttime awakenings can be caused by abdominal aches. A significant proportion of patients report nighttime gastrointestinal symptoms, but objective sleep abnormalities may be uncommon. In one study, no abnormalities in polysomnographic parameters, such as sleep efficiency, sleep latency, number of arousals, and percentage of NREM stages 3 and 4 sleep, were identified in patients with IBS.

Renal Disorders

Disturbances in sleep can be encountered in 60% to 80% of patients on maintenance hemodialysis for end-stage renal disease (ESRD). Common sleep complaints include insomnia, prolonged awakenings, early morning awakenings, excessive sleepiness, reversal of day-night sleep patterns, and disturbed nocturnal sleep (Box 9–11). There appears to be no differences in sleep characteristics between patients undergoing hemodialysis or continuous peritoneal dialysis.

Excessive daytime sleepiness is a major problem in some patients with ESRD. It can be due to metabolic disturbances (eg, uremia), dialysis treatments (with its accompany changes in serum electrolytes, osmolarity, and acid-base balance), parathyroid hormone excess, changes in levels of neurotransmitters, and the production of somnogenic substances, such as IL-1 and TNF-α during dialysis.

There is also a high prevalence of OSA, restless legs syndrome, and periodic limb movement disorder in this patient population. Sleep apnea is estimated to be 10 times more prevalent in patients with ESRD than in the general population and is improved by hemodialysis. In one study, 23% of patients with ESRD reported moderate to severe symptoms of restless legs syndrome.

Polysomnographic features of renal failure include an increase in sleep latency, decrease in sleep efficiency, increased sleep fragmentation, increase in frequency of awakenings, decrease in total sleep time, increase in NREM stages 1 and 2 sleep, decrease in NREM stages 3 and 4 sleep, and decrease in REM sleep (Box 9–11).

In one study, sleep quality in ESRD patients with anemia improved following therapy with recombinant human erythropoietin. Correction of anemia was associated with decreases in sleep fragmentation, arousals, and frequency of periodic limb movements during sleep, as well as an increase in daytime alertness. NREM stages 3 and 4 may increase.

Endocrine and Metabolic Disorders

The effects of selected endocrine and metabolic disorders on sleep are featured in Box 9–12.

Box 9–11. **Renal disorders and sleep**	End-stage renal disease
	Excessive sleepiness
	Insomnia
	Prolonged awakenings
	Reversal of day-night sleep patterns
	High prevalence of primary sleep disorders
	Obstructive sleep apnea
	Restless legs syndrome
	Periodic limb movement disorder
	Polysomnographic features
	↑ Sleep latency
	↓ Sleep efficiency
	↑ Frequency of awakenings
	↓ Total sleep time
	↑ NREM stages 1 and 2 sleep
	↓ NREM stages 3 and 4 sleep
	↓ REM sleep

Hypothyroidism

Patients with hypothyroidism may present with excessive sleepiness and fatigue. Polysomnography may reveal a decrease in NREM stages 3 and 4 sleep, which normalizes with thyroid hormone replacement.

A high incidence of OSA has been reported in patients with untreated hypothyroidism, especially when myxedema is present. Pathogenesis appears to involve obesity, myopathy, upper airway edema, and deposition of mucopolysaccharides in the upper airway. CSA secondary to an impaired central respiratory drive may also be present.

Indices of sleep apnea severity do not diminish significantly in all patients following attainment of a euthyroid state. Therapy of hypothyroidism with thyroxine in patients with OSA may be complicated by nocturnal angina and ventricular arrhythmias.

Acromegaly

Acromegaly is a condition resulting from excessive levels of growth hormone (GH). Polysomnographic features of acromegaly include a decrease in NREM stages 3 and 4 sleep (Box 9–12), which can increase following normalization of GH concentration.

Box 9-12.

Endocrine/ metabolic disorders and sleep

Hypothyroidism

    Excessive sleepiness

    High incidence of obstructive sleep apnea

    Central sleep apnea may also be present

    Polysomnographic features

        ↓ NREM stages 3 and 4 sleep (normalizes with thyroid hormone replacement)

Acromegaly

    Obstructive sleep apnea is common

    Central sleep apnea is also common

    Polysomnographic features

        ↓ NREM stages 3 and 4 sleep

        ↓ REM sleep

Cushing syndrome

    Insomnia

    Increase in incidence of obstructive sleep apnea

    Polysomnographic features

        ↑ Sleep fragmentation

        ↓ NREM stages 3 and 4 sleep

        ↓ REM sleep latency

        ↑ REM density

Addison Disease

    Insomnia

    Polysomnographic features

        ↓ NREM stages 3 and 4 sleep

Obstructive Sleep Apnea and Acromegaly

OSA is common in patients with acromegaly. The risk of developing OSA is increased with greater age, larger neck circumference, greater initial tongue volume, presence of abnormalities in cranio-facial dimensions (predominantly of the mandible), and upper airway narrowing due to changes in pharyngeal soft tissues. Other factors that may contribute to the development of OSA are facial bone deformity, mucosal edema, hypertrophy of the pharyngeal and laryngeal cartilages, and presence of nasal polyps.

There appears to be no correlation between OSA and biochemical parameters of disease activity (eg, GH and insulin-like growth factor 1 [IGF-1] levels).

Improvements in indices of sleep apnea severity have been reported following therapy of acromegaly with bromocriptine, octreotide (a long-acting somatostatin analog), and pituitary surgery (adenomectomy or hypophysectomy). Nonetheless, sleep apnea may persist despite normalization of GH levels during therapy.

Central Sleep Apnea and Acromegaly

CSA is also common in patients with acromegaly. Possible mechanisms for the development of central apneas include reflex inhibition of the respiratory center due to narrowing of the upper airways, or increase in ventilatory response to carbon dioxide. CSA is associated with higher levels of GH and IGF-1 than in obstructive apnea.

Cushing Syndrome

Patients with Cushing syndrome or Cushing disease have an excess of adrenocorticosteroid hormones. Sleep complaints, including insomnia, are common. There is an increased incidence of OSA with a prevalence of approximately 32% in patients with Cushing syndrome and Cushing disease. Fat accumulation in the parapharyngeal area may be important in the pathogenesis of OSA. In addition, changes in sleep architecture, including a decrease in sleep efficiency, an increase in sleep fragmentation, poorer sleep continuity, a decrease in NREM stages 3 and 4 sleep, a decrease in REM latency, and an increase in REM density, have been described.

Addison Disease

Patients with Addison disease (primary adrenal insufficiency) may present with complaints of weakness, fatigue, anorexia, gastrointestinal symptoms, weight loss, hyperpigmentation, and hypotension. Sleep disturbances in patients with Addison disease include sleep onset insomnia, repeated awakenings, and early morning awakenings. Polysomnographic features include a decrease in NREM stages 3 and 4 sleep.

Administration of hydrocortisone at bedtime in patients with Addison disease can lead to a decrease in REM latency, an increase in REM sleep, and greater WASO.

Other Endocrine Disorders

An increase in the frequency of periodic breathing or central apneas during sleep can develop in patients with diabetes mellitus. Insomnia can complicate the course of hyperthyroidism. Finally, deficiency of GH can lead to a reduction in NREM stages 3 and 4 sleep.

Infectious Diseases

HIV infection

Patients with human immunodeficiency virus (HIV) disease (acquired immunodeficiency syndrome [AIDS]) may present with complaints of insomnia, recurrent nighttime arousals, excessive sleepiness, and an increased tendency to nap (Box 9–13). An estimated 35% of HIV-infected

Box 9–13.	Insomnia
HIV infection and sleep	Excessive sleepiness

Insomnia

Excessive sleepiness

Recurrent arousals

Antiviral therapy for HIV infection can also lead to sleep disturbance

Efavirenz is associated with

Insomnia

Nocturnal awakenings

Vivid dreams

↑ Sleep latency

↓ NREM stages 3 and 4 sleep

Zidovudine is associated with insomnia

Polysomnographic features

↓ Sleep latency

↓ Sleep efficiency

↑ Frequency of awakenings and arousals

↑ Wake time after sleep onset

↓ NREM stage 2 sleep

↑ NREM stages 3 and 4 sleep (↓ in terminal stages)

patients have alterations in their sleep-wake patterns. Sleep disturbance may be a manifestation of an underlying encephalopathy. Sleep disturbances are also common in HIV-infected children. Increase in WASO, increase in frequency and longer duration of awakenings, and more frequent napping have been observed.

Sleep quality is related to the duration of HIV disease and HIV-related symptoms as well as to the presence of depression, anxiety, daytime sleepiness, fatigue, and pain. Impaired functional status is associated with worse sleep quality. Sleep quality is also influenced by immune status because lower T-cytotoxic/suppressor (CD3+CD8+) cell counts are associated with greater sleep disturbances.

Antiviral therapy for HIV infection can also lead to sleep disturbance (Box 9–13). Efavirenz therapy is associated with an increase in sleep latency and decrease in NREM stages 3 and 4 sleep. It can also give rise to a number of neuropsychiatric adverse reactions (eg, vivid dreams, nocturnal awakenings, and insomnia). Zidovudine can give rise to insomnia.

Polysomnographic Features

Alterations in sleep architecture may be present in patients with HIV disease (Box 9–13). A decrease in sleep latency, decrease in sleep efficiency, increase in frequency of arousals, decrease in NREM stage 2 sleep, and increase in NREM stages 3 and 4 sleep are often present. Sleep fragmentation with frequent arousals, and a decrease in NREM stages 3 and 4 sleep are typical in advanced disease.

Lyme Disease

Lyme disease is a multisystem disorder with rheumatologic, neurologic, and dermatologic features. It is caused by *Borrelia burgdorferi*. Human disease is transmitted via tick bites.

Sleep-related complaints are common in patients with Lyme disease and include sleep-onset insomnia, frequent awakenings, excessive daytime sleepiness, restless legs, and nocturnal leg jerking (Box 9–14). Sleep disturbances can persist for several years in patients with previous Lyme disease, especially in those who either had facial palsy or did not receive antibiotics for acute neuroborreliosis.

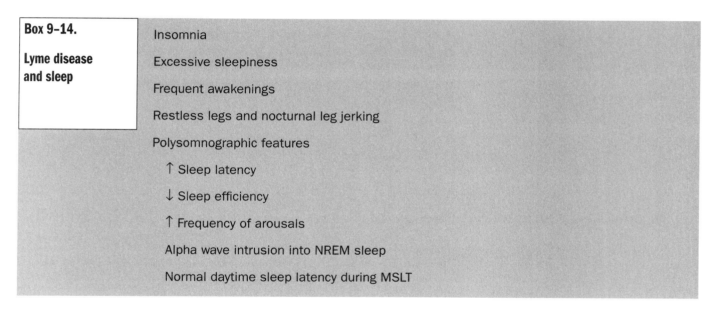

Box 9–14.

Lyme disease and sleep

Insomnia

Excessive sleepiness

Frequent awakenings

Restless legs and nocturnal leg jerking

Polysomnographic features

↑ Sleep latency

↓ Sleep efficiency

↑ Frequency of arousals

Alpha wave intrusion into NREM sleep

Normal daytime sleep latency during MSLT

Polysomnography may demonstrate an increased sleep latency, decreased sleep efficiency, increased arousals, and greater sleep fragmentation. Some patients may have alpha wave intrusion into NREM sleep. Mean sleep onset latency during multiple sleep latency testing is typically normal.

Sleeping Sickness

Sleeping sickness, or human African trypanosomiasis, is a parasitic disease caused by the protozoan *Trypanosoma brucei* or *Trypanosoma rhodesiense*. It is endemic in certain regions of intertropical Africa. Diagnosis is confirmed by demonstrating the infecting organisms in body fluids (eg, blood or cerebrospinal fluid) or tissues (eg, bone marrow or lymph node aspirates).Following the bite of a tsetse fly, human disease evolves through two stages. The hemolymphatic stage is characterized by fever, cervical adenopathy, skin lesions, facial edema and cardiac symptoms with arrhythmias. This is followed, after a variable period of time, by increasing neurologic symptoms in the meningoencephalitic stage with excessive daytime sleepiness, headaches, sensory deficits, and abnormal reflexes and movements. Insomnia is not uncommon. If untreated, the infection culminates in altered consciousness, cachexia, coma, and eventually death.

An important feature of trypanosomiasis is disruption of the circadian rhythm (eg, reversal of the sleep-wake periods and altered levels of cortisol and prolactin) (Box 9–15).

Box 9–15. **Sleeping sickness**	Excessive sleepiness
	Insomnia is not uncommon
	Reversal of sleep-wake periods
	Polysomnographic features
	Scarcity of vertex sharp waves, sleep spindles, and K complexes
	↓ REM sleep latency
	Sleep-onset REM periods

Nocturnal polysomnographic recordings have demonstrated decreased REM sleep latency with sleep-onset REM periods. Sleep stage scoring may be difficult due to the scarcity of vertex sharp waves, spindles, and K complexes (Box 9–15).

    Successful antiparasitic therapy can reverse the alterations of sleep and wakefulness.

Infectious Mononucleosis

Some patients may develop excessive sleepiness along with fatigue.

Fibromyalgia and Pain Syndromes

Acute Pain

Acute pain can give rise to sleep disruption (Box 9–16). Conversely, poor sleep can magnify perception of pain intensity. Patients with acute pain syndromes often complain of insomnia including early morning awakenings. Polysomnographic studies of patients with acute pain may reveal sleep fragmentation, and decrease in both NREM stages 3 and 4 sleep and REM sleep.

Chronic Pain Syndromes

Many causes of chronic nighttime pain, such as neoplastic diseases or rheumatologic disorders, can interfere with sleep. Patients with chronic pain may report poor sleep, insomnia, and early morning awakenings (Box 9–17). Development of depression in patients with chronic pain can further disturb sleep.

Box 9–16. **Acute pain and sleep**	Insomnia
	Sleep disruption
	Polysomnographic features
	↓ NREM stages 3 and 4 sleep
	↓ REM sleep

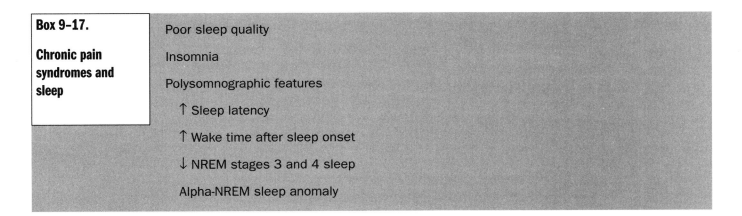

Box 9-17.

Chronic pain syndromes and sleep

Poor sleep quality

Insomnia

Polysomnographic features

   ↑ Sleep latency

   ↑ Wake time after sleep onset

   ↓ NREM stages 3 and 4 sleep

   Alpha-NREM sleep anomaly

Polysomnographic findings in patients with chronic pain consist of an increase in sleep latency, increase in wake time after sleep onset, and decrease in NREM stages 3 and 4 sleep (Box 9–17). An alpha frequency rhythm superimposed onto NREM sleep or "alpha-NREM sleep anomaly" (refer to section on fibromyalgia) may be present.

Management of pain includes pharmacotherapy (eg, oral long-acting opioids and implantable epidural or intrathecal delivery systems) and psychologic/behavioral therapy. Because administration of high-potency opioids can cause CSA, the presence of central apneas should be screened for in patients on chronic opioid therapy.

Fibromyalgia

Fibromyalgia (FM) is a syndrome characterized by chronic diffuse musculoskeletal pain and tenderness, physical discomfort, and fatigue. The American College of Rheumatology defined FM as the presence of widespread pain in combination with tenderness at 11 or more of 18 specific tender point sites. The tender points have a widespread distribution, are bilateral, occur above and below the waist, include axial sites (ie, neck, chest, and back), and have caused pain for at least 3 months. FM can be classified as primary (when there are no underlying or concomitant medical conditions) or secondary (when other rheumatologic disorders, such as rheumatoid arthritis, are present).

The onset of symptoms of FM can be acute or insidious and typically occurs during early adulthood. The condition is most prevalent in individuals between 30 and 50 years of age. The course is often chronic. FM affects women more frequently than men.

The etiology of FM is believed to involve a generalized heightened pain sensitivity arising from pathologic nociceptive processing within the central nervous system. Pain can be aggravated by poor sleep, stress, and a cold environment, and it can be relieved by rest, warm baths, heat, and relaxation.

Sleep in Fibromyalgia

Sleep in FM is often described as light, unrefreshing, or nonrestorative. Nonrestorative sleep is reported by 76% of FM patients. Sleep complaints can include insomnia and early morning awakenings (Box 9–18). Excessive daytime sleepiness is usually not prominent.

Primary sleep disorders, especially sleep apnea, restless legs syndrome and periodic limb movements of sleep may also be found in patients with FM. However, although sleep apnea is found in select patients with FM, it does not appear to be responsible for FM symptoms.

There may be a relationship between poor sleep quality, pain intensity, and perception of pain in patients with FM. Pain intensity in patients with FM appears to correlate with sleep quality; poor sleepers tend to report significantly more pain, and those with more daytime pain have poorer

Box 9-18.	Nonrestorative sleep
Fibromyalgia and sleep	Insomnia and early morning awakenings

Primary sleep disorders (eg, sleep apnea, restless legs syndrome, and periodic limb movements of sleep) may be present

Polysomnographic features

↑ Sleep latency

↓ Sleep efficiency

↓ Total sleep time

↑ Frequency of arousals

↑ Wake time after sleep onset

↑ NREM stage 1 sleep

↓ Sleep spindles during NREM stage 2 sleep

↓ NREM stages 3 and 4 sleep

↓ REM sleep

Alpha-NREM sleep anomaly

Spectral EEG analyses

↓ Delta frequency power

↓ Alpha frequency bands

nighttime sleep. One study found that fatigue in patients with FM was directly related to wake time after sleep onset and inversely related to sleep efficiency.

Polysomnographic Features of Fibromyalgia

Polysomnographic features of FM include an increase in sleep latency, decrease in sleep efficiency, decrease in total sleep time, increase in frequency of arousals and awakenings, increase in wake time after sleep onset, increase in NREM stage 1 sleep, decrease in sleep spindles during NREM stage 2 sleep, and decrease in both NREM stages 3 and 4 sleep and REM sleep (Box 9–18).

An alpha frequency rhythm, referred to as an alpha-NREM sleep anomaly ("alpha intrusion" or "alpha-delta"), has been described. Alpha activity (8–13 Hz), which is typically present only during relaxed wakefulness or brief arousals, is superimposed onto all stages NREM sleep. This sleep anomaly is proposed to be associated with increased vigilance during sleep and the subjective experience of unrefreshing sleep.

Spectral electroencephalographic (EEG) analyses of patients with FM have demonstrated a decreased delta frequency power and an increased power in alpha frequency bands (Box 9–18). Three patterns of alpha EEG sleep have been described: phasic alpha (episodic and simultaneous with delta activity), tonic alpha (continuous throughout NREM sleep), and low alpha activity. A phasic alpha sleep activity has been correlated with more nonrestorative sleep, less total sleep time, lower sleep efficiency, less NREM stages 3 and 4 sleep, worsening of pain after sleep, post-sleep increase in the number of tender points, and longer duration of pain compared to the other patterns of alpha intrusion. The alpha-NREM sleep anomaly is not specific for FM and it has been observed in those with other chronic pain syndromes (eg, chronic fatigue syndrome or rheumatoid arthritis), depression, psychophysiologic insomnia, febrile illness, and even in healthy individuals. In one study, fewer than 40% of subjects with this anomaly had pain syndromes, and the majority of subjects exhibiting this anomaly had a nonpainful medical or psychiatric condition. Alpha rhythm intrusion into NREM sleep can also be seen in some individuals taking sedative-hypnotic agents. Furthermore, the alpha-NREM sleep anomaly is not universally present in patients with FM.

Management of Sleep Disturbance in Fibromyalgia

There is no consensus regarding optimal management of sleep disturbances in patients with fibromyalgia. Treatment strategies should be individualized. Therapy is often of limited success.

Intermittent use of nonbenzodiazepine benzodiazepine receptor agonists may be useful for patients presenting with acute insomnia. However, although nonbenzodiazepine benzodiazepine receptor agonists improve subjective sleep and reduce excessive daytime sleepiness, they do not alter the alpha-NREM sleep anomaly or pain scores. Nonpharmacologic therapy includes maintenance of good sleep hygiene (eg, keeping a regular sleep-wake schedule; ensuring adequate sleep time; and avoiding alcohol, caffeine, and nicotine, which can interfere with sleep), exercise, and cognitive-behavioral therapy.

Effect of Pharmacotherapy for Fibromyalgia on Sleep

1. Amitriptyline improves sleep symptom scores, but the effect is not long lasting.

2. Chlorpromazine decreases alpha-delta frequencies, and, in one study, it reduced pain and trigger point tenderness.

3. Fluoxetine improves sleep scores but not pain scores or the number of tender points. Treatment with both amitriptyline and fluoxetine significantly improves sleep scores among patients with FM and appears to be superior to either drug alone.

4. Sodium oxybate reduces pain and fatigue symptoms, and it improves sleep quality in patients with FM. Therapy also significantly decreases sleep latency, duration of REM sleep, and the amount of alpha-NREM; in addition, it increases NREM stages 3 and 4 sleep.

5. Trazodone increases NREM stages 3 and 4 sleep, but it does not alter sleep latency, sleep efficiency, or percentage of wake time. Alpha activity is reduced.

Patients with FM should be evaluated for primary sleep disorders, including OSA and restless legs syndrome. In one study, fatigue, pain, sleep problems and disability improved following nasal CPAP therapy in patients with FM who had inspiratory flow limitation associated with arousals.

Sleep in the Intensive Care Unit

Patients in the intensive care unit (ICU) may complain of insomnia and/or hypersomnia. ICU patients often report that their sleep is poorer compared to their sleep at home and that sleep quality does not change significantly over the course of their ICU stay. Poor sleep quality does not appear to be related to gender, age, or duration of ICU stay. There is also an increased tendency for patients to sleep more during the day and less at night.

A variety of factors, operating either singly or, more often, in combination, contribute to the genesis of sleep disruption in the ICU. These include factors related to the patient, therapeutic and/or diagnostic interventions, and the ICU environment itself (Table 9–2).

Table 9–2. Etiology of sleep disruption in the intensive care unit

Patient factors	Diagnostic/Therapeutic interventions	Environmental factors
Acute illness (eg, myocardial infarction, respiratory failure)	Medication administration Nursing interventions (eg, measurements of vital signs)	Noises (eg, ventilators, cardiac monitors, pulse oximeter alarms, loud staff conversations)
Underlying chronic disease (eg, CHF, COPD)	Surgical procedures including dressing changes	Constant lighting Extremes of temperature
Pain	Respiratory treatments	Unpleasant odors
Anxiety, fear, and psychological stress	Routine care (eg, bathing, bed changes)	Uncomfortable beds or clothing Interactions with hospital staff

Patient Factors Causing Sleep Disturbance in the Intensive Care Unit

Patients in the ICU can have multiple medical and surgical problems, both acute and chronic, which could produce disturbances in sleep quality and continuity.

Following an acute myocardial infarction, sleep can be significantly disrupted in the ICU with a decrease in sleep efficiency, increase in frequency of awakenings, increase in wake time after sleep onset, increase in sleep stage shifts, and decrease in REM sleep compared with sleep in the medical ward.

Patients with CSR secondary to CHF are prone to fragmented sleep with frequent arousals and sleep stage changes. They may have a decrease in total sleep time along with an increase in frequency of awakenings, increase in NREM stage 1 sleep, and decrease in NREM stages 3 and 4 sleep.

Patients with acute respiratory failure have been found to have a significant decrease in total sleep time, decrease in percent nighttime sleep, increase in NREM stage 1 sleep, and decrease in NREM stage 4 sleep and REM sleep.

Diagnostic/Therapeutic Procedures Causing Sleep Disturbance in the Intensive Care Unit

Some diagnostic and therapeutic procedures are commonly performed round-the-clock in the ICU. Although interrupting the patients' sleep at night for these procedures may, at times, be unavoidable, often they can be performed at specifically scheduled times to allow maximum opportunities for sleep at night.

Surgical procedures have been reported to cause a decrease in total sleep time, increase in wake time after sleep onset, and decrease in NREM stages 3 and 4 sleep and REM sleep. Delirium is not uncommon following surgery and its incidence appears to be correlated to decreased sleep duration.

Many medications commonly prescribed in the ICU can disrupt sleep. These agents include opiates (increase in frequency of arousals, increase in NREM stage 1 sleep, and decrease in REM sleep); benzodiazepines (decrease in NREM stages 3 and 4 sleep); beta-blockers (decrease in REM sleep); and clonidine (decrease in total sleep time and REM sleep).

Environmental Noise in the Intensive Care Unit

The average noise level in the ICU ranges from 53 to 59 dB (peak of 83 dB) during the day and 42 to 56 dB (peak of 79 dB) at night. Most of the noise is from equipments in the ICU and loud staff conversations. In comparison, the noise level at a busy street corner is 72 dB and in a quite bedroom at night is 20 to 30 dB. Noise levels less than 35 to 45 dB are generally required to enable a person to fall asleep easily. The Environmental Protection Agency has recommended that hospital noise levels not exceed 45 dB during the day and 35 dB at night. Noise levels in the ICU clearly exceed these standards.

The Intensive Care Unit Syndrome

The ICU syndrome is characterized by reversible mental status changes, including delirium, among patients 3 to 7 days after admission to the ICU. Other features include fear, anxiety, depression, disorientation, and hallucinations. The ICU syndrome usually resolves within 48 hours of ICU discharge.

Sleep deprivation is one of the major causes of the ICU syndrome. Other factors such as age, severity of illness, type of surgical procedure, fever, and fluid and electrolyte imbalances can all contribute to the development of this condition.

Polysomnographic Features of Patients in the Intensive Care Unit

Polysomnography of patients in the ICU have demonstrated a number of sleep disturbances, including sleep fragmentation, increase in sleep latency, decrease in sleep efficiency, decrease in total sleep time, increase in frequency of arousals, increase in NREM stage 1 sleep, and decrease in NREM stages 3 and 4 sleep and REM sleep (Box 9–19).

The sleep of patients in the ICU can be measured using subjective techniques (eg, nursing assessment and charting), objective tests, or both. Daily sleep assessment and charting by nurses are commonly employed to subjectively assess sleep in the ICU. However, in one study, nursing observations overestimated sleep time compared to objective data obtained with polysomnography. Although objective measures of sleep with polysomnography or wrist actigraphy can provide more accurate estimates of sleep duration and continuity, they are rarely indicated in an ICU setting.

Improving Sleep of Patients in the Intensive Care Unit

Aided by regular assessment of ICU patients' sleep by the hospital staff, simple measures such as decreasing ambient lights and noise levels at night, limiting nighttime visiting hours and procedures (laboratory tests or radiology tests) unless urgently indicated, and judicious use of analgesics and sedative-hypnotic agents may be of value.

Miscellaneous Medical Disorders

Sleep may also be adversely affected by other medical disorders and the medications prescribed for them. Patients with these medical disorders may present with complaints of excessive sleepiness, insomnia or nighttime awakenings (Table 9–3).

Box 9–19. **Sleep in the intensive care unit**	Insomnia and/or excessive sleepiness
	Sleep disturbance
	Tendency for more sleep during the day and less at night
	ICU syndrome
	Polysomnographic features in ICU patients
	↑ Sleep latency
	↓ Sleep efficiency
	↑ Frequency of arousals and awakenings
	↓ Total sleep time
	↑ NREM stage 1 sleep
	↓ NREM stages 3 and 4 sleep
	↑ REM sleep latency
	↓ REM sleep

Table 9–3.   Disorders that adversely affect sleep

Medical disorder	Sleep disturbance
Anemia (severe)	Excessive sleepiness
Anorexia nervosa	Insomnia and early morning awakenings; sleep improves after weight gain Polysomnographic features include decreases in total sleep time and NREM stages 3 and 4 sleep
Chronic fatigue syndrome	Fatigue; nighttime awakenings
Dermatologic conditions	Insomnia secondary to pruritus
Diabetes mellitus	Excessive sleepiness and disturbed sleep
Epstein-Barr virus infection	Insomnia and nonrestorative sleep Polysomnography may reveal alpha-NREM sleep anomaly
Hepatic failure	Excessive sleepiness secondary to encephalopathy
Hereditary hemorrhagic telangiectasia	Excessive sleepiness
Paroxysmal nocturnal hemoglobinuria	Nighttime awakenings
Sickle cell disease	Nocturnal hypoxemia; nighttime awakenings

References

General References

American Academy of Sleep Medicine. *The International Classification of Sleep Disorders: Diagnostic and Coding Manual.* 2nd ed. Westchester, IL: American Academy of Sleep Medicine, 2005.

Ballard RD. Sleep and medical disorders. *Sleep Medicine.* Primary Care: Clinics in Office Practice. Elsevier Saunders, 2005.

Bowman TJ. *Review of Sleep Medicine.* Burlington, MA: Butterworth-Heinemann, 2002.

Berry RB. *Sleep Medicine Pearls.* 2nd ed. Philadelphia, PA: Hanley & Belfus, 2002.

Berry RB, Harding SM. Sleep and medical disorders. *Sleep Disorders.* Medical Clinics of North America. Elsevier Saunders, 2004.

Chokroverty S. *Clinical Companion to Sleep Disorders Medicine.* 2nd ed. Butterworth-Heinemann, 2000.

Lavie P, Pillar G, Malhotra A. *Sleep Disorders Handbook.* New York, NY: Taylor & Francis, 2002.

Lee-Chiong TL, ed. *Sleep: A Comprehensive Handbook.* Hoboken, NJ: John Wiley & Sons, 2006.

Lee-Chiong TL, Sateia M, Carskadon M, eds. *Sleep Medicine.* Philadelphia, PA: Hanley & Belfus (Elsevier), 2002.

Perlis ML, Lichstein KL, eds. *Treating Sleep Disorders: Principles and Practice of Behavioral Sleep Medicine.* Hoboken, NJ: John Wiley & Sons, 2003.

Rechtschaffen A, Kales A. *A Manual of Standardized Terminology, Techniques and Scoring System for Sleep Stages of Human Subjects.* Los Angeles, CA: Brain Information Service/Brain Research Institute, University of California, 1968.

Reite M, Ruddy J, Nagel K. *Concise Guide to Evaluation and Management of Sleep Disorders.* 3rd ed. Arlington, VA: American Psychiatric Publishing, April 2002.

Sleep Disorders. Medical Clinics of North America. Philadelphia, PA: Elsevier Saunders, 2004.

Sleep Medicine. Primary Care: Clinics in Office Practice. Philadelphia, PA: Elsevier Saunders, 2005.

Sleep Research Society. *SRS Basics of Sleep Guide.* Westchester, IL: Sleep Research Society, 2005.

Respiratory Disorders

Amino A, Shiozawa Z, Nagasaka T, Shindo K, Ohashi K, Tsunoda S, et al. Sleep apnoea in well-controlled myasthenia gravis and the effect of thymectomy. *J Neurol.* 1998(Feb);245(2):77–80.

Arnulf I, Similowski T, Salachas F, Garma L, Mehiri S, Attali V, Behin-Bellhesen V, et al. Sleep disorders and diaphragmatic function in patients with amyotrophic lateral sclerosis. *Am J Respir Crit Care Med.* 2000(Mar);161(3 Pt 1):849–56.

Ballard RD, Irvin CG, Martin RJ, Pak J, Pandey R, White DP. Influence of sleep on lung volume in asthmatic patients and normal subjects. *J Appl Physiol.* 1990(May);68(5):2034–41.

Barbe F, Quera-Salva MA, McCann C, Gajdos P, Raphael JC, de Lattre J, et al. Sleep-related respiratory disturbances in patients with Duchenne muscular dystrophy. *Eur Respir J.* 1994(Aug);7(8):1403–8.

Bednarek M, Plywaczewski R, Jonczak L, Zielinski J. There is no relationship between chronic obstructive pulmonary disease and obstructive sleep apnea syndrome: a population study. *Respiration.* 2005(Mar–Apr);72(2):142–9.

Brezinova V, Catterall JR, Douglas NJ, et al. Night sleep of patients with chronic ventilatory failure and age matched controls: number and duration of the EEG episodes of intervening wakefulness and drowsiness. *Sleep.* 1982;5:123–130.

Brown LK. Sleep-related disorders and chronic obstructive pulmonary disease. *Respir Care Clin N Am.* 1998(Sep);4(3):493–512.

Bye PT, Issa F, Berthon-Jones M, Sullivan CE. Studies of oxygenation during sleep in patients with interstitial lung disease. *Am Rev Respir Dis.* 1984(Jan);129(1):27–32.

Calverley PM, Brezinova V, Douglas NJ, Catterall JR, Flenley DC. The effect of oxygenation on sleep quality in chronic bronchitis and emphysema. *Am Rev Respir Dis.* 1982(Aug);126(2):206–10.

Chan CS, Woolcock AJ, Sullivan CE. Nocturnal asthma: role of snoring and obstructive sleep apnea. *Am Rev Respir Dis.* 1988(Jun);137(6):1502–4.

Chaouat A, Weitzenblum E, Krieger J, Ifoundza T, Oswald M, Kessler R. Association of chronic obstructive pulmonary disease and sleep apnea syndrome. *Am J Respir Crit Care Med.* 1995(Jan);151(1):82–6.

Ciftci TU, Ciftci B, Guven SF, Kokturk O, Turktas H. Effect of nasal continuous positive airway pressure in uncontrolled nocturnal asthmatic patients with obstructive sleep apnea syndrome. *Respir Med.* 2005(May); 99(5):529–34.

Cirignotta F, Mondini S, Zucconi M, Barrot-Cortes E, Sturani C, Schiavina M, et al. Sleep-related breathing impairment in myotonic dystrophy. *J Neurol.* 1987(Dec);235(2):80–5.

Clark TJ, Hetzel MR. Diurnal variation of asthma. *Br J Dis Chest.* 1977(Apr);71(2):87–92.

Culebras A. Sleep disorders and neuromuscular disease. *Semin Neurol.* 2005(Mar);25(1):33–8.

Dean AC, Graham BA, Dalakas M, Sato S. Sleep apnea in patients with postpolio syndrome. *Ann Neurol.* 1998(May);43(5):661–4.

DeMarco FJ Jr, Wynne JW, Block AJ, Boysen PG, Taasan VC. Oxygen desaturation during sleep as a determinant of the "Blue and Bloated" syndrome. *Chest.* 1981(Jun);79(6):621–5.

Douglas NJ, Calverley PM, Leggett RJ, Brash HM, Flenley DC, Brezinova V. Transient hypoxaemia during sleep in chronic bronchitis and emphysema. *Lancet.* 1979(Jan 6);1(8106):1–4.

Edwards N, Middleton PG, Blyton DM, Sullivan CE. Sleep disordered breathing and pregnancy. *Thorax.* 2002(Jun);57(6):555–8.

Ferguson KA, Strong MJ, Ahmad D, George CF. Sleep-disordered breathing in amyotrophic lateral sclerosis. *Chest.* 1996(Sep);110(3):664–9.

Fleetham J, West P, Mezon B, Conway W, Roth T, Kryger M. Sleep, arousals, and oxygen desaturation in chronic obstructive pulmonary disease. The effect of oxygen therapy. *Am Rev Respir Dis.* 1982 (Sep);126(3):429–33.

Gajdos P, Quera Salva MA. Respiratory disorders during sleep and myasthenia. *Rev Neurol (Paris).* 2001(Nov);157(11 Pt 2):S145–7.

George CF, Kryger MH. Sleep in restrictive lung disease. *Sleep.* 1987(Oct);10(5):409–18.

Guilleminault C, Kurland G, Winkle R, Miles LE. Severe kyphoscoliosis, breathing, and sleep: the "Quasimodo" syndrome during sleep. *Chest.* 1981(Jun);79(6):626–30.

Hudgel DW, Martin RJ, Capehart M, Johnson B, Hill P. Contribution of hypoventilation to sleep oxygen desaturation in chronic obstructive pulmonary disease. *J Appl Physiol.* 1983(Sep);55(3):669–77.

Jankelowitz L, Reid KJ, Wolfe L, Cullina J, Zee PC, Jain M. Cystic fibrosis patients have poor sleep quality despite normal sleep latency and efficiency. *Chest.* 2005(May);127(5):1593–9.

Kales A, Beall GN, Bajor GF, Jacobson A, Kales JD. Sleep studies in asthmatic adults: relationship of attacks to sleep stage and time of night. *J Allergy.* 1968(Mar);41(3):164–73.

Khan Y, Heckmatt JZ. Obstructive apnoeas in Duchenne muscular dystrophy. *Thorax.* 1994(Feb);49(2):157–61.

Martin RJ. Nocturnal asthma: circadian rhythms and therapeutic interventions. *Am Rev Respir Dis.* 1993(Jun);147(6 Pt 2):S25–8.

Martin RJ, Cicutto LC, Smith HR, Ballard RD, Szefler SJ. Airways inflammation in nocturnal asthma. *Am Rev Respir Dis.* 1991(Feb);143(2):351–7.

Milross MA, Piper AJ, Norman M, Dobbin CJ, Grunstein RR, Sullivan CE, et al. Subjective sleep quality in cystic fibrosis. *Sleep Med.* 2002(May);3(3):205–12.

Montplaisir J, Walsh J, Malo JL. Nocturnal asthma: features of attacks, sleep and breathing patterns. *Am Rev Respir Dis.*1982(Jan);125(1):18–22.

Patakas D, Tsara V, Zoglopitis F, Daskalopoulou E, Argyropoulou P, Maniki E. Nocturnal hypoxia in unilateral diaphragmatic paralysis. *Respiration.* 1991;58(2):95–9.

Perez-Padilla R, West P, Lertzman M, Kryger MH. Breathing during sleep in patients with interstitial lung disease. *Am Rev Respir Dis.* 1985(Aug);132(2):224–9.

Piper A. Sleep abnormalities associated with neuromuscular disease: pathophysiology and evaluation. *Semin Respir Crit Care Med.* 2002;23(3):211–20.

Resta O, Foschino Barbaro MP, Bonfitto P, Giliberti T, Depalo A, Pannacciulli N, et al. Low sleep quality and daytime sleepiness in obese patients without obstructive sleep apnoea syndrome. *J Intern Med.* 2003(May);253(5):536–43.

Resta O, Foschino-Barbaro MP, Legari G, Talamo S, Bonfitto P, Palumbo A, et al. Sleep-related breathing disorders, loud snoring and excessive daytime sleepiness in obese subjects. *Int J Obes Relat Metab Disord.* 2001(May);25(5):669–75.

Resta O, Guido P, Picca V, Sabato R, Rizzi M, Scarpelli F,et al. Prescription of nCPAP and nBIPAP in obstructive sleep apnoea syndrome: Italian experience in 105 subjects. A prospective two centre study. *Respir Med.* 1998(Jun);92(6):820–7.

Santiago JR, Nolledo MS, Kinzler W, Santiago TV. Sleep and sleep disorders in pregnancy. *Ann Intern Med.* 2001(Mar 6);134(5):396–408.

Sawicka EH, Branthwaite MA. Respiration during sleep in kyphoscoliosis. *Thorax.* 1987(Oct);42(10):801–8.48,49,50.

Steljes DG, Kryger MH, Kirk BW, Millar TW. Sleep in postpolio syndrome. *Chest.* 1990(Jul);98(1):133–40.

Stradling JR, Warley AR. Bilateral diaphragm paralysis and sleep apnoea without diurnal respiratory failure. *Thorax.* 1988(Jan);43(1):75–7.

Turner-Warwick M. Epidemiology of nocturnal asthma. *Am J Med.* 1988(Jul 29);85(1B): 6–8.

Ververs CC, Van der Meche FG, Verbraak AF, van der Sluys HC, Bogaard JM. Breathing pattern awake and asleep in myotonic dystrophy. *Respiration.* 1996;63(1):1–7.

Cardiac Disorders

Becker HF, Jerrentrup A, Ploch T, Grote L, Penzel T, Sullivan CE, et al. Effect of nasal continuous positive airway pressure treatment on blood pressure in patients with obstructive sleep apnea. *Circulation*. 2003(Jan 7);107(1):68–73.

Franklin KA, Eriksson P, Sahlin C, Lundgren R. Reversal of central sleep apnea with oxygen. *Chest*. 1997(Jan);111(1):163–9.

Hanly PJ, Zuberi-Khokhar NS. Increased mortality associated with Cheyne-Stokes respiration in patients with congestive heart failure. *Am J Respir Crit Care Med*. 1996(Jan);153(1):272–6.

Hanly PJ, Millar TW, Steljes DG, Baert R, Frais MA, Kryger MH. Respiration and abnormal sleep in patients with congestive heart failure. *Chest*. 1989(Sep);96(3):480–8.

Harbison J, O'Reilly P, McNicholas WT. Cardiac rhythm disturbances in the obstructive sleep apnea syndrome: effects of nasal continuous positive airway pressure therapy. *Chest*. 2000(Sep);118(3):591–5.

Ip MS, Tse HF, Lam B, Tsang KW, Lam WK. Endothelial function in obstructive sleep apnea and response to treatment. *Am J Respir Crit Care Med*. 2004(Feb 1);169(3):348–53.

Ip MS, Lam B, Ng MM, Lam WK, Tsang KW, Lam KS. Obstructive sleep apnea is independently associated with insulin resistance. *Am J Respir Crit Care Med*. 2002(Mar 1);165(5):670–6.

Javaheri S, Parker TJ, Wexler L, Michaels SE, Stanberry E, Nishyama H, Roselle GA. Occult sleep-disordered breathing in stable congestive heart failure. *Ann Intern Med*. 1995(Apr 1);122(7):487–92.

Kaneko Y, Floras JS, Usui K, Plante J, Tkacova R, Kubo T, et al. Cardiovascular effects of continuous positive airway pressure in patients with heart failure and obstructive sleep apnea. *N Engl J Med*. 2003(Mar 27);348(13):1233–41.

Krachman SL, D'Alonzo GE, Berger TJ, Eisen HJ. Comparison of oxygen therapy with nasal continuous positive airway pressure on Cheyne-Stokes respiration during sleep in congestive heart failure. *Chest*. 1999(Dec);116(6):1550–7.

Lanfranchi PA, Braghiroli A, Bosimini E, Mazzuero G, Colombo R, Donner CF, et al. Prognostic value of nocturnal Cheyne-Stokes respiration in chronic heart failure. *Circulation*. 1999(Mar 23);99(11):1435–40.

Lanfranchi PA, Somers VK, Braghiroli A, Corra U, Eleuteri E, Giannuzzi P. Central sleep apnea in left ventricular dysfunction: prevalence and implications for arrhythmic risk. *Circulation*. 2003(Feb 11);107(5):727–32.

Lavie L, Vishnevsky A, Lavie P. Evidence for lipid peroxidation in obstructive sleep apnea. *Sleep*. 2004(Feb 1);27(1):123–8.

Lavie P, Herer P, Hoffstein V. Obstructive sleep apnoea syndrome as a risk factor for hypertension: population study. *BMJ*. 2000(Feb 19);320(7233):479–82.

Logan AG, Tkacova R, Perlikowski SM, Leung RS, Tisler A, Floras JS, et al. Refractory hypertension and sleep apnoea: effect of CPAP on blood pressure and baroreflex. *Eur Respir J*. 2003(Feb);21(2):241–7.

Mansfield DR, Gollogly NC, Kaye DM, Richardson M, Bergin P, Naughton MT. Controlled trial of continuous positive airway pressure in obstructive sleep apnea and heart failure. *Am J Respir Crit Care Med*. 2004(Feb 1);169(3):361–6. Epub 2003 Nov 3.

Narkiewicz K, Kato M, Phillips BG, Pesek CA, Davison DE, Somers VK. Nocturnal continuous positive airway pressure decreases daytime sympathetic traffic in obstructive sleep apnea. *Circulation*. 1999(Dec 7);100(23):2332–5.

Naughton M, Benard D, Tam A, Rutherford R, Bradley TD. Role of hyperventilation in the pathogenesis of central sleep apneas in patients with congestive heart failure. *Am Rev Respir Dis.* 1993(Aug); 148(2):330–8.

Nieto FJ, Young TB, Lind BK, Shahar E, Samet JM, Redline S, et al. Association of sleep-disordered breathing, sleep apnea, and hypertension in a large community-based study. Sleep Heart Health Study. *JAMA.* 2000(Apr 12);283(14):1829–36.

Peppard PE, Young T, Palta M, Skatrud J. Prospective study of the association between sleep-disordered breathing and hypertension. *N Engl J Med.* 2000(May 11);342(19):1378–84.

Pepperell JC, Ramdassingh-Dow S, Crosthwaite N, Mullins R, Jenkinson C, Stradling JR, et al. Ambulatory blood pressure after therapeutic and subtherapeutic nasal continuous positive airway pressure for obstructive sleep apnoea: a randomised parallel trial. *Lancet.* 2002(Jan 19); 359(9302):204–10.

Punjabi NM, Sorkin JD, Katzel LI, Goldberg AP, Schwartz AR, Smith PL. Sleep-disordered breathing and insulin resistance in middle-aged and overweight men. *Am J Respir Crit Care Med.* 2002(Mar 1);165(5):677–82.

Shahar E, Whitney CW, Redline S, Lee ET, Newman AB, Javier Nieto F, et al. Sleep-disordered breathing and cardiovascular disease: cross-sectional results of the Sleep Heart Health Study. *Am J Respir Crit Care Med.* 2001(Jan);163(1):19–25.

Shamsuzzaman AS, Winnicki M, Lanfranchi P, Wolk R, Kara T, Accurso V, et al. Elevated C-reactive protein in patients with obstructive sleep apnea. *Circulation.* 2002(May 28);105(21):2462–4.

Sin DD, Logan AG, Fitzgerald FS, Liu PP, Bradley TD. Effects of continuous positive airway pressure on cardiovascular outcomes in heart failure patients with and without Cheyne-Stokes respiration. *Circulation.* 2000;(Jul 4);102(1):61–6.

Solin P, Bergin P, Richardson M, Kaye DM, Walters EH, Naughton MT. Influence of pulmonary capillary wedge pressure on central apnea in heart failure. *Circulation.* 1999(Mar 30);99(12):1574–9.

Somers VK, Dyken ME, Clary MP, Abboud FM. Sympathetic neural mechanisms in obstructive sleep apnea. *J Clin Invest.* 1995(Oct);96(4):1897–904.

Suzuki M, Guilleminault C, Otsuka K, Shiomi T. Blood pressure "dipping" and "non-dipping" in obstructive sleep apnea syndrome patients. *Sleep.* 1996(Jun);19(5):382–7.

von Kanel R, Dimsdale JE. Hemostatic alterations in patients with obstructive sleep apnea and the implications for cardiovascular disease. *Chest.* 2003(Nov);124(5):1956–67.

Xie A, Skatrud JB, Puleo DS, Rahko PS, Dempsey JA. Apnea-hypopnea threshold for CO_2 in patients with congestive heart failure. *Am J Respir Crit Care Med.* 2002(May 1);165(9):1245–50.

Gastrointestinal Diseases

Castell DO, Murray JA, Tutuian R, Orlando RC, Arnold R. Review article: the pathophysiology of gastro-oesophageal reflux disease—oesophageal manifestations. *Aliment Pharmacol Ther.* 2004(Dec);20 Suppl 9:14–25.

Demeter P, Vardi VK, Magyar P. Correlations between gastroesophageal reflux disease and obstructive sleep apnea. *Orv Hetil.* 2004(Sep)12;145(37):1897–901.

Elsenbruch S, Harnish MJ, Orr WC. Subjective and objective sleep quality in irritable bowel syndrome. *Am J Gastroenterol.* 1999(Sep);94(9):2447–52.

Elsenbruch S, Thompson JJ, Harnish MJ, Exton MS, Orr WC. Behavioral and physiological sleep characteristics in women with irritable bowel syndrome. *Am J Gastroenterol.* 2002(Sep);97(9): 2306–14.

Fass R, Fullerton S, Tung S, Mayer EA. Sleep disturbances in clinic patients with functional bowel disorders. *Am J Gastroenterol.* 2000(May);95(5):1195–2000.

Freidin N, Fisher MJ, Taylor W, Boyd D, Surratt P, McCallum RW, et al. Sleep and nocturnal acid reflux in normal subjects and patients with reflux oesophagitis. *Gut.* 1991(Nov);32(11):1275–9.

Green BT, Broughton WA, O'Connor JB. Marked improvement in nocturnal gastroesophageal reflux in a large cohort of patients with obstructive sleep apnea treated with continuous positive airway pressure. *Arch Intern Med.* 2003(Jan 13);163(1):41–5.

Guda N, Partington S, Vakil N. Symptomatic gastro-oesophageal reflux, arousals and sleep quality in patients undergoing polysomnography for possible obstructive sleep apnoea. *Aliment Pharmacol Ther.* 2004(Nov 15);20(10):1153–9.

Ing AJ, Ngu MC, Breslin AB. Obstructive sleep apnea and gastroesophageal reflux. *Am J Med.* 2000(Mar 6);108 (Suppl 4a):120S–125S.

Kahrilas PJ, Quigley EM. Clinical esophageal pH recording: a technical review for practice guideline development. *Gastroenterology.* 1996(Jun);110(6):1982–96.

Kahrilas PJ, Dodds WJ, Dent J, Haeberle B, Hogan WJ, Arndorfer RC. Effect of sleep, spontaneous gastroesophageal reflux, and a meal on upper esophageal sphincter pressure in normal human volunteers. *Gastroenterology.* 1987(Feb);92(2):466–71.

Kerr P, Shoenut JP, Steens RD, Millar T, Micflikier AB, Kryger MH. Nasal continuous positive airway pressure. A new treatment for nocturnal gastroesophageal reflux? *J Clin Gastroenterol.* 1993(Dec);17(4):276–80.

Kim HN, Vorona RD, Winn MP, Doviak M, Johnson DA, Ware JC. Symptoms of gastro-oesophageal reflux disease and the severity of obstructive sleep apnoea syndrome are not related in sleep disorders center patients. *Aliment Pharmacol Ther.* 2005(May 1);21(9):1127–33.

Orr WC. Gastrointestinal functioning during sleep: a new horizon in sleep medicine. *Sleep Med Rev.* 2001(Apr);5(2):91–101.

Orr WC, Johnson LF. Responses to different levels of esophageal acidification during waking and sleep. *Dig Dis Sci.* 1998(Feb);43(2):241–5.

Orr WC, Johnson LF, Robinson MG. Effect of sleep on swallowing, esophageal peristalsis, and acid clearance. *Gastroenterology.* 1984(May);86(5 Pt 1):814–9.

Schneyer LH, Pigman W, Hanahan L, Gilmore RW. Rate of flow of human parotid, sublingual, and submaxillary secretions during sleep. *J Dent Res.* 1956(Feb);35(1):109–14.

Shaker R, Castell DO, Schoenfeld PS, Spechler SJ. Nighttime heartburn is an under-appreciated clinical problem that impacts sleep and daytime function: the results of a Gallup survey conducted on behalf of the American

Gastroenterological Association. *Am J Gastroenterol.* 2003(Jul);98(7):1487–93.

Sontag SJ. Gastroesophageal reflux disease and asthma. *J Clin Gastroenterol.* 2000(Apr);30(3 Suppl): S9–30.

Thurnheer R, Henz S, Knoblauch A. Sleep-related laryngospasm. *Eur Respir J.* 1997(Sep);10(9):2084–6.

Vege SS, Locke GR III, Weaver AL, Farmer SA, Melton LJ III, Talley NJ. Functional gastrointestinal disorders among people with sleep disturbances: a population-based study. *Mayo Clin Proc.* 2004(Dec);79(12):1501–6.

Renal Disorders

Benz RL, Pressman MR, Hovick ET, Peterson DD. A preliminary study of the effects of correction of anemia with recombinant human erythropoietin therapy on sleep, sleep disorders, and daytime sleepiness in hemodialysis patients (The SLEEPO study). *Am J Kidney Dis.* 1999(Dec);34(6):1089–95.

Hanly P. Sleep apnea and daytime sleepiness in end-stage renal disease. *Semin Dial.* 2004 (Mar–Apr);17(2):109–14.

Parker KP. Sleep disturbances in dialysis patients. *Sleep Med Rev.* 2003(Apr);7(2):131–43.

Strub B, Schneider-Helmert D, Gnirss F, Blumberg A. Sleep disorders in patients with chronic renal insufficiency in long-term hemodialysis treatment. *Schweiz Med Wochenschr.* 1982(Jun 5);112(23):824–8.

Walker S, Fine A, Kryger MH. Sleep complaints are common in a dialysis unit. *Am J Kidney Dis.* 1995(Nov);26(5):751–6.

Winkelman JW, Chertow GM, Lazarus JM. Restless legs syndrome in end-stage renal disease. *Am J Kidney Dis.* 1996(Sep);28(3):372–8.

Endocrine and Metabolic Disorders

Astrom C, Christensen L, Gjerris F, Trojaborg W. Sleep in acromegaly before and after treatment with adenomectomy. Neuroendocrinology. 1991(Apr);53(4):328–31.

Blanco Perez JJ, Blanco-Ramos MA, Zamarron Sanz C, Souto Fernandez A, Mato Mato A, et al. Acromegaly and sleep apnea. *Arch Bronconeumol.* 2004(Aug);40(8):355–9.

Buyse B, Michiels E, Bouillon R, Bobbaers H, Demedts M. Relief of sleep apnoea after treatment of acromegaly: report of three cases and review of the literature. *Eur Respir J.* 1997(Jun);10(6):1401–4.

Dostalova S, Sonka K, Smahel Z, Weiss V, Marek J, Horinek D. Craniofacial abnormalities and their relevance for sleep apnoea syndrome aetiopathogenesis in acromegaly. *Eur J Endocrinol.* 2001(May);144(5):491–7.

Fatti LM, Scacchi M, Pincelli AI, Lavezzi E, Cavagnini F. Prevalence and pathogenesis of sleep apnea and lung disease in acromegaly. *Pituitary.* 2001(Sep);4(4):259–62.

Garcia-Borreguero D, Wehr TA, Larrosa O, Granizo JJ, Hardwick D, Chrousos GP, et al. Glucocorticoid replacement is permissive for rapid eye movement sleep and sleep consolidation in patients with adrenal insufficiency. *J Clin Endocrinol Metab.* 2000(Nov);85(11):4201–6.

Grunstein RR, Sullivan CE. Sleep apnea and hypothyroidism: mechanisms and management. *Am J Med.* 1988(Dec);85(6):775–9.

Grunstein RR, Ho KY, Sullivan CE. Effect of octreotide, a somatostatin analog, on sleep apnea in patients with acromegaly. *Ann Intern Med.* 1994(Oct)1;121(7):478–83.

Grunstein RR, Ho KY, Sullivan CE. Sleep apnea in acromegaly. *Ann Intern Med.* 1991(Oct 1);115(7):527–32.

Grunstein RR, Ho KY, Berthon-Jones M, Stewart D, Sullivan CE. Central sleep apnea is associated with increased ventilatory response to carbon dioxide and hypersecretion of growth hormone in patients with acromegaly. *Am J Respir Crit Care Med.* 1994(Aug);150(2):496–502.

Herrmann BL, Wessendorf TE, Ajaj W, Kahlke S, Teschler H, Mann K. Effects of octreotide on sleep apnoea and tongue volume (magnetic resonance imaging) in patients with acromegaly. *Eur J Endocrinol.* 2004(Sep);151(3):309–15.

Lovas K, Husebye ES, Holsten F, Bjorvatn B. Sleep disturbances in patients with Addison's disease. *Eur J Endocrinol.* 2003(Apr);148(4):449–56.

Mestron A, Webb SM, Astorga R, Benito P, Catala M, Gaztambide S, et al. Epidemiology, clinical characteristics, outcome, morbidity and mortality in acromegaly based on the Spanish Acromegaly Registry (Registro Espanol de Acromegalia, REA). *Eur J Endocrinol.* 2004(Oct); 151(4):439–46.

Rosenow F, McCarthy V, Caruso AC. Sleep apnoea in endocrine diseases. *J Sleep Res.* 1998(Mar);7(1):3–11.

Shipley JE, Schteingart DE, Tandon R, Starkman MN. Sleep architecture and sleep apnea in patients with Cushing's disease. *Sleep.* 1992(Dec);15(6):514–8.

Weiss V, Sonka K, Pretl M, Dostalova S, Klozar J, Rambousek P, et al. Prevalence of the sleep apnea syndrome in acromegaly population. *J Endocrinol Invest.* 2000(Sep);23(8):515–9.

Ziemer DC, Dunlap DB. Relief of sleep apnea in acromegaly by bromocriptine. *Am J Med Sci.* 1988(Jan);295(1):49–51.

Infectious Diseases

Buguet A, Gati R, Sevre JP, Develoux M, Bogui P, Lonsdorfer J. 24 hour polysomnographic evaluation in a patient with sleeping sickness. *Electroencephalogr Clin Neurophysiol.* 1989(Jun);72(6):471–8.

Cruess DG, Antoni MH, Gonzalez J, Fletcher MA, Klimas N, Duran R, et al. Sleep disturbance mediates the association between psychological distress and immune status among HIV-positive men and women on combination antiretroviral therapy. *J Psychosom Res.* 2003(Mar);54(3):185–9.

Darko DF, McCutchan JA, Kripke DF, Gillin JC, Golshan S. Fatigue, sleep disturbance, disability, and indices of progression of HIV infection. *Am J Psychiatry.* 1992(Apr);149(4):514–20.

Darko DF, Mitler MM, White JL. Sleep disturbance in early HIV infection. *Focus.* 1995(Oct);10(11):5–6.

Diaz-Ruiz O, Navarro L, Mendez-Diaz M, Galicia O, Elder JH, Sanna PP, et al. Inhibition of the ERK pathway prevents HIVgp120-induced REM sleep increase. *Brain Res.* 2001(Sep 14);913(1):78–81.

Franck LS, Johnson LM, Lee K, Hepner C, Lambert L, Passeri M, et al. Sleep disturbances in children with human immunodeficiency virus infection. *Pediatrics.* 1999(Nov);104(5):e62.

Gallego L, Barreiro P, del Rio R, Gonzalez de Requena D, Rodriguez-Albarino A, Gonzalez-Lahoz J, et al. Analyzing sleep abnormalities in HIV-infected patients treated with Efavirenz. *Clin Infect Dis.* 2004(Feb 1);38(3):430–2. Epub 2004 Jan 9.

Greenberg HE, Ney G, Scharf SM, Ravdin L, Hilton E. Sleep quality in Lyme disease. *Sleep.* 1995(Dec);18(10):912–6.

Kalish RA, Kaplan RF, Taylor E, Jones-Woodward L, Workman K, Steere AC. Evaluation of study patients with Lyme disease, 10–20-year follow-up. *J Infect Dis.* 2001(Feb 1);183(3):453–60. Epub 2000 Dec 27.

Kaplan RF, Jones-Woodward L. Lyme encephalopathy: a neuropsychological perspective. *Semin Neurol.* 1997(Mar);17(1):31–7.

Lochet P, Peyriere H, Lotthe A, Mauboussin JM, Delmas B, Reynes J. Long-term assessment of neuropsychiatric adverse reactions associated with efavirenz. *HIV Med.* 2003(Jan);4(1):62–6.

Nokes KM, Kendrew J. Correlates of sleep quality in persons with HIV disease. J Assoc Nurses AIDS Care. 2001 Jan-Feb;12(1):17–22.

Norman SE, Chediak AD, Kiel M, Cohn MA. Sleep disturbances in HIV-infected homosexual men. *AIDS.* 1990(Aug);4(8):775–81.

Robbins JL, Phillips KD, Dudgeon WD, Hand GA. Physiological and psychological correlates of sleep in HIV infection. *Clin Nurs Res.* 2004(Feb);13(1):33–52.

Sanner BM, Buchner N, Kotterba S, Zidek W. Polysomnography in acute African trypanosomiasis. *J Neurol.* 2000(Nov);247(11):878–9.

Fibromyalgia and Pain Syndromes

Affleck G, Urrows S, Tennen H, Higgins P, Abeles M. Sequential daily relations of sleep, pain intensity, and attention to pain among women with fibromyalgia. *Pain.* 1996(Dec);68(2–3):363–8.

Anch AM, Lue FA, MacLean AW, Moldofsky H. Sleep physiology and psychological aspects of fibrositis (fibromyalgia) syndrome. *Can J Exp Psychol.* 1991;45:179–84.

Branco JC, Martini A, Palva T. Treatment of sleep abnormalities and clinical complaints in fibromyalgia with trazodone(abstract). *Arthritis Rheum.* 1996;39:591.

Drewes AM, Gade J, Nielsen KD, Bjerregard K, Taagholt SJ, Svendsen L. Clustering of sleep electroencephalopathic patterns in patients with the fibromyalgia syndrome. *Br J Rheumatol.* 1995;34:1151–6.

Fitzcharles MA, Costa DD, Poyhia R. A study of standard care in fibromyalgia syndrome: a favorable outcome. *J Rheumatol.* 2003(Jan);30(1):154–9.

Gold AR, Dipalo F, Gold MS, Broderick J. Inspiratory airflow dynamics during sleep in women with fibromyalgia. *Sleep.* 2004;27:459–66.

Goldenberg D, Mayskiy M, Mossey C, Ruthazer R, Schmid C. A randomized, double-blind crossover trial of fluoxetine and amitriptyline in the treatment of fibromyalgia. *Arthritis Rheum.* 1996;39:1852–9.

Harding SM. Sleep in fibromyalgia patients: subjective and objective findings. *Am J Med Sci.* 1998(Jun);315(6):367–76.

Heymann RE, Helfenstein M, Feldman D. A double-blind, randomized, controlled study of amitriptyline, nortriptyline and placebo in patients with fibromyalgia. An analysis of outcome measures. *Clin Exp Rheumatol.* 2001(Nov–Dec);19(6):697–702.

Landis CA, Frey CA, Lentz MJ, Rothermel J, Buchwald D, Shaver JL. Self-reported sleep quality and fatigue correlates with actigraphy in midlife women with fibromyalgia. *Nurs Res.* 2003(May–Jun);52(3):140–7.

Landis CA, Lentz MJ, Rothermel J, Buchwald D, Shaver JL. Decreased sleep spindles and spindle activity in midlife women with fibromyalgia and pain. *Sleep.* 2004(Jun 15);27(4):741–50.

Mahowald ML, Mahowald MW. Nighttime sleep and daytime functioning (sleepiness and fatigue) in less well-defined chronic rheumatic diseases with particular reference to the 'alpha-delta NREM sleep anomaly.' *Sleep Med.* 2000(Jul 1);1(3):195–207.

Moldofsky H, Lue FA. The relationship of alpha and delta EEG frequencies to pain and mood in 'fibrositis' patients treated with chlorpromazine and L-tryptophan. *Electroencephalogr Clin Neurophysiol.* 1980(Oct);50(1–2):71–80.

Moldofsky H, Lue FA, Mously C, Roth-Schechter B, Reynolds WJ. The effect of zolpidem in patients with fibromyalgia: a dose ranging, double blind, placebo controlled, modified crossover study. *J Rheumatol.* 1996(Mar);23(3):529–33.

Okifuji A, Turk DC. Stress and psychophysiological dysregulation in patients with fibromyalgia syndrome. *Appl Psychophysiol Biofeedback.* 2002(Jun);27(2):129–41.

O'Malley PG, Balden E, Tomkins G, Santoro J, Kroenke K, Jackson JL. Treatment of fibromyalgia with antidepressants: a meta-analysis. *J Gen Intern Med.* 2000(Sep);15(9):659–66.

Rains JC, Penzien DB. Sleep and chronic pain: challenges to the alpha-EEG sleep pattern as a pain specific sleep anomaly. *J Psychosom Res.* 2003(Jan);54(1):77–83.

Roehrs T, Roth T. Sleep and pain: interaction of two vital functions. *Semin Neurol.* 2005(Mar); 25(1):106–16.

Roizenblatt S, Moldofsky H, Benedito-Silva AA, Tufik S. Alpha sleep characteristics in fibromyalgia. *Arthritis Rheum.* 2001(Jan);44(1):222–30.

Schaefer KM. Sleep disturbances and fatigue in women with fibromyalgia and chronic fatigue syndrome. *JOGNN.* 1995;24:229–33.

Scharf MB, Baumann M, Berkowitz DV. The effects of sodium oxybate on clinical symptoms and sleep patterns in patients with fibromyalgia. *J Rheumatol.* 2003(May);30(5):1070–4.

Wilson KG, Watson ST, Currie SR. Daily diary and ambulatory activity monitoring of sleep in patients with insomnia associated with chronic musculoskeletal pain. *Pain.* 1998(Mar);75(1):75–84.

Wolfe F, Smythe HA, Yunus MB, Bennett RM, Bombardier C, Goldenberg DL,, et al. The American College of Rheumatology 1990 Criteria for the Classification of Fibromyalgia. Report of the Multicenter Criteria Committee. *Arthritis Rheum.* 1990(Feb);33(2):160–72.

Sleep in the Intensive Care Unit

Aurell J, Elmqvist D. Sleep in the surgical intensive care unit: continuous polygraphic recording of sleep in nine patients receiving postoperative care. *Br Med J.* 1985;290:1029–1032.

Bentley S, Murphy F, Dudley H. Perceived noise in surgical wards and an intensive care area: an objective analysis. *Br Med J.* 1977;2:1503–1506.

Broughton R, Baron R. Sleep patterns in the intensive care unit and on the ward after acute myocardial infarction. *Electroencephalogr Clin Neurophysiol.* 1978;45:348–360.

Buckle P, Pouliot Z, Millar T, et al. Polysomnography in acutely ill intensive care unit patients. *Chest.* 1992;102:288–291.

Easton C, MacKenzie F. Sensory-perceptual alterations: delirium in the intensive care unit. *Heart Lung.* 1988;17:229–237.

Findley LJ, Zwillich CW, Ancoli-Israel S, et al. Cheyne-Stokes breathing during sleep in patients with left ventricular heart failure. *Southern Medical Journal.* 1985;78:11–15.

Freedman NS, Gazendam J, Levan L, et al. Abnormal sleep/ wake cycles and the effect of environmental noise on sleep disruption in the intensive care unit. *Am J Respir Crit Care Med.* 2001;163:451–457.

Freedman NS, Kotzer N, Schwab RJ. Patient perception of sleep quality and etiology of sleep disruption in the intensive care unit. *Am J Respir Crit Care Med.* 1999;159:1155–1162.

Hanly PJ, Millar TW, Steljes Dg, et al. Respiration and abnormal sleep in patients with congestive heart failure. *Chest.* 1989;96:480–488.

Heller S, Kornfeld D. Psychiatric aspects of cardiac surgery. *Advances in Psychosomatic Medicine.* 1986;15:124–139.

Helton MC, Gordon SH, Nunnery SL. The correlation between sleep deprivation and the intensive care unit syndrome. *Heart Lung.* 1980;9:464–468.

Meyer TJ, Eveloff SE, Bauer MS, et al. Adverse environmental conditions in the respiratory and medical ICU settings. *Chest.* 1994;105:1211–1216.

Orr WC, Stahl ML. Sleep disturbances after open heart surgery. *Am J Cardiol.* 1977;39:196–201.

Schwab RJ. Disturbances of sleep in the intensive care unit. *Crit Care Clin.* 1994;10:681–694.

Walder B, Francioli D, Meyer JJ, et al. Effects of guidelines implementation in a surgical intensive care unit to control nighttime light and noise levels. *Crit Care Med.* 2000;28:2242–2247.

Sleep in Neurologic Disorders 10

Dementia

Alzheimer disease is the most common degenerative disorder of the central nervous system that causes dementia. Fragmentation and repetitive arousals/awakenings characterize the sleep of persons with dementia. Confusion, agitation, and wandering can occur at night ("sun downing"), further contributing to sleep disruption (Box 10–1). Sleep complaints may be due primarily to the underlying dementia or to related sleep-disordered breathing, periodic limb movements of sleep, or secondary depression. Reversal of the sleep-wake rhythms can be seen with patients complaining of nocturnal insomnia and excessive daytime sleepiness. Polysomnography may demonstrate decreases in rapid eye movement (REM) sleep time and REM density. Sleep efficiency is reduced.

Box 10-1. Dementia and sleep	Sleep fragmentation
	Repetitive arousals and awakenings
	"Sun downing"
	Reversal of the sleep-wake rhythms with nocturnal insomnia and excessive daytime sleepiness
	Polysomnographic features
	↓ Sleep efficiency
	↓ REM sleep
	↓ REM density

Management includes proper sleep hygiene practices (eg, avoiding caffeine, maintaining a regular sleep schedule, and eliminating daytime naps), and treatment of concurrent depression and medical disorders, including pain syndromes, that might contribute to sleep disturbance. Short-term use of hypnotics, such as zolpidem, zaleplon, or eszopiclone, may be tried for insomnia.

Neurodegenerative Disorders

The cerebral degenerative disorders constitute a large group of neurologic conditions that have, in common, abnormalities in movement and behavior. Included in this category are Huntington disease, dystonia, ataxia, olivopontocerebellar and spinocerebellar degeneration, spastic torticollis, and musculorum deformans. Muscular contractions and gross body movements are prominent during sleep. REM sleep behavior disorder may develop. Affected individuals may complain of both sleep-onset and sleep-maintenance insomnia. Polysomnographic features include an increase in frequency of awakenings as well as a decrease in non–rapid eye movement (NREM)stages 3 and 4 sleep and REM sleep. Sleep efficiency is diminished (Box 10–2).

Huntington Disease

Clinical features of Huntington disease consist of relentlessly progressive chorea and dementia. It is transmitted as an autosomal dominant disorder with the affected gene linked to the short arm of chromosome 4. Insomnia and sleep fragmentation are common in patients with advanced disease. Chorea can persist during NREM stages 1 and 2 sleep.

Box 10-2.

Neurodegenerative disorders and sleep

Muscular contractions and gross body movements occurring during sleep

REM sleep behavior disorder

Insomnia

Polysomnographic features

↓ Sleep efficiency

↑ Frequency of awakenings

↓ NREM stages 3 and 4 sleep

↓ REM sleep

SPECIFIC DISORDERS

1. Huntington disease–insomnia and sleep fragmentation

2. Progressive supranuclear palsy–sleep disruption and insomnia

3. Torsion dystonia–sleep deterioration and dystonia during sleep

Progressive Supranuclear Palsy

Progressive supranuclear palsy is characterized by impairment of eye movements, disturbances of gait, and dystonia. Sleep disruption and insomnia are common complaints.

Torsion Dystonia

In torsion dystonia (dystonia musculorum deformans), abnormally contorted, twisting, or jerking movements may occur. Sleep deteriorates as disease progresses. Dystonia may be observed during NREM stages 1 and 2 sleep, and, occasionally, during REM sleep as well.

Parkinson Disease

Patients with Parkinson disease characteristically present with rigidity, resting tremor, akinesia or bradykinesia (absent or diminished movements), and loss of postural reflexes. Pathologic features of Parkinson disease consist of intracytoplasmic eosinophilic inclusions (Lewy bodies), and loss of neurons in the substantia nigra. Poor sleep is a major complaint of persons with Parkinson disease, especially in advanced disease, and patients may describe either excessive sleepiness due to sleep fragmentation or insomnia (Box 10–3).

Sleep disturbance in Parkinson disease is multifactorial. The etiology is described in Box 10–3. Muscle spasms, decreased spontaneous body movements, painful leg cramps, repetitive body movements such as tremors, and difficulty with turning in bed secondary to rigidity can contribute to poor sleep quality. Tremors often diminish during sleep and reemerges during arousals from sleep. Circadian rhythm disorders including reversal of sleep-wake schedules have been described. Akathisia, myoclonus, frightening dreams, and dyskinesias (dystonic or choreiform) related to the use of antiparkinsonian medications can give rise to sleep fragmentation. Finally, sleep disturbance in patients with Parkinson disease may be associated with concurrent dementia, mood disorder, or

Box 10-3. **Parkinson disease and sleep**	Excessive sleepiness due to sleep fragmentation Insomnia Reversal of sleep-wake schedules **ETIOLOGY OF SLEEP DISTURBANCE:** 1. Muscle spasms, decreased spontaneous body movements, painful leg cramps, repetitive body movements such as tremors, and difficulty with turning in bed secondary to rigidity 2. Circadian rhythm disorders 3. Adverse effects of medications 4. Concurrent dementia, mood disorder, or other sleep disorders

other sleep disorders (eg, periodic limb movements of sleep, restless legs syndrome, and parasomnias such as REM sleep behavior disorder). Respiratory abnormalities such as obstructive and central apneas and hypopneas may develop, particularly in patients with autonomic dysfunction.

Sleep-Related Headaches

Although some headaches occur during both sleep and wakefulness (eg, migraine, cluster headache, and chronic paroxysmal hemicrania), others occur only during sleep (eg, hypnic headaches) (Table 10–1). Migraines, cluster headaches, and chronic paroxysmal hemicrania commonly have their onset during sleep. Headaches may either cause an awakening during the night or be experienced on awakening. Headaches can cause sleep disruption and insomnia. Morning headaches have been described in patients with obstructive sleep apnea. Polysomnography may demonstrate a decrease in total sleep time and increase in frequency of arousals (Box 10–4).

Table 10-1. Headache syndromes

Syndrome	Clinical features	Sleep disorder
Migraine headaches	Episodic headaches, often unilateral, associated with nausea/vomiting, photophobia and phonophobia An aura consisting of scintillating scotomas and homonymous visual field defects precedes a "classic migraine." An aura does not accompany a "common migraine." Can occur during sleep or wakefulness	Headaches can be triggered by changes in sleep patterns. Headaches can be associated with NREM stages 3 and 4 sleep or REM sleep.

Table 10-1. Headache syndromes—cont'd

Syndrome	Clinical features	Sleep disorder
Cluster headaches	Excruciating, unilateral (periorbital or temporal) headaches with a rapid onset and a peak within several minutes Occur more frequently among men. During cluster periods, one to three headache attacks occur daily, often at the same hour each day, over a 1- to 2-month period. Individual attacks typically last a few hours. Associated features include lacrimation, conjunctival injection, rhinorrhea or nasal stuffiness, miosis, ptosis, and increased ipsilateral forehead sweating.	Headaches tend to occur during sleep, particularly during REM sleep. Obstructive sleep apnea is a known trigger.
Chronic paroxysmal hemicrania	Severe unilateral headache (eg, temporal, orbital or supraorbital) Responsive to therapy with indomethacin	Most commonly associated with REM sleep
Hypnic headaches	Generalized or unilateral headaches that occur during sleep and awaken the patient Headaches occur more frequently among the elderly and can be accompanied by nausea but not autonomic manifestations. Respond to therapy with lithium	Most common during REM sleep and, less commonly, during NREM stage 3 and 4 sleep
Exploding head syndrome	Patient is awakened with a sound or sensation of explosion in the head. May represent a form of sleep start or hypnic jerk and is classified as a parasomnia	Occurs during the transition from wakefulness to sleep

Miscellaneous headaches	Many headaches occur during sleep or on awakening, including those related to:
	    Obstructive sleep apnea
	    Hypertension
	    Central nervous system tumors
	    Depression	

Box 10-4. **Headaches and sleep**	Sleep disruption and insomnia
	Onset of migraines, cluster headaches and chronic paroxysmal hemicrania commonly during sleep
	Migraine headaches during NREM stages 3 and 4 sleep or REM sleep
	Cluster headaches during sleep, particularly during REM sleep
	Association of chronic paroxysmal hemicrania with REM sleep
	Hypnic headaches during REM sleep and, less commonly, during NREM stage 3 sleep
	Exploding head syndrome during the transition from wakefulness to sleep
	Occurence of hypnic headaches only during sleep
	Morning headaches in patients with OSA

	Polysomnographic features of headache syndromes:
	    ↓ Total sleep time
	    ↑ Frequency of arousals

Sleep-Related Epilepsy

Seizures are characterized by recurrent, abnormal, and stereotypic events that are produced by discrete cortical neuronal discharges. Recurrent seizures are referred to as epilepsy. Seizures can be classified based on their onset as *partial* (ie, focal onset that may or may not subsequently generalize) or *generalized* (ie, arises simultaneously from both cerebral hemispheres).

Partial seizures (eg, frontal and temporal lobe epilepsies) are often evident during NREM sleep. They can be further subdivided into two subtypes:

1. Simple partial seizures occur without a change of consciousness.

2. Complex partial seizures occur with loss of consciousness. They commonly originate from the temporal or frontal lobes and can be associated with localized sensorimotor manifestations, wanderings, and automatisms, such as lip smacking, vocalization, or sleepwalking.

Generalized seizures can occur during awakenings from sleep. They consist of three major subtypes:

1. Generalized tonic-clonic seizures are characterized by both tonic (sustained muscle contraction) and clonic (muscle jerks) phases. Confusion and disorientation are commonly present in the period following seizures.

2. Absence seizures (petit mal) consist of periods of unconsciousness and blank staring with typical diffuse 3 to 4 Hz spike and wave electroencephalographic (EEG) discharges.

3. Juvenile myoclonic seizures present with muscle jerks after awakenings from sleep.

EEG activity consists of two separate phases: ictal (occurring during seizures) and interictal (occurring between periods of seizures). Ictal discharges can appear as spike waves, repetitive sharp waves, slowing, fast activity, or spike-wave patterns. Interictal discharges often manifests as isolated spike waves or spike waves followed by slow waves.

For more information about seizures, see Tables 10–2 and 10–3.

Table 10-2. Classification of seizures based on type

Continuous spike waves during NREM sleep	Formerly referred to as electrical status epilepticus of sleep Generalized continuous EEG spike and slow-wave complexes occur continuously throughout NREM sleep with or without any apparent movements or clinical complaints. EEG discharges decrease during REM sleep and disappear with awakening. It is seen in children, many of whom have an underlying seizure disorder. The disorder lasts for several months to years, and tends to resolve within three years with increasing age. Seizures typically have a favorable response to antiseizure medications. Complications include neurocognitive and motor impairment.
Benign epilepsy of childhood with centrotemporal spikes (benign rolandic epilepsy)	Perioral numbness and clonic focal twitching of the face and mouth occur during drowsiness and sleep. Secondarily generalized tonic-clonic seizures may develop. EEG demonstrates rolandic or centrotemporal spike and sharp waves. Interictal discharges (diphasic sharp waves) increase during sleep. Onset is during childhood, with spontaneous resolution during the teenage years or adulthood.
Juvenile myoclonic epilepsy	Bilateral massive myoclonic jerks occur soon after awakening. Episodes can be precipitated by sleep deprivation or alcohol use. The epilepsy generally develops during adolescence. Myoclonic jerks may precede seizures by 1 to 4 years. EEG can demonstrate symmetric and synchronous 4–6 Hz polyspike and wave discharges.
Nocturnal frontal lobe epilepsy	Characterized by abnormal behaviors (eg, sleep terrors or sleepwalking), arousals, or nocturnal paroxysmal dystonia. Because it may originate in deeper brain structures, there is typically no evident abnormal ictal or interictal EEG activity. Onset is generally during childhood. This condition can result in sleep disturbance and daytime sleepiness. A majority of affected individuals respond favorably to antiseizure medications, including carbamazepine.

Table 10-3. Classification of seizures based on location

Frontal lobe	Consciousness is maintained and postseizure confusion is minimal. There is often no abnormal interictal EEG discharges. They usually occur only during sleep. Clinical features vary depending on the location of the seizure focus: 1. "Jacksonian march," with seizure activity starting at the distal part of the extremity and moving proximally, is associated with onset in the posterior frontal lobes. 2. Onset from midline regions can give rise to complex motor activity, such as vocalizations and dystonic posturing. 3. Seizures starting from the cingulated gyrus can present with automatisms, staring, and autonomic features (eg, tachycardia and tachypnea).
Temporal lobe	Seizures occur often only during sleep and are generally accompanied by impaired consciousness and postictal confusion. They begin focally. Automatisms, including lip smacking and other facial, body, and extremity movements, are typical. Seizures are most common during NREM sleep; some can be observed at the NREM-REM sleep transition. Interictal discharges, consisting of spike waves, can be present.

Nocturnal Seizures

Sleep is a recognized precipitant of seizure activity. Sleep-related seizures have an estimated prevalence of 10% to 40%. It is estimated that about 25% of persons with epilepsy have their seizures mostly restricted to sleep.

There are two peaks in the occurrence of nocturnal seizures, the first about 2 hours after bedtime, and the second from 4:00 to 5:00 AM. Generally, sleep-related seizures occur more frequently during NREM sleep (most commonly in stages 1 and 2 sleep, and occasionally in stages 3 and 4 as well) than REM sleep. Seizure thresholds are greater during REM sleep compared to NREM sleep (Box 10–5).

Box 10–5. **Seizures and sleep**	Two peaks in the occurrence of nocturnal seizures, the first one about 2 hours after bedtime, and the second one from 4 to 5 am
	Occurence of sleep-related seizures more commonly during NREM sleep (most commonly in stages 1 and 2 sleep, and occasionally in stages 3 and 4 as well) than REM sleep
	Partial seizures (eg, frontal and temporal lobe epilepsies) during NREM sleep
	Generalized seizures during awakenings from sleep
	Insomnia, frequent nighttime awakenings or excessive sleepiness
	Precipitation or exacerbation of nocturnal seizures by sleep deprivation, irregular sleep schedules, or concurrent sleep disorders, such as obstructive sleep apnea
	Polysomnographic features: ↑ Sleep latency ↑ Wake time after sleep onset ↑ NREM stages 1 and 2 sleep ↓ NREM stages 3 and 4 sleep ↓ REM sleep

Certain seizures occur predominantly or exclusively during sleep. These include (1) continuous spike waves during NREM sleep, (2) benign epilepsy of childhood with centrotemporal spikes, (3) generalized tonic-clonic seizures, (5) juvenile myoclonic epilepsy, (5) nocturnal frontal lobe epilepsy, and (6) tonic seizures. In addition, some partial complex seizures (frontal and temporal lobe epilepsies) can present during sleep.

Clinical features suggestive of sleep-related seizures include abrupt awakenings, abnormal motor activity (eg, generalized tonic clonic movements, focal movements, automatisms, tongue biting, nocturnal wandering, vocalizations, or parasomnia-like events), and urinary incontinence. Confusion may be evident following episodes.

Nocturnal seizures may be clinically asymptomatic. In instances when repetitive seizures occur during sleep, insomnia due to frequent nighttime awakenings may result. Sleep fragmentation can also lead to excessive sleepiness. Nocturnal seizures can be precipitated or exacerbated by sleep deprivation, irregular sleep schedules, and concurrent sleep disorders, such as obstructive sleep apnea. Sleep deprivation can increase seizure discharges, particularly during the transition from wakefulness to sleep.

Differential Diagnosis

Differential diagnosis includes a variety of parasomnias such as disorders of arousal or REM sleep behavior disorder, rhythmic movement disorder, bruxism, periodic limb movements of sleep, and pseudoseizures. With a pseudoseizure, onset and termination of "out-of-phase" muscle movements are gradual, there is no postictal confusion, and ictal and interictal EEG discharges are absent.

Evaluation

Diagnosis of sleep-related seizures requires an expanded EEG montage, with additional electrodes over the frontal and temporal areas. Video-polysomnography aided by sleep technologist observations may facilitate diagnosis. At the usual polysomnography rate of 30 seconds per page, spikes often appear as upward vertical deflections with duration of about 20–70 milliseconds. Interictal discharges may be evident as repetitive sharp activity.

Ictal discharges are common during NREM sleep in partial seizures. For both partial and generalized seizures, interictal discharges are common during NREM sleep and rare during REM sleep. Interictal discharges in partial epilepsies appear as an increase in the frequency of spikes in a localized distribution during NREM stages 2 (most common), 3 and 4 sleep. Phasic arousals can accompany interictal discharges.

A crucial distinction is between seizure discharges and EEG artifacts such as electrode popping, both of which can give rise to high-amplitude sharp waves. Examining the EEG at a faster rate by changing from a 30-second page to a 10-second page polysomnography view can help distinguish these two conditions.

Polysomnography

Polysomnography may demonstrate both ictal and interictal EEG epileptiform activity. Nonetheless, a normal EEG does not exclude a diagnosis of seizures. A majority of seizures occur during NREM sleep, especially stages 1 and 2 sleep, and they are less common during REM sleep. Changes in sleep architecture associated with seizures include increases in sleep latency, wake time after sleep onset, and NREM stages 1 and 2 sleep, and decrease in both NREM stages 3 and 4 sleep and REM sleep (Box 10–5).

Neuromuscular Disorders

A variety of neuromuscular disorders, such as amyotrophic lateral sclerosis, myotonic dystrophy, poliomyelitis, postpolio syndrome, or proximal myotonic myopathy are associated with sleep disturbances, including insomnia, excessive sleepiness, sleep fragmentation, sleep-related hypoventilation, and sleep apnea syndromes (Box 10–6).

Box 10-6. **Neuromuscular disorders and sleep**	Sleep disturbances, including insomnia, excessive sleepiness, sleep fragmentation, sleep-related hypoventilation, and sleep apnea syndromes 1. Amyotrophic lateral sclerosis—excessive sleepiness secondary to sleep fragmentation, insomnia, and sleep-related breathing disorder 2. Myasthenia gravis—both obstructive and central apneas 3. Myotonic dystrophy—both obstructive and central apneas, as well as alveolar hypoventilation 4. Poliomyelitis and postpolio syndrome—sleep-related breathing disorder and hypoventilation

Patients with neuromuscular disorders may develop respiratory failure that requires either nocturnal or continuous ventilatory support (eg, positive or negative pressure ventilation). Upper airway obstruction may complicate therapy with negative pressure ventilation.

Amyotrophic Lateral Sclerosis

Patients with amyotrophic lateral sclerosis may complain of excessive sleepiness secondary to sleep fragmentation, or insomnia. Sleep-related breathing disorders can occur as a result of destruction of respiratory neurons (central apneas) or upper airway muscle dysfunction (obstructive apneas). Respiratory failure with hypoxemia and hypercapnia can develop in advanced disease.

Myasthenia Gravis

Both obstructive and central apneas can develop in patients with myasthenia gravis. Respiratory insufficiency can result in oxygen desaturation.

Myotonic Dystrophy

Sleep-related breathing disorders (obstructive and central sleep apnea), alveolar hypoventilation, and nocturnal hypoxemia can complicate the course of myotonic dystrophy, giving rise to sleep disturbance and excessive sleepiness.

Poliomyelitis and Postpolio Syndrome

Sleep disordered breathing can develop during acute poliomyelitis. Hypoventilation can complicate the course of postpolio syndrome.

Mental Retardation and Developmental Disorders

The effects of mental retardation and developmental disorders on sleep are presented in Box 10–7.

Box 10-7.	**MENTAL RETARDATION**
Mental retardation, developmental disorders, and sleep	Insomnia (sleep-onset and early morning awakenings) and frequent night wakings
	Polysomnographic features
	$\uparrow$ Frequency of arousals and awakenings
	DEVELOPMENTAL DISORDERS
	Asperger disorder
	Insomnia
	Polysomnographic features
	$\downarrow$ Sleep time during the first part of the night

(continued from page 368)
Box 10-7.

Mental retardation, developmental disorders, and sleep

Autistic disorder

    Subjective sleep complaints and objective sleep disturbances

Rett disorder

    Polysomnographic features

        ↑ Total sleep time

        ↑ Daytime sleep

        ↓ Nighttime sleep

Mental Retardation

In mental retardation, considerably below average intellect develops prior to 18 years of age. Sleep complaints include insomnia (sleep-onset and early morning awakenings) and frequent night wakings. The severity of sleep disturbance is correlated with the degree of intellectual impairment. Polysomnography demonstrates increase in frequency of arousals and awakenings.

Developmental Disorders

Developmental disorders, including Asperger disorder, autistic disorder, and Rett disorder, are characterized either by a delay or abnormal development of language skills and social interaction (Table 10–4). Associated features include stereotypical activities or behavior and a restricted range of interests. Symptoms commonly manifest early in life.

Table 10-4. Developmental disorders

Disorder	Characteristics	Sleep disturbances
Asperger disorder	Asperger syndrome is characterized by stereotypical activities and behavior that are associated with significant impairment in daytime functioning and social interaction. Cognitive and language development are normal. Men are affected more commonly than women.	Insomnia is common. Changes in sleep architecture consist of a decrease in sleep time during the first part of the night and REM sleep disruption.
Autistic disorder	Autistic individuals have delays or abnormal functioning in communicative skills and social interaction as well as a limited range of activities. Impairments start early in life, typically prior to 3 years of age.	Subjective sleep complaints and objective sleep disturbances may be present in some autistic individuals.
Rett disorder	Characterized by sleep disturbance, developmental delay, seizures, cognitive dysfunction, bruxism, and hyperventilation and breathholding while awake. Speech impairment starts within the first 18 months of age.	Associated sleep disturbances include an increase in total sleep time with an increase in daytime sleep and decrease in nighttime sleep.

Table 10–4.   Developmental disorders—cont'd

Disorder	Characteristics	Sleep disturbances
	Individuals with Rett syndrome develop a variety of deficits (eg, gait incoordination, psychomotor retardation, head growth deceleration, impairment of language development, and stereotypical hand motions) following a period of normal psychomotor development during the first few months after birth. Rett disorder has been reported only in females. Some cases are related to mutations in MECP2 gene in chromosome X.	

Abnormal Movements during Sleep

There is a progressive diminution of muscle tone from wakefulness, through NREM sleep, and reaching either maximum hypotonia or atonia during REM sleep. Similarly, reflexes, both mono-synaptic and polysynaptic, progressively diminish during NREM and REM sleep. These phenomena are due to motor neuron hyperpolarization during NREM sleep. During REM sleep, further hyperpolarization occurs with intermittent breakthrough evident as phasic REM sleep muscle activity.

A variety of movements can occur during sleep. These can be physiologic processes, such as episodic body movements and postural changes, or abnormal disorders including periodic limb movements of sleep. Movements are most common during sleep-wake transitions and NREM stages 1 and 2 sleep, and REM sleep; they appear to be least common during NREM stages 3 and 4 sleep (Table 10–5).

Other Central Nervous System Conditions

Many other central nervous system conditions are associated with sleep disturbances or can complicate the course of primary sleep disorders (Table 10–6).

Table 10-5.	Timing of occurrence	Sleep disorders
Occurrence of movements during sleep	Prior to sleep onset	Restless legs syndrome
	At sleep onset	Propriospinal myoclonus Rhythmic movement disorder Sleep starts
	First half of sleep	Disorders of arousal (sleepwalking, sleep terrors, confusional arousals)
	Later half of sleep	Nightmares REM sleep behavior disorder
	Throughout sleep	Bruxism Medication-induced movement disorders Neonatal sleep myoclonus Nocturnal leg cramps Obstructive sleep apnea Periodic limb movement disorder Physiologic and excessive fragmentary myoclonus Postural shifts Seizures and pseudoseizures Sleep talking

Table 10-6. Central nervous system conditions that disturb sleep

Cerebrovascular disease	Patients with stroke may complain of recurrent awakenings and insomnia. Subdural hematomas may give rise to excessive sleepiness. The presence of OSA increases the risk of cerebrovascular disease. Conversely, stroke may increase the risk of developing OSA. Ondine's curse has been described following brainstem strokes.
Central nervous system infections	West Nile virus infection, encephalitis, meningitis, trypanosomiasis and neurosyphilis may present with excessive sleepiness.
Central nervous system neoplasms	Tumors involving the CNS can give rise to either insomnia or excessive sleepiness. Daytime hypersomnolence may be secondary to increased intracranial pressure resulting from tumors involving midline structures (eg, hypothalamus or brainstem). Nocturnal seizure activity or abnormal movements and behavior may also be observed.
Encephalopathy	Wernicke encephalopathy is associated with excessive sleepiness.
Multiple sclerosis	Either excessive sleepiness or insomnia can occur.

Continued

Table 10-6. Central nervous system conditions that disturb sleep—cont'd

Multiple system atrophy	Previously referred to as Shy Drager syndrome, multiple system atrophy is a multisystemic neurodegenerative disorder characterized by progressive autonomic dysfunction or failure as well as cerebellar and extrapyramidal (eg, parkinsonism) symptoms. Onset is during adulthood. Sleep disorders include sleep-related respiratory abnormalities (obstructive and central apneas and hypopneas), insomnia, and REM sleep behavior disorder. Common polysomnographic features include: ↓ Sleep efficiency ↑ Frequent of awakenings ↓ Total sleep time ↓ NREM stages 3 and 4 sleep ↓ REM sleep
Spinal cord disease	High spinal cord disease can result in both excessive sleepiness and insomnia due to chronic pain or muscle spasms. Sleep-related breathing disorders such as obstructive sleep apnea can also give rise to excessive sleepiness.
Traumatic brain injury	Insomnia or excessive sleepiness can complicate traumatic brain injuries. Sleep apnea syndromes and circadian rhythm sleep disturbances (eg, delayed sleep phase syndrome) can also occur. Polysomnography can reveal a decrease in total sleep time and an increase in the frequency of awakenings.
Tourette syndrome	This is characterized by repetitive motor and verbal tics. It may be associated with parasomnias such as disorders of arousal (eg, confusional arousals, sleepwalking, and sleep terrors). Onset of the disorder is often during childhood. During polysomnography, tics may be observed during sleep, particularly NREM stages 1 and 2 sleep.

References

General References

American Academy of Sleep Medicine. *The International Classification of Sleep Disorders: Diagnostic and Coding Manual.* 2nd ed. Westchester, IL: American Academy of Sleep Medicine, 2005.

Bowman. *Review of Sleep Medicine.* Burlington, MA: Butterworth-Heinemann, 2002.

Berry RB. *Sleep Medicine Pearls.* 2nd ed. Philadelphia, PA: Hanley & Belfus, 2002.

Chokroverty S. *Clinical Companion to Sleep Disorders Medicine.* 2nd ed. Butterworth-Heinemann, 2000.

Hoyt BD. Sleep in patients with neurologic and psychiatric disorders. *Sleep Medicine.* Primary Care: Clinics in Office Practice. Elsevier Saunders, 2005.

Lavie P, Pillar G, Malhotra A. *Sleep Disorders Handbook.* New York, NY: Taylor & Francis, 2002.

Lee-Chiong TL, ed. *Sleep: A Comprehensive Handbook.* Hoboken, NJ: John Wiley & Sons, 2006.

Lee-Chiong TL, Sateia M, Carskadon M, eds. *Sleep Medicine*. Philadelphia, PA: Hanley & Belfus (Elsevier), 2002.

Perlis ML, Lichstein KL, eds. *Treating Sleep Disorders: Principles and Practice of Behavioral Sleep Medicine*. Hoboken, NJ: John Wiley & Sons, 2003.

Rechtschaffen A, Kales A. *A Manual of Standardized Terminology, Techniques and Scoring System for Sleep Stages of Human Subjects*. Los Angeles, CA: Brain Information Service/Brain Research Institute, University of California, 1968.

Reite M, Ruddy J, Nagel K. *Concise Guide to Evaluation and Management of Sleep Disorders*. 3rd ed. Arlington, VA: American Psychiatric Publishing, April 2002.

Sleep Disorders. Medical Clinics of North America. Philadelphia, PA: Elsevier Saunders, 2004.

Sleep Medicine. Primary Care: Clinics in Office Practice. Philadelphia, PA: Elsevier Saunders, 2005.

Sleep Research Society. *SRS Basics of Sleep Guide*. Westchester, IL: Sleep Research Society, 2005.

Dementia

Vitiello MV. Alzheimer's dementia. In: Lee-Chiong TL, ed. *Sleep: A Comprehensive Handbook*. Hoboken, NJ: John Wiley & Sons, 2006.

Neurodegenerative Disorders

Harper DG. Neurodegenerative disorders. In: Lee-Chiong TL, ed. *Sleep: A Comprehensive Handbook*. Hoboken, NJ: John Wiley & Sons, 2006.

Parkinson Disease

Chokroverty S. *Clinical Companion to Sleep Disorders Medicine*. 2nd ed. Butterworth-Heinemann, 2000.

Lee-Chiong TL, ed. *Sleep: A Comprehensive Handbook*. Hoboken, NJ: John Wiley & Sons, 2006.

Lee-Chiong TL, Sateia M, Carskadon M, eds. *Sleep Medicine*. Philadelphia, PA: Hanley & Belfus (Elsevier), 2002.

Silber MH. Parkinson's disease. In: Lee-Chiong TL, ed. *Sleep: A Comprehensive Handbook*. Hoboken, NJ: John Wiley & Sons, 2006.

Sleep-Related Headaches

Greenough GP. Headaches and sleep. In: Lee-Chiong TL, ed. *Sleep: A Comprehensive Handbook*. Hoboken, NJ: John Wiley & Sons, 2006.

Sleep-Related Epilepsy

Chokroverty S. *Clinical Companion to Sleep Disorders Medicine*. 2nd ed. Butterworth-Heinemann, 2000.

Lee-Chiong TL, ed. *Sleep: A Comprehensive Handbook*. Hoboken, NJ: John Wiley & Sons, 2006.

Lee-Chiong TL, Sateia M, Carskadon M, eds. *Sleep Medicine.* Philadelphia, PA: Hanley & Belfus (Elsevier), 2002.

Shouse MN. Seizures. In: Lee-Chiong TL, ed. *Sleep: A Comprehensive Handbook.* Hoboken, NJ: John Wiley & Sons, 2006.

Neuromuscular Disorders

Chokroverty S. *Clinical Companion to Sleep Disorders Medicine.* 2nd ed. Butterworth-Heinemann, 2000.

Lee-Chiong TL, ed. *Sleep: A Comprehensive Handbook.* Hoboken, NJ: John Wiley & Sons, 2006.

Lee-Chiong TL, Sateia M, Carskadon M, eds. *Sleep Medicine.* Philadelphia, PA: Hanley & Belfus (Elsevier), 2002.

Mental Retardation and Developmental Disorders

Chokroverty S. *Clinical Companion to Sleep Disorders Medicine.* 2nd ed. Butterworth-Heinemann, 2000.

Lee-Chiong TL, ed. *Sleep: A Comprehensive Handbook.* Hoboken, NJ: John Wiley & Sons, 2006.

Lee-Chiong TL, Sateia M, Carskadon M, eds. *Sleep Medicine.* Philadelphia, PA: Hanley & Belfus (Elsevier), 2002.

Abnormal Movements during Sleep

Chokroverty S. *Clinical Companion to Sleep Disorders Medicine.* 2nd ed. Butterworth-Heinemann, 2000.

Lee-Chiong TL, ed. *Sleep: A Comprehensive Handbook.* Hoboken, NJ: John Wiley & Sons, 2006.

Lee-Chiong TL, Sateia M, Carskadon M, eds. *Sleep Medicine.* Philadelphia, PA: Hanley & Belfus (Elsevier), 2002.

Other Central Nervous System Conditions

Castriotta RJ. Brain and spinal cord injury. In: Lee-Chiong TL, ed. *Sleep: A Comprehensive Handbook.* Hoboken, NJ: John Wiley & Sons, 2006.

Chokroverty S. *Clinical Companion to Sleep Disorders Medicine.* 2nd ed. Butterworth-Heinemann, 2000.

Lee-Chiong TL, ed. *Sleep: A Comprehensive Handbook.* Hoboken, NJ: John Wiley & Sons, 2006.

Lee-Chiong TL, Sateia M, Carskadon M, eds. *Sleep Medicine.* Philadelphia, PA: Hanley & Belfus (Elsevier), 2002.

Psychiatric and Behavioral Disorders

11

A complicated interface exists between psychiatric and sleep disorders—psychiatric symptoms are amplified and aggravated by sleep disruption, and the pathology of psychiatric disorders may contribute to worsening sleep quality. In addition, persons with insomnia are at higher risk of developing a new psychiatric disorder, particularly major depression, within a year of the onset of insomnia.

Psychiatric disorders can give rise to insomnia, excessive sleepiness, or parasomnias (eg, nightmares or sleep terrors) (Boxes 11–1 and 11–2).. It has been estimated that a third to a half of cases of chronic insomnia are associated with a psychiatric condition. Changes in sleep architecture include a decrease in rapid eye movement (REM) sleep latency that is seen with depressive episodes, schizophrenia, and borderline personality disorder.

Box 11–1.

Psychiatric disorders associated with insomnia[a]

Bipolar disorder

Depression

Generalized anxiety disorder

Obsessive-compulsive disorder

Panic disorder

Personality disorders

Post-traumatic stress disorder

Schizophrenia

[a] Insomnia (difficulty initiating or maintaining sleep, or nonrestorative sleep) with a duration of at least 1 month and associated with distress and functional impairments, including daytime fatigue.

Box 11–2.

Psychiatric disorders associated with excessive sleepiness[a]

Atypical depression

Seasonal affective disorder

[a]Excessive sleepiness (daytime sleep episodes or increase in duration of nighttime sleep episodes) with a duration of at least 1 month and associated with distress and functional impairments, including daytime fatigue.

Schizophrenia

Schizophrenia (psychosis) is a chronic psychiatric disorder characterized by both "positive symptoms" (eg, hallucinations, delusions, and disorganized speech and behavior) and "negative symptoms" (eg, affective flattening, avolition [limited goal-directed behavior], and alogia [restricted thought and speech production]). This disabling condition has a median age of onset between 15 and 25 years of age. Course is chronic with significant impairments in self-care, interpersonal interactions, and work performance.

Sleep disturbance is an integral symptom of schizophrenia and often markedly worsens during exacerbations of psychotic symptoms. Sleep disruption can aggravate psychosis; conversely, increased sensitivity to external stimuli in schizophrenia increases sleep disruption. Use of antipsychotic medications and poor sleep hygiene also contribute to the disturbed sleep seen in patients.

Insomnia is common in schizophrenia and can involve disturbances with either sleep onset or maintenance. Wakefulness can be maintained for prolonged periods and terminated only by exhaustion. In addition, there may be a reversal of the day-night sleep patterns, increase in sleep during the daytime, polyphasic sleep episodes, and alternating phases of sleeplessness and hypersomnolence. Rebound sleepiness with an increase in sleep efficiency can occur during the waning phase of schizophrenia or during residual schizophrenia. Furthermore, many antipsychotic medications can produce significant sedation. Patients with schizophrenia on long-term neuroleptic treatment can develop obstructive sleep apnea, mediated via the weight gain produced by such medications.

Schizophrenia has been mistakenly diagnosed in patients with narcolepsy with unusually prominent hypnagogic hallucinations. Psychotic-like symptoms have also been observed in patients with narcolepsy who were taking amphetamines; symptoms resolved when the dose of amphetamines was lowered or treatment was changed to modafinil.

Depression, which can complicate the course of schizophrenia, can also, itself, increase sleep disturbance. In one study of persons with schizophrenia, poor sleepers were more depressed and distressed, and they had more adverse effects to medications than good sleepers.

For more information about the association between schizophrenia and sleep, see Box 11–3.

Box 11–3. Schizophrenia and sleep	Worsening of sleep disturbances during exacerbations of psychotic symptoms Aggravation of psychosis by Sleep disruption Insomnia Reversal of day-night sleep patterns, increase in sleep during the daytime, polyphasic sleep episodes, and alternating phases of sleeplessness and hypersomnolence Rebound sleepiness with an increase in sleep efficiency during the waning phase of schizophrenia or during residual schizophrenia Obstructive sleep apnea due to weight gain following long-term neuroleptic treatment

Note: There is a reduction in total sleep time and duration of REM sleep during the waxing phase of the disease, which normalizes during the waning, postpsychotic and remission phases. Successful therapy may increase REM sleep latency. Some antipsychotic agents can cause sedation. Insomnia may develop during discontinuation of antipsychotic medications.

Polysomnographic Features

Patients with schizophrenia generally have a decrease in REM sleep latency and in percent REM sleep time. A decrease in non-rapid eye movement (NREM) stages 3 and 4 sleep can be seen as well as an increase in sleep latency, decrease in sleep efficiency, increase in wake time after sleep onset (WASO), and decrease in total sleep time (Box 11–4).

In patients with schizophrenia, the duration of the first REM sleep period and REM density show a negative correlation with performance. REM sleep latency in drug-free patients is also inversely correlated with negative schizophrenic symptoms. Slow-wave sleep deficits correlate inversely with negative symptoms but not with positive symptoms.

Following sleep deprivation, actively symptomatic patients with schizophrenia have a decrease in total REM sleep and percent REM sleep rebound. In some instances, they may fail to generate NREM stages 3 and 4 sleep rebound.

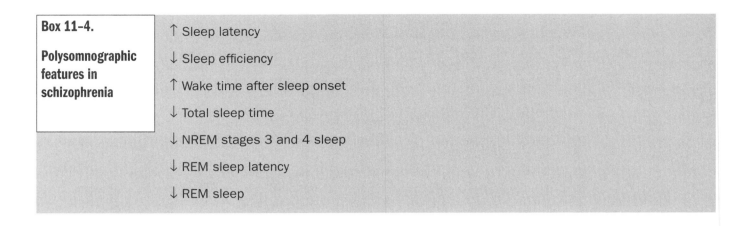

Box 11-4.

Polysomnographic features in schizophrenia

↑ Sleep latency

↓ Sleep efficiency

↑ Wake time after sleep onset

↓ Total sleep time

↓ NREM stages 3 and 4 sleep

↓ REM sleep latency

↓ REM sleep

Polysomnographic features vary over the course of schizophrenia, with a decrease in total sleep time and a disproportionately larger reduction in REM sleep during the waxing phase of the disorder; these parameters normalize during the waning phase and persists at normal levels during the post-psychotic and remission phases. Successful therapy may lead to a modest increase in REM sleep latency.

Effect of Medications on Sleep in Schizophrenia

Therapy of sleep disturbance in patients with schizophrenia consists of sedating antipsychotics and, occasionally, sedative hypnotics. Currently available antipsychotic medications can be divided into two groups: the "typical" (eg, chlorpromazine and haloperidol) and "atypical" (eg, olanzapine, risperidone, and clozapine) agents. The typical agents act by blocking dopaminergic transmission. The atypical antipsychotics have, in addition to their action on dopamine, significant activity on serotonin and other neurotransmitter systems.

Antipsychotic medications can improve sleep continuity and increase percent NREM stages 3 and 4 sleep. REM latency is increased. The atypical antipsychotics, olanzapine, risperidone, and clozapine, increase sleep efficiency, total sleep time, and NREM stage 2 sleep. Olanzapine and risperidone also increase NREM stages 3 and 4 sleep. The typical antipsychotics, haloperidol, thiothixene, and flupentixol, increase sleep efficiency, and decrease NREM stage 2 sleep latency. Compared with the typical agents, the atypical antipsychotics generate significantly more NREM stage 2 sleep and less NREM stage 1 sleep.

Some antipsychotic agents can cause considerable sedation that can be minimized by gradual dose escalation (Box 11–5).

Neuroleptic use can give rise to akathisia that has to be distinguished from restless legs or periodic limb movements of sleep; the latter have also been reported following administration of neuroleptics. Global deterioration of sleep can occur on withdrawal from neuroleptics.

Insomnia may develop during discontinuation of antipsychotic medications. Abrupt neuroleptic withdrawal may result in a transient reduction in total sleep time that will eventually stabilize within 2 to 4 weeks of withdrawal. Neuroleptic withdrawal can also decrease REM sleep, shorten REM sleep latency, and decrease total sleep time, sleep efficiency, and NREM sleep.

Mood Disorders

Insomnia is common among persons suffering from depression. Generally, there is a correlation between the severity of the mood disorder and insomnia. Sleep disturbance is accompanied by distress and impaired daytime functioning. Daytime sleepiness along with an increase in total sleep

Box 11-5. **Antipsychotic agents with sedative properties**	Chlorpromazine
	Clozapine
	Loxapine
	Olanzapine
	Perphenazine
	Quetiapine
	Risperidone
	Thioridazine
	Ziprasidone

time may develop during the depressive phase of a bipolar disorder, seasonal affective disorder, or atypical depression.

Selected mood episodes and their associated sleep disturbances are described in Table 11–1. Other mood disorders are described in Table 11–2. The sleep characteristics of mood disorders are presented in Box 11–6.

Table 11-1. Mood episodes

Episode	Clinical features	Sleep disturbance
Major depressive episode	Period of at least 2 weeks characterized by depressed mood and anhedonia (ie, absence of pleasure or interest in most activities), accompanied by significant functional impairment. Depressed mood is present almost daily and throughout most of the day.	Up to 90% of patients with major depression may complain of sleep disturbance. The most common sleep complaint is insomnia (eg, sleep-onset disturbance, frequent or prolonged awakenings, or early morning awakening). Less commonly, excessive sleepiness or prolonged sleep periods may be present. Polysomnographic features: ↓ Sleep efficiency ↑ Sleep latency ↓ Total sleep time ↑ Wakefulness after sleep onset ↑ NREM stage 1 sleep ↓ NREM stages 3 and 4 sleep ↓ REM sleep latency ↑ REM density The duration of REM sleep is increased early during sleep. There is often a delay in NREM stages 3 and 4 sleep from the first NREM cycle to the second. Multiple Sleep Latency Test does not reveal severe sleepiness.

Continued

Table 11-1. Mood episodes—cont'd

Episode	Clinical features	Sleep disturbance
		Note: Sleep disturbances and changes in sleep architecture may both precede or persist after remission of major depressive episodes.
Manic episode	Period of at least one week with a marked and persistent elevation of mood. Clinical features include irritability and euphoria. This abnormally expansive mood may be of any duration if hospitalization is required.	A manic episode is associated with a decrease in both amount of and requirement for sleep. Patients may complain of insomnia, which can be severe. Polysomnographic features: ↑ Awakenings ↓ NREM stages 3 and 4 sleep ↓ REM sleep latency ↑ REM density
Hypomanic episode	Period of persistently elevated, expansive, or irritable mood accompanied by a change in a person's usual functioning lasting at least 4 days. There is typically no distress or functional impairment. Less severe than a manic episode	Patients report diminished requirement for sleep or may complain of insomnia.
Mixed episode	Period during which mood rapidly alternates Features of both major depressive and manic episodes occur during most days and last at least 1 week.	Sleep disturbances include insomnia with a decrease in sleep duration.

Major Depressive Disorder

Individuals with major depressive disorder present with at least one major depressive episode without any manic, hypomanic, or mixed episodes. Sleep complaints include insomnia or excessive sleepiness, both of which occur almost daily. The severity of sleep disturbance may parallel the severity of major depression.

Insomnia in patients with major depressive disorder may be treated with psychotherapy and pharmacotherapy (selective serotonin reuptake inhibitors [SSRIs], tricyclic antidepressants [TCAs], monoamine oxidase (MAO) inhibitors, venlafaxine, or trazodone). The drugs bupropion, nefazodone, and mirtazapine may also be used. Except for bupropion and nefazodone, which increase REM sleep, antidepressants generally increase REM sleep latency and decrease REM sleep. MAO inhibitors are the most potent REM sleep inhibitors. Either adding low doses of trazodone or a nonbenzodiazepine benzodiazepine receptor agonist hypnotic agent (eg, eszopiclone, zolpidem or zaleplon) or switching to another antidepressant such as mirtazapine or nefazodone can manage insomnia induced by SSRIs.

Dysthymic Disorder

This chronic (ie, occurring during most of the day and on most days) depressed mood persists for at least 2 years, during which asymptomatic intervals are less than 2 months in duration.

Table 11–2.   Other mood disorders

Disorder	Features
Seasonal affective disorder	The appearance of mood disorders (eg, depressive, manic and hypomanic episodes) is closely associated with certain seasons of the year.
	Individuals commonly have major depressive episodes during the fall and winter. Patients may present with atypical features such as decreased energy levels and activity, as well as increased appetite with subsequent weight gain. Daytime sleepiness and fatigue may be accompanied by an increase in total sleep time.
	Depression is absent during spring and summer, at which time some patients may experience hypomanic symptoms, including increases in activity levels and sleep requirements.
	No polysomnographic features are distinctive for this disorder. An increase in total sleep time and decreased REM latency have been described.
	Therapy involves appropriately timed bright light exposure and, occasionally, medications (eg, antidepressants).
Atypical depression	Unlike major depressive episodes, patients may present with lethargy, increase in appetite, weight gain, leaden paralysis (sensation of heaviness in the extremities), and sensitivity to rejection.
	Sleep complaints include excessive sleepiness.
	Polysomnographic features: ↑ Total sleep time ↓ REM sleep latency

Box 11–6.

Mood disorders and sleep

Insomnia among persons suffering from depression

Daytime sleepiness along with an increase in total sleep time during the depressive phase of a bipolar disorder, seasonal affective disorder, or atypical depression

MAJOR DEPRESSIVE EPISODE

Insomnia or, less commonly, excessive sleepiness

Polysomnographic features:

↓ Sleep efficiency

↑ Sleep latency

↓ Total sleep time

↑ Wakefulness after sleep onset

↑ NREM stage 1 sleep

↓ NREM stages 3 and 4 sleep

↓ REM sleep latency

↑ REM density

MANIC EPISODE

Decreased in both amount of and requirement for sleep

(continued from page 381)
Box 11-6.

Mood disorders and sleep

Polysomnographic features:

↑ Awakenings

↓ NREM stages 3 and 4 sleep

↓ REM sleep latency

↑ REM density

HYPOMANIC EPISODE

Insomnia

MIXED EPISODE

Insomnia with a decrease in sleep duration

Patients may complain of decreased energy levels, poor concentration, changes in appetite, and diminished self-esteem. Sleep complaints include excessive sleepiness, fatigue, and sleep-onset or sleep-maintenance insomnia. In some, polysomnography may demonstrate decreases in NREM stages 3 and 4 sleep and REM sleep latency, as well as an increase in REM density.

Therapy consists of psychotherapy and antidepressant agents.

Bipolar Disorders

Excessive sleepiness may occur during the depressive episodes of bipolar disorder. During this phase, polysomnography may demonstrate an increase in total sleep time and decrease in REM sleep latency. During the acute manic phase of the disorder, total sleep time is reduced and patients report increased levels of energy. Manic episodes can be precipitated by sleep deprivation as well as antidepressant medications in patients with bipolar disorder.

Therapy may include lithium, divalproex, neuroleptics (eg, olanzapine), carbamazepine, or benzodiazepines.

Bipolar I

The disorder is defined by the occurrence of at least one manic, hypomanic, or mixed episode. Some individuals may also have one or more major depressive episodes. Patients with manic or hypomanic episodes do not complain of excessive sleepiness despite a shortened duration of sleep. When a major depressive episode is present, patients may present with excessive sleepiness.

Bipolar II

The disorder is characterized by the occurrence of at least one major depressive episode with at least one hypomanic episode. Manic and mixed episodes are absent.

Anxiety Disorders

Anxiety disorders can give rise to complaints of insomnia, frequent nighttime awakenings, recurring anxiety dreams, or excessive daytime sleepiness (Table 11–3). Some patients may report early morning awakenings. The characteristic sleep features of anxiety disorders are listed in Box 11–7. Polysomnographic features consist of an increase in sleep latency, decrease in sleep efficiency, increase in wake time after sleep onset, and decrease in total sleep time. There is an increase in NREM stages 1 and 2 sleep, and a decrease in NREM stages 3 and 4 as well as REM sleep. REM sleep latency can either be normal or prolonged (Box 11–7).

Table 11-3. Anxiety disorders

Disorder	Characteristics	Sleep disturbances
Acute stress disorder	Intense anxiety develops within 4 weeks following exposure to a traumatic experience. Features include reexperiencing of the traumatic event, dissociative symptoms (eg, detachment, depersonalization and derealization), and avoidance of factors that might lead to recall of the inciting event.	Insomnia is a frequent complaint.
Generalized anxiety disorder	Excessive anxiety about a variety of events or activities that occurs for most days during a period of at least 6 months. Chronic worry is associated with easy fatigability, irritability, restlessness, muscle tension, difficulty with concentration, and sleep disturbance. Treatment of generalized anxiety disorder includes behavioral therapy and pharmacotherapy (eg, benzodiazepines or TCAs).	Insomnia and nonrestorative sleep are common. Polysomnographic findings: ↓ Sleep efficiency ↑ Sleep latency ↓ Total sleep time ↑ Wake time after sleep onset ↓ NREM stages 3 and 4 sleep Note: Insomnia due to GAD should be distinguished from *psychophysiological insomnia,* in which anxiety is restricted primarily to issues related to insomnia.
Panic disorder	Recurrent panic attacks (ie, sudden onset of extreme fear or anxiety unrelated to real imminent danger) and the concerns and worries related to them. Panic attacks are associated with autonomic features (tachypnea, tachycardia, palpitations, and sweating). Panic disorders may respond to antidepressants (eg, SSRIs) or benzodiazepines (eg, alprazolam).	Patients may present with complaints of sleep-onset and sleep-maintenance insomnia. Panic attacks can occur during sleep, often during the transition from NREM stage 2 sleep to NREM stages 3 and 4 sleep. Occasionally, panic attacks may arise from REM sleep. Awakenings can be accompanied by sympathetic activation (eg, tachycardia, chest discomfort, dyspnea, and diaphoresis). Patients can often recall the preceding panic attack during awakenings. Return to sleep can be delayed.

Continued

Table 11–3. Anxiety disorders—cont'd

Disorder	Characteristics	Sleep disturbances
Post-traumatic stress disorder	Chronic hyperarousal (heightened startle response) and anxiety associated with preoccupation and repetitive reexperiencing (eg, flashbacks) of a severely traumatic or life-threatening event that develops following a physical attack, accident, or natural disaster Duration is over 1 month. Affected patients may actually directly experience, witness, or learn about a traumatic event. They often actively avoid stimuli that would evoke memories of the trauma. Numbing of general responsiveness, feelings of fear, helplessness or detachment, irritability, amnesia for aspects of the traumatic event, difficulty with concentration, and diminished range of affect and interest in usual activities can be present. It can be complicated by depression and substance and alcohol abuse Therapy includes counseling, psychotherapy, or pharmacotherapy, including SSRIs (eg, sertraline), TCAs, MAOIs, carbamazepine, lithium, or valproic acid.	Hyperarousal gives rise to sleep disturbance and chronic insomnia (difficulty falling or staying asleep). Polysomnographic features: There are no consistent abnormalities in sleep architecture. Some studies have described: ↓ Sleep efficiency ↓ Total sleep time ↑ Frequency of awakenings (with frightening dreams) ↓ NREM stages 3 and 4 sleep ↓ REM sleep ↑ Body movements or Periodic limb movements during sleep Reexperiences of the original event can occur through frequent distressing dreams, nightmares, and sleep terrors Dreams occur during both NREM and REM sleep, and they are often accompanied by vocalizations. Full alertness and recall of the preceding dream are typical after awakenings.

| Box 11-7.

Anxiety disorders and sleep | Insomnia, frequent nighttime awakenings, recurring anxiety dreams, or excessive daytime sleepiness

Polysomnographic features

　　↑ Sleep latency

　　↓ Sleep efficiency

　　↑ Wake time after sleep onset

　　↓ Total sleep time

　　↑ NREM stages 1 and 2 sleep

　　↓ NREM stages 3 and 4 sleep

　　↓ REM sleep

ACUTE STRESS DISORDER

　　Insomnia

GENERALIZED ANXIETY DISORDER

　　Insomnia or nonrestorative sleep |

(continued from page 384)

Box 11–7.

Anxiety disorders and sleep

PANIC DISORDER

Insomnia

Awakenings accompanied by sympathetic activation and delayed return to sleep

POST-TRAUMATIC STRESS DISORDER

Insomnia

Reexperiences of the original event through frequent distressing dreams, nightmares, and sleep terrors

Panic Disorders

Panic attacks occur repetitively (at least four episodes over a 4-week period) in patients with panic disorder. Attacks of extreme anxiety typically begin spontaneously without an identifiable precipitating factor. Patients may report dyspnea or a sensation of choking, chest discomfort, tachycardia, palpitations, nausea, flushing, lightheadedness, dizziness, tremulousness, paresthesia, or diaphoresis. There is often a feeling of depersonalization. Agoraphobia may be present as well. Patients may report a profound fear of dying.

A number of sleep disturbances may be encountered in persons with panic disorder, including insomnia and sleep panic attacks (Box 11–8). Although most panic attacks occur while the patient is awake, nocturnal panic attacks can disrupt sleep. Sleep panic attacks consist of abrupt awakenings with subsequent sustained wakefulness and, less commonly, sleep-onset attacks. Patients are immediately alert after each panic attack. Sleep panic attacks may be triggered by sleep deprivation or relaxation.

Differential diagnosis includes nightmares, sleep terrors, and obstructive sleep apnea. Unlike sleep panic attacks, nightmares are accompanied by terrifying dreams.

Polysomnographic findings may either be normal or consist of an increase in sleep latency and decrease in sleep efficiency (Box 11–8). An increase in frequency of panic attacks occurs during the transition from NREM stage 2 sleep to NREM stage 3 sleep.

Therapy for sleep-related panic attacks includes behavioral therapy (eg, relaxation) or pharmacotherapy (eg, SSRIs, TCAs, or benzodiazepines).

Box 11–8.

Panic disorders and sleep

Insomnia and sleep panic attacks

Sleep panic attacks triggered by sleep deprivation or relaxation

Polysomnographic features

↑ Sleep latency

↓ Sleep efficiency

May be normal

Alcoholism

Acute consumption of alcohol close to bedtime decreases wakefulness during the first several hours of sleep. However, the frequency of awakenings increases as alcohol is metabolized by the body and its serum levels fall during the last 2 to 3 hours of sleep.

Frequent awakenings are also commonly encountered with chronic use of alcohol or during early abstinence. Profound sleeplessness often accompanies delirium tremens. Abnormal sleep patterns persist in some persons despite prolonged abstinence.

The incidence of anxiety dreams, enuresis, sleep terrors, and sleepwalking may increase with alcohol consumption. Snoring may intensify and obstructive sleep apnea may worsen. Alcoholism and its effects on sleep are described in Box 11–9.

Box 11–9. Alcoholism and sleep	Frequent awakenings
	Sleeplessness, often accompanying delirium tremens
	Possible increase in anxiety dreams, enuresis, sleep terrors, and sleepwalking
	Possible worsening of snoring and obstructive sleep apnea

Attention Deficit Hyperactivity Disorder

Attention deficit hyperactivity disorder (ADHD) is characterized by inattention, hyperactivity, and/or impulsivity, with some symptoms developing prior to 7 years of age. Patients may present with significant functional impairments at school, home, or work. Patients with ADHD appear to have greater rates of sleep disorders including obstructive sleep apnea and periodic limb movement disorder. Clinical improvements in attention and impulse control following therapy of an underlying obstructive sleep apnea, if present, have been described.

Attention-deficit hyperactivity disorder and sleep

Greater rates of obstructive sleep apnea and periodic limb movement disorder

Personality Disorders

This is a group of disorders that is characterized by chronic, stable and enduring patterns of behavior, cognition, emotional response, impulse control and interpersonal and social relationships that differ from usual cultural expectations. This results in distress and functional impairment. Onset is often during adolescence or early adulthood. There are numerous specific types of personality disorders, including paranoid, schizoid, schizotypal, antisocial, borderline, histrionic, narcissistic, avoidant, dependent, and obsessive-compulsive personality disorders. For more information about obsessive-compulsive disorder, see Table 11–4.

Polysomnography may reveal an increase in sleep latency, decrease in sleep efficiency, decrease in total sleep time, increase in wake time after sleep onset, and decrease in REM sleep latency among patients with borderline personality disorder (Box 11–10). There may be an increase in NREM stages 3 and 4 sleep in patients with antisocial personality disorder.

Table 11–4. Personality disorder

Disorder	Characteristics	Sleep disturbances
Obsessive-compulsive disorder	It is characterized by obsessions (persistent or recurrent intrusive thoughts) and compulsions (repetitive intentional behaviors or actions related to obsessions) that cause functional impairment Treatment involves either psychotherapy, behavior therapy (eg, cognitive therapy or desensitization), or pharmacotherapy (eg, SSRIs, MAO inhibitors, or TCAs).	Sleep may be delayed by compulsive behaviors. Polysomnographic features: ↓ Sleep efficiency ↓ Total sleep time ↑ Frequency of awakenings ↓ NREM stages 3 and 4 sleep ↓ REM sleep latency ↑ REM density

Box 11–10. **Personality disorders and sleep**	Polysomnographic features of obsessive-compulsive disorder: ↓ Sleep efficiency ↓ Total sleep time ↑ Frequency of awakenings ↓ NREM stages 3 and 4 sleep ↓ REM sleep latency ↑ REM density Polysomnographic features of borderline personality disorder: ↑ Sleep latency ↓ Sleep efficiency ↓ Total sleep time ↑ Wake time after sleep onset ↓ REM sleep latency Polysomnographic features of antisocial personality disorder: ↑ NREM stages 3 and 4 sleep

Somatization Disorder

This group is characterized by multiple recurring physical complaints or symptoms (ie, pain, gastrointestinal, sexual, or pseudoneurologic) that appear to be related to, yet are not explained fully by, a medical or neurologic condition, or a medication. These symptoms are not deliberately produced or contrived, commonly begin before 30 years of age, occur over several years, and can give rise to functional impairments as well as sleep initiation and sleep maintenance insomnia.

Differential diagnosis includes generalized anxiety disorder, psychosis, and malingering.

Eating Disorders

Insomnia may develop in patients with anorexia nervosa, whereas excessive sleepiness can occur in bulimia (Box 11–11). Eating disorders may respond to psychotherapy or drug therapy (eg, SSRIs).

Box 11-11. Eating disorders and sleep	Insomnia in anorexia nervosa Excessive sleepiness in bulimia

References

General References

American Academy of Sleep Medicine. The International Classification of Sleep Disorders: Diagnostic and Coding Manual. 2nd ed. American Academy of Sleep Medicine, 2005.

Bowman TJ. Review of Sleep Medicine. Burlington, MA: Butterworth-Heinemann, 2002.

Berry RB. Sleep Medicine Pearls. 2nd ed. Philadelphia, PA: Hanley & Belfus, 2002.

Chokroverty S. Clinical Companion to Sleep Disorders Medicine. 2nd ed. Butterworth-Heinemann, 2000.

Hoyt BD. Sleep in patients with neurologic and psychiatric disorders. Sleep Medicine. Primary Care: Clinics in Office Practice. Elsevier Saunders, 2005.

Lavie P, Pillar G, Malhotra A. Sleep Disorders Handbook. New York, NY: Taylor & Francis, 2002.

Lee-Chiong TL, ed. Sleep: A Comprehensive Handbook. Hoboken, NJ: John Wiley & Sons, 2006.

Lee-Chiong TL, Sateia M, Carskadon M, eds. Sleep Medicine. Philadelphia, PA: Hanley & Belfus (Elsevier), 2002.

Perlis ML, Lichstein KL, eds. Treating Sleep Disorders: Principles and Practice of Behavioral Sleep Medicine. Hoboken, NJ: John Wiley & Sons, 2003.

Rechtschaffen A, Kales A. A Manual of Standardized Terminology, Techniques and Scoring System for Sleep Stages of Human Subjects. Los Angeles, CA: Brain Information Service/Brain Research Institute, University of California, 1968.

Reite M, Ruddy J, Nagel K. Concise Guide to Evaluation and Management of Sleep Disorders. 3rd ed. Arlington, VA: American Psychiatric Publishing, April 2002.

Sleep Disorders. Medical Clinics of North America. Philadelphia, PA: Elsevier Saunders, 2004.

Sleep Medicine. Primary Care: Clinics in Office Practice. Philadelphia, PA: Elsevier Saunders, 2005.

Sleep Research Society. SRS Basics of Sleep Guide. Westchester, IL: Sleep Research Society, 2005.

Schizophrenia

Hiatt JF, Floyd TC, Katz PH, Feinberg I. Further evidence of abnormal non-rapid-eye-movement sleep in schizophrenia. Arch Gen Psychiatry. 1985(Aug);42(8):797–802.

Kajimura N, Kato M, Okuma T, Sekimoto M, Watanabe T, Takahashi K. A quantitative sleep-EEG study on the effects of benzodiazepine and zopiclone in schizophrenic patients. Schizophr Res. 1995(May);15(3):303–12.

Keshavan MS, Reynolds CF III, Miewald JM, Montrose DM. A longitudinal study of EEG sleep in schizophrenia. Psychiatry Res. 1996(Jan 31);59(3):203–11.

Kupfer DJ, Wyatt RJ, Scott J, Snyder F. Sleep disturbance in acute schizophrenic patients. Am J Psychiatry. 1970(Mar);126(9):1213–23.

Luby ED, Caldwell DF. Sleep deprivation and EEG slow wave activity in chronic schizophrenia. Arch Gen Psychiatry. 1967(Sep);17(3):361–4.

Monti JM, Monti D. Sleep in schizophrenia patients and the effects of antipsychotic drugs. Sleep Med Rev. 2004(Apr);8(2):133–48.

Ritsner M, Kurs R, Ponizovsky A, Hadjez J. Perceived quality of life in schizophrenia: relationships to sleep quality. Qual Life Res. 2004(May);13(4):783–91.

Tandon R, Shipley JE, Taylor S, Greden JF, Eiser A, DeQuardo J, et al. Electroencephalographic sleep abnormalities in schizophrenia. Relationship to positive/negative symptoms and prior neuroleptic treatment. Arch Gen Psychiatry. 1992(Mar);49(3):185–94.

Taylor SF, Goldman RS, Tandon R, Shipley JE. Neuropsychological function and REM sleep in schizophrenic patients. Biol Psychiatry. 1992(Sep 15);32(6):529–38.

Thaker GK, Wagman AM, Kirkpatrick B, Tamminga CA. Alterations in sleep polygraphy after neuroleptic withdrawal: a putative supersensitive dopaminergic mechanism. Biol Psychiatry. 1989(Jan);25(1):75–86.

Vourdas A, Shneerson JM, Gregory CA, Smith IE, King MA, Morrish E, et al. Narcolepsy and psychopathology: is there an association? Sleep Med. 2002(Jul);3(4):353–60.

Wetter TC, Lauer CJ, Gillich G, Pollmacher T. The electroencephalographic sleep pattern in schizophrenic patients treated with clozapine or classical antipsychotic drugs. J Psychiatr Res. 1996(Nov–Dec);30(6):411–9.

Winkelman JW. Schizophrenia, obesity, and obstructive sleep apnea. J Clin Psychiatry. 2001(Jan);62(1):8–11.

Zarcone V, Azumi K, Dement W, Gulevich G, Kraemer H, Pivik T. REM phase deprivation and schizophrenia II. Arch Gen Psychiatry. 1975(Nov);32(11):1431–6.

Mood Disorders

Hoyt BD. Sleep in patients with neurologic and psychiatric disorders. Sleep Medicine. Primary Care: Clinics in Office Practice. Elsevier Saunders, 2005.

Nowell P. Sleep in patients with mood disorders. In: Lee-Chiong TL, Sateia M, Carskadon M, eds. Sleep Medicine. Philadelphia, PA: Hanley & Belfus (Elsevier), 2002.

Anxiety Disorders

Hoyt BD. Sleep in patients with neurologic and psychiatric disorders. Sleep Medicine. Primary Care: Clinics in Office Practice. Elsevier Saunders, 2005.

Mellman TA. Anxiety disorders and sleep. In: Lee-Chiong TL, Sateia M, Carskadon M, eds. Sleep Medicine. Philadelphia, PA: Hanley & Belfus (Elsevier), 2002.Panic Disorders

American Academy of Sleep Medicine. The International Classification of Sleep Disorders: Diagnostic and Coding Manual. 2nd ed. American Academy of Sleep Medicine, 2005.

Hoyt BD. Sleep in patients with neurologic and psychiatric disorders. Sleep Medicine. Primary Care: Clinics in Office Practice. Elsevier Saunders, 2005.

Alcoholism

American Academy of Sleep Medicine. The International Classification of Sleep Disorders: Diagnostic and Coding Manual. 2nd ed. American Academy of Sleep Medicine, 2005.

Hoyt BD. Sleep in patients with neurologic and psychiatric disorders. Sleep Medicine. Primary Care: Clinics in Office Practice. Elsevier Saunders, 2005.

Attention Deficit Hyperactivity Disorder

American Academy of Sleep Medicine. The International Classification of Sleep Disorders: Diagnostic and Coding Manual. 2nd ed. American Academy of Sleep Medicine, 2005.

Reite M, Ruddy J, Nagel K. Concise Guide to Evaluation and Management of Sleep Disorders. 3rd ed. American Psychiatric Publishing, April 2002.

Personality Disorders

American Academy of Sleep Medicine. The International Classification of Sleep Disorders: Diagnostic and Coding Manual. 2nd ed. American Academy of Sleep Medicine, 2005.

Reite M, Ruddy J, Nagel K. Concise Guide to Evaluation and Management of Sleep Disorders. 3rd ed. American Psychiatric Publishing, April 2002.

Somatization Disorder

Reite M, Ruddy J, Nagel K. Concise Guide to Evaluation and Management of Sleep Disorders. 3rd ed. American Psychiatric Publishing, April 2002.

Eating Disorders

Hoyt BD. Sleep in patients with neurologic and psychiatric disorders. Sleep Medicine. Primary Care: Clinics in Office Practice. Elsevier Saunders, 2005.

Miscellaneous Sleep Disorders 12

Benign Sleep Myoclonus of Infancy

This disorder is characterized by recurrent, massive myoclonic jerks involving large muscle groups (ie, entire body, trunk, or extremities) that occur only during sleep (predominantly during quiet sleep) among infants during the first year of life, usually from birth to 6 months of age. The muscle jerks are not associated with arousals or awakenings.

Prevalence is unknown but is believed to be rare. There is no difference between genders. It has a self-limited course, with resolution by 6 months of age in most infants. No specific therapy is necessary. Pathogenesis has been postulated to involve a possible developmental abnormality of the reticular activating system.

Video-electroencephalography (EEG) and electromyography (EMG) monitoring during polysomnography demonstrate muscle activity with a frequency of four to five jerks per second, occurring in clusters lasting 3 to 15 minutes. It is generally observed during non–rapid eye movement (NREM) sleep but can sometimes occur during rapid eye movement (REM) sleep. No seizure activity is present on EEG tracings.

Environmental Sleep Disorder

In environmental sleep disorder, the sleep disturbance is directly related to adverse environmental conditions such as excessive noise, noxious odors, extremes of ambient temperature or bright lights. Individuals complain of either insomnia or daytime sleepiness. Its exact prevalence is not known. Because the elderly are more sensitive to environmental disturbances compared with younger individuals, older people have a greater risk of developing this type of sleep disturbance.

When the environmental disturbances are replicated during laboratory polysomnography, or if ambulatory sleep studies are performed in the usual bedroom environment, decreases in sleep efficiency, total sleep time, NREM stages 3 and 4 sleep, and REM sleep may be observed. Normal sleep architecture and sleep duration are restored after removal of the causative agent.

Fragmentary Myoclonus

Fragmentary myoclonus is characterized by asynchronous, asymmetric, and brief contractions of the muscles of the face, trunk, and extremities appearing at the onset of sleep and continuing throughout the night. They may also be present during wakefulness. Episodes last from 10 minutes to over an hour. Affected individuals are typically unaware of these movements, with the fragmentary myoclonus being merely an incidental EMG finding during polysomnography.

Excessive fragmentary myoclonus may be seen in association with obstructive and central sleep apnea, hypoventilation syndromes, narcolepsy, insomnia, periodic limb movement disorder, restless legs syndrome, and Niemann-Pick disease type C disease. Fragmentary myoclonus can be exacerbated by excessive sleepiness.

This rare disorder occurs predominantly among males. Onset is typically in adulthood. Course is generally benign, but excessive sleepiness secondary to sleep disruption and frequent arousals may develop in some individuals.

Differential diagnosis includes physiologic phasic REM sleep muscle twitching. Polysomnography demonstrates brief EMG potentials in various muscle groups, with more than five potentials per minute for at least 20 minutes of NREM stages 2, 3, or 4 sleep. Although muscle twitches may accompany EMG discharges, no movements may be evident. Muscle twitches occur predominantly during NREM sleep and persist into REM sleep. No accompanying EEG changes are present.

Hypnagogic Foot Tremor and Alternating Leg Muscle Activation

The International Classification of Sleep Disorders (second edition) grouped the two entities, hypnagogic foot tremor and alternating leg muscle activation, together because of similarities in many of their clinical features.

Hypnagogic Foot Tremor

In hypnagogic foot tremor (HFT), rhythmic tremors of the feet or toes occur during the transition between wakefulness and sleep or during NREM stages 1 and 2 sleep. HFT appears to be a common and usually incidental finding noted during polysomnography performed for other reasons. Most cases involve middle-aged adults, and both genders are affected equally. Course is generally benign.

Polysomnographic findings consist of repetitive leg or foot EMG bursts or movements lasting several seconds to minutes and occurring during drowsy wakefulness or light stages of sleep.

Alternating Leg Muscle Activation

As the name alternating leg muscle activation (ALMA) implies, brief activity of the anterior tibialis muscle of one leg alternates with activity of the same muscle in the other leg, usually prior to or following an arousal or awakening. ALMA can also occur without any associated arousals from sleep. It diminishes gradually with return to sleep.

ALMA is most common among middle-aged adults. There is a male predominance. It is likely a benign condition and complications have not been described.

Polysomnography demonstrates repetitive, brief, and alternating activations of the anterior tibialis EMGs. Each activation has a duration of 0.1 to 0.5 seconds, with at least 4 muscle activations occurring in sequence lasting from 1 to 30 seconds and with less than 2 seconds between activations.

Long Sleeper

There is continuum in normal sleep duration ranging from one extreme in the long sleeper to the other end in the short sleeper. The sleep of a long sleeper is substantially lengthier than is typical for his or her age group, often consistently greater than 10 hours during a 24-hour period for a young adult. Patients may present with complaints of daytime sleepiness if they habitually obtain less than this amount of sleep. Onset is generally during childhood. It has an unrelenting, chronic course.

This condition has to be distinguished from other causes of excessive sleepiness such as idiopathic hypersomnia, insufficient sleep syndrome, narcolepsy, and obstructive sleep apnea. Sleep logs kept over several days aid in diagnosis.

Polysomnography documents normal sleep efficiency, an increase in total sleep time (ie, 10 hours or longer), normal amounts of NREM stages 3 and 4 sleep, and increases in NREM stage 2 and REM sleep (Box 12–1). Mean sleep latency on the Multiple Sleep Latency Test (MSLT) is normal if the patient had obtained the usual amount of nighttime sleep prior to the test.

Propriospinal Myoclonus at Sleep Onset

Patients with this condition exhibit spontaneous sudden muscle jerks that occur typically during relaxed wakefulness in the transition from wakefulness to sleep. The jerks start in the abdominal

Box 12-1. Polysomnographic features of a long sleeper	Normal sleep efficiency
	↑ Total sleep time
	Normal NREM stages 3 and 4 sleep
	↑ NREM stage 2 sleep
	↑ REM sleep

and truncal muscles and then spread slowly rostrally and caudally to the proximal limb and neck muscles. Nonperiodic trunk flexion (more common) and extension disappear at sleep onset or with mental activation.

This is likely a rare disorder with an unknown etiology. Its prevalence appears higher among adult men. Onset is generally during adulthood with a chronic course. Sleep-onset insomnia may develop. Propriospinal myoclonus should be distinguished from sleep starts that occur at sleep onset, periodic limb movements of sleep, and rhythmic movement sleep disorder.

Polysomnographic features include brief, recurring myoclonic EMG activity associated with alpha EEG rhythms that disappear with EEG desynchronization and remain absent during sleep.

Short Sleeper

Habitual sleep duration in a short sleeper is, as its name aptly describes, less than is customary for a similarly aged person, often averaging 5 hours or less daily in an adult younger than 60 years of age. Sleep is otherwise unremarkable with normal sleep initiation, quality, continuity and consolidation. Sleep is restorative despite its brevity. The final awakening is spontaneous and is constant regardless of opportunities or attempts to lengthen sleep.

This rare condition is not associated with daytime symptoms. Men and women are affected equally. It is uncommon among children, and prevalence may increase with age. It often begins in early adolescence or adulthood. Course is characteristically chronic and it persists life-long.

The condition should be distinguished from shortened sleep duration secondary to insomnia or voluntary restriction of sleep time (ie, insufficient sleep syndrome). Requirements for sleep may be reduced transiently during the manic phase of a bipolar disorder. Finally, frequent napping to make up for a restricted nocturnal sleep period should be excluded.

Polysomnographic features include a decrease in total sleep time accompanied by a decrease in sleep latency, NREM sleep stage 2, and REM sleep (Box 12–2). MSLT is invariably normal.

Despite the absence of any impairment in daytime functioning, short sleepers may seek medical evaluation because of concerns about their inability to sleep longer. Aside from reassurance, no specific therapy is required.

Box 12-2. Polysomnographic features of a short sleeper	↓ Sleep latency
	↓ Total sleep time
	↓ NREM sleep stage 2
	↓ REM sleep
	Normal MSLT

Sleep Hyperhidrosis

Diaphoresis or profuse sweating occurring during sleep may be seen in association with obstructive sleep apnea, pregnancy, or febrile illnesses. It has also been described in certain endocrine, autonomic, or neurologic disorders. Sleep hyperhidrosis can lead to awakenings from sleep.

Sleep-Related Abnormal Swallowing Syndrome

Persons with this disorder have difficulty swallowing their own saliva during sleep and have repeated transient arousals from sleep due to coughing, choking, or gagging. Abnormal swallowing mechanisms during sleep result in accumulation of saliva in the upper airway, with subsequent aspiration into the trachea leading to an arousal with coughing and a sensation of choking. A characteristic "gurgling" sound due to pooling of secretions in the oral cavity can be heard preceding each coughing spell. Possible causes include unusually large amounts of salivary production, impaired function of muscles associated with deglutition, or structural abnormality of the upper airway. Patients can present with complaints of insomnia, restless sleep, a sensation of choking or dyspnea occurring during sleep, or transient hoarseness following awakenings.

This condition is believed to be quite rare. Clinical course is unknown. Differential diagnosis includes obstructive sleep apnea, gastroesophageal reflux, sleep terrors, and sleep choking syndrome. An overnight polysomnography may aid in diagnosis.

Sleep-Related Choking Syndrome

Persons may complain of frequent, almost nightly, episodes of abrupt awakenings accompanied by a sensation of choking or being unable to breathe, fear, intense anxiety, sensation of dying, and tachycardia. These attacks are not accompanied by stridor, nightmares, or sleep terrors. Sleep choking syndrome may result in recurrent awakenings and may give rise to insomnia.

This syndrome is reportedly rare. It is most often seen during early to middle adulthood and occurs predominantly in females. Etiology is unknown.

Sleep-related choking syndrome should be distinguished from sleep-related laryngospasm, obstructive sleep apnea, nocturnal asthma, panic disorder, and gastroesophageal reflux.

Sleep-Related Laryngospasm

Severe breathlessness with an initial total or near-total cessation of airflow while asleep is followed by a sudden awakening with inspiratory stridor. Episodes are infrequent, and last from seconds to several minutes. Events may be accompanied by temporary hoarseness, tachycardia, cyanosis, anxiety, panic, or a sensation of dying. They tend to resolve spontaneously or may be relieved by drinking water. Spasm of the vocal cords, tracheal swelling, or muscle dysfunction has been described in some patients.

Sleep-related laryngospasm is probably rare. It is most prevalent among middle-aged adults and appears to be more common among males. Differential diagnosis includes obstructive sleep apnea, gastroesophageal reflux, nocturnal asthma, and seizure disorder.

Sleep-Related Neurogenic Tachypnea

This disorder is characterized by sustained tachypnea that starts at sleep onset, persists throughout sleep, and resolves on awakening. Sleep-related neurogenic tachypnea can give rise to excessive sleepiness due to sleep fragmentation; however, some affected individuals are completely asymptomatic. This condition is apparently rare, and may occur either in an idiopathic form or be due to a variety of central nervous system (CNS) lesions.

Sleep Starts

Sleep starts (hypnic jerks or hypnic myoclonia) consist of sudden muscle contractions of part or all of the body that occur at sleep onset. The individual may be startled out of sleep by a single, brief, body jerk accompanied by a sensation of "falling" or "dreaming." It can also present as visual (flashes of light or vivid imagery), auditory (loud bangs), or somesthetic (floating) phenomena. In rare cases, repetitive sleep starts can give rise to sleep-onset insomnia.

This condition may be seen in up to 60% to 70% of the population and can affect all age groups and both genders. It is a common experience among many normal individuals during the transition between wake and sleep and is most likely a normal physiologic phenomenon. Sleep starts are believed to be due to a sudden loss of muscle tone at sleep onset and the subsequent reflex muscle contraction to restore muscle tone. Although they are frequently spontaneous, sleep starts can also be triggered by external stimuli. Episodes may be precipitated by sleep deprivation, stress, excessive caffeine ingestion, stimulant use, or intense physical activity performed close to bedtime. Course is generally benign and sleep starts typically require no specific therapy.

Polysomnographic monitoring during the event would occasionally show an arousal or complete awakening from drowsiness or NREM stage 1 sleep related to brief EMG potentials.

Sleep Talking

Sleep talking or somniloquy refers to the vocalization or utterance of sounds, words, or sentences during sleep. It can occur in all stages of sleep but is most commonly described in NREM stages 1 and 2 sleep and REM sleep. The sleep talker is typically unaware of the event. Although often brief, sporadic and self-limited, episodes can, at times, be lengthy and recur nightly.

It is common in the general population and is of no apparent clinical or psychological significance. It affects all age groups with no gender difference. There is a substantial genetic influence in both childhood and adult sleep talking. A number of sleep disorders, including obstructive sleep apnea, REM sleep behavior disorder, sleep terrors, and confusional arousals can trigger sleep talking.

Subwakefulness Syndrome

This syndrome describes a rare condition in which an individual complains of a subjective sensation of constant daytime sleepiness in the absence of any objective evidence of excessive sleepiness. There is no history of frequent napping. Polysomnographic findings are normal. The condition has a chronic course.

Sudden Unexplained Nocturnal Death Syndrome

Sudden unexplained nocturnal death syndrome (SUNDS) is characterized by sudden death that occurs during sleep without any apparent cause. Victims are mostly healthy adult males from Southeast Asia between 25 and 44 years of age. SUNDS is referred to as "bangungut" in the Philippines, "pokkuri" in Japan, "non-laita" in Laos, and "Lai Tai" in northeastern Thailand. The incidence in the United States is approximately 90/100,000.

The pathogenesis of SUNDS is unknown. Proposed mechanisms include instability of physiologic systems, especially respiration, during sleep, nocturnal hypoxia, or a variety of cardiac anomalies (eg, unexplained cardiomegaly or conduction system abnormalities). Ventricular fibrillation has been described in cases of successful resuscitation or monitored death. However, some victims had no evidence of atherosclerotic coronary artery disease, myocarditis, cardiomyopathy, or congenital cardiac anomalies. Mutations in SCN5A, the gene known to cause Brugada syndrome, has been identified in some families with SUNDS. Both SUNDS and Brugada syndrome are associated with abnormal electrocardiograms with ST-segment elevation in leads V1-V3 and sudden death due to ventricular fibrillation.

Witnessed reports include descriptions of moaning, thrashing, screaming, violent motor activity, perspiration, and labored breathing that usually last for a few minutes prior to death. Resuscitated victims have reported sensations of airway obstruction, chest discomfort or pressure, and numb or weak limbs. They are unresponsive and are difficult to arouse during the event.

Terrifying Hypnagogic Hallucinations

Terrifying hypnagogic hallucinations manifest as nightmares occurring at sleep onset. A sudden awakening with intense fear from REM sleep is accompanied by vivid recollection of the preceding threatening dream. There is full alertness on awakening. This is a rare condition that has a benign course. It may occasionally produce difficulty in initiating sleep.

Toxin-Induced Sleep Disorder

Chronic poisoning with toxins such as heavy metals (eg, arsenic, copper, lead, mercury) or chemicals can give rise to either insomnia secondary to CNS excitation or to hypersomnolence due to CNS depression. Polysomnography may demonstrate an increase in sleep latency, decrease in sleep efficiency, and repetitive awakenings.

References

General References

American Academy of Sleep Medicine. *The International Classification of Sleep Disorders: Diagnostic and Coding Manual*. 2nd ed. Westchester, IL: American Academy of Sleep Medicine, 2005.

American Sleep Disorders Association. *International Classification of Sleep Disorders: Diagnostic and Coding Manual*, revised. Rochester, MN: American Sleep Disorders Association, 1997.

Bowman TJ. *Review of Sleep Medicine*. Burlington, MA: Butterworth-Heinemann, 2002.

Berry RB. *Sleep Medicine Pearls*. 2nd ed. Philadelphia, PA: Hanley & Belfus, 2002.

Chokroverty S. *Clinical Companion to Sleep Disorders Medicine*. 2nd ed. Butterworth-Heinemann, 2000.

Lavie P, Pillar G, Malhotra A. *Sleep Disorders Handbook*. New York, NY: Taylor & Francis, 2002.

Lee-Chiong TL, ed. *Sleep: A Comprehensive Handbook*. Hoboken, NJ: John Wiley & Sons, 2006.

Lee-Chiong TL, Sateia M, Carskadon M, eds. *Sleep Medicine*. Philadelphia, PA: Hanley & Belfus (Elsevier), 2002.

Perlis ML, Lichstein KL, eds. *Treating Sleep Disorders: Principles and Practice of Behavioral Sleep Medicine*. Hoboken, NJ: John Wiley & Sons, 2003.

Rechtschaffen A, Kales A. *A Manual of Standardized Terminology, Techniques and Scoring System for Sleep Stages of Human Subjects.* Los Angeles, CA: Brain Information Service/Brain Research Institute, University of California, 1968.

Reite M, Ruddy J, Nagel K. *Concise Guide to Evaluation and Management of Sleep Disorders.* 3rd ed. Arlington, VA: American Psychiatric Publishing, April 2002.

Sleep Disorders. Medical Clinics of North America. Philadelphia, PA: Elsevier Saunders, 2004.

Sleep Medicine. Primary Care: Clinics in Office Practice. Philadelphia, PA: Elsevier Saunders, 2005.

Sleep Research Society. *SRS Basics of Sleep Guide.* Westchester, IL: Sleep Research Society, 2005.

Other References

Baron RC, Thacker SB, Gorelkin L, Vernon AA, Taylor WR, Choi K. Sudden death among Southeast Asian refugees. An unexplained nocturnal phenomenon. *JAMA* 1983;250:2947–2951.

Brown WD. Other parasomnias. In: Lee-Chiong TL, Sateia M, Carskadon M, eds. *Sleep Medicine.* Philadelphia, PA: Hanley & Belfus (Elsevier), 2002:237–244.

Charoenpan P, Muntarbhorn K, Boongird P, Puavilai G, Ratanaprakarn R, Indraprasit S, et al. Nocturnal physiological and biochemical changes in sudden unexplained death syndrome: a preliminary report of a case control study. *Southeast Asian J Trop Med Public Health.* 1994(Jun);25(2):335–40.

Fusco L, Pachatz C, Cusmai R, Vigevano F. Repetitive sleep starts in neurologically impaired children: an unusual non-epileptic manifestation in otherwise epileptic subjects. *Epileptic Disord.* 1999(Mar);1(1):63–7.

Hublin C, Kaprio J, Partinen M, Koskenvuo M. Sleeptalking in twins: epidemiology and psychiatric co-morbidity. *Behavior Genetics.* 1998;28:289–298.

Kirschner RH, Eckner FA, Baron RC. The cardiac pathology of sudden, unexplained nocturnal death in Southeast Asian refugees. *JAMA.* 1986;(Nov 21);256(19):2700–5.

Pollanen MS, Chiasson DA, Cairns J, Young JG. Sudden unexplained death in Asian immigrants: Recognition of a syndrome in metropolitan Toronto. *Canadian Medical Association J.* 1996;155(5):537–540.

Reimao RN, Lefevre AB. Prevalence of sleep-talking in childhood. *Brain Dev.* 1980;2(4):353–7.

Tanchaiswad W. Is sudden unexplained nocturnal death a breathing disorder? *Psychiatry Clin Neurosci.* 1995(May);49(2):111–4.

Vatta M, Dumaine R, Varghese G, Richard TA, Shimizu W, et al. Genetic and biophysical basis of sudden unexplained nocturnal death syndrome (SUNDS), a disease allelic to Brugada syndrome. *Hum Mol Genet.* 2002(Feb 1);11(3):337–45.

Sleep in Infants, Children and Adolescents 13

In many instances, a child is not merely a small adult. This is particularly relevant with regards to sleep and sleep disorders in the infant, child, and adolescent, in whom there are many significant differences from that of the adult. Nonetheless, there are also many similarities in the clinical features, pathophysiology, evaluation and therapy of sleep disorders between children and adults. This chapter, rather than repeating what has been described in earlier sections that dealt with adults, will, instead, emphasize the differences between these two age groups.

Normal Human Sleep Across the Ages

The physiology, regulation, organization, architecture and distribution of sleep vary across the ages of one's lifetime, from early infancy to elderly adulthood.

Number of Sleep Phases

Sleep among newborns is *polyphasic* (occurring several times throughout the 24-hour day). In early childhood, typically between the ages of 3 to 5 years, sleep becomes *monophasic* (occurring only once, generally at night). Some adults continue to prefer a *biphasic* sleep pattern with an afternoon nap and a major nocturnal sleep period (Table 13–1).

Table 13-1.	Age group	Number of sleep phases
Number of sleep phases	< 3–5 years	Polyphasic
	> 3–5 years	Monophasic (biphasic in some)

Duration of Sleep

Newborn infants spend approximately 70% of their time in a 24-hour day asleep, whereas adults sleep about 25% to 35% of the 24-hour day sleeping.

Sleep Distribution

Sleep is distributed equally across the day and night in newborns. Nocturnal sleep consolidation and the ability to sleep through the night develop by 6 to 9 months of age (Table 13–2).

Sleep Electrophysiology

In the first 6 months of life, sleep is classified as either active sleep (REM sleep equivalent) or quiet sleep (NREM sleep equivalent). Specific sleep stages present in infants in the first 6 months of life

Table 13-2.	Age group	Distribution of sleep
Sleep distribution	< 6–9 months	Distributed equally across the day and night
	> 6–9 months	Consolidation of sleep to the night

include active sleep, quiet sleep, indeterminate sleep, and transitional sleep. The conventional adult sleep stages (NREM stages 1, 2, 3 and 4 sleep, and REM sleep) are used to describe sleep in infants older than 6 months of age. Sleep classification in infants as well as sleep stages and their characteristics are presented in Tables 13–3, 13–4, and 13–5.

The initial sleep episode is often REM sleep in young infants until the age of 3 months when the adult pattern of NREM sleep during sleep onset develops (Table 13–6).

The proportion of NREM and REM sleep are equal during early infancy. REM sleep declines throughout childhood. NREM stages 3 and 4 sleep are greatest during early childhood and progressively decline with aging (Table 13–7).

The percentage of REM sleep decreases with aging, from 50% of total sleep time (TST) in the newborn period to 20% to 25% of TST by adulthood. A marked reduction of REM sleep occurs during the first 6 months of life (Table 13–8).

During sleep, NREM sleep and REM sleep alternates in cycles every 50 minutes during infancy. Cycle length increases progressively during childhood. Adults have NREM-REM cycles of about 90 t0120 minutes. The relative proportion of NREM stages 3 and 4 sleep is greater early in the sleep period, whereas the proportion of REM sleep increases in the latter part of sleep (Table 13–9).

Specific electroencephalographic waveforms that are used to describe sleep in adults develop over the first 6 months of life (Table 13–10). Polysomnographic studies of sleep after 6 months of age are described in Table 13–11.

Table 13–3.	Age group	Sleep classification
Classification of sleep based on electrophysiology	< 6 months	Active or quiet sleep
	> 6 months	REM or NREM sleep

Table 13–4.	Age group	Specific sleep stages
Sleep stages	< 6 months	Active, quiet, intermediate, and transitional sleep
	> 6 months	NREM stages 1, 2, 3, and 4 sleep, and REM sleep

Table 13–5.	Active sleep	Presence of frequent body and facial twitches and jerks (including limb movements, sucking movements, grimaces, vocalizations, and tremors), rapid eye movements, and irregular breathing
Characteristics of sleep stages in the first 6 months of age		This is the first behavioral sleep state to appear and is the predominant sleep state in the newborn (accounts for 60% of sleep in the newborn, 30% of sleep in the 3-month-old infant, and 20% of sleep in the 2- to 6-year-old child).
	Quiet sleep	Characterized by minimal or no body movements and by regular breathing High-voltage, slow-wave EEG activity EEG pattern of *trace' alternant* in the newborn (*trace' alternant* disappears at about 1 month of age)

Continued

Table 13-5.	Intermediate sleep	Sleep that does not fully meet criteria for either active or quiet sleep
Characteristics of sleep stages in the first 6 months of age—cont'd	Transitional sleep	Sleep that occurs in the transition between active, quiet and intermediate sleep

Table 13-6.	Age group	Initial sleep episode
Initial sleep episode	< 3 months	REM sleep
	> 3 to 4 months	NREM sleep

Table 13-7.	Age group	Proportion of NREM-REM sleep
Proportion of non–rapid eye movement and rapid eye movement sleep	Infancy	50:50
	Adulthood	75:25

Table 13-8.	Age group	Percentage REM sleep time
Percentage of rapid eye movement sleep	Infancy	50%
	Adulthood	25%

Table 13-9.	Age group	NREM-REM cycle length
Ultradian sleep cycles	Infancy	≈ 50 minutes
	Childhood	≈ 60 to 70 minutes
	Adulthood	≈ 90 to 120 minutes

Table 13–10.

Developmental electrophysiological milestones

Electroencephalographic feature	Age at appearance
Trace' alternant pattern of quiet sleep	32 to 34 weeks gestation
Sleep spindles	After 4 weeks to 3 months of age
K-complexes	After 6 months of age
Slow wave activity	8 to 12 weeks of age
Development of distinct electroencephalographic features that allows differentiation of NREM sleep into four specific stages (ie, stages 1, 2, 3, and 4 sleep)	3 to 6 months of age

Table 13–11.   Sleep stages after 6 months of age

Polysomnography	Stage NREM 1	Stage NREM 2	Stages NREM 3/4	Stage REM
EEG	Desynchronized (low voltage, mixed frequency) activity	Rhythmic activity (eg, sleep spindles and K-complexes)	High voltage, slow (< 2 Hz) frequency activity	Desynchronized (low voltage, mixed frequency) activity
EOG	Absence of eye movements	Absence of eye movements	Absence of eye movements	Episodic rapid eye movements (phasic REM)
EMG	Low muscle tone	Low muscle tone	Low muscle tone	Absence of muscle tone
Other features	Regular respiration and heart rate	Regular respiration and heart rate	Regular respiration and heart rate	Irregular respiration and heart rate

Regulation of Sleep-Wake Rhythms

Processes regulating sleep homeostasis are present early in life. The suprachiasmatic nuclei, which control circadian processes, are functional *in utero*, with rhythms in body temperature apparent as early as 1 month of age, and nocturnal sleep consolidation developing shortly thereafter.

Sleep Behaviors During Infancy and Childhood

Five behavioral states have been described in young infants, namely quiet sleep, active sleep, quiet alertness, active alertness, and vocalization.

There is great individual variability in the age at which sleep-related developmental milestones, described in Table 13–12, occur. Whether a specific sleep behavior in a child is considered "normal-for-age" or "problematic" also depends on both cultural perceptions and parental expectations.

Table 13–12.	Sleep-related behavior	Age
Developmental sleep behavior milestones	Longest sleep period occurs at night (rather than sleep occuring randomly throughout the 24-hour day)	6 weeks
	Consolidation of daytime sleep into discrete naps	3 months
	Nocturnal sleep consolidation with ability to sleep through the night	Between 6 and 9 months
	Increase in frequency of wakings during the night ("night wakings")	Between 12 and 72 months
	Cessation of daytime napping	Between 3 and 5 years
	Development of circadian sleep phase preference ("eveningness" vs. morningness")	Between 6 and 12 years
	Development of sleep phase delay	Between 12 and 18 years (adolescence)

Normal Pediatric Sleep

Sleep architecture changes as a function of age, as shown in Table 13–13. Children gradually assume adult patterns of sleep with decreased duration of sleep, and longer NREM-REM ultradian cycles.

Pediatric Sleep Disorders

Sleep problems are present in an estimated 25% of children. Prevalence of sleep disturbance is greater among those with developmental disabilities, medical disorders (with multiple medications, medical procedures or hospitalizations), attention deficit hyperactivity disorder (ADHD), and sleep disorders (obstructive sleep apnea [OSA], periodic limb movement disorder [PLMD], or restless legs syndrome [RLS]). Sleep disorders can manifest as bedtime resistance, insomnia, problematic night wakings, nighttime fears, snoring, sleep apnea, parasomnias (enuresis, nightmares, sleep terrors), excessive sleepiness, behavioral problems, and academic difficulties. Examples of pediatric sleep disorders are listed in Table 13–14.

Sleep-Related Breathing Disorders

Snoring

The prevalence of snoring among children is estimated to be about 3% to 20%. Isolated snoring in children, unaccompanied by OSA, is associated with behavioral and academic problems, and excessive sleepiness. Snoring is believed to be related to significant adenotonsillar hypertrophy in about 60% of cases, and incidence peaks at the ages from 2 to 8 years, coinciding with the peak enlargement of the tonsils and adenoids.

Table 13–13. Sleep patterns as a function of age

Age group	Sleep characteristics	Common sleep disorders
Premature infant	From 24 to 26 weeks of gestation, no clearly definable sleep states are present. Active sleep (presence of eye movements, body movements, and irregular respiration) can be identified by 28 to 30 weeks of gestation and constitutes the majority of sleep at this stage. Quiet sleep (EEG pattern of *trace' discontineau* or *trace' alternant* can be noted by 32 weeks and 36 weeks of gestation, respectively. At the same conceptual age, premature and full-term infants attain similar EEG patterns. However, development of sleep spindles is advanced in premature infants compared to full-term infants.	Irregular sleep patterns
Neonate (newborn to 2 months)	Aggregate hours of sleep per day: 16 to 18 hours (higher among premature infants) Sleep periods, occurring throughout the 24-hour day with no clear diurnal-nocturnal pattern, range from 2 to 3 hours among breast-fed infants and 3 to 5 hours among bottle-fed infants. Sleep periods are separated by periods of wakefulness lasting 1 to 3 hours. Frequent awakenings from sleep (greater likelihood of awakening from active rather than quiet sleep) Regular sleep-wake rhythms develop by 2 to 4 months of age.	Irregular sleep patterns, including day-night reversal
Infant (2 to 12 months)	Aggregate hours of sleep per day: 12 to 16 (with naps accounting for 2 to 4 hours of sleep time) Progressive decrease in duration of nocturnal sleep and frequency of daytime napping as infant gets older (eg, 18 hours/day at birth; 14 to 15 hours/day at 6 months of age) Quiet sleep becomes the dominant sleep stage by 3 months of age. There is increasing use of transitional objects (eg, pacifier) during bedtime. Except for brief arousals (about four to five times each night), most infants are able to sleep through the night by 6 to 9 months of age. Most infants older than 6 months of age do not require night feedings (greater frequency of awakenings during the night for feeding among breast-fed infants compared to bottle-fed infants). Separation anxiety may be present at bedtime.	Difficulties with sleep onset Bedtime resistance Sleep-onset association disorder Rhythmic movement disorders Problematic night wakings
Toddler (1 to 3 years)	Aggregate hours of sleep per day: 11 to 12 Progressive decrease in duration of nocturnal sleep and frequency of daytime napping as child gets older Naps decrease to once per day by 18 months of age. Increasing mobility and independence	Difficulties with sleep onset Bedtime resistance Limit-setting sleep disorder Sleep-onset association disorder Rhythmic movement disorders Problematic night wakings

Continued

Table 13-13. Sleep patterns as a function of age—cont'd

Age group	Sleep characteristics	Common sleep disorders
Preschool (3 to 5 years)	Aggregate hours of sleep per day: 10 to 12 Most children stop napping by the age of 3 to 5 years. Gradual reduction of REM sleep	Obstructive sleep apnea Bedtime resistance Limit-setting sleep disorder Sleep-onset association disorder Disorders of arousal (sleep terrors, confusional arousals, sleepwalking) Problematic night wakings Nighttime fears/nightmares
Preadolescent (5 to 14 years)	Aggregate hours of sleep per day: 8 to 11 Progressive decrease in duration of nocturnal sleep Daytime sleepiness is less common than during adolescence. Circadian sleep-wake rhythm preference ("morningness" or "eveningness") starts to become manifest.	Snoring Obstructive sleep apnea Disorders of arousal (sleep terrors, confusional arousals, sleepwalking) Insufficient sleep syndrome Inadequate sleep hygiene Bruxism
Adolescent (14 to 18 years)	Aggregate hours of sleep per day: 7 to 9 Increase in daytime sleepiness at puberty Phase delay in circadian sleep-wake rhythms occurs in some at puberty.	Snoring Obstructive sleep apnea Delayed circadian phase sleep syndrome Excessive sleepiness Narcolepsy Inadequate sleep hygiene Insomnia

Apnea of Prematurity

Infants less than 37 weeks of gestational age may develop central pauses in respiration lasting at least 20 seconds as well as briefer events associated with bradycardia, hypoxemia, or need for caregiver intervention. The most common type of respiratory event is a mixed apnea. Obstructive and central apneas occur less frequently. These respiratory events are due to immaturity of respiratory control systems. Apnea of prematurity resolves with maturation.

Infant Sleep Apnea

Infant sleep apnea is similar to apnea of prematurity but is seen is infants greater than 37 weeks of gestation. Both obstructive and central sleep apneas or hypopneas can occur during infancy. Central respiratory events appear to be more common than obstructive apneas. Respiratory events can be associated with hypoxemia, brady-tachycardia, and arousals. These occur more frequently during REM sleep. Factors increasing the risk and severity of infant sleep apnea include low birth weight, comorbid medical disorders (anemia, lung disease, gastroesophageal reflux, metabolic derangements, or infection), neurologic disorders, and medication use, including anesthesia.

Infant sleep apnea is *not* an independent risk factor for sudden infant death syndrome (SIDS).

Table 13–14.	Sleep-related breathing disorders	Snoring
Pediatric sleep disorders		Apnea of prematurity
		Infant sleep apnea
		Childhood sleep apnea
	Insomnia	Psychophysiologic insomnia
		Inadequate sleep hygiene
		Bedtime resistance
		Limit-setting sleep disorder
		Sleep-onset association disorder
		Night wakings
		Nighttime fears
		Separation anxiety
		Adjustment sleep disorder
		Food allergy insomnia
	Excessive sleepiness	Insufficient sleep syndrome
		Narcolepsy
		Idiopathic hypersomnia
	Parasomnia	Disorders of arousal
		Confusional arousals
		Sleepwalking
		Sleep terrors
		Enuresis
		Rhythmic movement disorder
		Bruxism
		Nocturnal eating (drinking) syndrome
	Movement disorders	Restless legs syndrome
		Periodic limb movement disorder
	Circadian rhythm sleep disorders	Delayed sleep phase syndrome
		Advanced sleep phase syndrome
		Irregular sleep-wake pattern
		Non–24-hour sleep-wake syndrome
	Sleep associated with medical disorders	Colic
		Allergies
		Atopic dermatitis
		Asthma
		Cystic fibrosis
		Congenital central hypoventilation syndrome
		Otitis media
		Irritable bowel syndrome
		Gastroesophageal reflux
		Chronic renal failure
		Sickle cell disease
		Juvenile rheumatoid arthritis
		Chronic fatigue syndrome
		Fibromyalgia
		Achondroplasia
		Down syndrome
		Prader-Willi syndrome
		Williams syndrome
		Mucopolysaccharidoses

Continued

Table 13-14.		Fragile X syndrome
Pediatric sleep disorder—cont'd		Smith-Magenis syndrome
		Angelman syndrome
		San Filippo syndrome
		Burns
		Hospitalization
	Sleep associated with neurologic and developmental disorders	Autism
		Blindness
		Mental retardation
		Rett syndrome
		Asperger syndrome
		Neuromuscular disorders
		Meningomyelocele
		Traumatic brain injury
		Migraines
		Tuberous sclerosis
		Seizures
	Sleep associated with psychiatric and behavioral disorders	Mood disorder
		Bipolar disorder
		Anxiety disorder
		Post-traumatic stress disorder
		Adjustment disorder
		Attention deficit hyperactivity disorder

Childhood Sleep Apnea

OSA is present in an estimated 1% to 5% of children.

Risk factors for childhood sleep apnea include the following:

1.   Adenotonsillar enlargement—most important risk factor for OSA in children

2.   Other craniofacial features (please refer to Table 13–15)

Table 13-15.	Risk factor	Characteristics
Risk factors for childhood obstructive sleep apnea	Craniofacial features	Choanal stenosis
		Nasal polyps
		Midfacial hypoplasia
		Achondroplasia
		Apert syndrome
		Crouzon syndrome
		Down syndrome
		Macroglossia
		Cleft palate repair (pharyngeal flap operations)
		Micrognathia
		Mandibular hypoplasia
		Cornelia de Lange syndrome
		Cri du chat
		Down syndrome
		Pierre-Robin sequence
		Treacher-Collins syndrome
		Laryngomalacia
		Subglottic stenosis

Table 13-15.	Risk factor	Characteristics
Risk factors for childhood obstructive sleep apnea—cont'd	Medical and neurologic syndromes	Arnold-Chiari malformation Beckwith-Wiedemann syndrome Brainstem injury or masses Cerebral palsy Gastroesophageal reflux Goldenhar syndrome Hallerman-Streiff syndrome Hypothyroidism Hypotonic cerebral palsy Klippel-Feil syndrome Meningomyelocele Mobius syndrome Mucopolysaccharidoses Muscular dystrophies Myasthenia gravis Neuromuscular diseases Pfeiffer syndrome Sickle cell disease

3. Gender—no gender difference prior to puberty; increase in prevalence among boys after puberty

4. Obesity—although excess body weight is a risk factor, most children with OSA are not overweight

5. Ethnicity—prevalence of OSA is higher among African-American children compared to Caucasian children

6. Age—childhood OSA peaks between 2 and 5 years of age, which coincides with the peak ages of adenotonsillar enlargement; a second peak in prevalence may be seen during adolescence

7. Down syndrome—increased risk of OSA in patients with Down syndrome due to hypotonia, midfacial and mandibular hypoplasia, glossoptosis, and associated obesity or hypothyroidism

8. Prader-Willi syndrome—increased likelihood of OSA due to obesity and hypotonia; clinical features include obesity, hyperphagia, short stature, short extremities, upsloping palpebral fissures, high-arched palate, hypotonia, mental retardation, hypogonadism, excessive sleepiness, daytime hypercapnia, and abnormal ventilatory response to hypercapnia and hypoxemia; due to a mutation on chromosome 5

9. Medical and neurologic syndromes (refer to Table 13–15)

Although many children with OSA may present with excessive sleepiness, others may not. It has been estimated that only about 30% of children with OSA complain of excessive sleepiness. Childhood OSA may manifest as behavioral problems and academic difficulties (Table 13–16).

Evaluation

Polysomnography Evaluation of children with suspected OSA requires formal polysomnography (Box 13–1). In addition to the usual measurements obtained for adult patients, many pediatric sleep centers routinely monitor end-tidal or transcutaneous CO_2.

Table 13-16. Manifestations of childhood sleep apnea

Clinical features	Associated features	Physical features
Excessive sleepiness	Growth retardation and failure to thrive	Adenotonsillar enlargement
Habitual snoring	Developmental delay	(however, the size of the
Witnessed apneas	Attention deficit/hyperactivity disorder	tonsils and adenoids do
Labored breathing during sleep	Increase in frequency of parasomnias	not necessarily correlate
Nocturnal dyspnea	(disorders of arousal such as	with the presence or
Sleep disturbance (increase in	sleepwalking or sleep terrors)	severity of OSA)
frequency of arousals)	Increase in frequency of body	Mouth breathing
Bedtime resistance	movements during sleep	Paradoxical respiration
Problematic night wakings	Intellectual impairment with delay in	Thoracic retractions
Irritability	language development	Hyponasal speech/nasal
Behavioral problems (inattentiveness,	Hypoxemia and hypercapnia	congestion
hyperactivity, aggressiveness,	Sinus arrhythmia and other cardiac	Unusual positions during
impulsivity, social withdrawal)	arrhythmias	sleep (hyperextension of
Neurocongnitive impairment (memory,	Pulmonary hypertension or cor	neck, or sleeping seated
executive function, attention,	pulmonale	or being propped up by
vigilance, reaction time, motor skills)	Systemic hypertension	pillows)
Poor school performance	Secondary enuresis	Note: Physical examination
Nighttime sweating	Congestive heart failure	may be completely
Morning headaches	Decreased quality of life	normal.
Mood disorder (depression, anxiety)		

Multiple Sleep Latency Test Sleep latency is often normal.

Radiologic Studies Lateral cephalometric radiographs may be useful in children with significant craniofacial abnormalities or for those in whom more extensive surgeries for OSA are being contemplated.

Differences Between Childhood and Adult Obstructive Sleep Apnea

OSA in children differs from the disorder in adults in several ways. Excessive sleepiness, which is common among adults, is encountered less frequently in children. Rather, children may demonstrate behavioral problems, including hyperactivity and restlessness. There are no gender differences in prevalence among children, whereas adult OSA is more often seen among men. Finally, adenotonsillar enlargement is the most important risk factor for childhood OSA, and adenotonsillectomy is the most common therapy for this age group. Differences between childhood and adult OSA are presented in Table 13–17.

Therapy

Adenotonsillectomy Because a majority of childhood OSA is due to significant adenotonsillar enlargement, adenotonsillectomy is the first-line and most common therapy for children with OSA. It is effective in most cases of uncomplicated childhood OSA (ie, without craniofacial anomalies, choanal atresia, macroglossia, or hypotonia). In patients with complicated cases of

Box 13-1. **Polysomnographic features**	Obstructive apneas or hypopneas
	Pauses in breathing or reduction in airflow (> 30% to 50% compared to baseline) lasting 2 normal respiratory cycles or longer
	One or more scoreable respiratory events per hour of sleep is considered significant
	Oxygen desaturation and hypercapnia related to respiratory events
	Oxygen desaturation nadir < 92%; or change in oxygen desaturation nadir from baseline > 4%
	Maximal end-tidal CO_2 > 53 to 55 mm Hg
	Increase in end-tidal CO_2 > 45 mm Hg for greater than 60% of total sleep time (TST)
	Increase in end-tidal CO_2 > 50 mm Hg for greater than 10% of TST
	Paradoxical rib cage–abdominal wall excursions
	Increasingly negative esophageal pressure swings
	Electroencephalographic arousals may or may not occur following apneas
	Occur predominantly during REM sleep
	Obstructive hypoventilation
	Prolonged periods of hypoventilation, with hypercapnia and hypoxemia, due to persistent but partial upper airway obstruction
	Can occur with or without arousals
	Upper airway resistance syndrome
	Increasingly negative esophageal pressure swings without significant airflow limitation
	Usually normal sleep architecture

Table 13-17. Differences between childhood and adult obstructive sleep apnea

Manifestation	Childhood OSA	Adult OSA
Excessive sleepiness	Less frequent	More frequent
Hyperactivity and restlessness	More common	Less common
Gender ratio	Equal	More prevalent among men
Usual cause/s	Adenotonsillar enlargement	Obesity, narrow oropharynx
Polysomnographic features	Normal sleep architecture Few respiratory event-related arousals Less oxygen desaturation	Decrease in NREM stages 3 and 4, and REM sleep Respiratory events are often associated with arousals Greater oxygen desaturation
Usual therapy	Adenotonsillectomy	Continuous positive airway pressure therapy

OSA, a postoperative polysomnogram following adenotonsillectomy is recommended to assess the efficacy of the procedure. OSA may recur during adolescence in children with initial success with adenotonsillectomy.

Continuous Positive Airway Pressure Therapy   Indications for continuous positive airway pressure (CPAP) for children with OSA include:

1.   When adenotonsillectomy is not indicated or contraindicated

2.   When significant symptoms persist following adenotonsillectomy

3.   During the perioperative period in children with severe disease

CPAP titration should be repeated periodically to account for the age-related changes in upper airway and craniofacial dimensions.

Oral Devices   Oral appliances may be considered in older adolescents when growth of craniofacial bones and upper airway soft tissues is largely complete.

Insomnia

Developmental milestones influence the occurrence of sleep disturbance in children. Different types of insomnia may develop during various stages of childhood. Both the child's self report of his/her sleep quality and the parents' report of their child's sleep quality may be unreliable, and objective measures using polysomnography or actigraphy may offer useful clues in some patients. The various types of insomnia in children are listed in Box 13–2.

Inadequate Sleep Hygiene

Inadequate sleep hygiene is among the most common causes of sleep-initiation and sleep-maintenance insomnia. It involves practices by the child that increase arousal (stimulating activities too close to bedtime, poor bedroom environmental control, or caffeine intake) or practices that decrease sleep propensity (irregular sleep-wake schedule, excessive time in bed, frequent use of the bed and bedroom for non–sleep-related activities [television or computer use], or late afternoon/early evening napping). Inadequate sleep hygiene can also give rise to problematic night wakings and excessive sleepiness. Polysomnographic features of inadequate sleep hygiene are listed in Box 13–3.

Psychophysiologic Insomnia

Psychophysiologic insomnia, with learned sleep-preventing associations, greater somatized tension, and conditioned arousal to the bedroom environment, can occur in children. Clinical features, underlying pathophysiology, and treatment options are similar to that of adults.

Bedtime Resistance

Bedtime resistance commonly starts during the toddler years, associated with the development of independence and autonomy. Behavioral treatment of bedtime resistance is described in Box 13–4.

Box 13–2. **Etiology of insomnia in children**	Insufficient sleep (can give rise to hyperarousal)
	Psychophysiologic insomnia
	Behavioral disorders
	Inadequate sleep hygiene
	Limit-setting sleep disorder
	Sleep-onset association disorder
	Primary sleep disorders
	Obstructive sleep apnea
	Restless legs syndrome
	Periodic limb movement disorder
	Parasomnias
	Nightmares
	Circadian rhythm sleep disorder
	Delayed sleep phase syndrome
	Night awakenings
	Separation anxiety
	Nighttime fears

Box 13–3. **Polysomnographic features of inadequate sleep hygiene**	↑ Increased sleep latency
	↓ Reduced sleep efficiency
	Frequent arousals
	Early-morning awakenings
	Excessive sleepiness on Multiple Sleep Latency Test

Box 13–4. **Behavioral treatment of bedtime resistance**	Parental education
	Maintenance of consistent bedtimes and appropriate nighttime activities
	Establishment of optimal bedroom environment
	Extinction procedures
	Faded bedtime
	Positive bedtime routines

Polysomnographic features of limit setting sleep disorder	Normal duration, timing and quality of sleep when appropriate limits are instituted by the caregiver

Limit-Setting Sleep Disorder

Children with limit-setting sleep disorder repetitively refuse to go to sleep at an appropriate time when requested to do so because of inadequate enforcement of bedtimes by the caregiver. In order to stay up later, they often stall going to bed. If the caretaker recognizes the child's attempts to delay his or her bedtime, and when limits to further activity are strictly enforced, sleep comes naturally and quickly. This disorder affects an estimated 5% to 30% of children, typically 2 years of age or older, with a slightly greater prevalence among boys.

Differential diagnosis includes a variable sleep schedule, childhood fears of darkness or being left alone in their room, separation anxiety, inadequate sleep hygiene, psychophysiologic insomnia, delayed sleep-phase syndrome, or RLS.

Treatment is behavioral (Box 13–5).

Sleep-Onset Association Disorder

Children with sleep-onset association disorder are incapable of falling asleep or returning to sleep after an awakening, without the presence of certain desired, but inappropriate, conditions or objects (eg, feeding bottle, pacifier, or intervention by caregiver, such as being held). In addition to sleep-initiation insomnia, these children may have recurrent awakenings. Duration, timing, and quality of sleep are normal when the desired associations are present.

Sleep-onset association disorder is generally diagnosed in children between the ages of 6 months and 3 years; in this age group, it is estimated to be present in 15% to 30% of children. There may be a slight male predominance in prevalence. It commonly remits by age 3 to 4 years. Occasionally, it may persist into adulthood.

Differential diagnosis includes separation anxiety and nighttime fears. Polysomnographic features of sleep-onset association disorder are listed in Box 13–6. Behavioral treatment of sleep-onset association disorder is described in Box 13–7.

Box 13–5. Behavioral treatment of limit-setting sleep disorder	Parental education
	Consistent and predictable parental limit-setting behavior
	Age-appropriate bedtime (bedtimes should be reasonably set and should not be enforced at an inappropriately early time)
	Faded bedtime
	Positive and consistent bedtime routines
	Establishment of optimal bedroom environment
	Appropriate use of transitional objects (eg, doll, blanket)

Box 13-6.
 	
Polysomnographic features of sleep-onset association disorder
	When the associations are absent:
	  ↑ Sleep latency
	  ↑ Frequency of awakenings
	When the associations are present:
	    Normal duration, timing and quality of sleep

Box 13-7. **Behavioral treatment of sleep-onset association disorder**	Parental education Age-appropriate bedtime Faded bedtime Positive and consistent bedtime routines Establishment of optimal bedroom environment Appropriate use of transitional objects (eg, doll, blanket) Extinction procedures

Nighttime Awakenings

Most infants are capable of sleeping through the night by 6 months of age. However, arousals occur normally four to six times each night. Certain conditions, such as co-sleeping, colic, otitis media, and breast-feeding, may increase the frequency of arousals. Whether these spontaneous arousals are brief or prolonged depend, in part, on the infants' ability to soothe themselves back to sleep without the need for parental intervention. Problematic and prolonged night wakings are commonly encountered in those who are unable to fall asleep at bedtime or return to sleep during arousals at night unless certain sleep onset associations are present. The practice of putting infants to bed while drowsy but still awake appears to be associated with the development of the capacity to self-soothe. Conversely, immediate parental intervention during night wakings may reinforce the need for repeated parental-child interactions during the night. Behavioral treatment of nighttime awakenings is described in Box 13–8.

Box 13-8. **Behavioral treatment of nighttime awakenings**	Parental education Establishment of optimal bedroom environment Extinction procedures Scheduled awakenings

Nighttime Fears

Nighttime fears of the dark or being left alone can result in significant bedtime resistance and problematic night wakings. Prevalence peaks between 3 and 6 years of age. Many of these fears are benign age-appropriate behaviors, respond to reassurance, and resolve spontaneously by 5 to 6 years of age. Parents should be instructed to avoid reacting excessively because this may reinforce their child's fears. Differential diagnosis includes post-traumatic stress disorder, anxiety disorder, bipolar disorder, schizophrenia, and separation anxiety.

Separation Anxiety

Separation anxiety can give rise to sleep-initiation insomnia or problematic awakenings. It must be distinguished from sleep-onset association disorder and nighttime fears.

Adjustment Sleep Disorder

Transient insomnia can be related to acute stress or change in the bedroom environment. Sleep improves once the stressor resolves or if adaptation to the stress develops.

Food Allergy Insomnia

Insomnia and sleep disturbance, with frequent awakenings, can result from allergy to cow's milk. This condition is usually seen in the first 2 to 4 years of life.

Behavioral Treatment of Childhood Insomnia

General Recommendations

1. Selection of age-appropriate bedtimes

2. Consistent bedtime routines (minimal stimulating activities) and sleep schedules

3. Teaching a child to fall asleep independently by placing the child in bed sleepy but still awake, both at bedtime and during nighttime awakenings beginning at 2 to 4 months of age

4. Transitioning the infant to a final sleep environment (eg, crib in infant's room) by 3 months of age

5. Proper use of transitional objects (eg, blanket or stuffed animal) at bedtime

6. Discontinuation of nighttime feedings in children 6 months of age or older.

    American Academy of Sleep Medicine recommendations for the behavioral treatment of children with sleep problems are described in Box 13–9.

Scheduled Awakenings

With scheduled awakenings, the parent wakes up the child slightly before the usual time of awakening, reassures the child, and then permits the child to return to sleep. The frequency of scheduled

Box 13-9.	1. Behavioral interventions are recommended for treating bedtime problems and night wakings in young children (standard).

Box 13-9.

American Academy of Sleep Medicine (AASM) recommendations regarding behavioral treatment of bedtime problems and night wakings in infants and young children

1. Behavioral interventions are recommended for treating bedtime problems and night wakings in young children (standard).

2. Behavioral interventions are effective in improving the child's daytime functioning and parental well-being in children with bedtime problems and night wakings (guideline).

3. Effective interventions recommended for treating bedtime problems and night wakings in young children include:

   - Unmodified extinction, and extinction of undesired behavior with parental presence (standard)

   - Parent education and prevention (standard)

   - Graduated extinction of undesired behavior (guideline)

   - Delayed bedtime with removal from bed, and positive bedtime routines (guideline)

   - Scheduled awakenings (guideline)

4. There is insufficient evidence to formulate recommendations on any single therapy over another, or on combination interventions over single therapies (option).

Source: Adapted and modified from Morgenthaler TI, Owens J, Alessi C, et al. Practice parameters for behavioral treatment of bedtime problems and night wakings in infants and young children. Sleep 2006;29(10):1277-1281.

AASM definition of terms:

Standard	Generally accepted practice with a high level of clinical certainly
Guideline	Practice associated with a moderate degree of clinical certainty
Option	Practice of uncertain clinical use

awakenings is then progressively reduced until they are discontinued completely when the child is able to sleep through the night. Treatment time is often longer than that of extinction procedures, occasionally requiring several weeks. Another disadvantage is that children are not taught sleep initiation skills. Nonetheless, scheduled awakenings may be preferable to extinction procedures for children who demand parental attention by engaging in self-injurious behaviors or for those who have failed extinction procedures.

Extinction Techniques

There are three general types of extinction techniques, namely the fast approach, gradual approach, and the parental presence approach.

1. Fast approach (absolute extinction)—this involves having the parent put the child in bed, leaving the child alone in his/her room, and ignoring inappropriate child behavior until the next morning. Parents must try to distinguish unreasonable demands from true dangers or medical emergencies. It is usually effective within 3 to 7 days. However, an extinction burst (worsening of attention-seeking behavior) may occur between 5 to 30 days from starting this technique.

2. Gradual approach (graduated extinction)—this involves having the parent put the child in bed, leaving the child alone in his/her room, and responding to the child's inappropriate demands in a gradually decreasing fashion (eg, longer duration between interventions, shorter period of intervention, or lesser physical contact with the child) until parental intervention is finally stopped.

3.   Extinction with parental presence—the parent is allowed to sleep in a separate bed in the child's bedroom for about a week but is instructed to ignore any inappropriate behavior by the child.

Faded Bedtime

Bedtime is delayed for about 30 minutes later than usual. If the child remains awake, bedtime is delayed for another 30 minutes before the child is placed back in bed. This is continued until the child is able to rapidly fall asleep. Subsequent bedtimes are then advanced or delayed in 30-minute increments or decrements depending on how easily the child is able to sleep, until the desired bedtime is reached.

Positive Bedtime Routines

Positive bedtime routines include selecting a proper age-appropriate bedtime (including temporarily delaying bedtime to decrease sleep latency, and advancing bedtime gradually until the desired bedtime is attained), and establishing relaxing pre-bedtime activities.

Cognitive-Behavioral Therapy

Sleep restriction, stimulus control, and cognitive therapy can be provided following principles used for adult patients with insomnia. With sleep restriction, sleep should not be reduced to less than 6 hours in children.

Pharmacologic Treatment of Childhood Insomnia

No hypnotic agents are currently approved by the U.S. Food and Drug Administration (FDA) for use in children, and their efficacy and safety in this age group are not established. Use of the following agents, which generally shorten sleep latency and reduce the frequency of night wakings, have been described in children with insomnia:

1.   Antihistamines (first-generation agents)

2.   Chloral hydrate

3.   Benzodiazepines and nonbenzodiazepine benzodiazepines receptor agonists (zolpidem, zaleplon, eszopiclone)

4.   Trazodone

5.   Melatonin

6.   Clonidine (particularly in children with ADHD or neurologic impairment)

Sleepiness

Sleepiness in children can manifest as increased likelihood of falling asleep at inappropriate times and situations, behavioral problems (irritability, impulsiveness or ADHD) and cognitive impairment (inattentiveness or academic difficulties). Daytime napping in a child 5 to 10 years of age or older is unusual and may indicate the presence of excessive sleepiness.

Etiology of sleepiness in children include inadequate sleep duration; sleep fragmentation (eg, OSA or PLMD); alteration in circadian sleep-wake rhythms (eg, delayed sleep phase syndrome); medical, neurologic, and psychiatric disorders (eg, narcolepsy or idiopathic hypersomnia); or the use and abuse of substances or medications (eg, alcohol, use of sedative agents, or withdrawal from stimulants). The consequences of sleepiness in children are outlined in Box 13–10.

Box 13–10. **Consequences of sleepiness in children**	Impaired vigilance Difficulty waking in the morning Fatigue and lethargy Changes in mood (irritability, depression, anxiety, low frustration tolerance, emotional lability) Behavioral problems (inattentiveness, distractibility, poor impulse control, hyperactivity, aggression, disinhibition, oppositional behavior, risk-taking behavior) Neurocognitive impairment (memory, concentration, learning, creativity, verbal fluency, problem solving, executive functions) Deficits in academic performance Unplanned daytime napping Increase in accidents Family and social disruption Negative impact on cardiovascular, metabolic, endocrine, and immune function

Insufficient Sleep

In insufficient sleep syndrome, the child has a sleep duration that is regularly shorter than is expected for age. This is the most common cause of excessive sleepiness in children.

If performed over the child's habitual sleep period, polysomnography reveals a decrease in sleep latency, increase in sleep efficiency, and decrease in wake time after sleep onset. Decrease in sleep latency can also be noted during MSLT. Sleepiness secondary to insufficient sleep duration generally resolves following a trial of sleep extension.

Narcolepsy

Narcolepsy often manifests initially as excessive sleepiness (eg, resumption of daytime napping) during the second decade of life. Cataplexy, sleep paralysis, hypnagogic hallucinations, and sleep-onset REM periods may not be present in young children. In addition, unlike the repetitive short naps that can be seen in adult patients, children with narcolepsy may have prolonged sleep periods.

Because of the evolving nature of narcolepsy in children, several polysomnographic studies performed over several months to years may be required for diagnosis. Multiple Sleep Latency Test (MSLT) parameters have not been standardized for children younger than 8 years of age.

No medications for narcolepsy are currently approved by the FDA for use in children younger than 16 years of age. The efficacy and safety of any drugs for narcolepsy have not been well established in children.

Idiopathic Hypersomnia

Onset of idiopathic hypersomnia is usually during adolescence or early adulthood. Many children with narcolepsy, who might not have yet developed cataplexy, sleep paralysis, hypnagogic hallucinations or REM-sleep abnormalities during MSLT, may initially be diagnosed as having idiopathic hypersomnia.

Evaluation of the Sleepy Child

Excessive sleepiness should be considered in any child older than 5 years of age who continues to nap, especially if unplanned, during the day, or who sleep 2 or more hours on weekends compared to weekdays ("weekend oversleep").

There are no universally accepted norms for the MSLT in children. It is not uncommon for children to have an average sleep latency of 20 to 25 minutes.

Parasomnia

Disorders of Arousal

Disorders of arousal (eg, confusional arousals, sleepwalking, and sleep terrors) are more common among children than in adults. These parasomnias occur predominantly during NREM stages 3 and 4 sleep. Onset of sleepwalking is commonly between 4 and 6 years of age, with a peak in prevalence between 4 and 6 years of age. Sleep terrors typically start between 4 and 10 years of age.

Therapy includes proper sleep hygiene and avoidance of sleep deprivation. Pharmacologic agents (short-acting benzodiazepines or tricyclic antidepressants) or behavioral therapy (scheduled awakenings approximately 15 to 30 minutes prior to the time the first parasomnia of the night typically occurs) may be indicated for cases that are frequent, violent, potentially injurious, or disruptive of the sleep of the patient or family members.

Most cases of sleepwalking and sleep terrors spontaneously resolve by adolescence along with the decrease in NREM stages 3 and 4 sleep.

Enuresis

Enuresis is considered primary if it persists in a child older than 5 years of age without any associated medical, neurologic, psychiatric, or urologic disorders, or secondary if it recurs after 6 months to 1 year of dry nights. Although enuresis occurs most commonly during the first third of the night, it can occur throughout the evening and during all sleep stages.

The likelihood of enuresis may be related to genetic predisposition (higher concordance rates in monozygotic compared to dizygotic twins, and increasing prevalence of enuresis correlated with the number of affected parents), decrease in ease of arousability during sleep, lower nocturnal secretion of antidiuretic hormone, or a reduced urinary bladder capacity.

The treatment of enuresis is outlined in Box 13–11.

Box 13–11. Treatment of enuresis	Parent education
	Evaluation and treatment of secondary causes of enuresis
	Avoidance of coercive toilet training or punitive punishment
	Limiting fluid intake close to bedtime
	Bell and pad therapy (approximately 70% effective)
	Relaxation and mental imagery
	Pharmacotherapy (desmopressin or imipramine) when acute control is desired, such as during sleepovers

Rhythmic Movement Disorder

Children with developmental, neurologic, or psychiatric disorders, or those who are blind, may manifest with rhythmic movement disorder (headbanging, headrolling, or body rolling). This condition appears to be more common in boys than in girls. Course is typically transient with complete resolution as the child gets older. Child abuse or neglect should be considered in persistent cases.

Bruxism

Nocturnal teeth grinding may begin during childhood or adolescence. Prevalence is similar in boys and girls.

Nocturnal Eating (Drinking) Syndrome

A child with nocturnal eating (drinking) syndrome wakes up repeatedly during the night and is unable to return to sleep without first eating or drinking. This condition is diagnosed in children older than 2 months of age and is most common during infancy and early childhood. Prevalence appears to be greater in children who were breast-fed than those who were bottle-fed.

Nocturnal eating (drinking) syndrome must be differentiated from sleep-onset association disorder or limit-setting sleep disorder. Therapy involves gradually increasing the duration between feedings, or reducing the amount of feedings during the night.

Benign Neonatal Sleep Myoclonus

Benign sleep myoclonus is a self-limited disorder that consists of repetitive, brief, asynchronous muscle jerks occurring in clusters during quiet sleep. The movements involve the body and/or extremities and are not accompanied by arousals. Its onset is typically in the first week of life.

Restless Legs Syndrome and Periodic Limb Movement Disorder

Among children, RLS and PLMD may present as bedtime refusal, insomnia, recurrent night arousals, problematic night wakings, restlessness during sleep, excessive sleepiness or behavioral problems (eg, ADHD). The prevalence of RLS and PLMD in the pediatric population is unknown.

Evaluation may be hindered by the inability of children to fully articulate the sensations they experience.

Criteria for the diagnosis of "definite" RLS in children are presented in Box 13–12. Criteria for the diagnosis of "probable" and "at risk" RLS are presented in Boxes 13–13 and 13–14, respectively. Criteria for the diagnosis of periodic limb movement disorder in children are presented in Box 13–15.

Box 13-12. **Criteria for the diagnosis of "definite" restless legs syndrome in children**	*Either* Presence of all four adult criteria for RLS, namely: 1. An urge to move the legs, usually accompanied or caused by uncomfortable and unpleasant sensations (paresthesias or dysesthesias) in the limbs. The arms or other body parts may be involved as well. Occasionally, the urge to move is unaccompanied by uncomfortable sensations, and 2. The urge to move or unpleasant sensations: · Begin or worsen during periods of rest or inactivity (eg, lying or sitting) · Are partially or totally relieved by movement (eg, walking or stretching), at least during the time of the activity · Are worse in the evening or night than during the day, or only occur in the evening or night And description consistent with leg discomfort in the child's own words *Or* 1. Presence of all four adult criteria for RLS, and 2. Presence of at least 2 of the following supportive criteria, namely: · Sleep disturbance · Biological parent or sibling with definite RLS · Periodic leg movement index of five or more per hour of sleep during polysomnography. *Source: Adapted and modified from NIH/RLS Foundation Workshop. RLS: Diagnosis and Diagnostic and Epidemiological Tools. May 2002.*

Although therapy using dopaminergic agents, benzodiazepines, opiates, anticonvulsants, and clonidine have been described for adult patients with RLS and/or PLMD, limited information is currently available on the use of these agents for RLS or PLMD among children.

Circadian Rhythm Sleep Disorders

Children with circadian rhythm sleep disorders have sleep periods occurring at inappropriate times relative to the desired, conventional, or socially acceptable bedtimes. Sleep, once it occurs, is generally of normal duration and quality.

Delayed Sleep-Phase Syndrome

In delayed sleep-phase syndrome (DSPS), the major nocturnal sleep period is chronically delayed in relation to the desired bedtime, with an inability to advance sleep onset to an earlier time.

Box 13–13.

Criteria for the diagnosis of "probable" restless legs syndrome in children

Either

Presence of all four adult criteria for RLS, except criterion 2 (ie, urge to move or sensation worse in the evening than during the day), *and*

Biological parent or sibling with definite RLS

Or

Observed leg discomfort worse during rest and inactivity, accompanied and relieved by movement, and worse at night, *and*

Biological parent or sibling with definite RLS

Source: Adapted and modified from NIH/RLS Foundation Workshop. RLS: Diagnosis and Diagnostic and Epidemiological Tools. May 2002.

Box 13–14.

Criteria for the diagnosis of "at risk" for restless legs syndrome in children

Diagnosis of periodic limb movement disorder, *and*

Presence of biological parent or sibling with definite RLS

Note: Child does not meet criteria for definite or probable childhood RLS

Source: Adapted and modified from NIH/RLS Foundation Workshop. RLS: Diagnosis and Diagnostic and Epidemiological Tools. May 2002.

Box 13–15.

Criteria for the diagnosis of periodic limb movement disorder in children

Periodic leg movement index of 5 or more per hour of sleep during polysomnography, *and*

Sleep disturbance (eg, sleep-onset or sleep-maintenance insomnia, or excessive sleepiness) *and*

Leg movements are not due to sleep-disordered breathing or medication effect.

Source: Adapted and modified from NIH/RLS Foundation Workshop. RLS: Diagnosis and Diagnostic and Epidemiological Tools. May 2002.

Sleep onset occurs at about the same delayed time each night. The patient may "sleep in" until the late morning or early afternoon especially on weekends.

Onset of DSPS often occurs during adolescence, but cases starting during childhood have been described. It has a prevalence of about 2% to 10% among children and adolescents. It appears to be more common among males in this younger age group. DSPS may be associated with academic difficulties with chronic tardiness or absenteeism, behavioral problems, and depression.

Advanced Sleep-Phase Syndrome

Advanced sleep-phase syndrome (ASPS) is characterized by an advance in the major nocturnal sleep period in relation to the desired bedtime and an inability to delay sleep onset at night. Although ASPS is not associated with impairment of daytime academic work, it can give rise to difficulty with nighttime homework or extracurricular activities due to excessive early evening sleepiness. The preadolescent child often has a mild degree of phase-advancement in his/her sleep schedules.

Irregular Sleep-Wake Pattern

This disorder is defined by variable periods of sleep and wakefulness throughout the 24-hour day. This sleep-wake variability is common among newborn infants and is not considered pathologic until after 6 months of age when consolidation of nighttime sleep develops.

Non–24-Hour Sleep-Wake Syndrome

In non-24-hour sleep-wake syndrome, the sleep-wake schedule relies entirely on endogenous circadian rhythms. This results in incremental delays in the major sleep period. This condition is more commonly observed in blind children but may also be encountered in children with mental retardation, or with severely schizoid or avoidant personality disorder, and, rarely, in sighted individuals. Given the extreme variability in sleep-wake schedules, children with this condition are generally unable to attend school.

Therapy

Chronotherapy, appropriately timed light exposure and proper sleep hygiene measures are often prescribed for children with circadian rhythm sleep disorders. Neither the efficacy nor safety of melatonin among children has been established.

Sleep in Children with Medical Disorders

A number of medical conditions commonly encountered in children can give rise to sleep disturbance (Table 13–18).

Sudden Infant Death Syndrome

The sudden infant death syndrome (SIDS) is defined by an abrupt unexpected death in an apparently healthy infant, the cause of which is not determined by history, postmortem examination, and death scene investigation. A majority of victims are believed to have died during their sleep.

Table 13-18. Childhood sleep and medical disorders

Medical disorder	Characteristics
Colic	Colic is defined as repeated, sustained episodes of crying (> 3 hours), irritability, or fussing, with no apparent reason. It has been reported in up to 20% of infants, beginning generally at about 3 weeks of age. Colic usually resolves by 3 to 4 months of age. Colic can give rise to insomnia. Compared with infants without colic, affected infants often have shorter reported sleep duration and slightly greater prevalence of REM sleep-related obstructive apneas on polysomnography.

Table 13-18. Childhood sleep and medical disorders—cont'd

Medical disorder	Characteristics
Allergies	Insomnia Chronic allergic rhinitis can increase upper airway resistance and exacerbate obstructive sleep apnea
Atopic dermatitis	Atopic dermatitis, with frequent scratching, can influence sleep duration and quality (even in children whose condition is in remission). Sleep disruption related to atopic dermatitis may be associated with insomnia or excessive sleepiness. Polysomnographic features in children with atopic dermatitis: ↑ Sleep latency ↓ Total sleep time ↑ Frequency of awakenings
Asthma	Children with asthma may have worsening of their symptoms at night. Coughing and dyspnea can give rise to sleep disturbance, insomnia, and excessive sleepiness. Polysomnographic features in children with nocturnal asthma: ↓ Sleep efficiency ↓ Total sleep time ↑ Frequency of awakenings ↓ NREM stages 3 and 4 sleep Psychological problems, decrements in cognition and memory, and poor academic performance have been described in asthmatic children with poor sleep. Symptoms are often accompanied by a decrease in forced expiratory volume in 1 second (FEV_1) and peak expiratory flow (PEF). Oxygen desaturation may also be present.
Cystic fibrosis	Increase in sleep disturbance ↓ Sleep efficiency ↑ Frequency of arousals Greater risk of obstructive sleep apnea Nocturnal hypoxemia
Congenital central hypoventilation syndrome	Hypoventilation, with hypoxemia and hypercapnia, may first manifest in newborn infants.
Otitis media	Pain from acute otitis media can lead to insomnia and sleep disturbance.
Irritable bowel syndrome	Increase in sleep disturbance
Gastroesophageal reflux disease	Sleep-related gastroesophageal reflux (GER) can have a negative impact on sleep and give rise to insomnia, arousals, and nighttime awakenings. It can cause nocturnal coughing, bronchoconstriction, aspiration, or heartburn. GER may be exacerbated by comorbid obstructive sleep apnea
Chronic renal failure	Daytime sleepiness Greater frequency of periodic limb movements of sleep or restless legs syndrome
Chronic pain syndromes	Daytime sleepiness and fatigue Sleep fragmentation Polysomnographic features of children with chronic pain syndromes: ↑ Sleep latency ↓ Total sleep time ↑ Frequency of awakenings

Continued

Table 13-18. Childhood sleep and medical disorders—cont'd

Medical disorder	Characteristics
Sickle cell disease	Sleep disturbance during painful crises Increased risk of obstructive sleep apnea due to adenotonsillar hypertrophy Conversely, oxygen desaturation secondary to obstructive sleep apnea can lead to more painful crises.
Juvenile rheumatoid arthritis	Sleep disruption secondary to recurrent pain may be associated with sleep fragmentation, increase in frequency of night wakings, and excessive sleepiness. Prevalence of other sleep disorders, including obstructive sleep apnea, restless legs syndrome, and periodic limb movement disorder, may be increased in children with juvenile rheumatoid arthritis.
Chronic fatigue syndrome	Children with chronic fatigue syndrome can present with complaints of insomnia, or daytime sleepiness and fatigue.
Fibromyalgia	Polysomnographic features of children with fibromyalgia: ↑ Sleep latency ↓ Sleep efficiency ↑ Frequency of arousals ↑ Frequency of periodic limb movements of sleep
Achondroplasia	Children with achondroplasia have a higher risk of developing obstructive sleep apnea.
Down syndrome	There is an increased likelihood of obstructive and central sleep apnea, insomnia, and periodic limb movements of sleep.
Prader-Willi syndrome	Children with Prader-Willi syndrome may complain of excessive sleepiness. There is increased risk of obstructive sleep apnea secondary to obesity and ventilatory abnormalities, including hypoventilation.
Williams syndrome	Frequency of periodic limb movements of sleep is increased.
Mucopolysaccharidoses	Greater risk of obstructive sleep apnea
Fragile X syndrome	Greater risk of obstructive sleep apnea
Smith-Magenis syndrome	Increased sleep disturbance
Angelman syndrome	Insomnia may complicate the course of the disorder.
San Filippo syndrome	Insomnia is a clinical feature.
Burns	Burn victims may develop sleep disturbance due to pain or pruritus. Excessive sleepiness and nightmares are also common. Polysomnographic features: ↑ Sleep latency ↑ Frequency of arousals ↓ NREM stages 3 and 4 sleep
Hospitalization	Insomnia (sleep-initiation and sleep-maintenance) and sleep fragmentation can develop during hospitalization. Polysomnographic features: ↑ Sleep latency ↑ Frequency of arousals ↓ NREM stages 3 and 4 sleep

It is more prevalent in males and occurs predominantly in children younger than 6 months of age. The risk of SIDS is elevated with prematurity, prone (and to a lesser extent side) sleeping position, pre- and postnatal exposure to tobacco smoke, maternal substance abuse, multiple births, teenage pregnancy, siblings with SIDS, lower socioeconomic group, and the occurrence of apnea of infancy.

The incidence of SIDS is reduced by having infants sleep on their backs.

Sleep in Children with Neurologic and Developmental Disorders

Sleep in children with neurodevelopmental disorders are described in Table 13–19.

Table 13-19. Childhood sleep and neurodevelopmental disorders

Developmental disorder	Characteristics
Autism	Severe sleep disturbance can be present in as many as 50% to 70% of children with autism and autistic spectrum disorders, such as Asperger syndrome. Specific sleep disorders include insomnia, problematic night wakings, and circadian rhythm sleep disorders (delayed sleep phase syndrome or irregular sleep-wake pattern), Asperger syndrome may be associated with Kleine-Levin syndrome. Polysomnographic features: ↑ Sleep latency ↓ Total sleep time ↑ Frequency of awakenings
Blindness	Compared to sighted children, blind children tend to have less total sleep time and greater prevalence of circadian sleep-wake rhythm disturbances, insomnia, problematic night wakings, and excessive sleepiness.
Mental retardation	Over half of children with severe mental retardation may experience significant sleep disturbances.
Cerebral palsy	Increased likelihood of having obstructive sleep apnea is seen in children with cerebral palsy.
Rett syndrome	Insomnia and problematic night wakings can develop. Polysomnographic features: ↑ Sleep latency ↓ Total sleep time ↑ Frequency of awakenings
Neuromuscular disorders	Children with neuromuscular disorders may complain of excessive sleepiness and sleep disturbance. There is an increased likelihood of having upper airway obstruction, obstructive sleep apnea, decreased ventilatory drive, and respiratory failure. Obstructive sleep apnea may develop secondary to weakness of the upper airway muscles. Hypoventilation, with hypoxemia and hypercapnia, due to diaphragm weakness or paralysis, or abnormal respiratory drive has been described.

Continued

Table 13-19. Childhood sleep and neurodevelopmental disorders—cont'd

Developmental disorder	Characteristics
	Neuromuscular disorders include Duchenne muscular dystrophy, myotonic dystrophy, myopathies, and Charcot-Marie-Tooth disease. Oxygen desaturation is most pronounced during REM sleep. Polysomnographic features: ↓ Sleep efficiency ↓ Total sleep time
Meningomyelocele	Risk of upper airway obstruction and sleep disordered breathing is increased. Central apneas and central hypoventilation syndrome may develop in cases of meningomyelocele associate with type II Arnold-Chiari malformation.
Traumatic brain injury	NREM stages 3 and 4 sleep are increased immediately following brain injury.
Migraines	Insomnia and increased frequency of sleepwalking may develop in patients with migraine headaches.
Tuberous sclerosis	Insomnia can develop in persons with tuberous sclerosis.
Seizures	Sleep disruption and excessive sleepiness have been described in patients with nocturnal seizures. Sleep deprivation can trigger seizures. Nocturnal seizures are more common in NREM stages 1 and 2 sleep or during sleep-wake transitions.

Sleep in Children with Psychiatric and Behavioral Disorders

Sleep disturbances are common in psychiatric and behavioral disorders, including mood disorder, anxiety disorder, post-traumatic stress disorder, and ADHD (Table 13–20). Conversely, sleep disturbance and sleep deprivation can adversely influence the course of psychiatric and behavioral disorders. Finally, psychotropic medications often have a significant negative impact on sleep.

Table 13-20. Childhood sleep and psychiatric and behavioral disorders

Psychiatric disorder	Characteristics
Mood disorder	The following sleep disturbances have been described in children with mood disorder: Insomnia (major depressive disorder or dysthymia) Irregular sleep-wake patterns Nightmares Problematic night wakings Nonrestorative sleep Excessive sleepiness Early morning awakening (depression)

Table 13-20. Childhood sleep and psychiatric and behavioral disorders—cont'd

Psychiatric disorder	Characteristics
Bipolar disorder	Nightmares and circadian rhythm sleep-wake disorders (delayed sleep phase syndrome) have been described in children with bipolar disorder. There is often a decrease in sleep requirements and total sleep time during the manic phase of bipolar disorder. Sleep deprivation may precipitate a manic or hypomanic episode.
Anxiety disorder	Insomnia (sleep-initiation and sleep-maintenance) can develop.
Post-traumatic stress disorder	The following sleep disturbances have been described in children with post-traumatic stress disorder: Insomnia Bedtime resistance Nightmares and nighttime fears Nonrestorative sleep Excessive sleepiness
Adjustment disorder	The following sleep disturbances have been reported in children with adjustment disorder: Insomnia Bedtime resistance Problematic night wakings
Attention deficit hyperactivity disorder	Children with attention deficit hyperactivity disorder are more likely to have difficulty settling, difficulty going to sleep, and sleep disruption compared with those without this condition. The following sleep disturbances have been described in children with attention deficit hyperactivity disorder: Excessive sleepiness Bedtime resistance Insomnia Problematic night wakings Early morning awakenings Polysomnographic features (inconsistent): ↑ Sleep latency ↓ Total sleep time ↑ Frequency of awakenings Symptoms of attention deficit hyperactivity disorders may be exacerbated by sleep disruption.

References

General References

American Academy of Sleep Medicine. *The International Classification of Sleep Disorders: Diagnostic and Coding Manual*. 2nd ed. Westchester, IL: American Academy of Sleep Medicine, 2005.

Bowman TJ. *Review of Sleep Medicine*. Burlington, MA: Butterworth-Heinemann, 2002.

Berry RB. *Sleep Medicine Pearls*. 2nd ed. Philadelphia, PA: Hanley & Belfus, 2002.

Capp PK, Pearl PL, Lewin D. Pediatric sleep disorders. *Sleep Medicine*. Primary Care: Clinics in Office Practice. Elsevier Saunders, 2005.

Chokroverty S. *Clinical Companion to Sleep Disorders Medicine*. 2nd ed. Butterworth-Heinemann, 2000.

Lavie P, Pillar G, Malhotra A. *Sleep Disorders Handbook*. New York, NY: Taylor & Francis, 2002.

Lee-Chiong TL, ed. *Sleep: A Comprehensive Handbook*. Hoboken, NJ: John Wiley & Sons, 2006.

Lee-Chiong TL, Sateia M, Carskadon M, eds. *Sleep Medicine*. Philadelphia, PA: Hanley & Belfus (Elsevier), 2002.

Perlis ML, Lichstein KL, eds. *Treating Sleep Disorders: Principles and Practice of Behavioral Sleep Medicine*. Hoboken, NJ: John Wiley & Sons, 2003.

Rechtschaffen A, Kales A. *A Manual of Standardized Terminology, Techniques and Scoring System for Sleep Stages of Human Subjects*. Los Angeles, CA: Brain Information Service/Brain Research Institute, University of California, 1968.

Reite M, Ruddy J, Nagel K. *Concise Guide to Evaluation and Management of Sleep Disorders*. 3rd ed. Arlington, VA: American Psychiatric Publishing, April 2002.

Sleep Disorders. Medical Clinics of North America. Philadelphia, PA: Elsevier Saunders, 2004.

Sleep Medicine. Primary Care: Clinics in Office Practice. Philadelphia, PA: Elsevier Saunders, 2005.

Sleep Research Society. *SRS Basics of Sleep Guide*. Westchester, IL: Sleep Research Society, 2005.

Basic Pediatric Sleep Medicine

Anders T, Emde R, Parmelee A, eds. *A Manual of Standardized Terminology, Techniques and Criteria for Scoring of States of Sleep and Wakefulness in Newborn Infants*. UCLA Brain Information Service, NINDS Neurological Information Network, 1971.

Anders TF, Keener M. Developmental course of nighttime sleep-wake patterns in full term and premature infants during the first years of life. *Sleep*. 1985;8:173.

Dreyfus-Brisac C. Sleep ontogenesis in early human prematurity from 24 to 27 weeks of conceptual age. *Develop Psychobiol*. 1968;1:62.

Dreyfus-Brisac C. Ontogenesis of sleep in human prematures after 32-weeks of conceptual age. *Dev Psychobiol*. 1970;3:91.

Metcalf D. The ontogenesis of sleep-awake states from birth to 3 months. *Electroenceph Clin Neurophysiol*. 1979;28:421.

Sheldon S. Sleep in infants and children. In: Lee-Chiong TL, ed. *Sleep: A Comprehensive Handbook*. Hoboken, NJ: John Wiley & Sons, 2006.

Normal Human Sleep Across the Ages

Capp PK, Pearl PL, Lewin D. Pediatric sleep disorders. *Sleep Medicine*. Primary Care: Clinics in Office Practice. Elsevier Saunders, 2005.

Mindell JA, Owens JA. *A Clinical Guide to Pediatric Sleep: Diagnosis and Management of Sleep Problems*. Lippincott Williams & Wilkins, 2003.

Sheldon S. Sleep in infants and children. In: Lee-Chiong TL, ed. *Sleep: A Comprehensive Handbook*. Hoboken, NJ: John Wiley & Sons, 2006.

Regulation of Sleep-Wake Rhythms

Capp PK, Pearl PL, Lewin D. Pediatric sleep disorders. *Sleep Medicine*. Primary Care: Clinics in Office Practice. Elsevier Saunders, 2005.

Mindell JA, Owens JA. *A Clinical Guide to Pediatric Sleep: Diagnosis and Management of Sleep Problems*. Lippincott Williams & Wilkins, 2003.

Sheldon S. Sleep in infants and children. In: Lee-Chiong TL, ed. *Sleep: A Comprehensive Handbook*. Hoboken, NJ: John Wiley & Sons, 2006.

Sleep Behaviors During Infancy and Childhood

Capp PK, Pearl PL, Lewin D. Pediatric sleep disorders. *Sleep Medicine*. Primary Care: Clinics in Office Practice. Elsevier Saunders, 2005.

Mindell JA, Owens JA. *A Clinical Guide to Pediatric Sleep: Diagnosis and Management of Sleep Problems*. Lippincott Williams & Wilkins, 2003.

Sheldon S. Sleep in infants and children. In: Lee-Chiong TL, ed. *Sleep: A Comprehensive Handbook*. Hoboken, NJ: John Wiley & Sons, 2006.

Normal Pediatric Sleep

Capp PK, Pearl PL, Lewin D. Pediatric sleep disorders. *Sleep Medicine*. Primary Care: Clinics in Office Practice. Elsevier Saunders, 2005.

Mindell JA, Owens JA. *A Clinical Guide to Pediatric Sleep: Diagnosis and Management of Sleep Problems*. Lippincott Williams & Wilkins, 2003.

Sheldon S. Sleep in infants and children. In: Lee-Chiong TL, ed. *Sleep: A Comprehensive Handbook*. Hoboken, NJ: John Wiley & Sons, 2006.

Pediatric Sleep Disorders

American Academy of Sleep Medicine. *The International Classification of Sleep Disorders: Diagnostic and Coding Manual*. 2nd ed. American Academy of Sleep Medicine, 2005.

Sleep-Related Breathing Disorders

American Academy of Sleep Medicine. *The International Classification of Sleep Disorders: Diagnostic and Coding Manual*. 2nd ed. American Academy of Sleep Medicine, 2005.

Bandla P, Marcus CL. Obstructive sleep apnea in children. In: Lee-Chiong TL, ed. *Sleep: A Comprehensive Handbook*. Hoboken, NJ: John Wiley & Sons, 2006.

Insomnia

Garcia J, Wills L. Sleep disorders in children and teens; helping parents and their families get some rest. *Postgraduate Medicine*. 2000;107:161–4,170–1,175–8.

Mindell JA. Empirically supported treatments in pediatric psychology: Bedtime refusal and night wakings in young children. *Journal of Pediatric Psychology*. 1999;24:465–481.

Moorcroft WH. The sleepless child. In: Lee-Chiong TL, ed. *Sleep: A Comprehensive Handbook.* Hoboken, NJ: John Wiley & Sons, 2006.

National Sleep Foundation. Children and sleep. *Sleep in America* 2004 (P011)http://www.sleep-foundation.org/polls/2004SleepPollFinalReport.pdf

Stein MA, Mendelsohn J, Obermeyer WH, Amromin, J, Benca R. Sleep and behavior problems in school-aged children. *Pediatrics.* 2001;107:e60.

Thiedke CC. Sleep disorders and sleep problems in childhood. *American Family Physician.* 2001;63:277–84.

Ward T, Mason TBA. Sleep disorders in children. *Nursing Clinics of North America.* 2002;37: 693–706.

Wiggs L, France K. Behavioral treatments for sleep problems in children and adolescents with physical illness, psychological problems or intellectual disabilities. *Sleep Medicine Reviews.* 2000;4:299–314.

Sleepiness

Fallone G, Owens J, Deane J. Sleepiness in children and adolescents: clinical implications. *Sleep Med Reviews.* 2002;287–306.

Iglowstein I, Jenni O, Molinari L, Largo R. Sleep duration from infancy to adolescence: Reference values and generational trends. *Pediatrics.* 2003;111:302–307.

Rosen G. The sleepy child. In: Lee-Chiong TL, ed. *Sleep: A Comprehensive Handbook.* Hoboken, NJ: John Wiley & Sons, 2006.

Parasomnia

American Academy of Sleep Medicine. *The International Classification of Sleep Disorders: Diagnostic and Coding Manual.* 2nd ed. American Academy of Sleep Medicine, 2005.

Restless Legs Syndrome and Periodic Limb Movement Disorder

American Academy of Sleep Medicine. *The International Classification of Sleep Disorders: Diagnostic and Coding Manual.* 2nd ed. American Academy of Sleep Medicine, 2005.

NIH/RLS Foundation Workshop. *RLS: Diagnosis and Diagnostic and Epidemiological Tools.* May 2002.

Circadian Rhythm Sleep Disorders

Miles LE, Wilson MA. High incidence of cyclic sleep-wake disorders in the blind. *Sleep Res.* 1977;6:192

Weber AL, Cary MS, Conner N, Keyes P. Human non-24-hour sleep-wake cycles in an everyday environment. *Sleep.* 1980;2:347–354.

Sleep in Children with Medical Disorders

Dahl RE, et al. Sleep disturbances in children with atopic dermatitis. *Arch Pediatr Adolesc Med.* 1995;149:856–60.

Fitzpatrick MF, et al. Morbidity in nocturnal asthma: sleep quality and daytime cognitive performance. *Thorax.* 1991;46:569–73.

Kahn A, et al. Arousals induced by proximal esophageal reflux in infants. *Sleep.* 1991;14:39–42.

Kirjavainen J, et al. Infants with colic have a normal sleep structure at 2 and 7 months of age. *J Pediatr.* 2001;138:218–23.

Miser AW, et al. Pain as a presenting symptom in children and young adults with newly diagnosed malignancy. *Pain.* 1987;29:85–90.

Morgan AD, et al. Breathing patterns during sleep in patients with nocturnal asthma. *Thorax.* 1987;42:600–3.

Reuveni H, et al. Sleep fragmentation in children with atopic dermatitis. *Arch Pediatr Adolesc Med.* 1999;153:249–53.

Stores G, et al. Sleep and psychological disturbance in nocturnal asthma. *Arch Dis Child.* 1998;78:413–9.

Strunk RC, et al. Nocturnal awakening caused by asthma in children with mild-to-moderate asthma in the childhood asthma management program. *J Allergy Clin Immunol.* 2002;110: 395–403.

Sleep in Children with Neurological and Developmental Disorders

Leger D, et al. Sleep disorders in children with blindness. *Ann Neurol.* 1999;46:648–51.

Quine L. Sleep problems in children with mental handicap. *J Ment Defic Res.* 1991;35:269–90.

Wiggs L, Stores G. Sleep patterns and sleep disorders in children with autistic spectrum disorders: insights using parent report and actigraphy. *Dev Med Child Neurol.* 2004;46:372–80.

Sleep in Older Adults 14

Normal Sleep in Aging

Although the requirements for sleep do not appear to decline with aging, the ability to sleep and achieve consolidated sleep may decrease in some older adults. Approximately 50% of older adults complain of sleep disturbance. Older adults often take longer to fall asleep, have lower sleep efficiencies, and have more nighttime awakenings. They are also sleepier during the day than younger adults. Compared to elderly men, women are better able to maintain satisfactory sleep with aging.

Changes in Sleep Architecture With Aging

Aging is associated with changes in sleep architecture (Box 14–1). Greater nighttime sleep disturbance may lead to daytime sleepiness and more frequent daytime napping.

Sleep Disturbance With Aging

Significant disturbances may occur during sleep with aging (Table 14–1).

Etiology of Sleep Disturbance With Aging

Although some of the observed changes can be attributed to normal aging itself (eg, age-related alterations in circadian rhythms), most are due to comorbid medical, neurologic, psychiatric, and primary sleep disorders.

Box 14–1. **Changes in sleep architecture related to aging**	↓ Sleep efficiency ↑ Time in bed ↑ Sleep latency ↓ Total sleep time ↑ Frequency of awakenings and sleep stage shifts ↑ Duration of nighttime awakenings ↑ NREM stage 1 sleep ↓ Frequency of sleep spindles ↓ NREM stages 3 and 4 sleep (↓ number and amplitude of delta waves) ↓ NREM stages 3 and 4 sleep during the first NREM sleep episode ↓ REM sleep latency ↑ Duration of the first REM sleep episode ↓ Total REM sleep ↓ Daytime sleep latency on multiple sleep latency test ↑ Frequency of naps

Table 14-1. Sleep changes associated with aging

Sleep complaints	Increase in frequency of sleep complaints (eg, insomnia)
Neuroendocrine parameters	Decrease in melatonin levels Change in relationship between sleep-wake rhythms and timing of melatonin output with sleep onset and offset occurring earlier relative to melatonin secretion

Circadian rhythms of sleep-wake	Dampening of circadian sleep-wake rhythms
	Advancement in phase of circadian rhythms
	   Increase in likelihood of early morning awakenings
	   Compared to younger adults, zone of increased alertness occur earlier after the nadir of the core body temperature

Sleep disorders	Greater sleep fragmentation Decreased strength of homeostatic sleep drive Greater prevalence of insomnia, obstructive sleep apnea, periodic limb movements of sleep, restless legs syndrome, and REM sleep behavior disorder Increase in risk of developing advanced sleep phase syndrome Decrease in arousal threshold with greater sensitivity to adverse environmental factors, such as noise

Elderly adults often complain of sleep disturbances caused by a number of factors, including:

1. Primary sleep disorders

2. Medical, neurologic, and psychiatric illnesses and the adverse effects on sleep of medications used to treat them

3. Chronic pain syndromes

4. Menopause (associated with hot flashes, insomnia, increase in sleep latency, decrease in sleep efficiency, decrease in total sleep time, increase in wake time after sleep onset, and, possibly, decrease in rapid eye movement [REM] sleep; there is also an increased prevalence of obstructive sleep apnea associated with the post-menopausal state)

5. Nocturia (frequent voiding during the night), which may be due to age-related physiologic changes such as decrease in urinary bladder capacity, greater urine production (decrease in urinary concentrating ability), prostatic enlargement (in men), and detrusor overactivity

6. Alterations in the consolidation and timing (eg, phase advancement) of sleep

7. Stress (eg, loss of spouse or retirement)

Consequences of Sleep Disturbance With Aging

Sleep disturbance among older adults can give rise to several consequences, including daytime sleepiness; mood disorders; increased risk of accidents; and decrease in quality of life, alertness, vigilance, and cognitive functions (eg, memory, attention, response time, and concentration).

Aging and Circadian Rhythms

There is an age-related reduction in the amplitude of the circadian sleep-wake rhythms, melatonin secretion, and core body temperature. The diminished sleep-wake rhythm amplitude gives rise to greater sleepiness during the daytime and reduced nocturnal sleep efficiency. Nocturnal levels of melatonin are reduced. Other hormonal changes related to aging include a diminished release of growth hormone during sleep and increase in the circadian nadir of cortisol level.

Phase advancement of the circadian rhythms of sleep and wakefulness as well as body temperature also occurs with aging. Phase advancement of the sleep-wake circadian rhythm may be related to several mechanisms, including a weakening of the circadian pacemaker itself or the entrainment mechanisms (eg, reduced morning light exposure or diminished retinal sensitivity to photic stimuli). This causes an onset of sleep earlier in the evening as well as an earlier awakening in the morning. Furthermore, phase advancement of body temperature results in a rising temperature during the second half of sleep that also contributes to earlier awakening.

Caution should be exercised when using bright light therapy for circadian sleep disorders in elderly adults with macular degeneration.

Aging and Primary Sleep Disorders

Insomnia

Insomnia is the most common sleep complaint among older adults. Increasing age is associated with a higher prevalence of insomnia and a greater likelihood that insomnia will become chronic. Prevalence of insomnia in older adults is estimated to be between 20% and 40%.

Among the elderly, the prevalence of insomnia is higher in women. There is a weaker correlation between subjective complaints and objective sleep parameters in older women compared to men.

In contrast to younger individuals who present more commonly with sleep-onset insomnia, older adults complain primarily of sleep-maintenance insomnia. Other complaints include difficulty with sleep initiation and early morning awakenings.

Causes of insomnia in the older adult include changes in circadian sleep-wake rhythms (phase advancement and dampening of circadian amplitude); sleep disorders (obstructive sleep apnea and restless legs syndrome); medical disorders (acute and chronic pain syndromes, fibromyalgia, chronic obstructive pulmonary disease, ischemic heart disease, congestive heart failure, gastroesophageal reflux and nocturia); neurologic disorders (Parkinson disease, dementia, and stroke); psychiatric disorders (depression and anxiety); medications; substance use (alcohol and caffeine); and psychologic stressors (retirement and bereavement). Rarely is insomnia in the elderly due exclusively to aging itself.

Consequences of insomnia and sleep disturbance in the older adult include diminished quality of life, excessive sleepiness, fatigue, changes in mood (depression and anxiety), and neuro-cognitive impairment (attention, memory, concentration and reaction time). Balance may be affected. Insomnia may also be related to early institutionalization. The use of hypnotic agents in elderly patients with insomnia is associated with excessive sleepiness (with long-acting agents), anterograde amnesia, increased frequency of accidents and falls, and possibly greater mortality risk. Nonbenzodiazepine benzodiazepine receptor agonists (eg, eszopiclone, zaleplon, and zolpidem) appear to be safer in the older adult compared to benzodiazepine hypnotic agents.

Behavioral therapy of insomnia in the elderly is similar to recommendations given to younger adults. Instructions on proper sleep hygiene should include avoiding alcohol, caffeine, and medications that might affect sleep; limiting the amount of liquid intake in the evening; maintaining a regular schedule of wake-, bed- and meal times; increasing daytime activity, including exercise; and avoiding prolonged daytime naps, especially in the late afternoon or early evening.

Obstructive Sleep Apnea

Compared with younger age groups, older adults have a significantly greater prevalence of obstructive sleep apnea (OSA) based on polysomnographic criteria. Nevertheless, unlike younger adults, the presence of clinical symptoms associated with OSA, such as excessive daytime sleepiness, appears to be less common, and, if present, is less severe.

Most of the increase in prevalence of OSA among older adults occurs prior to 65 years of age, with the prevalence remaining relatively stable thereafter. Interestingly, the apnea-hypopnea index remains relatively unchanged when measured over time in the same population group.

Male predominance in prevalence persists even in this age group. The risk of developing OSA among women increases after menopause, possibly due to decreasing levels of estrogen and progesterone. Hormone replacement therapy in women 50 years of age or older has been shown to decrease the prevalence of OSA.

Obstructive sleep apnea in older adults can manifest with reduced sleep quality, repetitive awakenings, sleep fragmentation, increased daytime sleepiness, impaired neurocognitive function (eg, memory and concentration), mood disorders (eg, depression), and nocturia. The increased risk of cardiopulmonary diseases appears to be less pronounced in the elderly population compared with younger individuals; however, increase in mortality among elderly patients with concurrent ischemic heart disease or stroke has been described.

Unlike in younger individuals, excess body weight, snoring and witnessed apneas are less consistent indicators for the presence of OSA in older adults. In addition, body habitus as a risk factor for OSA is less important with advancing age than in younger adults. Age-specific changes in respiratory drive, respiratory muscle strength, upper airway muscle tone, and airway size might contribute to the increased risk of OSA seen with aging.

Polysomnography is the gold standard diagnostic method for OSA. However, normative data on the apnea-hypopnea index for elderly patients is lacking, as is the appropriate threshold for clinically significant disease.

Therapy for OSA is similar for both young and older adults. Positive airway pressure (PAP) remains the treatment of choice, but nonadherence continues to be problematic. Mandibular advancement devices are a viable alternative for patients with mild to moderate OSA who are unable to tolerate PAP therapy, but these cannot be used in edentulous patients.

Periodic Limb Movements of Sleep

The prevalence of periodic limb movements during sleep (PLMS) increases with aging. It has been estimated that up to 45% of older adults may have PLMS. The many conditions that are associated with PLMS, including rheumatologic conditions, diabetes mellitus, renal insufficiency, vasculopathy, neuropathy, and Parkinson disease are also more common in older adults.

Rapid Eye Movement Sleep Behavior Disorder

REM sleep behavior disorder generally develops in the sixth or seventh decade of life, and its prevalence increases with advancing age.

Sleep in the Institutionalized Older Adult

Institutionalized older adults often have significant disturbances in sleep-wake cycles, with frequent awakenings interrupting nighttime sleep. Repetitive napping commonly occurs throughout the day. Some residents may demonstrate a polyphasic sleep pattern with several brief sleep episodes distributed randomly across the day and night that replaces the major nocturnal sleep period.

Causes of Sleep Disturbance in the Institutionalized Older Adult

Various factors can contribute to sleep disturbance among institutionalized older adults. Nursing home residents may suffer from chronic pain syndromes, respiratory distress from an underlying pulmonary or cardiac condition, nocturia, neurologic disorders such as Parkinson disease and dementia, and primary sleep disorders (eg, OSA) that can disrupt sleep. Patients with dementia may have worsening confusion at night accompanied by abnormal behaviors ("sun downing"). Age-related changes in the phase and amplitude of the circadian sleep-wake rhythm results in decreased nighttime sleep efficiency and early morning awakenings (Box 14–2). Lastly, sleep disturbance can arise from medication use.

The nursing home environment may not be conducive to nighttime sleep. Many patients nap frequently or remain relatively inactive in the daytime with limited light exposure. At night, excessive noise and nursing interventions can interrupt sleep continuity.

Box 14–2. **Polysomnographic features of dementia**	↓ Sleep efficiency ↑ Wake time after sleep onset ↑ NREM stage 1 sleep ↓ NREM stages 3 and 4 sleep ↓ REM sleep

Therapy of Sleep Disturbance in the Institutionalized Older Adult

Interventions designed to improve nighttime sleep in the institutionalized elderly should be individualized. Patients may benefit from increased daytime physical activity (including exercise); reduced napping (limited to 1 hour or less in the afternoon); decreased time in bed during the day; greater light exposure during the day; regular bedtime, arising, and meal times; avoidance of alcohol and caffeinated beverages; and optimizing the nursing home environment. Sleep disorders should be identified and addressed appropriately.

References

General References

American Academy of Sleep Medicine. *The International Classification of Sleep Disorders: Diagnostic and Coding Manual.* 2nd ed. Westchester, IL: American Academy of Sleep Medicine, 2005.

Avidan AY. Sleep disorders in the older patient. *Sleep Medicine. Primary Care: Clinics in Office Practice.* Elsevier Saunders, 2005.

Ayalon L, Liu L, Ancoli-Israel S. Diagnosing and treating sleep disorders in the older adult. *Sleep Disorders.* Medical Clinics of North America. Elsevier Saunders, 2004.

Bowman TJ. *Review of Sleep Medicine.* Burlington, MA: Butterworth-Heinemann, 2002.

Berry RB. *Sleep Medicine Pearls.* 2nd ed. Philadelphia, PA: Hanley & Belfus, 2002.

Chokroverty S. *Clinical Companion to Sleep Disorders Medicine.* 2nd ed. Burlington, MA: Butterworth-Heinemann, 2000.

Lavie P, Pillar G, Malhotra A. *Sleep Disorders Handbook.* New York, NY: Taylor & Francis, 2002.

Lee-Chiong TL, ed. *Sleep: A Comprehensive Handbook.* Hoboken, NJ: John Wiley & Sons, 2006.

Lee-Chiong TL, Sateia M, Carskadon M, eds. *Sleep Medicine.* Philadelphia, PA: Hanley & Belfus (Elsevier), 2002.

Perlis ML, Lichstein KL, eds. *Treating Sleep Disorders: Principles and Practice of Behavioral Sleep Medicine.* Hoboken, NJ: John Wiley & Sons, 2003.

Rechtschaffen A, Kales A. *A Manual of Standardized Terminology, Techniques and Scoring System for Sleep Stages of Human Subjects.* Los Angeles, CA: Brain Information Service/Brain Research Institute, University of California, 1968.

Reite M, Ruddy J, Nagel K. *Concise Guide to Evaluation and Management of Sleep Disorders.* 3rd ed. Arlington, VA: American Psychiatric Publishing, April 2002.

Sleep Disorders. Medical Clinics of North America. Philadelphia, PA: Elsevier Saunders, 2004.

Sleep Medicine. Primary Care: Clinics in Office Practice. Philadelphia, PA: Elsevier Saunders, 2005.

Sleep Research Society. *SRS Basics of Sleep Guide.* Westchester, IL: Sleep Research Society, 2005.

Normal Sleep in Aging

Avidan AY. Sleep disorders in the older patient. *Sleep Medicine. Primary Care: Clinics in Office Practice.* Elsevier Saunders, 2005.

Ayalon L, Liu L, Ancoli-Israel S. Diagnosing and treating sleep disorders in the older adult. *Sleep Disorders.* Medical Clinics of North America. Elsevier Saunders, 2004.

Sleep Disturbance With Aging

Ali A, Snape J. Nocturia in older people: a review of causes, consequences, assessment and management. *International Journal of Clinical Practice.* 2004;58:366–373.

Ancoli-Israel S. Insomnia in the elderly: a review for the primary care practitioner. *Sleep.* 2000;23: S23-S30.

Woodward S, Freedman RR. The thermoregulatory effects of menopausal hot flashes on sleep. *Sleep.* 1994;17:497–501.

Changes in Sleep Architecture With Aging

Prinz PN, Vitiello MV, Raskind MA, Thorpy MJ. Geriatrics: Sleep disorders and aging. *N Engl J Med.* 1990;323:520–526.

Wauquier A. Aging and changes in phasic events during sleep. *Physiol Behav.* 1993;54:803.

Weitzman ED. Sleep and aging. In: Katzman R, Terry RD, eds. *The Neurology of Aging.* Philadelphia, PA: F.A. Davis, 1983;167–188.

Etiology of Sleep Disturbance With Aging

Avidan AY. Sleep disorders in the older patient. *Sleep Medicine. Primary Care: Clinics in Office Practice*. Elsevier Saunders, 2005.

Ayalon L, Liu L, Ancoli-Israel S. Diagnosing and treating sleep disorders in the older adult. *Sleep Disorders*. Medical Clinics of North America. Elsevier Saunders, 2004.

Consequences of Sleep Disturbance With Aging

Avidan AY. Sleep disorders in the older patient. *Sleep Medicine. Primary Care: Clinics in Office Practice*. Elsevier Saunders, 2005.

Ayalon L, Liu L, Ancoli-Israel S. Diagnosing and treating sleep disorders in the older adult. *Sleep Disorders*. Medical Clinics of North America. Elsevier Saunders, 2004.

Aging and Circadian Rhythms

Myers BL, Badia P. Changes in circadian rhythms and sleep quality with aging—mechanisms and interventions. *Neurosci Biobehav Rev*. 1995;19:553–571.

Aging and Primary Sleep Disorders

Ancoli-Israel S. Insomnia in the elderly: a review for the primary care practitioner. *Sleep*. 2000;23(suppl 1):S23–30.

Ancoli-Israel S, Klauber MR, Stepnowsky C, Estline E, Chinn A, Fell R. Sleep-disordered breathing in African-American elderly. *Am J Respir Crit Care Med*. 1995;152:1946–1949.

Ancoli-Israel S, Kripke DF, Klauber MR, Mason WJ, Fell R, Kaplan O. Sleep-disordered breathing in community-dwelling elderly. *Sleep*. 1991;14:486–495.

Ancoli-Israel S, Kripke DF, Klauber MR, Fell R, Stepnowsky C, Estline E, et al. Morbidity, mortality and sleep-disordered breathing in community dwelling elderly. *Sleep*. 1996;19:277–282.

Ancoli-Israel S, Kripke DF, Klauber MR, Parker L, Stepnowsky C, Kullen A, et al. Natural history of sleep disordered breathing in community dwelling elderly. *Sleep*. 1993;16:S25–29.

Avidan AY. Sleep changes and disorders in the elderly patient. *Current Neurology and Neuroscience Reports*. 2002;2:178–185.

Benca RM, Ancoli-Israel S, Moldofsky H. Special considerations in insomnia diagnosis and management: depressed, elderly, and chronic pain populations. *J Clin Psychiatry*. 2004;65 (suppl 8):26–35.

Bixler E, Vgontzas A, Ten H, T, Tyson K, Kales A. Effects of age on sleep apnea in men: I. Prevalence and severity. Am J Resp Crit Care Med 1998;157:144–148.Bliwise DL. Normal aging. In: Kryger MH, Roth T, Dement WC, eds. *Principles and Practice of Sleep Medicine*. 3rd ed. Philadelphia, PA: W.B. Saunders,, 2000;26–42.

Bliwise DL, Adelman CL, Ouslander JG. Polysomnographic correlates of spontaneous nocturnal wetness episodes in incontinent geriatric patients. *Sleep*. 2004;27:153–157.

Buysse DJ. Insomnia, depression and aging. Assessing sleep and mood interactions in older adults. *Geriatrics*. 2004;59:47–51.

Buysse DJ, Reynolds CF III, Monk TH, Hoch CC, Yeager AL, Kupfer DJ. Quantification of subjective sleep quality in healthy elderly men and women using the Pittsburgh Sleep Quality Index (PSQI). *Sleep.* 1991;14:331–338.

Endeshaw YW, Johnson TM, Kutner MH, Ouslander JG, Bliwise DL. Sleep-disordered breathing and nocturia in older adults. *J Am Geriatr Soc.* 2004;52:957–60.

Enright PL, Newman AB, Wahl PW, Manolio TA, Haponik EF, Boyle PJ. Prevalence and correlates of snoring and observed apneas in 5,201 older adults. *Sleep.* 1996;19:531–538.

Foley DJ, Monjan AA, Simonsick EM, Wallace RB, Blazer DG. Incidence and remission of insomnia among elderly adults: an epidemiologic study of 6,800 persons over three years. *Sleep.* 1999;22:S366–72.

Krieger J, Sforza E, Boudewijns A, Zamagni M, Petiau C. Respiratory effort during obstructive sleep apnea: role of age and sleep state. *Chest.* 1997;112:875–884.

Kripke DF, Garfinkel L, Wingard DL, Klauber MR, Marler MR. Mortality associated with sleep duration and insomnia. *Arch Gen Psychiatry.* 2002;59:131–6.

Middelkoop HA, Smilde-van den Doel DA, Neven AK, Kamphuisen HA, Springer CP. Subjective sleep characteristics of 1,485 males and females aged 50–93: effects of sex and age, and factors related to self-evaluated quality of sleep. *J Gerontol A Biol Sci Med Sci.* 1996;51:M108–15.

Nieto FJ, Young TB, Lind BK, Shahar E, Samet JM, Redline S, et al. Association of sleep-disordered breathing, sleep apnea, and hypertension in a large community-based study. Sleep Heart Health Study. *JAMA.* 2000;283:1829–1836.

Peker Y, Hedner J, Kraiczi H, Loth S. Respiratory disturbance index: an independent predictor of mortality in coronary artery disease. *Am J Respir Crit Care Med.* 2000;162:81–86.

Phillips BA, Berry DT, Schmitt FA, Magan LK, Gerhardstein DC, Cook YR. Sleep-disordered breathing in the healthy elderly. Clinically significant? *Chest.* 1992;101:345–349.

Redline S, Kirchner HL, Quan SF, Gottlieb DJ, Kapur V, Newman A. The effects of age, sex, ethnicity, and sleep-disordered breathing on sleep architecture. *Arch Intern Med.* 2004;164:406–418.

Russo-Magno P, O'Brien A, Panciera T, Rounds S. Compliance with CPAP therapy in older men with obstructive sleep apnea. *J Am Geriatr Soc.* 2001;49:1205–1211.

Sateia MJ, Doghramji K, Hauri PJ, Morin CM. Evaluation of chronic insomnia. An American Academy of Sleep Medicine review. *Sleep.* 2000;23:243–308.

Schubert CR, Cruickshanks KJ, Dalton DS, Klein BEK, Klein R, Nondahl DM. Prevalence of sleep problems and quality of life in an older population. *Sleep.* 2002;25:48–52.

Shahar E, Whitney CW, Redline S, Lee ET, Newman AB, Javier Nieto F, et al. Sleep-disordered breathing and cardiovascular disease: cross-sectional results of the Sleep Heart Health Study. *Am J Respir Crit Care Med.* 2001;163:19–25.

Tishler PV, Larkin EK, Schluchter MD, Redline S. Incidence of sleep-disordered breathing in an urban adult population: the relative importance of risk factors in the development of sleep-disordered breathing. *JAMA.* 2003;289:2230–2237.

Umlauf MG, Chasens ER, Greevy RA, Arnold J, Burgio KL, Pillion DJ. Obstructive sleep apnea, nocturia and polyuria in older adults. *Sleep.* 2004;27:139–144.

Vitiello MV, Larsen LH, Moe KE. Age-related sleep change. Gender and estrogen effects on the subjective-objective sleep quality relationships of healthy, noncomplaining older men and women. *J Psychosom Res.* 2004;56:503–510.

Vitiello MV, Moe KE, Prinz PN. Sleep complaints cosegregate with illness in older adults: clinical research informed by and informing epidemiological studies of sleep. *J Psychosom Res.* 2002;53: 555–559.

Young T, Shahar E, Nieto FJ, Redline S, Newman AB, Gottlieb DJ, et al. Predictors of sleep-disordered breathing in community-dwelling adults: the Sleep Heart Health Study. *Arch Intern Med.* 2002;162:893–900.

Sleep in the Institutionalized Older Adult

Ancoli-Israel S, Klauber MR, Kripke DF, Parker L, Cobarrubias M. Sleep apnea in female patients in a nursing home: increased risk of mortality. *Chest.* 1989;96(5):1054–1058.

Bliwise DL. Review: sleep in normal aging and dementia. *Sleep.* 1993;16:40–81.

Bliwise DL, Bevier WC, Bliwise NG, Edgar DM, Dement WC. Systemic 24-hour behavior observations of sleep and wakefulness in a skilled-care nursing facility. *Psychology and Aging.* 1990;15:16–24.

Friedman JH, Chou KL. Sleep and fatigue in Parkinson's disease. *Parkinsonism and Related Disorders.* 2004;10:S27-S35.

Gehrman PR, Martin JL, Shochat T, Nolan S, Corey-Bloom J, Ancoli-Israel S. Sleep disordered breathing and agitation in institutionalized adults with Alzheimer's disease. *American Journal of Geriatric Psychiatry.* 2003;11:426–433.

Martin J, Marler MR, Shochat T, Ancoli-Israel S. Circadian rhythms of agitation in institutionalized patients with Alzheimer's Disease. *Chronobiol Intl.* 2000;17:405–418.

Pat-Horenczyk R, Klauber MR, Shochat T, Ancoli-Israel S. Hourly profiles of sleep and wakefulness in severely versus mild-moderately demented nursing home patients. *Aging Clin Exp Res.* 1998;10:308–315.

Sleep in Women 15

Sleep can be affected by changes in reproductive cycles across the lifespan of women. Levels of estrogen and progesterone vary throughout the reproductive years, with a monthly cyclic pattern associated with menstruation, increasing during pregnancy, returning to preconception levels after delivery, and declining during perimenopause and menopause. Compared with men, women generally have more subjective complaints of insufficient or nonrestorative sleep while reporting a greater need for sleep.

Sleep During the Menstrual Cycle

The usual 28- to 30-day menstrual cycle is divided into two phases, each lasting about 14 to 15 days. The initial follicular phase starts on the first day of menses. Estrogen is the predominant hormone during this phase. The second luteal phase begins at ovulation, with the peak of the surge in levels of luteinizing hormone brought about by rising levels of estrogen and progesterone. The subsequent menstruation is preceded by withdrawal of estrogen and progesterone. Mean daily body temperatures are lower by about 0.4°C during the follicular phase when compared with the luteal phase. Regular menstrual cycles start at menarche and end at menopause.

Poorer sleep quality has been described immediately prior to and during the first several days of menstruation. Subjective sleep disturbance appears to be most severe during the premenstrual period. Nocturnal sleep duration is longer before menstruation than during ovulation. Sleep disturbance is related to a variety of complaints, including abdominal cramping, headaches, breast tenderness, sensation of bloating, and mood changes. Subjective sleepiness increases during the luteal phase. Compared with the follicular phase, the luteal phase is associated with a longer sleep latency and lower sleep efficiency. Despite subjective complaints of sleep disturbance, women's sleep architecture and circadian rhythms (serum or salivary melatonin levels) remain relatively stable across their menstrual cycle (Table 15–1).

Oral Contraceptives and Sleep

Oral contraceptives contain either estrogen and progesterone (combined agents), or progestin only ("minipills"). Changes in sleep architecture related to oral contraceptive use include an increase in non–rapid eye movement (NREM) stage 2 sleep, no change or decrease in NREM stages 3 and 4 sleep, decrease in rapid eye movement (REM) sleep latency, and no change in REM sleep. The use of oral contraceptives is associated with increases in mean levels of melatonin and body temperature during sleep. No changes in daytime alertness or reaction times have been observed.

Table 15–1.   Changes in sleep architecture during the menstrual cycle

Follicular phase	Sleep efficiency (compared with the luteal phase)
Luteal phase	↑ NREM stage 2 sleep ↑ Sleep spindles and ≈ 14 Hz frequency electroencephalogram power density during NREM sleep (compared with the follicular phase) ↓ REM sleep (compared with the follicular phase)
Menstruation	↑ Latency to NREM stages 3 and 4 sleep

Menstrual Cycle Disorders

Sleep may be disrupted by menstrual cycle disorders, including dysmenorrhea, endometriosis, premenstrual syndrome, and premenstrual dysphoric disorder. Dysmenorrhea, defined as painful uterine cramps that occur during menstruation, can give rise to reduced sleep quality, decreased sleep efficiency, decrease in REM sleep (during the luteal phase and menstruation), and increase in daytime fatigue. Pain secondary to endometriosis, characterized by the presence of endometrial tissue outside the uterus (eg, abdomen and pelvis), can also disrupt sleep.

Premenstrual Syndrome

Women with premenstrual syndrome complain of abdominal bloating, increased irritability, poor sleep, and fatigue that occur late in the luteal phase prior to menstruation. Symptoms remit with menses. Sleep complaints include insomnia, decrease subjective sleep quality, frequent awakenings, increase in body movements during sleep, unpleasant dreams or nightmares, unrefreshing sleep, and excessive sleepiness and fatigue. There are no significant changes in sleep efficiency or sleep architecture.

Premenstrual Dysphoric Disorder

Premenstrual dysphoric disorder is a severe form of premenstrual syndrome. Patients generally present with fatigue, changes in mood, and functional impairment. Reduced sleep quality can give rise to sleep complaints, including excessive sleepiness or insomnia. Polysomnographic features include a decrease in sleep efficiency, increase in NREM stage 2 sleep, and decrease in REM sleep. There is diminished nocturnal levels of melatonin and a later onset of nocturnal melatonin secretion during the luteal phase.

Premenstrual Parasomnia

Repeated sleep terrors and sleepwalking occurring primarily during the luteal phase have been described.

Menstrual-Associated Sleep Disorder

Both menstrual-associated insomnia and excessive sleepiness unrelated to menstrual cycle disorders (eg, premenstrual syndrome) have been described. Anxiety, abdominal cramping and bloating, and headaches can contribute to insomnia. Excessive sleepiness may be accompanied by anorexia. By definition, these complaints occur primarily during the late luteal phase and are present for at least three consecutive months. Affected patients are asymptomatic between episodes. Both conditions appear to be rare. Therapy consists of using oral contraceptives to suppress ovulation.

Sleep During Pregnancy and the Postpartum Period

Pregnancy and the immediate postpartum period have profound effects on sleep quality. Pregnant women may complain of sleep disturbance as early as the first trimester. Disturbances include frequent awakenings, increase in wake time after sleep onset, and decrease in sleep duration. The frequency of napping increases during the first trimester. Sleep quality typically improves during the second trimester. Sleep is most disrupted during the third trimester of pregnancy, which is also associated with more frequent napping. Sleep disruption can give rise to fatigue and excessive sleepiness.

During the postpartum period, in particular on the first month following delivery, women may complain of poor sleep quality. Disturbances include significant sleep loss, excessive sleepiness, neurocognitive impairment, and mood changes.

Etiology of Sleep Disturbance

Sleep can be disrupted by the direct effects of the growing fetus as well as by changes in anatomic and physiologic variables related to pregnancy (Table 15–2).

Table 15–2. Causes of sleep disturbance during pregnancy

Trimester	Causes of sleep disturbance
First	Anxiety Back pain Breast tenderness Increase in progesterone levels (resulting in excessive sleepiness) Nausea and vomiting Urinary frequency
Second and third	Anxiety Back pain Difficulty with turning or changing positions during sleep Dyspnea Fetal movements Heartburn and gastroesophageal reflux Leg cramps Nausea and vomiting Nightmares and terrifying dreams Pruritus Restless legs syndrome Snoring Urinary frequency

Endocrine System

There is an increase in progesterone, estrogen, and prolactin levels during pregnancy. The increase in levels of progesterone during pregnancy can give rise to excessive sleepiness (sedative effect) and urinary frequency (smooth muscle inhibitory effect). Estrogen decreases REM sleep.

Respiratory System

The cephalad displacement of the diaphragm by the enlarging uterus and changing hormonal milieu related to pregnancy can significantly affect respiratory patterns. Pregnant women often complain of dyspnea. Reduction in tidal volume, increase in respiratory rate, greater minute ventilation, and reduction in functional residual capacity, as well as respiratory alkalosis, are generally present. Gas exchange worsens further during a supine position. Nonetheless, oxygen saturation remains relatively stable during sleep in most women who have no significant sleep-related breathing disorders.

Renal System

A reduction in urinary bladder capacity due to downward displacement of the uterus during late pregnancy can contribute to urinary frequency. Fluid retention during pregnancy can result in pedal edema and nasal congestion.

Gastrointestinal System

The enlarging uterus can give rise to gastroesophageal reflux and accompanying complaints of nocturnal heartburn.

Changes in Sleep Architecture Related to Pregnancy, Labor, and the Postpartum Period

Changes in sleep architecture can occur during pregnancy, including an increase in wake time after sleep onset and decrease in NREM stages 3 and 4 sleep. There is no significant change in REM sleep. See Table 15–3 for more information.

Sleep Disorders Related to Pregnancy and the Postpartum Period

Pregnancy increases the risk of snoring, obstructive sleep apnea, restless legs syndrome, periodic limb movement disorder, and nocturnal leg cramps (Table 15–4).

Table 15-3. Sleep during pregnancy, labor, and the postpartum period

Period	Sleep characteristics
Pregnancy	Changes in sleep architecture during pregnancy, include: ↓ Sleep efficiency ↑ Total sleep time (decreases by late pregnancy) ↑ Frequency of awakenings ↑ Wake time after sleep onset ↑ NREM stage 1 and 2 sleep ↓ or no change in NREM stages 3 and 4 sleep No change in REM sleep except perhaps for a decrease during late pregnancy Increase in daytime napping
Labor and delivery	Shorter nighttime sleep duration (< 6 h) in the period before labor and delivery is associated with longer labor and increased likelihood of cesarean delivery compared with longer nighttime sleep duration (> 7 h).
Postpartum period	Postpartum period is generally defined as the first 6 months following birth of the infant. Increase in frequency of napping Changes in sleep architecture include: ↓ Sleep efficiency ↓ Total sleep time ↑ Frequency of awakenings ↑ Wake time after sleep onset ↓ NREM stages 1 and 2 sleep ↑ NREM stages 3 and 4 sleep (returning to baseline prepregnancy levels at 1–3 months postpartum) ↓ REM sleep latency No change in REM sleep

Continued

Table 15-3. Sleep during pregnancy, labor, and the postpartum period—cont'd

Period	Sleep characteristics
	In the postpartum period, primiparas (first-time mothers) have greater sleep disruption, more interrupted sleep, less total sleep time, and lower sleep efficiency than multiparas. Sleep disruption is also more severe after delivery by cesarean section as compared with vaginal delivery. Awakenings are frequently related to the infant's intrinsic schedule of sleep-wakefulness and feeding.
Breast-feeding	No change in subjective perceptions of sleep quality Changes in sleep architecture include: ↓ or no change in total sleep time ↓ NREM stages 1 and 2 sleep ↑ NREM stages 3 and 4 sleep (compared with bottle-feeding) ↑ REM sleep in some mothers; no change in REM sleep in others
Cosleeping with infant	Changes in sleep architecture include: ↑ Frequency of arousals (but possibly shorter duration of arousals) ↓ NREM stages 3 and 4 sleep No significant change in sleep efficiency or total sleep time compared with sleeping alone

Sleep During Perimenopause and Postmenopause

Menopause is defined as the cessation of menstruation. Perimenopause, the transition period during which changes in the frequency and duration of the menstrual cycle secondary to declining levels of estrogen and progesterone starts to develop, may last for several years prior to menopause. There is a shift in circulating estrogen from estradiol to estrone. During perimenopause, menstruation starts to become irregular. Common complaints during this period include hot flashes, night sweats, weight gain, diminished sex drive, fatigue, excessive sleepiness, headaches, vaginal dryness, and urinary frequency.

Hot Flashes

Hot flashes are characterized by episodes of warmth in the face and chest associated with sweating and skin flushing. They affect a majority of perimenopausal and postmenopausal women, and they may continue for several years after menopause.

Hot flashes occurring at night can significantly disturb sleep, leading to a decrease in sleep efficiency, increase in frequency of awakenings, and decrease in subjective sleep quality. The frequency of hot flashes is influenced by environmental temperature prior to bedtime (more frequent in warmer environments and less frequent in cooler environments).

Sleep Disturbance During Perimenopause and Postmenopause

Compared with men, healthy older women are more likely to complain of insomnia (difficulty with sleep initiation or maintenance, or early morning awakening), poor sleep quality, insufficient

Table 15–4.   Sleep disorders related to pregnancy and the postpartum period

Sleep disorder	Characteristics
Sleep-related breathing disorders	Snoring and obstructive sleep apnea can develop in women who have risk factors for sleep-related breathing disorders prior to pregnancy or can worsen in pregnant women with preexisting disorders. Factors responsible for the increased incidence of snoring and obstructive sleep apnea during pregnancy include weight gain and upper airway congestion (related to estrogen). Conversely, progesterone, a respiratory stimulant, may protect against worsening sleep apnea. Sleep-related breathing disorders during pregnancy are related to higher rates of maternal hypertension, preeclampsia, intrauterine growth retardation, and low birth weight.
Restless legs syndrome and periodic limb movements of sleep	Pregnancy can precipitate or aggravate an existing periodic limb movement disorder or restless legs syndrome (RLS). Periodic limb movements of sleep can be noted in up to a third of pregnant women. The prevalence of RLS peaks during the third trimester when it can affect approximately 20% of women. RLS improves following delivery. The risk of developing RLS is greater among women who have experienced similar complaints during previous pregnancies as well as in those with low serum ferritin and folate levels.
Nocturnal leg cramps	The prevalence of leg cramps causing awakenings from sleep is greater during pregnancy than before or after conception. The risk of developing leg cramps is increased among women who have twin pregnancies compared with those who have single pregnancies. The frequency of leg cramps progressively increases during the first, second, and third trimesters.
Hypertension	Preeclampsia, or pregnancy-induced hypertension, is characterized by the presence of high blood pressure, proteinuria, pedal edema, and headaches. Women who develop preeclampsia have been observed to have a higher frequency of snoring, greater neck circumference, more restricted airflow secondary to narrower upper airways, increase frequency of arousals, and a higher prevalence of periodic limb movements of sleep when compared with healthy pregnant women.
Postpartum depression	Major depression can develop during pregnancy and the postpartum period. Postpartum depression is associated with reduced sleep efficiency, decrease in total sleep time, and shorter REM sleep latency. Reports of insomnia are common.

or nonrestorative sleep, and need for daytime naps. Older women also report that their sleep is more easily disrupted and a greater use of sedative-hypnotic agents. There appears to be an increase in NREM stage 1 sleep during perimenopause and postmenopause. Unlike men, no significant decrease in NREM stages 3 and 4 sleep with aging has been described in healthy women. There is greater NREM stages 3 and 4 sleep during perimenopause than in premenopause.

Several factors are related to sleep disturbance among older women. These include menopause itself, presence of comorbid medical (chronic pain syndromes), psychiatric (depression) and primary sleep (obstructive sleep apnea and insomnia) conditions, decrease in daytime physical activity, weight gain, stress, significant life events, and caregiving responsibilities.

Insomnia

The prevalence of subjective sleep disturbance appears to be higher during menopause than in the premenopausal period. Insomnia during menopause may be due to hot flashes, mood changes (eg, depression and anxiety), primary sleep disorders such as obstructive sleep apnea, or other medical conditions. Menopausal and postmenopausal women may have more subjective complaints of sleep disturbance compared with premenopausal women but may actually have better objective sleep parameters, with increase in total sleep time, decrease in wake time after sleep onset, and increase in NREM stages 3 and 4 sleep.

Endocrine Changes During Perimenopause

Endocrine changes during the perimenopausal period include a reduction in estradiol secretion, decrease in testosterone and androstenedione levels, and increase in follicle-stimulating hormone and luteinizing hormone levels. These changes in hormone levels appear to be responsible, at least in part, for the sleep disturbance during the perimenopausal period.

  Hormone replacement therapy (HRT; eg, oral synthetic estrogens and medroxyprogesterone) has been shown to increase sleep duration and to improve subjective sleep quality in both asymptomatic women during perimenopause as well as in those with climacteric symptoms (eg, hot flashes) (Box 15–1). Administration of progesterone is associated with a decrease in wake time after sleep onset. Women receiving estrogen therapy report less insomnia and sleep disturbance. HRT is also associated with a decreased prevalence of obstructive sleep apnea and hot flashes. Cessation of this therapy can give rise to recurrence of hot flashes and insomnia.

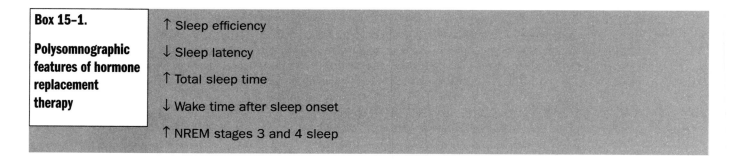

Box 15–1. **Polysomnographic features of hormone replacement therapy**	↑ Sleep efficiency ↓ Sleep latency ↑ Total sleep time ↓ Wake time after sleep onset ↑ NREM stages 3 and 4 sleep

Sleep-Related Breathing Disorders in Women

Anatomy and Physiology of the Upper Airway

Compared with men, women have less neck soft tissue volume, a shorter pharyngeal airway, a lower pharyngeal compliance during sleep, and decreased neck circumference. All these factors might be responsible for the decreased susceptibility to upper airway collapse during sleep among women. There is no significant gender difference in pharyngeal cross-sectional area, upper airway resistance, and hypoxic and hypercapnic ventilatory response during NREM sleep.

Obstructive Sleep Apnea

Obstructive sleep apnea is more common in men than in premenopausal women. There are also gender differences in clinical presentation of obstructive sleep apnea, with fewer reports of snoring as well as more frequent reports of daytime sleepiness, fatigue, and insomnia by women.

The risk of obstructive sleep apnea appears to be increased in women during menopause compared to the premenopausal period. REM sleep–related respiratory events are more frequent during the follicular phase compared with the luteal phase among premenopausal women. Possible mechanisms for the increased risk of obstructive sleep apnea during the perimenopausal and menopausal period include increased age, changes in hormone levels (decrease in progesterone which is a respiratory stimulant), weight gain with greater visceral adiposity (increase in waist:hip circumference ratio), and alterations in ventilatory drive.

The prevalence of obstructive sleep apnea is less among postmenopausal women who use HRT compared to those who do not use HRT. However, current published literature does not conclusively support the use of HRT as therapy for obstructive sleep apnea among postmenopausal women.

Polycystic Ovarian Syndrome

In polycystic ovarian syndrome, increased production of androgens by the ovaries gives rise to irregular or absent menstrual cycles, infertility, weight gain, hirsutism, and greater likelihood of obstructive sleep apnea. Apnea-hypopnea indices appear to correlate with serum levels of testosterone.

Central Sleep Apnea

Central sleep apnea is less common in premenopausal women compared with men. This may be due to a lower hypocapnic apneic threshold among women in whom a more pronounced fall in $PaCO_2$ is necessary for central sleep apneas to develop.

Polysomnography

Compared with men, women tend to demonstrate less supine position dependency in respiratory events and lower apnea-hypopnea indices especially during NREM sleep (when matched for body weight).

References

General References

American Academy of Sleep Medicine. *The International Classification of Sleep Disorders: Diagnostic and Coding Manual.* 2nd ed. Westchester, IL: American Academy of Sleep Medicine, 2005.

Bowman TJ. *Review of Sleep Medicine.* Burlington, MA: Butterworth-Heinemann, 2002.

Berry RB. *Sleep Medicine Pearls.* 2nd ed. Philadelphia, PA: Hanley & Belfus, 2002.

Chokroverty S. *Clinical Companion to Sleep Disorders Medicine.* 2nd ed. Burlington, MA: Butterworth-Heinemann, 2000.

Driver HS, Baker FC. Menstrual factors in sleep. *Sleep Med Rev.* 1998;2:213–229.

Lavie P, Pillar G, Malhotra A. *Sleep Disorders Handbook.* New York, NY: Taylor & Francis, 2002.

Lee-Chiong TL, ed. *Sleep: A Comprehensive Handbook.* Hoboken, NJ: John Wiley & Sons, 2006.

Lee-Chiong TL, Sateia M, Carskadon M, eds. *Sleep Medicine.* Philadelphia, PA: Hanley & Belfus (Elsevier), 2002.

Moline ML, Broch L, Zak R. Sleep in women across the life cycle from adulthood through menopause. *Sleep Disorders. Medical Clinics of North America.* Elsevier Saunders, 2004.

Perlis ML, Lichstein KL, eds. *Treating Sleep Disorders: Principles and Practice of Behavioral Sleep Medicine.* Hoboken, NJ: John Wiley & Sons, 2003.

Reite M, Ruddy J, Nagel K. *Concise Guide to Evaluation and Management of Sleep Disorders.* 3rd ed. Arlington, VA: American Psychiatric Publishing, April 2002.

Sleep Disorders. Medical Clinics of North America. Philadelphia, PA: Elsevier Saunders, 2004.

Sleep Medicine. Primary Care: Clinics in Office Practice. Philadelphia, PA: Elsevier Saunders, 2005.

Sleep Research Society. *SRS Basics of Sleep Guide.* Westchester, IL: Sleep Research Society, 2005.

Sleep During the Menstrual Cycle

Baker FC, Driver HS. Self-reported sleep across the menstrual cycle in young, healthy women. *J Psychosom Res.* 2004;56:39–243.

Baker FC, Waner JI, Vieira EF, Taylor SR, Driver HS, Mitchell D. Sleep and 24-hour body temperatures: a comparison in young men, naturally-cycling women, and in women taking hormonal contraceptives. *J Physiol.* 2001;530:565–574.

Driver HS, Baker FC. Menstrual factors in sleep. *Sleep Med Rev.* 1998;2:213–229.

Driver HS, Dijk D-J, Werth E, Biedermann K, Borbély A. Menstrual cycle effects on sleep EEG in young healthy women. *J Clin Endocrinol Metab.* 1996;81:728–735.

Ito M, Kohsaka M, Fukuda N, Honma K, Honma S, Katsuno Y, et al. Effects of menstrual cycle on plasma melatonin level and sleep characteristics. *Japanese Journal of Psychiatry & Neurology.* 1993;47:478–9.

Moline ML, Broch L, Zak R, Gross V. Sleep in women across the life cycle from adulthood through menopause. *Sleep Med Rev.* 2003;7:155–178.

National Sleep Foundation. (1998). *Women and sleep poll.* Available: http://www.sleepfoundation. org/publications/1998womenpoll.html [1999].

Parry BL, Mendelson WB, Duncan WC, Sack DA, Wehr TA. Longitudinal sleep EEG, temperature, and activity measurements across the menstrual cycle in patients with premenstrual depression and in age-matched controls. *Psychiatry Research.* 1989;30:285–303.

Oral Contraceptives and Sleep

Baker FC, Waner JI, Vieira EF, Taylor SR, Driver HS, Mitchell D. Sleep and 24-hour body temperatures: a comparison in young men, naturally-cycling women, and in women taking hormonal contraceptives. *J Physiol.* 2001;530:565–574.

Menstrual Cycle Disorders

Baker FC, Driver HS, Rogers G, Paiker J, Mitchell D. High nocturnal body temperatures and disturbed sleep in women with primary dysmenorrhea. *Am J Physiol.* 1999;277:E1013–E1021.

Bamford CR. Menstrual-associated sleep disorder: an unusual hypersomniac variant associated with both menstruation and amenorrhea with a possible link to prolactin and metoclopramide. *Sleep.* 1993;16:484–6.

Billiard M, Guilleminault C, Dement WC. A menstruation-linked periodic hypersomnia. Kleine-Levin syndrome or new clinical entity? *Neurology.* 1975;25:436–43.

Bootzin RR, Bamford CR. Premenstrual insomnia: a case study. *Sleep Research.* 1990;19:196.

Chuong CJ, Kim SR, Taskin O, Karacan I. Sleep pattern changes in menstrual cycles of women with premenstrual syndrome: a preliminary study. *Am J Obste Gynecol.* 1997;177:554–8.

Sleep During Pregnancy and the Postpartum Period

Baratte-Beebe KR, Lee K. Sources of mid-sleep awakenings in childbearing women. *Clinical Nursing Research.* 1999;8:386–397.

Blyton DM, Sullivan CE, Edwards N. Lactation is associated with an increase in slow-wave sleep in women. *J Sleep Res.* 2002;11:297–303.

Botez MI, Lambert B. Folate deficiency and restless legs syndrome in pregnancy (letter). *New Engl J Med.* 1977;297:670.

Coble PA, Reynolds CF, Kupfer DJ, Houck PR, Day NL, Giles DE. Childbearing in women with and without a history of affective disorder. II. Electroencephalographic sleep. *Comp Psychiatry.* 1994;35:215–224.

Driver HS, Shapiro CM. A longitudinal study of sleep stages in young women during pregnancy and postpartum. *Sleep.* 1992;15:449–453.

Edwards N, Middleton PG, Blyton DM, Sullivan CE. Sleep disordered breathing and pregnancy. *Thorax.* 2002;57:555–558.

Edwards N, Blyton DM, Kirjavainen T, Kesby GJ, Sullivan CE. Nasal continuous positive airway pressure reduces sleep-induced blood pressure increments in preeclampsia. *Am J Respir Crit Care Med.* 2000;162:252–257.

Ekholm EM, Polo O, Rauhala ER, Ehblad UU. Sleep quality in preeclampsia. *Am J Obstet Gynecol.* 1992;167:1262–1266.

Franklin KA, Holmgren PA, Jönsson F, Poromaa N, Stenlund H, Svanborg E. Snoring, pregnancy-induced hypertension, and growth retardation of the fetus. *Chest.* 2000;117:137–141.

Gay CL, Lee KA, Lee S. Sleep patterns and fatigue in new mothers and fathers. *Biological Research for Nursing.* 2004;5:311–318.

Greenwood KM, Hazendonk KM. Self-reported sleep during the third trimester of pregnancy. *Behavioral Sleep Medicine.* 2004;2:191–204.

Hedman C, Pohjasvaara T, Tolonen U, Suhonen-Malm AS, Myllyla VV. Effects of pregnancy on mothers' sleep. *Sleep Medicine.* 2002;3:37–42.

Herrmann WM, Beach RC. Experimental and clinical data indicating the psychotropic properties of progestogens. *Postgrad Med J.* 1978;54:82–7.

Karacan I, Heine W, Agnew HW, Williams RL, Webb WB, Ross JJ. Characteristics of sleep patterns during late pregnancy and postpartum periods. *Am J Obstet & Gynecol.* 1968;101: 579–586.

Kennedy HP, Beck CT, Driscoll JW. A light in the fog: caring for women with postpartum depression. *J Midwifery & Women's Health.* 2002;47:318–330.

Lee KA. Alterations in sleep during pregnancy and postpartum: a review of 30 years of research. *Sleep Med Rev.* 1998;2:231–242.

Lee KA, McEnany G, Zaffke, ME. REM sleep and mood state in childbearing women: sleepy or weepy? *Sleep.* 2000;23:877–885.

Lee KA, Zaffke ME, Barette-Beebe K. Restless legs syndrome and sleep disturbance during pregnancy: the role of folate and iron. *J Women's Health and Gender-Based Med.* 2001;10:335–341.

Lee KA, Zaffke ME, McEnany G. Parity and sleep patterns during and after pregnancy. *Obstetrics & Gynecology.* 2000;95:14–18.

Maasilta P, Bachour A, Teramo K, Polo O, Laitinen LA. Sleep-related disordered breathing during pregnancy in obese women. *Chest.* 2000;120:1448–1454.

McKenna JJ, Thoman EB, Anders TF, Sadeh A, Schechtman VL, Glotzbach SF. Infant-parent co-sleeping in an evolutionary perspective: implications for understanding infant sleep development and the sudden infant death syndrome. *Sleep.* 1993;16:263–282.

Moline ML, Broch L, Zak R, Gross V. Sleep in women across the life cycle from adulthood through menopause. *Sleep Med Rev.* 2003;7:155–178.

Nishihara K, Horiuchi S, Eto, H, Uchida S. Comparisons of sleep patterns between mothers in post-partum from 9 to 12 weeks and non-pregnant women. *Psychiatry and Clinical Neurosciences.* 2001;55:227–228.

Petre-Quadens I, DeLee C. Sleep-cycle alterations during pregnancy, postpartum and the menstrual cycle. In: Ferin M, Halberg F, Richart RM, Van Wiele RL, eds. *Biorhythms and Human Reproduction.* New York, NY: John Wiley & Sons, 1974:335–351.

Pien GW, Schwab RJ. Sleep disorders during pregnancy. *Sleep.* 2004;27:1405–1417.

Quillan SI. Infant and mother sleep patterns during 4th postpartum week. *Iss Comprehens Pediatric Nurs.* 1997;20:115–123.

Romito P, Saurel-Cubizolles MJ, Cuttini M. Mothers' health after the birth of the first child: the case of employed women in an Italian city. *Women & Health.* 1994;21:1–22.

Sahota PK, Jain SS, Dhand R. Sleep disorders in pregnancy. *Curr Opin Pulm Med.* 2003;9:477–4ç83.

Schutte S, Del Conte A, Doghramji K, Gallagher K, Gallagher E, Oliver R, et al. Snoring during pregnancy and its impact on fetal outcome. *Sleep Research.* 1994;23:325.

Schweiger MS. Sleep disturbance in pregnancy. *Am J Obstet Gynecol.* 1972;114:879–882.

Suga M, Ibuka E. The prevalence of restless legs syndrome among pregnant women in Japan and the relationship between restless legs syndrome and sleep problems. *Sleep.* 2003;26:673–677.

Suzuki K, Ohida T, Sone T, Takemura S, Yokoyama E, Miyake T, et al. Nursing diagnoses for the postpartum woman. *J Obstet Gynecol Neonatal Nurs.* 1988;17:410–417.

Wambach KA. Maternal fatigue in breastfeeding primiparae during the first 9 weeks postpartum. *J Human Lactation.* 1998;14:219–229.

Wilkie G, Shapiro CM. Sleep deprivation and the postnatal blues. *J Psychosomatic Research.* 1992;36:309–316.

Wolfson AR, Crowley SJ, Anwer U, Bassett JL. Changes in sleep patterns and depressive symptoms in first-time mothers: last trimester to one-year postpartum. *Behavioral Sleep Medicine.* 2003;1:54–67.

Zaffke ME, Lee KA. Sleep architecture in a postpartum sample: a comparative analysis. *Sleep Research.* 1992;21:327.

Sleep During Perimenopause and Postmenopause

Baker A, Simpson S, Dawson D. Sleep disruption and mood changes associated with menopause. *Journal of Psychosomatic Research.* 1997;43(4):359–69.

Baldwin CM, Kapur VK, Holberg CJ, Rosen C, Nieto FJ. Associations between gender and measures of daytime somnolence in the Sleep Heart Health Study. *Sleep.* 2004;27:305–311.

Barnabei VAM, Grady D, Stovall DW, Cauley JA, Lin F, Stuenkel CA, et al. Menopausal symptoms in older women and the effects of treatment with hormone therapy. *Obstet Gynecol.* 2002;100:1209–1218.

Dennerstein L, Dudley EC, Hopper JL, Guthrie JR, Burger HG. A prospective population-based study of menopausal symptoms. *Obstetrics & Gynecology.* 2000;96(3):351–8.

Foley DJ, Monjan AA, Brown SL, Simonsick EM, Wallace RB, Blazer DG. Sleep complaints among elderly persons: an epidemiologic study of three communities. *Sleep.* 1995;18:425–432.

Grady D, Ettinger B, Tosteson ANA, Pressman A, Macer JL. Predictors of difficulty when discontinuing postmenopausal hormone therapy. *Obstet Gynecol.* 2003;102:1233–1239.

Kravitz HM, Ganz PA, Bromberger J, Powell LH, Sutton-Tyrrell K, Meyer PM. Sleep difficulty in women at midlife: a community survey of sleep and the menopausal transition. *Menopause.* 2003;10(1):19–28.

Krystal AD, Edinger J, Wohlgemuth W, Marsh GR. Sleep in peri-menopausal and post-menopausal women. *Sleep Med Rev.* 1998;2:243–254.

Kuh DL, Wadsworth M, Hardy R. Women's health in midlife: the influence of the menopause, social factors and health in earlier life. *British Journal of Obstetrics & Gynaecology.* 1997;104(8):823–33.

Middelkoop HAM, Smilde-van den Doel DA, Knuistingh Neve A, Kamphuisen HAC, Springer CP. Subjective sleep characteristics of 1,485 males and females aged 50–93: effects of sex and age, and factors related to self-evaluated quality of sleep. *J Gerontol Med Sci.* 1996;51A:M108–M115.

Moe KE. Reproductive hormones, aging, and sleep. *Seminars in Reproductive Endocrinology.* 1999;17(4):339–348.

Moline ML, Broch L, Zak R, Gross V. Sleep in women across the life cycle from adulthood through menopause. *Sleep Med Rev.* 2003;7:155–178.

Redline S, Kirchner HL, Quan SF, Gottlieb DJ, Kapur V, Newman A. The effects of age, sex, ethnicity, and sleep-disordered breathing on sleep architecture. *Arch Intern Med.* 2004;164:406–418.

Reynolds CF III, Monk TH, Hoch CC, Jennings JR, Buysse DJ, Houck PR, et al. Electroencephalographic sleep in the healthy "old old": a comparison with the "young old" in visually scored and automated measures. *J Gerontol Med Sci.* 1991;46:M39–46.

Sutton DA, Moldofsky H, Badley EM. Insomnia and health problems in Canadians. *Sleep.* 2001;24:665–670.

Vgontzas AN, Zoumakis E, Bixler EO, Lin H-M, Follett H, Chrousos GP. Healthy young women compared to men are more resilient to sleep loss and sleep disturbance than age-matched men: potential protective role of estrogen. In: The Endocrine Society Conference; 2003;2003.

Vitiello MV, Larsen LH, Moe KE. Age-related sleep change. Gender and estrogen effects on the subjective-objective sleep quality relationships of healthy, noncomplaining older men and women. *Journal of Psychosomatic Research.* 2004;56:503–510.

Wiklund I, Karlberg J, Mattsson LA. Quality of life of postmenopausal women on a regimen of transdermal estradiol therapy: a double-blind placebo-controlled study. *American Journal of Obstetrics & Gynecology.* 1993;168(3 Pt 1):824–30.

Sleep-Related Breathing Disorders in Women

Baldwin CM, Griffith KA, Nieto FJ, O'Connor GT, Walsleben JA, Redline S. The association of sleep-disordered breathing and sleep symptoms with quality of life in the Sleep Heart Health Study. *Sleep*. 2001;24:96–105.

Berthon-Jones M, Sullivan CE. Ventilatory and arousal responses to hypoxia in sleeping humans. *Am Rev Respir Dis*. 1982;125:632–639.

Bixler EO, Vgontzas AN, Ten Have T, Tyson K, Kales A. Effects of age on sleep apnea in men. I. Prevalence and severity. *Am J Respir Crit Care Med*. 1998;157:144–148.

Bixler EO, Vgontzas AN, Lin HM, Ten Have T, Rein J, Vela-Bueno A, et al. Prevalence of sleep-disordered breathing in women: effects of gender. *Am J Respir Crit Care Med*. 2001;163:608–613.

Brown IG, Zamel N, Hoffstein V. Pharyngeal cross-sectional area in normal men and women. *J Appl Physiol*. 1986;61:890–895.

Carr MC. The emergence of the metabolic syndrome with menopause. *J Clin Endocrinol Metab*. 2003;88:2404–2411.

Chervin RD. Sleepiness, fatigue, tiredness, and lack of energy in obstructive sleep apnea. *Chest*. 2000;118:372–379.

Cistulli PA, Barnes DJ, Grunstein RR, Sullivan CE. Effect of short-term hormone replacement in the treatment of obstructive sleep apnoea in postmenopausal women. *Thorax*. 1994;49(7):699–702.

Douglas NJ, White DP, Weil JV, Pickett CK, Zwillich CW. Hypercapnic ventilatory response in sleeping adults. *Am Rev Respir Dis*. 1982;126:758–762.

Douglas NJ, White DP, Weil JV, Pickett CK, Martin RJ, Hudgel DW, et al. Hypoxic ventilatory response decreases during sleep in normal men. *Am Rev Respir Dis*. 1982;125:286–289.

Edwards N, Wilcox I, Sullivan C. Haemodynamic responses to obstructive sleep apnoeas in premenopausal women. *J Hypertens*. 1999;17:603–610.

Fogel RB, Malhotra A, Pillar G, Pittman SD, Dunaif A, White DP. Increased prevalence of obstructive sleep apnea syndrome in obese women with polycystic ovary syndrome. *J Clin Endocrinol Metab*. 2001;86:1175–1180.

Gopal M, Duntley S, Uhles M, Attarian H. The role of obesity in the increased prevalence of obstructive sleep apnea syndrome in patients with polycystic ovarian syndrome. *Sleep Medicine*. 2002;3:401–404.

Malhotra A, Huang Y, Fogel RB, Pillar G, Edwards JK, Kikinis R, et al. The male predisposition to pharyngeal collapse: importance of airway length. *Am J Respir Crit Care Med*. 2002;166:1388–1395.

Martin SE, Mathur R, Marshall I, Douglas NJ. The effect of age, sex, obesity and posture on upper airway size. *Eur Respir J*. 1997;10:2087–2090.

Mohsenin V. Gender differences in the expression of sleep-disordered breathing: role of upper airway dimensions. *Chest*. 2001;120:1442–1447.

O'Connor C, Thornley KS, Hanly PJ. Gender differences in the polysomnographic features of obstructive sleep apnea. *Am J Respir Crit Care Med*. 2000;161:1465–1472.

Pillar G, Malhotra A, Fogel R, Beauregard J, Schnall R, White DP. Airway mechanics and ventilation in response to resistive loading during sleep: influence of gender. *Am J Respir Crit Care Med*. 2000;162:1627–1632.

Rowley JA, Sanders CS, Zahn BK, Badr MS. Gender differences in upper airway compliance during NREM sleep: role of neck circumference. *J Appl Physiol*. 2002;92:2535–2541.

Rowley JA, Zhou ZS, Vergine I, Shkoukani BS, Badr MS. The influence of gender on upper airway mechanics: upper airway resistance and Pcrit. *J Appl Physiol.* 2001;91:2248–2254.

Schwab RJ, Gefter WB, Hoffman EA, Gupta KP, Pack AI. Dynamic upper airway imaging during awake respiration in normal subjects and patients with sleep disordered breathing. *Am Rev Respir Dis.* 1993;148:1385–1400.

Sin DD, Fitzgerald F, Parker JD, Newton G, Floras JS, Bradley TD. Risk factors for central and obstructive sleep apnea in 450 men and women with congestive heart failure. *Am J Respir Crit Care Med.* 1999;160:1101–1106.

Thurnheer R, Wraith PK, Douglas NJ. Influence of age and gender on upper airway resistance in NREM and REM sleep. *J Appl Physiol.* 2001;90:981–988.

Trinder J, Kay A, Kleiman J, Dunai J. Gender differences in airway resistance during sleep. *J Appl Physiol.* 1997;83:1986–1997.

Vgontzas AN, Legro RS, Bixler EO, Grayev A, Kales A, Chrousos GP. Polycystic ovary syndrome is associated with obstructive sleep apnea and daytime sleepiness: role of insulin resistance. *J Clin Endocrinol Metab.* 2001;86:517–520.

Ware JC, McBrayer RH, Scott JA. Influence of sex and age on duration and frequency of sleep apnea events. *Sleep.* 2000;23:165–170.

White DP, Douglas NJ, Pickett CK, Weil JV, Zwillich CW. Hypoxic ventilatory response during sleep in normal premenopausal women. *Am Rev Respir Dis.* 1982;126:530–533.

Whittle AT, Marshall I, Mortimore IL, Wraith PK, Sellar RJ, Douglas NJ. Neck soft tissue and fat distribution: comparison between normal men and women by magnetic resonance imaging. *Thorax.* 1999;54:323–328.

Zhou XS, Shahabuddin S, Zahn BK, Babcock MA, Badr MS. Effect of gender on the development of hypocapnic apnea/hypopnea during NREM sleep. *J Appl Physiol.* 2000;89:192–199.

Medications and Their Effects on Sleep

16

Many medications affect the central nervous system (CNS) and can alter the patterns of sleep and wakefulness. Others can induce sleep disorders (eg, nightmares, periodic limb movements of sleep or restless legs syndrome) or exacerbate them (eg, obstructive sleep apnea). Some agents can cause both insomnia and excessive sleepiness in different individuals, or in the same individual under different circumstances. These can be a primary therapeutic effect of the drug, a withdrawal effect, or an adverse reaction. Each medication possesses class- and agent-specific effects on sleep.

Alcohol

Alcohol's effect on arousal and sleep is biphasic. Alcohol has both stimulatory effects (at low doses and on the rising phase of alcohol levels) and sedative effects (at high doses and on the falling phase of alcohol levels). Metabolism of alcohol occurs at a constant rate of 10 to 20 mg/dl per hour.

Alcohol's sedating effect can be additive with other agents such as benzodiazepines. Acute ingestion decreases sleep latency, increases non–rapid eye movement (NREM) stages 3 and 4 sleep, and reduces rapid eye movement (REM) sleep during the first half of the sleep period (Table 16–1). It is metabolized quickly, and alcohol causes a rebound increase in the frequency of arousals and awakenings and an increase in REM sleep during the second part of the night. Nightmares and vivid dreams can occur. In addition, alcohol ingestion can cause worsening of snoring and obstructive sleep apnea by increasing upper airway resistance due to a decrease in pharyngeal dilator muscle tone.

Table 16–1.   Alcohol use, withdrawal, and abstinence

Acute ingestion	Acute withdrawal	Chronic abstinence
↓ Sleep latency	↑ Sleep latency	↓ Total sleep time
Total sleep time (increase total sleep time in some patients)	↓ Total sleep time ↑ Wake time after sleep onset	↑ Frequency of arousals ↑ NREM stage 1 sleep
↓ Wake time after sleep onset	↓ NREM stages 3 and 4 sleep	↓ NREM stages 3 and 4 sleep
↑ NREM stages 3 and 4 sleep during the first half of the sleep period	↓ REM sleep latency ↑ Frequency of REM episodes	↑ REM density
↑ REM sleep latency	↓ Duration of NREM-REM cycles	Note: Sleep disturbance can persist for several years following cessation of alcohol use.
↓ REM sleep during the first half of the sleep period	↑ REM sleep (rebound)	
Note: During the second half of the sleep period, sleep fragmentation with increase in arousals develops. REM sleep rebound is present, and NREM stages 3 and 4 sleep are reduced.	Note: Delirium tremens is associated with a markedly decreased total sleep time.	Predictors of alcohol relapse among alcoholics include: ↓ NREM stages 3 and 4 sleep ↓ REM sleep latency ↑ REM sleep ↑ REM density
Nightmares and disorders of arousal may occur. Alcohol can exacerbate obstructive sleep apnea and restless legs syndrome.		

During alcohol withdrawal, there is a decrease in total sleep time, and increase in sleep latency, wake time after sleep onset, and REM sleep. REM sleep latency is decreased. NREM stages 3 and 4 sleep are reduced (Table 16–1).

During alcohol abstinence, sleep disturbance, including insomnia, can persist. Total sleep time and NREM stages 3 and 4 sleep are reduced (Table 16–1).

Alcohol-Dependent Sleep Disorder

Persons with alcohol-dependent sleep disorder do not exhibit other patterns of behavior compatible with overt alcoholism, and they appear to use alcohol only for its sedative effects. However, habitual use of alcohol prior to anticipated bedtime in an attempt to enhance sleep onset could paradoxically lead to insomnia. As serum levels of alcohol decline in the latter half of the night, individuals can awaken repeatedly with headaches and diaphoresis.

Attempts to terminate alcohol use abruptly can precipitate profound insomnia with frequent awakenings. Virtual absence of sleep can occur during delirium tremens.

Antidepressants

Some antidepressants can disrupt sleep and cause daytime sleepiness. Others are sedating and improve sleep. See Table 16–2 for a list of sedating and nonsedating antidepressants.

Table 16-2.	Sedating antidepressants	Nonsedating antidepressants
Sedating and nonsedating antidepressants	Amitriptyline Doxepin Mirtazapine Trazodone	Selective serotonin reuptake inhibitors (some) Tricyclic antidepressants (some) Monoamine inhibitors (some)

Administration of certain monoamine oxidase inhibitors (MAOIs), tricyclic antidepressants (TCAs) and selective serotonin reuptake inhibitors (SSRIs) can result in insomnia. TCAs and SSRIs can precipitate or worsen periodic limb movement disorder (Table 16–3).

Antidepressants (except nefazodone, bupropion, and mirtazapine) decrease REM sleep and increase REM sleep latency. Sudden discontinuation of REM-suppressant antidepressants can lead to a rebound in REM sleep (Table 16–3).

Mirtazapine, nefazodone, TCAs, trazodone, and lithium increase NREM stages 3 and 4 sleep, whereas SSRIs either decrease or have no significant effect on NREM stages 3 and 4 sleep. Bupropion and nefazodone increase REM sleep (Table 16–3).

Sedative-Hypnotics

This class includes barbiturates, chloral hydrate, benzodiazepines, as well as nonbenzodiazepine benzodiazepine receptor agonists such as eszopiclone, zaleplon and zolpidem. Unlike the earlier sedative-hypnotic agents such as barbiturates, benzodiazepine receptor agonists possess less abuse liability and risk for dependency. Sedation is dose dependent.

Generally, benzodiazepines decrease both NREM stages 3 and 4 as well as REM sleep. Eszopiclone, zaleplon and zolpidem have minimal effects on sleep architecture.

Table 16–3.   Antidepressants

Agent	Mechanism of action	Effect on sleep
Amoxapine	Serotonin and histamine receptor blocker; norepinephrine uptake inhibitor	Excessive sleepiness
Bupropion	Dopamine and norepinephrine reuptake inhibitor	Alerting Insomnia and impairment of cognitive and psychomotor function Polysomnographic features: ↓ NREM stage 2 sleep ↑ NREM stages 3 and 4 sleep ↓ REM sleep latency ↑ REM sleep Note: No effect on periodic leg movements of sleep (PLMS)
Lithium	Antidepressant	Excessive sleepiness Impairment of cognitive and psychomotor functions Polysomnographic features: ↑ Total sleep time ↓ NREM stage 1 sleep ↑ NREM stage 2 sleep ↑ NREM stages 3 and 4 sleep ↑ REM sleep latency ↓ REM sleep (variable) Note: Abrupt withdrawal may cause REM sleep rebound.
Maprotiline	Norepinephrine uptake inhibitor; histamine receptor blocker	Excessive sleepiness Polysomnographic features: ↑ NREM stages 3 and 4 sleep ↓ REM sleep
Mirtazapine	Serotonin and alpha 2-receptor blocker; histamine receptor blocker; norepinephrine blocker	Excessive sleepiness Polysomnographic features: ↓ Sleep latency ↑ Total sleep time ↑ Sleep efficiency ↓ Wake time after sleep onset ↓ NREM stage 1 sleep ↑ NREM stages 3 and 4 sleep ↑ REM sleep latency No significant change in REM sleep Note: Can cause abnormal dreams and nightmares
Monoamine oxidase inhibitors	Inhibition of enzymes involved in the metabolism of norepinephrine, dopamine and serotonin Note: Classified as either classic agents that cause irreversible enzyme inhibition (eg, phenelzine and tranylcypromine), or newer reversible agents (eg, brofaromine and moclobemide)	Insomnia; can also cause excessive sleepiness Polysomnographic features: ↓ Total sleep time ↑ Wake time after sleep onset No change in NREM stages 3 and 4 sleep ↑ REM sleep latency ↓ REM sleep Notes: 1. MAO inhibitors are the most potent REM inhibitors. 2. REM sleep rebound can occur during drug withdrawal. 3. MAO inhibitors can cause abnormal dreams and nightmares.

Table 16-3. Antidepressants—cont'd

Agent	Mechanism of action	Effect on sleep
Nefazodone	Serotonin reuptake inhibitor and serotonin-2 antagonist	Excessive sleepiness Polysomnographic features: ↑ Sleep efficiency ↑ Total sleep time ↓ Wake time after sleep onset ↑ NREM stages 3 and 4 sleep Note: 1. Does not increase REM sleep latency or decrease REM sleep 2. May increase REM sleep and REM density
Selective serotonin reuptake inhibitors (eg, citalopram, fluoxetine, fluvoxamine, paroxetine, and sertraline)	Serotonin reuptake inhibitor	Excessive sleepiness Insomnia (citalopram, fluoxetine) Polysomnographic features: ↑ Sleep latency ↑ Frequency of awakenings ↑ Wake time after sleep onset ↓ Sleep efficiency ↓ Total sleep time ↑ NREM stages 1 and 2 sleep ↓ NREM stages 3 and 4 sleep (inconsistent) ↑ REM sleep latency ↓ REM sleep ↑ REM density Note: 1. Fluvoxamine and paroxetine are among the most sedating SSRIs. 2. SSRIs can precipitate or worsen periodic limb movements of sleep and restless legs syndrome. 3. SSRIs can increase movement disorders during sleep. 4. SSRIs can cause REM sleep behavior disorder. 5. SSRIs can increase eye movements during NREM sleep. Abnormal slow eye movements during sleep following ingestion of fluoxetine ("Prozac eyes") can occur. 6. SSRIs can increase electromyographic (EMG) (submental and anterior tibialis) activity during REM sleep.
Trazodone	Blocks serotonin, alpha 1 and histamine receptors; serotonin reuptake inhibitor; serotonin-2 antagonist	Sedating Excessive sleepiness and impairment of performance Polysomnographic features: ↓ Sleep latency ↑ Sleep efficiency ↑ Total sleep time ↓ Wake time after sleep onset ↑ NREM stages 3 and 4 sleep ↑ REM sleep latency ↓ REM sleep (inconsistent)

Continued

Table 16–3. **Antidepressants—cont'd**

Agent	Mechanism of action	Effect on sleep
		Note: 1. Trazodone is a sedating antidepressant that has been used to treat insomnia. 2. Trazodone can cause postural hypotension and priapism.
Tricyclic antidepressants (eg, amitriptyline, clomipramine, desipramine, doxepin, imipramine, nortriptyline, protriptyline, and trimipramine)	Inhibition of norepinephrine and serotonin uptake; blockade of histamine and acetylcholine Note: Some agents have considerable anticholinergic effects	*Tertiary amines* (eg, amitriptyline, clomipramine, doxepin, and imipramine) Excessive sleepiness and impairment of cognition and psychomotor performance Polysomnographic features of tertiary amines: ↓ Sleep latency ↑ Increase in sleep efficiency ↑ Total sleep time ↓ Frequency of arousals ↑ NREM stage 1 and 2 sleep ↓ NREM stages 3 and 4 sleep ↑ REM sleep latency ↓ REM sleep ↑ REM density *Secondary amines* (eg, desipramine and protriptyline) Activating Polysomnographic features of secondary amines: ↑ Sleep latency ↓ Sleep efficiency ↑ Wake time after sleep onset No change in NREM stages 3 and 4 sleep ↑ REM sleep latency ↓ REM sleep ↑ REM density Notes: 1. Due to their sedating properties, TCAs have been used to treat insomnia. 2. TCAs may precipitate or exacerbate periodic limb movements of sleep or restless legs syndrome. 3. TCAs can cause abnormal dreams and nightmares. 4. Amitriptyline and desipramine can increase NREM stages 3 and 4 sleep. Trimipramine can increase REM sleep latency. 5. Protriptyline may enhance upper airway muscle tone. 6. Sudden drug withdrawal can produce REM sleep rebound and insomnia.
Venlafaxine	Serotonin and norepinephrine reuptake inhibitor	Insomnia or excessive sleepiness Polysomnographic features: ↓ Sleep efficiency ↓ Total sleep time (increase in sleep time in some cases) ↑ Wake time after sleep onset ↑ REM sleep latency ↓ REM sleep Note: Can cause or increase periodic leg movements of sleep

Benzodiazepines act via the gamma-aminobutyric acid (GABA)-A receptor complex, which consists of several receptors, including BZ1, BZ2 and BZ3. The receptor primarily related to sedation is the BZ1. Eszopiclone, zaleplon and zolpidem also act via the BZ1 receptor.

Chronic use of benzodiazepines can lead to tolerance and/or dependency. During abrupt drug withdrawal of benzodiazepines, insomnia, sleep fragmentation, and REM sleep rebound (with nightmares) may develop.

Rebound insomnia related to sudden discontinuation of chronic benzodiazepine use is characterized by difficulty in both initiating and maintaining sleep that lasts for several days and appears to be more severe in drugs with short half-lives compared to longer-acting agents.

Hypnotic-Dependent Sleep Disorder

Habitual use of hypnotic agents (eg, benzodiazepines and barbiturates) may give rise to either insomnia during abrupt withdrawal of the medication, or residual excessive daytime sleepiness if the dose is escalated to compensate for increasing tolerance. Hypnotics may also precipitate or aggravate sleep-related breathing disorders. For information about specific hypnotics, see Table 16–4. Half-lives of selected benzodiazepines are presented in Table 16–5.

Table 16–4.   Hypnotic agents

Agent	Mechanism of action	Effect on sleep
Barbiturates (eg, pentobarbital and phenobarbital)	Act via GABA receptors	Excessive sleepiness Polysomnographic features: ↓ Sleep latency ↑ Sleep continuity ↑ Total sleep time ↓ Wake time after sleep onset ↑ NREM stage 2 sleep (increase in spindle density) ↓ NREM stages 3 and 4 sleep ↑ REM sleep latency ↓ REM sleep Notes: 1. May worsen obstructive sleep apnea 2. Drug withdrawal can cause rebound insomnia
Benzodiazepines (eg, alprazolam, clonazepam, diazepam, estazolam, flurazepam, lorazepam, midazolam, oxazepam, temazepam, and triazolam)	Act via GABA receptors	Excessive sleepiness Polysomnographic features: ↓ Sleep latency ↑ Total sleep time ↓ Frequency of arousals ↓ Wake time after sleep onset ↑ or ↓ NREM stage 1 sleep ↑ NREM stage 2 sleep ↓ NREM stages 3 and 4 sleep ↑ REM sleep latency ↓ REM sleep Notes: 1. ↑ Spindle (12–14 cycles per second) density 2. ↑ "Pseudospindles" (14–18 cycles per second) Multiple Sleep Latency Test: ↓ Daytime sleep latency

Table 16-4. Hypnotic agents—cont'd

Agent	Mechanism of action	Effect on sleep
		Notes: 1. With shorter-acting agents, sleep is improved in the first part of the night, but sleep disruption and fragmentation occur in the second part of the night due to drug withdrawal. Excessive sleepiness is more pronounced with long-acting agents. 2. Insomnia (↓ total sleep time) and REM rebound can occur following sudden drug discontinuation. 3. Benzodiazepines can reduce upper airway muscle tone and worsen obstructive sleep apnea. 4. Benzodiazepines can depress respiration and should be used cautiously in patients with COPD. 5. Reduce severity of symptoms of restless legs syndrome.
Chloral hydrate	Act via the GABA receptor complex Note: Short half-life	Polysomnographic features: ↓ Sleep latency ↑ Total sleep time
Melatonin	A hormone secreted by the pineal gland during darkness that can induce sleep Peak levels at sleep onset at night. Levels are low during the day.	Excessive sleepiness Polysomnographic features: ↓ Sleep latency
Zaleplon	Act via the GABA receptor complex Note: Short half-life Note: Tolerance and withdrawal are rare.	Polysomnographic features: ↓ Sleep latency Note: Minimal effect on NREM stages 3 and 4 sleep as well as REM sleep
Zolpidem and eszopiclone	Act via the GABA receptor complex at a different site than the benzodiazepines Note: No significant effect on respiratory function	Polysomnographic features: ↓ Sleep latency ↓ Wake time after sleep onset ↔ or ↑ NREM stage 2, 3 and 4 sleep ↔ or ↓ REM sleep

Table 16–5.	Agent	Elimination half-life (hours)
Half-lives of benzodiazepines	Triazolam	1.5 to 5.5
	Estazolam	10 to 24
	Temazepam	8 to 20
	Clonazepam	18 to 40
	Chlordiazepoxide	24 to 100
	Flurazepam	70 to 90

Stimulants

Stimulants increase wakefulness and alertness, and they decrease sleepiness. CNS stimulants include amphetamines (dextroamphetamine and methamphetamine), caffeine, cocaine, ephedrine, fenfluramine, mazindol, methylphenidate, modafinil, nicotine, pemoline, phentermine, phenylpropanolamine, and theophylline. Their mechanism of action involves elevating levels of monoamines in the neural synaptic cleft. Psychomotor stimulants are listed in Box 16–1.

Box 16–1.	Amphetamine
Psychomotor stimulants	Caffeine
	Cocaine
	Methylphenidate
	Modafinil
	Nicotine

Polysomnography typically demonstrates an increase in sleep latency, decrease in total sleep time, increase in NREM stage 1 sleep, decrease in NREM stages 3 and 4 sleep, increase in REM sleep latency, and decrease in REM sleep. Hypersomnia accompanied by a decrease in sleep latency, increase in total sleep time, decrease in REM sleep latency, and REM sleep rebound can develop during drug withdrawal.

Caffeine

Caffeine increases alertness and vigilance, and it reverses sleepiness. It is the most commonly used psychostimulant worldwide, being ingested as coffee, tea, caffeinated beverages, or caffeine tablets. Ingestion of caffeine can give rise to insomnia. Tolerance to the stimulating effects of caffeine can develop.

Chemically classified as a methylxanthine, caffeine acts by antagonizing CNS adenosine receptors located on the basal forebrain cholinergic neurons. Adenosine is a sleep-promoting neurotransmitter. Caffeine may also increase cortical release of acetylcholine and affect the GABAergic neurons located in the posterior hypothalamus.

Modafinil

Modafinil is an atypical psychostimulant whose precise mechanism of action remains incompletely understood. It has been suggested that modafinil may alter neurotransmission of hypocretin neurons in the perifornical region, histaminergic neurons in the tuberomammillary nucleus, and hypothalamic centers associated with sleep and waking.

Modafinil is indicated for excessive sleepiness secondary to narcolepsy and shift work sleep disorders. It is also used for residual sleepiness in patients with obstructive sleep apnea who are being treated with continuous positive airway pressure (CPAP) therapy. Compared with the other stimulating compounds, modafinil appears to possess no major addiction potential.

Stimulant-Dependent Sleep Disorder

A decrease in sleepiness or complaints of insomnia may develop whenever stimulant therapy is started, especially when the medication is taken close to bedtime, or during dosage escalations. Excessive sleepiness occurs with abrupt drug withdrawal. See Table 16–6 for information about specific stimulants.

Table 16–6.   Stimulants

Agent	Mechanism of action	Effect on sleep

Amphetamines	Increase the availability of the monoamine neurotransmitters norepinephrine, dopamine, and serotonin at the neural synapse, either by increasing their presynaptic release or blocking their reuptake	Enhance wakefulness and alertness
		Can produce insomnia
		During amphetamine use:
		  ↓ Sleepiness
		  ↑ Sleep latency
		  ↓ Sleep efficiency
		  ↑ Wake time after sleep onset
		  ↓ Total sleep time
		  ↑ Sleep fragmentation
		  ↓ NREM stages 3 and 4 sleep
		  ↑ REM sleep latency
		  ↓ REM sleep
		During amphetamine discontinuation:
		  ↑ Sleepiness
		  ↑ NREM stages 3 and 4 sleep
		  ↑ REM sleep
		Notes:
		1. They are indicated for the therapy of narcolepsy and attention deficit hyperactivity disorder (ADHD).
		2. Amphetamine administration can give rise to complaints of insomnia.
		3. Its elimination half-life is 12 hours.
		4. Amphetamines have a high abuse potential.
		5. Dependency and tolerance can develop.

Caffeine	Adenosine receptor antagonist Adenosine, which increases in the CNS with prolonged wakefulness, is involved with sleep promotion. By blocking the effect of adenosine, caffeine produces cortical arousal.	Increases wakefulness and alertness, and it decreases drowsiness during sleep deprivation Insomnia following ingestion of large quantities of caffeine Excessive sleepiness during withdrawal from chronic large-quantity caffeine use

Table 16-6. Stimulants—cont'd

Agent	Mechanism of action	Effect on sleep
		Polysomnographic features: ↑ Sleep latency ↓ Total sleep time ↑ Frequency of arousals ↑ NREM stage 1 sleep ↓ NREM stages 3 and 4 sleep ↓ REM sleep Note: Caffeine may exacerbate symptoms of restless legs syndrome.
Cocaine	Potentiates effect of epinephrine and norepinephrine	Increase in alertness Polysomnographic features are similar to amphetamines During cocaine use ↓ Total sleep time ↓ REM sleep Daytime stimulation: increases arousal and improves reaction time in sleep-deprived persons During initial cocaine discontinuation ↑ Total sleep time ↑ REM sleep Multiple Sleep Latency Test ↓ Sleep latency Presence of sleep onset REM periods During chronic cocaine abstinence: Persistent insomnia Disturbance in REM sleep Notes: 1. It has an elimination half-life of 50 to 75 minutes. 2. Withdrawal can give rise to excessive sleepiness and REM sleep rebound. 3. High abuse liability
Ecstasy	Chemically related to methamphetamine	Increase in wakefulness Polysomnographic features: ↓ REM sleep
Methylphenidate	Piperidine derivative structurally similar to amphetamine	Polysomnographic features are similar to amphetamines During methylphenidate use ↓ Sleepiness ↓ Sleep efficiency ↓ Total sleep time ↑ Wake time after sleep onset ↓ NREM stages 3 and 4 sleep ↑ REM sleep latency ↓ REM sleep

Continued

Table 16–6. Stimulants—cont'd

Agent	Mechanism of action	Effect on sleep
		During methylphenidate discontinuation: ↓ Sleep latency on the Maintenance of Wakefulness Test (MWT) ↑ REM sleep Notes: 1. It is indicated for the therapy of narcolepsy and ADHD. 2. Its elimination half-life is 2 to 4 hours.
Modafinil	Unknown mechanism of action Possible mechanisms: 1. Decrease release of gamma-aminobutyric acid 2. Increase activity of histaminergic and hypocretin containing neurons	Increases alertness Can cause insomnia if taken close to bedtime Polysomnographic features: ↓ Total sleep time Notes: 1. Does not produce sleep rebound with drug discontinuation
Pemoline	Dopamine agonist Note: Withdrawn from the market due to concerns regarding serious liver toxicity	Increases alertness; can cause insomnia Polysomnographic features: ↓ Total sleep time ↑ Wake time after sleep onset ↓ NREM stages 3 and 4 sleep ↓ REM sleep

Antipsychotics

Antipsychotics (neuroleptics) are indicated for the treatment of schizophrenia. Typical polysomnographic features during antipsychotic administration include a shortened sleep latency, increase in sleep efficiency, decrease in wake time after sleep onset, increase in total sleep time, and decrease in REM sleep (higher doses) (Table 16–7).

Table 16–7. Antipsychotics

Agent	Mechanism of action	Effect on sleep
Chlorpromazine	Typical antipsychotic	Polysomnographic features: ↓ Sleep latency ↑ Sleep efficiency ↑ Total sleep time No consistent changes in NREM stages 3 and 4 sleep ↑ REM sleep latency
Clozapine	Atypical antipsychotic	Sedating Polysomnographic features: ↓ Sleep latency ↓ Wake time after sleep onset ↑ Sleep efficiency ↑ Total sleep time ↑ NREM stage 2 sleep ↓ NREM stages 3 and 4 sleep No change in REM sleep

Table 16-7. Antipsychotics—cont'd

Agent	Mechanism of action	Effect on sleep
Haloperidol	Typical antipsychotic	Polysomnographic features: ↓ Sleep latency ↑ Sleep efficiency ↑ Total sleep time No consistent changes in NREM stages 3 and 4 sleep ↑ REM sleep latency
Olanzapine	Atypical antipsychotic	Polysomnographic features: ↓ Sleep latency ↓ Wake time after sleep onset ↑ Sleep efficiency ↑ Total sleep time ↓ NREM stage 1 sleep ↑ NREM stage 2 sleep ↑ Increase in NREM stages 3 and 4 sleep ↑ REM sleep latency ↓ REM sleep ↑ REM density
Risperidone	Atypical antipsychotic	Polysomnographic features: ↓ Frequency of awakenings ↑ NREM stages 3 and 4 sleep No change in REM sleep latency ↓ REM sleep Note: Can cause or increase periodic leg movements of sleep
Quetiapine	Atypical antipsychotic	Polysomnographic features: ↓ Sleep latency ↓ Wake time after sleep onset ↑ Sleep efficiency ↑ Total sleep time ↑ NREM stage 2 sleep No change in NREM stages 3 and 4 sleep No change in REM sleep latency ↓ REM sleep No change in REM density Can cause or increase periodic leg movements of sleep
Thioridazine	Typical antipsychotic	Sedating and causes excessive sleepiness Polysomnographic features: ↓ Sleep latency ↑ Total sleep time ↑ NREM stages 3 and 4 sleep ↓ REM sleep
Thiothixene	Typical antipsychotic	Polysomnographic features: ↓ Sleep latency ↑ Sleep efficiency ↑ Total sleep time No consistent changes in NREM stages 3 and 4 sleep ↑ REM sleep latency

Other Central Nervous System Active Medications

Table 16–8 presents information about the effect of these drugs on sleep.

Table 16–8. Other central nervous system active medications

Agent	Effect on Sleep

Anticonvulsants
  Carbamazepine
  Ethosuximide
  Felbamate
  Gabapentin
  Lamotrigine
  Phenobarbital
  Phenytoin
  Primidone
  Tiagibine
  Topiramate
  Valproic acid
  Viagabatrin
	Agents causing excessive sleepiness:
	  Carbamazepine
	  Gabapentin
	  Felbamate
	  Lamotrigine
	  Phenobarbital
	  Phenytoin
	  Primidone
	  Tiagibine
	  Topiramate
	  Valproic acid
	  Viagabatrin
	Polysomnographic features:
	  ↓ Sleep latency
	  ↑ Total sleep time
	  ↓ Wake time after sleep onset
	  ↑ NREM stage 2 sleep
	  ↑ NREM stages 3 and 4 sleep (carbamazepine, phenytoin, and possibly valproic acid)
	  ↓ NREM stages 3 and 4 sleep (phenobarbital and, possibly, valproic acid)
	  ↓ REM sleep (carbamazepine, ethosuximide, phenobarbital, and phenytoin)
	Multiple sleep latency test:
	  ↓ Daytime sleep latency (carbamazepine and phenobarbital)
	Notes:
	1. Sedation secondary to anticonvulsants is dose-dependent. Tolerance to this effect may develop with chronic use.
	2. Ethosuximide, felbamate, and lamotrigine can cause insomnia.

Antiparkinsonian drugs
  Dopamine agonists (bromocriptine, pergolide, pramipexole, ropinirole)
  Dopamine precursors (levodopa)
  Anticholinergics (benztropine)
  Selegiline
	Insomnia (amantadine, benztropine, bromocriptine, levodopa, pergolide, pramipexole, and selegiline)
	Excessive sleepiness (pramipexole and ropinirole)
	High-dose levodopa can cause sleep disruption.
	Polysomnographic features of levodopa:
	  ↓ NREM stages 3 and 4 sleep
	  ↑ REM sleep latency
	Polysomnographic features of benztropine:
	  ↑ NREM stages 3 and 4 sleep
	  ↓ REM sleep latency
	Notes:
	1. Pramipexole and ropinirole can cause hallucinations and sudden sleep episodes.
	2. Amantadine and levodopa can cause nightmares.
	3. Benztropine can cause hallucinations.

Buspirone (Anxiolytic)	Unlike other anxiolytics, buspirone is not sedating.

Table 16-8.   Other central nervous system active medications—cont'd

Agent	Effect on Sleep
Donepezil (Acetylcholinesterase inhibitor)	Polysomnographic features: ↑ Wake time after sleep onset ↑ REM sleep Note: Can cause vivid dreams
Gamma-hydroxybutyrate (GHB)	Enhances sleep quality Decreases daytime sleepiness, cataplexy, hypnagogic hallucinations, and sleep paralysis in patients with narcolepsy
Nicotine (Present in cigarettes and other tobacco products)	Nicotine increases alertness and decreases sleepiness. It enhances cortical cholinergic neurotransmission. Used close to bedtime, it can cause disrupted nonrestorative sleep. Produces mild sedation in low blood concentrations Drowsiness can occur during nicotine withdrawal. Polysomnographic features (with smoking close to bedtime): ↑ Sleep latency ↓ Sleep efficiency ↓ Total sleep time ↑ Wake time after sleep onset ↓ REM sleep Polysomnographic features (during withdrawal): ↑ Wake time after sleep onset (first few days of smoking cessation) Multiple sleep latency test: ↑ Daytime sleep latency Notes: 1. Bupropion, an agent used to aid smoking cessation, can give rise to insomnia. 2. Nicotine gum reduces slow-wave sleep. Nicotine patch reduces sleep efficiency (time asleep/time in bed) and prolongs sleep onset latency. 3. Nicotine can increase restless legs symptoms. 4. Nicotine increases risk of sleep-related breathing disorders. 5. Nicotine withdrawal may result in disrupted sleep and daytime somnolence.
Opiates (eg, codeine, heroin, methadone, morphine, oxycodone, and propoxyphene) (Primarily used for analgesia)	Excessive sleepiness Polysomnographic features: During opioid use: ↓ Sleep efficiency ↑ Sleep fragmentation ↓ Total sleep time ↓ NREM stages 3 and 4 sleep ↓ REM sleep ↑ Daytime sleepiness During opioid discontinuation: Sleep disturbance Insomnia Nightmares (abrupt drug withdrawal)

Continued

Table 16-8.   Other central nervous system active medications—cont'd

Agent	Effect on Sleep
	Notes:
	1. Opiates can cause sedation and permit sleep in people with acute and chronic pain syndromes.
	2. Insomnia may develop during opiate withdrawal.
	3. Opiates may exacerbate obstructive sleep apnea
	4. Opiates improve symptoms of restless legs syndrome
	5. Opiates have a high abuse potential, with development of both psychological and physical dependency.
Tetrahydrocannabinol (THC) (one of the active constituents found in marijuana.)	Administration of THC at low doses results in mild sedation; higher doses can produce hallucinations.
	During THC use:
	Low doses (mild sedative action)
	↑ Total sleep time
	↑ NREM stages 3 and 4 sleep
	↓ REM sleep (slight)
	High doses (hallucinatory action)
	↓ NREM stages 3 and 4 sleep
	↓ REM sleep
	During THC discontinuation:
	↓ Total sleep time
	↑ Sleep latency
	↑ REM sleep

Cardiovascular Drugs

This category includes antihypertensive agents, antiarrhythmics, and antilipidemic drugs (Table 16–9). Calcium channel blockers and angiotensin-converting enzyme inhibitors generally do not affect sleep.

Table 16-9.   Cardiovascular drugs

Agent	Mechanism of action	Effect on sleep
Amiodarone	Antiarrhythmic	Insomnia
Beta-adrenergic blockers Note: Can be either lipid soluble (eg, labetalol, oxprenolol, propranolol, and timolol) or nonlipid soluble (eg, atenolol, nadolol, and sotalol)	Antihypertensive, antiarrhythmic	Excessive sleepiness and daytime fatigue; insomnia; can cause nightmares, sleep terrors, and hallucinations Polysomnographic features (drug specific): ↑ Wake time after sleep onset ↑ NREM stage 1 sleep ↑ REM sleep latency ↓ REM sleep (except atenolol and metoprolol)
Carvedilol	Alpha and beta antagonist	Excessive sleepiness
Cholestyramine	Antilipidemic agent	Insomnia

Table 16-9. **Cardiovascular drugs—cont'd**

Agent	Mechanism of action	Effect on sleep
Clofibrate	Antilipidemic agent	Excessive sleepiness
Clonidine	Alpha 2 agonist antihypertensive agent	Excessive sleepiness Can cause nightmares Polysomnographic features: ↓ Sleep latency ↑ Total sleep time ↓ Wake time after sleep onset ↑ NREM stage 2 sleep ↑ NREM stages 3 and 4 sleep ↑ REM sleep latency ↓ REM sleep
Colestipol	Antilipidemic agent	Insomnia
Diltiazem	Calcium channel blocker	Insomnia (in some)
Flecainide	Antiarrhythmic	Insomnia
Gemfibrozil	Antilipidemic agent	Excessive sleepiness
Hydralazine	Vasodilator	Insomnia
Labetalol	Alpha and beta antagonist	Excessive sleepiness
Losartan	Angiotensin II receptor blocker	Insomnia
Lovastatin	Antilipidemic agent	Insomnia
Methyldopa	Alpha 2 antagonist antihypertensive	Excessive sleepiness or insomnia May cause nightmares Polysomnographic features: ↑ Total sleep time ↓ NREM stages 3 and 4 sleep ↑ or ↓ REM sleep
Mexelitine	Antiarrhythmic agent	Excessive sleepiness or insomnia
Monoxidine	Imidazoline agonist	Excessive sleepiness
Prazosin	Alpha 1 antagonist	Excessive sleepiness Can cause nightmares
Reserpine	Depletes catecholamines	Excessive sleepiness Can cause nightmares Polysomnographic features: ↓ Sleep latency ↓ REM sleep latency ↑ REM sleep
Ritanserin	5-hydroxytryptamine antagonist	Insomnia
Simvastatin	Antilipidemic agent	Insomnia
Spironolactone	Diuretic	Excessive sleepiness
Terazosin	Alpha 1 antagonist	Excessive sleepiness

Miscellaneous Agents

A variety of drug classes cause sleep disturbances (Table 16–10).

Table 16–10. **Miscellaneous agents**

Medication class	Agents	Sleep disturbance
Antihistamines	Activation of histaminergic neurons located in the posterior hypothalamus gives rise to wakefulness There are two types of histamine receptor antagonists: histamine 1 (H_1) and histamine 2 (H_2) antagonists. H_1 antagonists are commonly used for allergies. First-generation H_1 antagonists (eg, chlorpheniramine, clemastine, diphenhydramine, hydroxyzine, and triprolidine) are lipophilic and easily cross the blood-brain barrier. Second-generation H_1 antagonists (eg, cetirizine, fexofenadine, loratadine, and terfenadine) are hydrophilic and do not cross the blood-brain barrier. H_2 antagonists (eg, cimetidine, famotidine, and ranitidine) are used for peptic ulcer disease. They do not readily cross the blood-brain barrier. Note: Cyproheptadine (serotonin antagonist) possesses antihistaminergic activity.	Histamine 1(H_1) antagonists: First-generation H_1 antagonists can induce sedation and cause excessive sleepiness; multiple sleep latency studies reveal a decrease in daytime sleep latency. Second-generation H_1 antagonists are generally not sedating and do not impair performance; however, they may produce sedation at high doses. Cetirizine can decrease sleep latency and cause sedation. Polysomnographic features of H_1 antagonists: ↑ NREM stages 2, 3, and 4 sleep ↓ REM sleep Note: Cyproheptadine can cause nightmares. H_2 antagonists: Do not generally produce sedation. Can cause insomnia. Excessive sleepiness has been reported in the elderly and in patients with renal impairment. Cimetidine increases NREM stages 3 and 4 sleep.
Antitussives	Benzoate Dextromethorphan	Excessive sleepiness
Bronchodilators	Albuterol Salmeterol	Insomnia Polysomnographic features of salmeterol: ↓ NREM stages 1 and 2 sleep ↑ NREM stages 3 and 4 sleep
Corticosteroids	Dexamethasone Hydrocortisone	Can cause insomnia and nightmares Polysomnographic features: ↑ NREM stage 2 sleep ↓ NREM stages 3 and 4 sleep ↓ REM sleep
Decongestants	Phenylpropanolamine Pseudoephedrine	Possess central nervous system stimulating effects Can cause insomnia Polysomnographic features: ↑ Sleep latency ↑ Wake time after sleep onset

Table 16-10. Miscellaneous agents—cont'd

Medication class	Agents	Sleep disturbance
Dietary supplements and herbal preparations		Intoxication with vitamin A is associated with excessive sleepiness Herbal preparations reported to cause sedation include chamomile, kava-kava, marjoram, poppy seeds, rosemary, and valerian.
Hormonal agents	Estrogen Progesterone	Polysomnographic features of estrogen: ↓ Sleep latency ↑ Total sleep time ↓ REM sleep latency ↑ REM sleep Polysomnographic features of progesterone: ↑ REM sleep latency ↓ REM sleep
Theophylline	Respiratory stimulant and bronchodilator that is chemically related to caffeine	Produces sleep disruption and may result in complaints of insomnia Polysomnographic features: ↑ Sleep latency ↑ Wake time after sleep onset ↑ NREM stage 1 sleep ↓ REM sleep

Additional Tables About Changes in Sleep Architecture Related to Medications

Tables 16–11 and 16–12 and Boxes 16–2 through 16–13 present specific information about the effects of various drugs on sleep and sleep architecture.

Table 16-11. Medications that can cause insomnia

Drug classification	Agents
Anorexiants/anorectics	Dexfenfluramine Phentermine
Antidepressants	Bupropion Selective serotonin reuptake inhibitors Tricyclic antidepressants Venlafaxine
Antiepileptics	Ethosuximide Ethotoin Felbamate Lamotrigine

Continued

Table 16–11.   Medications that can cause insomnia—cont'd

Drug classification	Agents
Antilipidemics	Cerivastatin Cholestyramine Colestipol Fluvastatin Lovastatin Simvastatin
Antimicrobials/antivirals	Abacavir Amantadine Amphotericin B Ciprofloxacin Levofloxacin
Antiparkinsonian drugs	Benztropine Bromocriptine Levodopa Pergolide Pramipexole Selegiline
Antipsychotics	Haldol
Bronchodilators	Albuterol Metaproterenol Salmeterol Theophylline
Cardiovascular drugs	Amiodarone Antiarrhythmic agents Beta-blockers Diltiazem Flecainide Hydralazine Losartan Methyldopa Mexelitine Ritanserin
Corticosteroids	Dexamethasone Hydrocortisone
Decongestants	Phenylpropanolamine Pseudoephedrine
Ethanol (withdrawal from)	
Stimulants	Amphetamines Caffeine Cocaine Ecstasy Methylphenidate Modafinil Pemoline Theophylline

Table 16-12. Medications that can cause excessive sleepiness

Drug classification	Agents
Analgesic agents	Aspirin Diclofenac Ibuprofen Ketorolac Naproxen Sumatriptan Tramadol
Anticonvulsants	Carbamazepine Ethosuximide Gabapentin Lamotrigine Phenobarbital Phenytoin Primidone Tiagibine Topiramate Valproic acid Viagabatrin
Antidepressants	Amitriptyline Amoxapine Brofaromine Clomipramine Desipramine Doxepin Fluvoxamine Imipramine Lithium Maprotiline Meclobemide Mirtazapine Nefazodone Nortriptyline Paroxetine Phenelzine Tranylcypromine Trazodone Venlafaxine
Antiemetics	Domperidone Metoclopramide Ondansetron Phenothiazines Prochlorperazine Scopolamine
Antihistamines	Cetirizine Chlorpheniramine Clemastine Diphenhydramine Doxylamine Hydroxyzine

Continued

Table 16–12. Medications that can cause excessive sleepiness—cont'd

Drug classification	Agents
Antiparkinsonian drugs	Pramipexole Ropinirole
Antipsychotics	Chlorpromazine Clozapine Haloperidol Thioridazine
Antitussives	Benzonatate Dextromethorphan
Cardiovascular agents	Beta-blockers Carvedilol Clofibrate Clonidine Gemfibrozil Labetalol Methyldopa Mexiletine Monoxidine Prazosin Reserpine Spironolactone Terazosin
Herbal compounds	Chamomile Kava kava Marjoram Poppy seeds Rosemary Valerian
Hypnotics	Barbiturates Benzodiazepines Chloral hydrate Eszopiclone Zaleplon Zolpidem
Muscle relaxants	Baclofen Carisoprodol Cyclobenzaprine
Narcotics	Codeine Methadone Morphine Oxycodone Propoxyphene
Neuroleptics	Phenothiazine

Box 16–2. **Medications that can cause abnormal dreams**	Amantadine Diltiazem Felodipine Levodopa Mirtazapine

Box 16–3. **Medications that can cause night terrors**	Alcohol ingestion Beta-blockers

Box 16–4. **Medications that can cause nightmares**	Alcohol ingestion (during the REM rebound portion of the night Amantadine Amiodarone Antipsychotics (eg, clozapine, risperidone) Antidepressants (selective serotonin reuptake inhibitors, tricyclic antidepressants) Beta-blockers, lipophilic (eg, propranolol) Clonidine Clozapine Corticosteroids (eg, dexamethasone, hydrocortisone) Cyproheptadine Levodopa Methyldopa Narcotic analgesics Nicotine Phenelzine Prazosin Reserpine Temazepam

Box 16-5. **Medications that can cause periodic limb movement disorder**	Lithium Selective serotonin reuptake inhibitors Tricyclic antidepressants

Box 16-6. **Medications that can cause rapid eye movement sleep behavior disorder**	Alcohol withdrawal Barbiturates Caffeine Fluoxetine Monoamine oxidase inhibitors Selegiline Tricyclic antidepressants Venlafaxine

Box 16-7. **Medications that can increase non-rapid eye movement stage 2 sleep**	Barbiturates Benzodiazepines Zolpidem Zopiclone

Box 16–8.

Medications that can increase rapid eye movement sleep latency

Alcohol (acute ingestion)

Amphetamine

Barbiturates

Benzodiazepines

Chlorpromazine

Clonidine

Doxepin

Haloperidol

Levodopa

Lithium

Loxapine

Methylphenidate

Mirtazapine

Phenelzine

Progesterone

Scopolamine

Selective serotonin reuptake inhibitors

Trazodone

Tricyclic antidepressants

Trifluoperazine

Box 16–9.

Medications that can decrease rapid eye movement sleep latency

Estrogen

Reserpine

Box 16–10.

Medications that can increase rapid eye movement sleep[a]

Acetylcholine

Acute withdrawal from REM suppressants

Alcohol (withdrawal)

Bupropion

Carbachol

Estrogen

Methyldopa

Nefazodone

Physostigmine

Reserpine

Yohimbine

[a]REM sleep is enhanced by cholinergic medications.

Box 16–11.

Medications that can decrease rapid eye movement sleep[a]

Alcohol (acute ingestion)

Amphetamines

Antihistamines

Atropine

Barbiturates

Benzodiazepines

Benztropine

Beta-blockers

Caffeine

Carbamazepine

Chlorpromazine

Clonidine

Corticosteroids

Ethosuximide

Haloperidol

Lithium

Loxapine

(continued from page 486)
Box 16–11.

Medications that can decrease rapid eye movement sleep[a]

Maprotiline

Metoclopramide

Narcotic agents (morphine)

Nicotine

Phenelzine

Phenytoin

Progesterone

Scopolamine

Selective serotonin reuptake inhibitors (fluoxetine)

Selegiline

Stimulants

Tricyclic antidepressants (except trimipramine)

Trifluoperazine

Trihexyphenidyl

Venlafaxine

---

[a]*REM sleep is suppressed by monoaminergic medications.*

Box 16–12.

Medications that can increase non–rapid eye movement stages 3 and 4 sleep

Adenosine agonists

Alcohol (acute ingestion)

Antihistamines

Apomorphine

Benztropine

Carbamazepine

Clonidine

Interleukin-1

Lithium

(continued from page 487)
Box 16-12.

Medications that can increase non-rapid eye movement stages 3 and 4 sleep

L-Tryptophan

Maprotiline

Mirtazapine

Phenytoin

Ritanserin

Trazodoneh

Tricyclic antidepressants

Trihexyphenidyl

Box 16-13.

Medications that can decrease non-rapid eye movement stages 3 and 4 sleep

Adenosine antagonists

Alcohol (withdrawal)

Barbiturates

Benzodiazepines

Beta-adrenergic blockers

Caffeine (during first half of the sleep period)

Corticosteroids

Levodopa

Methyldopa

Prostaglandin E$_2$

Selective serotonin reuptake inhibitors

Selegiline

Stimulants

References

General References

American Academy of Sleep Medicine. *The International Classification of Sleep Disorders: Diagnostic and Coding Manual.* 2nd ed. Westchester, IL: American Academy of Sleep Medicine, 2005.

Bowman TJ. *Review of Sleep Medicine.* Burlington, MA: Butterworth-Heinemann, 2002.

Berry RB. *Sleep Medicine Pearls.* 2nd ed. Philadelphia, PA: Hanley & Belfus, 2002.

Chokroverty S. *Clinical Companion to Sleep Disorders Medicine.* 2nd ed. Butterworth-Heinemann, 2000.

Lavie P, Pillar G, Malhotra A. *Sleep Disorders Handbook.* Taylor & Francis, 2002.

Lee-Chiong TL, ed. *Sleep: A Comprehensive Handbook.* Hoboken, NJ: John Wiley & Sons, 2006.

Lee-Chiong TL, Sateia M, Carskadon M, eds. *Sleep Medicine.* Philadelphia, PA: Hanley & Belfus (Elsevier), 2002.

Pagel JF. Medications and their effects on sleep. *Sleep Medicine. Primary Care: Clinics in Office Practice.* Elsevier Saunders, 2005.

Perlis ML, Lichstein KL, eds. *Treating Sleep Disorders: Principles and Practice of Behavioral Sleep Medicine.* Hoboken, NJ: John Wiley & Sons, 2003.

Qureshi A, Lee-Chiong T. Medications and their effects on sleep. *Sleep Disorders. Medical Clinics of North America.* Elsevier Saunders, 2004.

Rechtschaffen A, Kales A. *A Manual of Standardized Terminology, Techniques and Scoring System for Sleep Stages of Human Subjects.* Los Angeles, CA: Brain Information Service/Brain Research Institute, University of California, 1968.

Reite M, Ruddy J, Nagel K. *Concise Guide to Evaluation and Management of Sleep Disorders.* 3rd ed. Arlington, VA: American Psychiatric Publishing, April 2002.

Sleep Disorders. Medical Clinics of North America. Philadelphia, PA: Elsevier Saunders, 2004.

Sleep Medicine. Primary Care: Clinics in Office Practice. Philadelphia, PA: Elsevier Saunders, 2005.

Sleep Research Society. *SRS Basics of Sleep Guide.* Westchester, IL: Sleep Research Society, 2005.

Alcohol

Obermeyer W, Benca R. Effects of Drugs on Sleep. *Neurologic Clinics.* 1996;14(4):827–840.

Strading JR. Recreational drugs and sleep. ABC of sleep disorders. *BMJ.* 1993;306:575–576.

Antidepressants

Bech P, Ciadella P. Citalopram in depression: meta-analysis of intended and unintended effects. *Int Clin Psychopharmacol.* 1992;6(S5):45–54.

Eisen J, MacFarlane J, Shapiro CM. Psychotropic drugs and sleep. ABC of sleep disorders. *BMJ.* 1993;306:1331–1334.

Feighner J. Mechanism of action of antidepressant medications. *J Clin Psychiatry*. 1999;60(S4):4–11.

Haria M, Fitton A, McTavish D. Trazodone: a review of its pharmacology, therapeutic use in depression and therapeutic potential in other disorders. *Drugs Aging*. 1994;4:331–355.

Kupfer DJ, Bowers MB Jr. REM sleep and central monoamine oxidase inhibition. *Psychopharmacologia*. 1972;27:183–190.

Luthringer R, Toussaint M, Schaltenbrand N, Bailey P, Danjou PH, Hackett D, et al. A double blind, placebo controlled evaluation of the effects of orally administered venlafaxine on sleep in inpatients with major depression. *Psychopharmacol Bull*. 1996;32:637–646.

Nofzinger EA, Reynolds CF III, Thase ME, Frank E, Jennings JR, Fasiczka AL, et al. REM sleep enhancement by bupropion in depressed men. *Am J Psychiatry*. 1995; 152:274–276.

Nutt D. Mitrazipine: pharmacology in relation to adverse effects. *Acta Psychiatr Scand Suppl*. 1997;391:31–37.

Obermeyer W, Benca R. Effects of drugs on sleep. *Neurologic Clinics*. 1996;14(4):827–840.

Rickles K, Schweizer E. Clinical overview of serotonin reuptake inhibitors. *J Clin Psychiatry*. 1990;51(B):9–12.

Salin-Pascual RJ, Galicia-Polo L, Drucker-Colin R. Sleep changes after 4 consecutive days of venlafaxine administration in normal volunteers. *J Clin Psychiatry*. 1997;58:348–350.

Schneerson JM. Drugs and sleep. In: Schneerson JM. *Handbook of Sleep Medicine*. Malden, MA: Blackwell Science Ltd: 2000:33–58.

Van Laar MW, van Willigenburg APP, Volkerts ER. Acute and subacute effects of nefazodone and imipramine on highway driving, cognitive functions and daytime sleepiness in healthy adult and elderly subjects. *J Clin Psychopharmacol*. 1995;15:30–40.

Sedative-Hypnotics

Eisen J, MacFarlane J, Shapiro CM. Psychotropic drugs and sleep. ABC of sleep disorders. *BMJ*. 1993;306:1331–1334.

Gillin JC. The long and the short of sleeping pills. *N Engl J Med*. 1991;324:1735–1736.

Guilleminault C. Benzodiazepines, breathing and sleep. *Am J Med*. 1990;88(3A):25S-28S.

Obermeyer W, Benca R. Effects of drugs on sleep. *Neurologic Clinics*. 1996;14(4):827–840.

Schnabel T. Evaluation of the safety and side effects of anti anxiety agents. *Am J Med*.1987;82(5a):7–13.

Schweitzer PK. Drugs that disturb sleep and wakefulness. In: Kryger MH, Roth T, Dement WC, eds. *Principles and Practice of Sleep Medicine*. 3rd ed. Philadelphia, PA: WB Saunders 2000:441–461.

Zhdanova IV, Lynch HJ, Wurtman RJ. Melatonin. A sleep-promoting hormone. *Sleep*. 1997;20:899–907.

Stimulants

Buguet A, Montmayeur A, Pigeau R, Naithoh P. Modafinil, d-amphetamine and placebo during 64 hours of sustained mental work. II. Effects on two nights of recovery sleep. *J Sleep Res*. 1995;4:229–241.

Eisen J, MacFarlane J, Shapiro CM. Psychotropic drugs and sleep. ABC of sleep disorders. *BMJ*. 1993;306:1331–1334.

Obermeyer W, Benca R. Effects of drugs on sleep. *Neurologic Clinics*. 1996;14(4):827–840.

Post RM, Gillin JC, Wyatt RJ, Goodwin FK. The effect of orally administered cocaine on sleep of depressed patients. *Psychopharmacology.* 1974;37:59.

Schneerson JM. Drugs and sleep. In: Schneerson JM. *Handbook of Sleep Medicine.* Malden, MA: Blackwell Science Ltd, 2000:33–58.

Strading JR. Recreational drugs and sleep. ABC of sleep disorders. *BMJ.* 1993;306:575–576.

Antipsychotics

Casey DE. The relationship of pharmacology to side effects. *J Clin Psychiatry.* 1997; 58:(S10):55–62.

Eisen J, MacFarlane J, Shapiro CM. Psychotropic drugs and sleep. ABC of sleep disorders. *BMJ.* 1993;306:1331–1334.

Gerlach J, Peacock L. New antipsychotics: the present status. *Int Clin Psychopharmacol.* 1995:10(S3):39–48.

Other Central Nervous System Active Medications

Brodie MJ, Dichter MA. Established antiepileptic drugs. *Seizure.* 1997;6:159–174.

Cooper JA, Sagar HJ, Dohertty SM, et al. Different effects of dopaminergic and anticholinergics therapies on cognitive and motor function in Parkinson's disease. *Brain.* 1992;115:1701–1725.

Cumming JL. Behavioral complications of drug treatment of Parkinson's disease. *J Am Geriatr Soc.* 1991;39:708–716.

Ferrendelli JA. Pharmacology of antiepileptic drugs. *Epilepsia.* 1987;28(S3):S14-S16.

Nausieda PA, Weiner WJ, Kaplan LR, Weber S, Klawans HL. Sleep disruption in the course of chronic levodopa therapy: an early feature of levodopa psychosis. *Clin Neuropharmacol.* 1982;5:183–194.

Obermeyer W, Benca R. Effects of drugs on sleep. *Neurologic Clinics.* 1996;14(4):827–840.

Rogvi-Hansen B, Gram L. Adverse effects of established and new antiepileptic drugs: an attempted comparison. *Pharmacol Ther.* 1995;68:425–434.

Sammaritano M, Sherwin A. Effects of anticonvulsants on sleep. *Neurology.* 2000;54(5S):S16-S24.

Cardiovascular Drugs

Gleiter CH, Deckert J. Adverse CNS effects of beta adrenoceptor blockers. *Pharmacopsychiatry.* 1996;29:201–211.

Idzikowski C, Shapiro C. Non psychotropic drugs and sleep. ABC of sleep disorders. *BMJ.* 1993;306:1118–1121.

Kuyer WB, Hickman JR Jr. Medication induced performance decrements: cardiovascular medications. *J Occup Med.* 1990;32:342–349.

Michelson EL, Dreifus LS. Newer antiarrhythmic drugs: cardiovascular pharmacotherapy II. *Med Clin North Am.* 1988;72:275–319.

Monti J. Minireview: disturbances of sleep and wakefulness associated with the use of antihypertensive agents. *Life Sci.* 1987;41:1979–1988.

Paykel ES, Fleminger R, Watson JP. Psychiatric side effects of antihypertensive drugs other than reserpine. *J Clin Psychopharmacol.* 1982;2:14–39.

Webster J, Koch HF. Aspects of tolerability of centrally acting antihypertensive drugs. *J Cardiovasc Pharmacol.* 1996;27(S3):S49-S54.

Wesnes K, Simpson PM, Jansson B, Grahnen A, Weimann HJ, Kuppers H. Moxonidine and cognitive function: interactions with moclobemide and lorazepam. *Eur J Clin Pharmacol.* 1997;52:351–358.

Miscellaneous Agents

Berlin RG. Effects of H2-receptor antagonists on the central nervous system. *Drug Dev Res.* 1989;17:97–108.

Donnelly F, Rihoux JP, DeVos C. Sedative effects of antihistamines: safety, performance, learning and quality of life. *Clin Ther.* 1998;20:365–372.

Lipsy RJ, Fennerty B, Fagan T. Clinical review of histamine 2 receptor antagonists. *Arch Intern Med.* 1990;150:745–751.

Ramaekers GJ, Uiterwijk MM, O'Hanlon JF. Effects of loratadine and cetirizine on actual driving and psychometric test performance, and EEG during driving. *Eur J Clin Pharmacol.* 1992;42:363–369.

Roehrs T, Merlotti L, Halpin D, Rosenthal L, Roth T: Effects of Theophylline on nocturnal sleep and daytime sleepiness/alertness. *Chest.* 1995;108:382–387.

Roth T, Roehrs T, Koshorek G, Sicklesteel J, Zorick F. Sedative effects of antihistamines. *J Allergy Clin Immunol.* 1987;80:94–98.

Schentag JJ. Cimetidine associated mental confusion: further studies in 36 severely ill patients. *Ther Drug Monit.* 1980;78:791–795.

Wiegand L, Mende CN, Zaidel G, et al. Salmeterol vs theophylline: sleep and efficacy outcomes in patients with nocturnal asthma. *Chest.* 1999;115(6):1525–1532.

Highlights of the Manual of Standardized Terminology, Techniques, and Scoring System for Sleep Stages of Human Subjects[a]

1. General notes:

   - Designed for *adult* humans

   - Designation of electrode placements uses the Ten Twenty Electrode System of the International Federation

   - Sleep is polysomnographically defined as stages 1, 2, 3, 4, and REM based on EEG, EOG, and EMG changes

   - NREM (non-REM) sleep—consists of stages 1, 2, 3, and 4

     ◦ Delta or slow wave sleep—consists of stages 3 and/or 4

2. Scoring by epochs:

   - The polygraph record is divided into segments of equal size (eg, epoch length of 300 mm and duration of 30 s [10 mm/s]).

   - A single stage score is assigned to each epoch—when more than one stage is present in an epoch, the stage score of the epoch is determined by the stage that takes up the greatest portion of the epoch.

3. Stage W (wakefulness):

   - EEG: alpha activity and/or low voltage, mixed frequency activity

   - EOG: rapid eye movements (REMs) and eye blinks

   - EMG: usually relatively high tonic EMG

4. Stage 1:

   - EEG: relatively low voltage, mixed frequency

     ◦ Prominence of activity in the 2–7 cps range

     ◦ Decrease in the amount, amplitude, and frequency of alpha activity

     ◦ Absence of K-complexes and sleep spindles

     ◦ Vertex sharp waves may appear, often in conjunction with high amplitude 2–7 cps activity. The amplitude of the vertex sharp wave is occasionally as high as 200 µV.

   - EOG: slow eye movements

     ◦ No rapid eye movements

   - EMG: tonic EMG levels are typically below that of relaxed wakefulness

5. Stage 2:

   - EEG: relatively low voltage, mixed frequency:

     ◦ Presence of sleep spindles and/or K-complexes

     ◦ Sleep spindle—activity between 12 and 14 cps of at least 0.5 second duration

     ◦ K-complexes—negative sharp wave immediately followed by a positive component with a total duration of over 0.5 second

     ◦ Long periods may intervene between sleep spindles and K complexes.

- ◦ "3-minute rule"—if < 3 minutes of record meeting requirements for stage 1 occur between sleep spindles and/or K-complexes in the absence of movement arousals or pronounced increases in muscle tone, intervening epochs are considered stage 2. The intervening epochs are scored as stage 1 if the interval without sleep spindles or K-complexes lasts ≥ 3 minutes.

  - ◦ Absence of sufficient high-amplitude, slow activity that defines stages 3 and 4

6. Stage 3:

  - EEG: ≥ 20% but < 50% of the epoch consists of 2 cps or slower waves having amplitudes > 75 μV from peak to peak

7. Stage 4:

  - EEG: > 50% of the epoch consists of 2 cps or slower waves having amplitudes > 75 μV peak to peak

8. Stage REM

  - EEG: relatively low voltage, mixed frequency

    - ◦ Resembles stage 1

    - ◦ Vertex sharp waves are not prominent

    - ◦ "Saw-tooth" waves may be seen

    - ◦ Absence of sleep spindles and K-complexes

    - ◦ When sleep spindles are present in a background of relatively low voltage, mixed frequency EEG activity and the EMG remains at the stage REM level throughout, Any section contiguous with stage REM is scored stage REM regardless of whether REMs are present if there are no intervening movement arousals.

  - EOG: episodic REMs

  - EMG: Low amplitude

    - ◦ Tonic mental-submental EMG tracing almost always reaches its lowest levels

    - ◦ A relatively elevated tonic EMG precludes the scoring of stage REM

9. Stage REM rules—start of stage REM:

  - if sleep spindles and K-complexes stop and the EEG changes to a relatively low voltage, mixed frequency for one or more epochs before REMs start;

  - If the EMG during the epochs before REMs is at the same level as after REMs and if there has been no intervening movement arousal, score as stage REM all the records from the last sleep spindle or K-complex;

  - If the EMG remains at a relatively high level for some portion of this interval before it drops to the stage REM level, score as stage REM from the point where the EMG amplitude dropped (if REMs occur before any additional sleep spindles or K-complexes appear);

  - If there is a movement arousal during these epochs, score as stage REM from the point following the movement arousal at which the EMG tracing is reduced to stage REM level (score as stage 1 for those epochs following the movement arousal during which EMG is relatively elevated).

- Score as stage 2 if the interval between the cessation of sleep spindles and K-complexes and the movement arousal is < 3 min. Score as stage REM if the interval is ≥ 3 min.

10. Stage REM Rules—end of Stage REM:

- score as Stage REM any period of relatively low voltage, mixed frequency EEG without eye movements that follows contiguously from an unambiguous stage REM, if the EMG tracing remains at stage REM level and no intervening sleep spindles, K-complexes, or movement arousals are present.

- In this period, if the EMG is initially at stage REM level but becomes elevated later in the interval, score as stage REM up to the point of EMG augmentation, and as stage 1 thereafter.

- In this period, score as stage REM if a movement arousal transiently interrupts the continuity of stage REM, and (1) the mental-submental EMG quickly reverts to the stage REM level following the movement arousal; (2) the EEG remains relatively low voltage, mixed frequency; (3) there is a resumption of REMs or change to stage 2 on one or more epochs following the movement arousal; and (4) there are no or only very minimal signs of stage 1 following the movement arousal.

11. Movement time (MT)—polygraph record is obscured by movements of the subject

- Use Score "MT" when the EEG and EOG tracings are obscured in more than half of the epoch by muscle tension and/or amplifier blocking artifacts due to movements of the subject in epochs which immediately precede or follow sleep stages.

- Score MT is not counted with either sleep or wake time.

- Score as stage W when an epoch is obscured by muscle tension and/or amplifier blocking artifacts but is immediately preceded and followed by stage W.

12. Movement arousal: any increase in EMG accompanied by a change in pattern on any additional channel, including:

- EMG—increase EMG signal amplitude, or amplifier blocking artifact

- EOG—presence of EMG activity, amplifier blocking artifacts, or blink artifacts

- EEG—presence of EMG activity, amplifier blocking artifacts, decrease in amplitude, increase in alpha activity, or paroxysmal burst of high voltage activity

13. Monitoring techniques: EEG recording

- When EEG information is limited to one derivation, the recommended derivation is C4/A1 or C3/A2 (C = central; A = ear or mastoid).

- A minimum paper speed of 10 mm/s, a minimal pen deflection of 7.5–10 mm for 50 microvolts (μV), time constants greater than 0.3s, and a electrode resistances not exceeding 10,000 ohms at the beginning of the recording are recommended.

14. Monitoring techniques: eye movement recording

- At least two channels are necessary.

  ○ First channel—electrode is placed approximately 1 cm above and slightly lateral to the outer canthus of one eye and a reference electrode on either the homolateral ear lobe or mastoid.

  ○ Second channel—electrode is placed 1 cm below and slightly lateral to the outer canthus of the other eye referred to the contralateral ear or mastoid (ie, both eyes are referred to the same ear or mastoid electrode).

- This electrode arrangement produces out-of-phase deflections on the two channels for almost all eye movements

    ◦ Apparatus artifacts register as in-phase deflections on the two channels (artifacts from the reference electrode) or deflections on one channel only (artifacts from one of the outer canthus electrodes)

- Minimum gain of 7.5 mm for 50 µV and time constants less than 0.3 are recommended.

15. Monitoring techniques: EMG (mental, submental) recording: high gains (20 µV/cm or higher), minimal high frequency filtering, and time constants of 0.15 or faster are recommended.

ªSource: Modified and adapted from Rechtschaffen A, Kales A. A Manual of Standardized Terminology, Techniques and Scoring System for Sleep Stages of Human Subjects. Brain Information Service/Brain Research Institute, University of California, 1968.
Note: Electroencephalography (EEG), Electromyography (EMG), Electrooculography (EOG), non- rapid eye monument (NREM), rapid eye movement (REM), wakefulness (W).

2007 American Academy of Sleep Medicine Sleep Scoring Guidelines

The following tables describe and summarize the recommendations of the American Academy of Sleep Medicine* regarding the scoring of sleep stages, arousals, respiratory events, cardiac events, and movement events.

Table 1. Electrode and sensor placements

Measurement	Recommended	Alternative	Comments
Electro-encephalography (EEG)	F4M1 C4M1 O2M1	FzCz CzOz C4M1	Based on the International 10-20 system
	Backup electrodes: F3M2 C3M2 O1M2	Backup electrodes: FpzC3 C3O1 C3M2	F: frontal C: central O: occipital M: mastoid
			Odd numbers: left Even numbers: right Z: midline
Electro-oculography (EOG)	E1M2 E2M1	E1Fpz E2Fpz	M1: left mastoid process M2: right mastoid process Z: midline
	E1: 1 cm below the left outer canthus E2: 1 cm above the right outer canthus	E1: 1 cm below and 1 cm lateral to the left outer canthus E2: 1 cm below and 1 cm lateral to the right outer canthus	For children: may reduce electrode distance to 0.5 cm
Electro-myography (EMG)	Three chin EMG electrodes: 1. Midline, 1 cm above the inferior edge of the mandible 2. 2 cm to the right of midline and 2 cm below the inferior edge of the mandible 3. 2 cm to the left of midline and 2 cm below the inferior edge of the mandible		Derivation consists of either of the inferior electrodes (below the mandible) referred to the electrode placed above the mandible The other inferior electrode can be used as a back-up if the initial electrodes fail For children: may reduce electrode distance to 1 cm
Electro-cardiography (EKG)	Modified lead II (electrodes placed below the right clavicle and the left 6th or 7th intercostal space)		
Airflow (apnea)	Oronasal thermal sensor	Nasal air pressure transducer End tidal PCO_2, or summed calibrated inductance plethysmography (for children)	

Table 1. Electrode and sensor placements—cont'd

Measurement	Recommended	Alternative	Comments
Airflow (hypopnea)	Nasal air pressure transducer	Inductance plethysmography, or oronasal thermal sensor	
Respiratory effort	Esophageal manometry, or inductance plethysmography	Diaphragmatic or intercostal EMG	
Blood oxygen	Pulse oximetry		
Alveolar hypoventilation (in children)	Transcutaneous or end-tidal PCO_2 monitoring		Minimum acceptable signal averaging time is 3 seconds

Table 2. Technical specifications

Electrode	Desirable sampling rate (Hz)	Minimal sampling rate (Hz)	High frequency filter (Hz)	Low frequency filter (Hz)	Maximum impedance (K ohms)
EEG	500	200	35	0.3	5
EOG	500	200	35	0.3	5
EMG	500	200	100	10	
EKG	500	200	70	0.3	
Snoring	500	200	100	10	
Respiration			15	0.1	
Airflow	100	25			
Nasal pressure	100	25			
Esophageal pressure	100	25			
Oximetry	25	10			
Chest and abdominal movements	100	25			
Body position	1	1			

Minimum digital resolution: 12 bits per sample

Table 3. Scoring rules for sleep stages (Adults)

Sleep Stage	Scoring Rules
	Sleep stages are scored in 30-second epochs; each epoch is assigned a sleep stage that comprises the greatest percentage of the epoch
W (wakefulness)	> 50% of epoch has alpha (8-13 Hz) EEG waves over the occipital region with eye closure; or If alpha waves are absent, the presence of any of the following: 1. Conjugate vertical eye blinks (0.5-2 Hz) 2. Reading eye movements consisting of a conjugate slow movement followed by a rapid movement in the opposite direction 3. Voluntary rapid open eye movements
N1	Presence of any of the following: 1. Alpha EEG waves are replaced by low amplitude, mixed frequency (4-7 Hz) waves occupying > 50% of the epoch 2. In those who do not generate alpha waves, the start of: a. 4-7 Hz waves with slowing of background activity by ≥ 1 Hz compared to stage W b. Vertex sharp waves with duration of < 0.5 seconds that are maximal over the central regions c. Slow eye movements
N2	The start of stage N2 is defined by the presence of K complexes (not associated with arousals) or sleep spindles during the first half of the epoch or during the last half of the previous epoch if criteria for stage N3 are absent The continuation of stage N2 is defined by the presence of low amplitude, mixed frequency EEG rhythms, and if the epoch contains, or is preceded, by K complexes (not associated with arousals) or sleep spindles The end of stage N2 is defined by the presence of any of the following: 1. Transition to stage W, N1, N3 or R 2. Arousal 3. Major body movement *not* followed by low amplitude, mixed frequency EEG rhythms containing K complexes (not associated with arousals) or sleep spindles
N3	Replaces Rechtschaffen and Kales NREM stages 3 and 4 sleep ≥ 20% of the epoch is occupied by slow wave (0.5-2 Hz and > 75 μV) EEG activity over the frontal regions
R (REM)	Presence of all of the following: 1. EEG: low amplitude, mixed frequency activity 2. EOG: rapid eye movements 3. Chin EMG: low tone (lowest level in the study or at least no higher than the other sleep stages) The continuation of stage R is defined by the presence of low amplitude, mixed frequency EEG activity, low chin EMG tone, and no K complexes or sleep spindles in epochs that either contain rapid eye movements or that are preceded by stage R The end of stage R is defined by presence of any of the following: 1. Transition to stage W, N3 2. Criteria for N1 *plus* increase in chin EMG tone 3. An arousal followed by low amplitude, mixed frequency EEG activity and slow eye movements 4. Major body movement followed by low amplitude, mixed frequency EEG rhythms containing K complexes (not associated with arousals) or sleep spindles and the presence of slow eye movements 5. Absence of eye movements and the presence of K complexes (not associated with arousals) or sleep spindles in the first half of the epoch

Table 3.   Scoring rules for sleep stages (Adults)—cont'd

Sleep Stage	Scoring Rules
Major body movements	A major body movement is defined by the presence of movement or muscle artifact that obscures the EEG for > 50% of the epoch An epoch with a major body movement is scored the same stage as the epoch that follows it except as follows: 1. It is scored as stage W if alpha rhythm is present 2. It is scored as stage W if it is preceded or followed by a stage W epoch

Table 4.   Scoring rules for sleep stages (Children [≥ 2 Months Post-term])

Sleep Stage	Scoring Rules
W (wakefulness)	Alpha activity is replaced by dominant posterior rhythm

N1	Presence of any of the following:
	1. Dominant posterior EEG rhythm is replaced by low amplitude, mixed frequency (4-7 Hz) waves occupying > 50% of the epoch
	2. In those who do not generate a dominant posterior rhythm, the start of:
	  a. 4-7 Hz waves with slowing of the background activity by ≥ 1-2 Hz compared to stage W
	  b. Vertex sharp waves
	  c. Slow eye movements
	  d. Rhythmic anterior theta activity
	  e. Hypnagogic hypersynchrony
	  f. Diffuse or occipital predominant high amplitude 3-5 Hz rhythmic activity

N2	Same as adult scoring rules
N3	Same as adult scoring rules
N (NREM)	If K complexes, sleep spindles and slow wave activity are absent in all epochs of NREM sleep
R (REM)	Same as adult scoring rules

Table 5.   Scoring rules for arousals

Arousal Event	Scoring Rules
During NREM sleep	Abrupt EEG frequency shift (eg, alpha, theta or frequencies > 16 Hz but not spindles) lasting ≥ 3 seconds and preceded by ≥ 10 seconds of stable sleep
During REM sleep	Abrupt EEG frequency shift (eg, alpha, theta or frequencies > 16 Hz but not spindles) lasting ≥ 3 seconds and preceded by ≥ 10 seconds of stable sleep, accompanied by an increase in chin EMG that is ≥ 1 second in duration

Table 6. Scoring rules for respiratory events (Adults)

Respiratory Event	Scoring Rules
Apnea	Decrease in peak thermal sensor amplitude by ≥ 90% from baseline for a duration of at least 10 seconds (≥ 90% of the duration of each event must meet the criteria for minimum thermal sensor amplitude reduction from baseline) Score as an *obstructive* event if inspiratory effort is present throughout the entire period; Score as a *central* event if inspiratory effort is absent throughout the entire period; and Score as a *mixed* event if absent inspiratory effort in the initial part of the period is followed by the presence of inspiratory effort
Hypopnea	Decrease in nasal pressure by ≥ 30% of baseline for a duration of at least 10 seconds accompanied by ≥ 4% oxygen desaturation (≥ 90% of the duration of each event must meet the criteria for minimum nasal pressure amplitude reduction from baseline)
Respiratory effort-related arousal	Breaths associated with increasing respiratory efforts or flattening of the nasal pressure waveform with a duration ≥ 10 seconds and preceding an arousal, but not meeting criteria for either apnea or hypopnea
Hypoventilation	≥ 10 mmHg increase in $PaCO_2$ during sleep compared to supine awake values
Cheyne Stokes breathing (CSB)	≥ 3 consecutive cycles of crescendo-decrescendo amplitude in respiration *plus* either duration of CSB of at least 10 consecutive minutes *or* ≥ 5 central apneas/hypopneas per hour of sleep

Table 7. Scoring rules for respiratory events (Children [< 18 Years of Age])

Respiratory Event	Scoring Rules
Apnea	Score as an *obstructive* event if inspiratory effort is present throughout the entire period associated with a ≥ 90% fall in signal amplitude lasting ≥ 2 missed breaths (≥ 90% of the duration of each event must meet the criteria for minimum amplitude reduction from baseline) Score as a *central* event if inspiratory effort is absent throughout the entire period associated with a ≥ 90% fall in signal amplitude lasting ≥ 20 seconds in duration, or ≥ 2 missed breaths (associated with arousal, awakening or ≥3% oxygen desaturation) in duration Score as a *mixed* event if absent inspiratory effort in the initial part of the period is followed by the presence of inspiratory effort associated with a ≥ 90% fall in signal amplitude lasting ≥ 2 missed breaths (≥ 90% of the duration of each event must meet the criteria for minimum amplitude reduction from baseline)
Hypopnea	≥ 50% reduction in nasal pressure amplitude compared to baseline, associated with arousal, awakening or ≥3% oxygen desaturation, lasting for a duration of ≥ 2 missed breaths (≥ 90% of the duration of each event must meet the criteria for minimum nasal pressure amplitude reduction from baseline)

Table 7. Scoring rules for respiratory events (Children [< 18 Years of Age])—cont'd

Respiratory Event	Scoring Rules
Respiratory effort related arousal	Presence of either: a. When a nasal pressure sensor is used, a decrease in sensor signal < 50% of baseline levels, associated with flattening of the waveform, snoring, increase in end-tidal or transcutaneous PCO_2, or visible increase in work of breathing lasting ≥ 2 breath cycles, is present b. When an esophageal pressure sensor is used, a progressive increase in inspiratory effort accompanied by snoring, increase in end-tidal or transcutaneous PCO_2, or visible increase in work of breathing lasting ≥ 2 breath cycles, is present
Hypoventilation	CO_2 > 50 mmHg in > 25% of total sleep time
Periodic breathing	> 3 episodes of central apneas with a duration of > 3 seconds separated by ≤ 20 seconds of normal respiration

Table 8. Scoring rules for cardiac events

Cardiac Event	Scoring Rules
Asystole	Cardiac pause > 3 seconds (for patients 6 years and older)
Bradycardia	Heart rate (HR) < 40 beats per minute (for patients 6 years and older)
Atrial fibrillation	Irregularly irregular rhythm with variable P wave morphologies
Sinus tachycardia	HR > 90 beats per minute (for adult patients); sinus rates are faster in children compared to adults
Wide-complex tachycardia	HR > 100 beats per minute; ≥ 3 consecutive beats with QRS duration ≥ 120 msec
Narrow-complex tachycardia	HR > 100 beats per minute; ≥ 3 consecutive beats with QRS duration < 120 msec

Table 9. Scoring rules for movement events

Movement Event	Scoring Rules
Periodic limb movements in sleep	≥ 4 consecutive leg movements (each 0.5 to 10 seconds in duration with an amplitude ≥ 8 μV above resting EMG) characterized by period lengths of between 5 and 90 seconds between onsets of consecutive movements Leg movements on different legs are counted as one movement if they are separated by < 5 seconds between movement onsets
Alternating leg muscle activation	≥ 4 EMG bursts, 0.5 to 3.0 Hz in frequency, alternating between legs with a duration of 100 to 500 msec *Note: May be a benign movement event*

Continued

Table 9. Scoring rules for movement events—cont'd

Movement Event	Scoring Rules
Hypnagogic foot tremor	≥ 4 EMG bursts, 0.3 to 4.0 Hz in frequency, with a duration of 250 to 1000 msec *Note: May be a benign movement event*
Excessive fragmentary myoclonus	≥ 5 EMG potentials (each with a usual maximum duration of 150 msec) per minute occurring during at least 20 minutes of NREM sleep *Note: May be a benign movement event*
Bruxism	Presence of any of the following: Increase in chin EMG activity that are ≥ twice the background EMG tone, separated by ≥ 3 seconds of stable EMG, and that are either: a. Brief episodes (0.25-2 seconds in duration occurring in a sequence of ≥ 3 episodes) b. Sustained episodes (> 2 seconds in duration) ≥ 2 audible bruxism episodes per night
REM sleep behavior disorder	Presence of either sustained chin EMG muscle activity, or excessive transient chin or limb EMG muscle activity, or both during REM sleep
Rhythmic movement disorder	≥ 4 individual movements, each with a frequency of 0.5-2 Hz and an amplitude ≥ 2 times above resting EMG

Modified and adapted from Iber C, Ancoli-Israel S, Chesson A and Quan SF for the American Academy of Sleep Medicine. The AASM Manual for the Scoring of Sleep and Associated Events: Rules, Terminology and Technical Specifications, 1st ed.: Westchester, Illinois: American Academy of Sleep Medicine, 2007

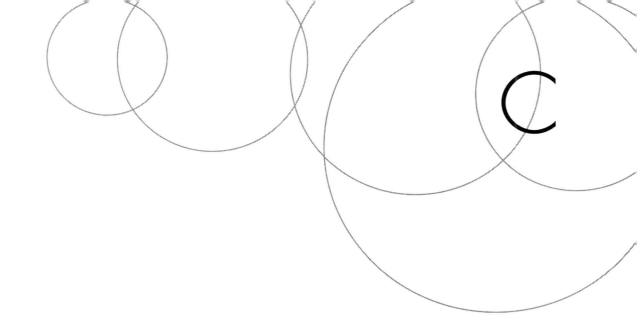

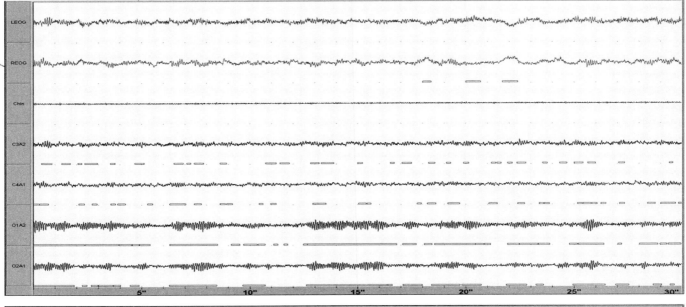

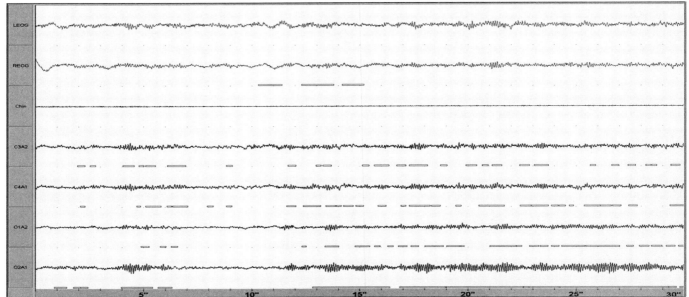

Figures A-1 and A-2.

Stage wake. Electroencephalography demonstrates low-voltage, high-frequency activity when a person is alert and the eyes are open; lower frequency activity when a person is relaxed; and prominent alpha (8–13 Hz) activity, occupying greater than 50% of the epoch, when a person is drowsy and the eyes are closed. Electro-oculography shows either blinking or rapid eye movements when a person is awake and alert, or slow rolling eye movements when a person is drowsy and the eyes are closed. There is high chin electromyographic amplitude.

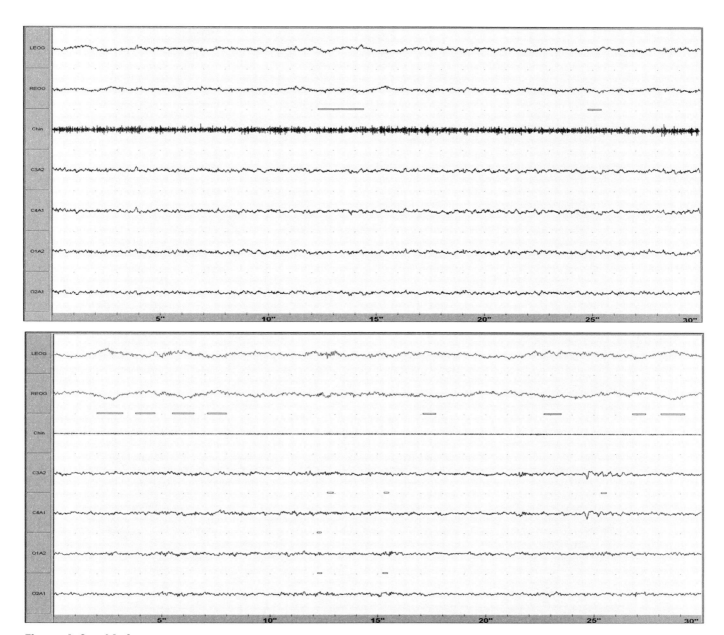

Figures A–3 and A–4.
Stage 1 sleep. Electroencephalography demonstrates a low-voltage, mixed-frequency activity with prominent theta activity. Alpha activity occupies less than 50% of the epoch. Beta rhythms may be present. Sleep spindles and K-complexes are absent. Electro-oculography may show occasional slow rolling eye movements but no rapid eye movements. There is high chin muscle activity (high chin EMG amplitude) that is less than or equal to that during wakefulness.

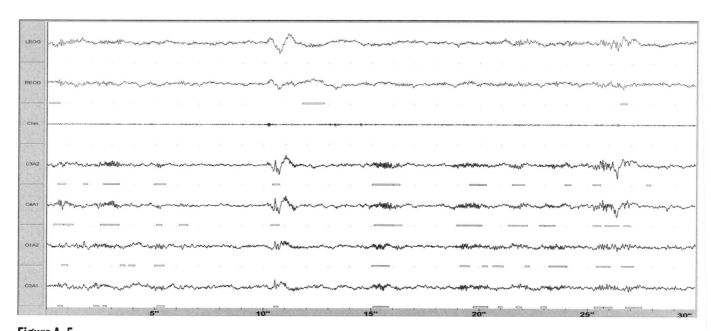

Figure A–5.

Stage 2 sleep. Electroencephalography reveals low-voltage, mixed-frequency activity and the presence of sleep spindles and K-complexes. Delta activity, if present, occupies less than 20% of the epoch. No movements are evident on electro-oculography. There is low chin muscle electromyographic activity.

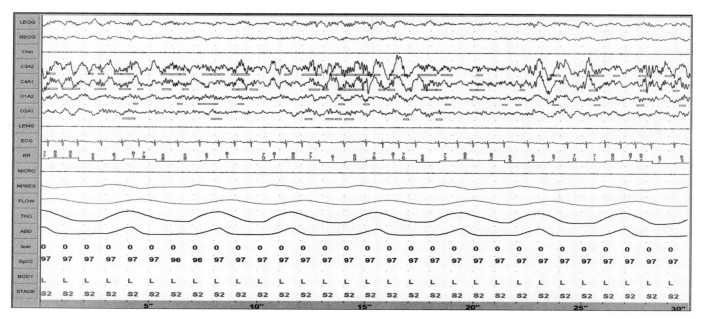

Figure A–6.

Stage 3 sleep. Delta activity occupies between 20% and 50% of the epoch in the electroencephalographic leads. Sleep spindles may be present. Electro-oculography demonstrates no movements. Low chin electromyographic muscle activity is generally less than that in seen in sleep stages 1 or 2.

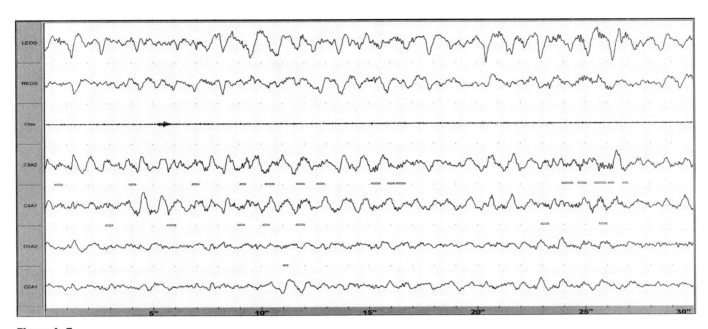

Figure A–7.
Stage 4 sleep. Electroencephalography shows that delta activity occupies more than 50% of the epoch. Sleep spindles may be present during this stage of sleep. Electro-oculography demonstrates no movements. There is low chin electromyographic muscle activity.

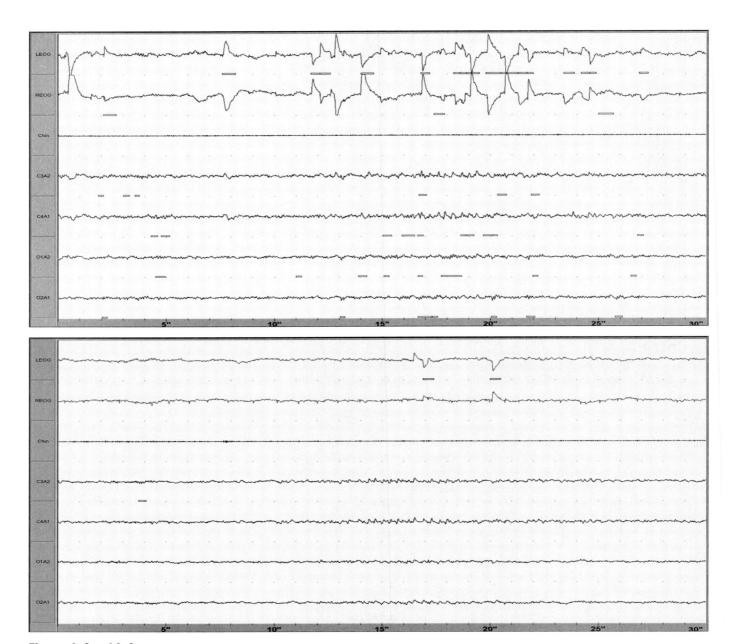

Figures A-8 and A-9.

Stage REM sleep. There is low-voltage, mixed-frequency electroencephalographic activity consisting of theta and beta rhythms. Alpha waves are 1–2 Hz slower than those occurring during wakefulness and NREM stage 1 sleep. Electro-oculography shows either no movements (tonic REM sleep) or bursts of conjugate (out-of-phase) rapid eye movements (phasic REM sleep). The amplitude of chin electromyographic activity is reduced or absent (ie, at least equal to or, more commonly, lower than the lowest amplitude during NREM sleep).

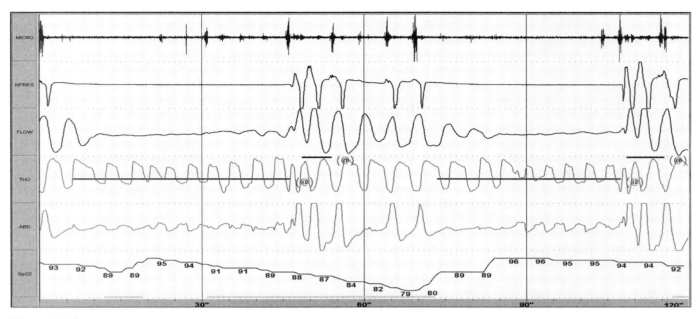

Figures A-10.

Obstructive apnea. An obstructive apnea is characterized by a cessation or nasal and oral airflow for at least 10 seconds that occurs despite the persistence of ventilatory efforts.

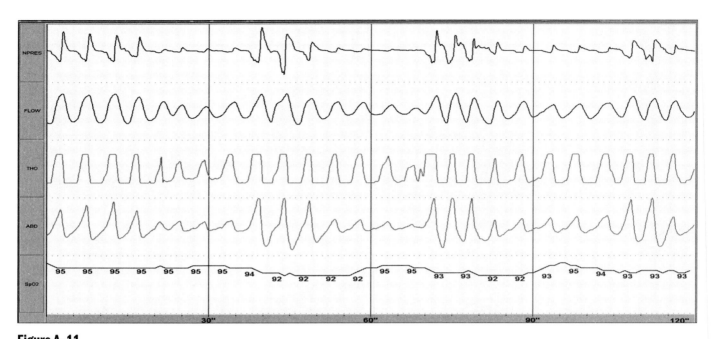

Figure A-11.

Obstructive hypopnea. An obstructive hypopnea is defined by a reduction of airflow or amplitude of thoracoabdominal movement of at least 30% from baseline, that lasts for at least 10 seconds. and is accompanied by oxyhemoglobin desaturation of 4% or more.

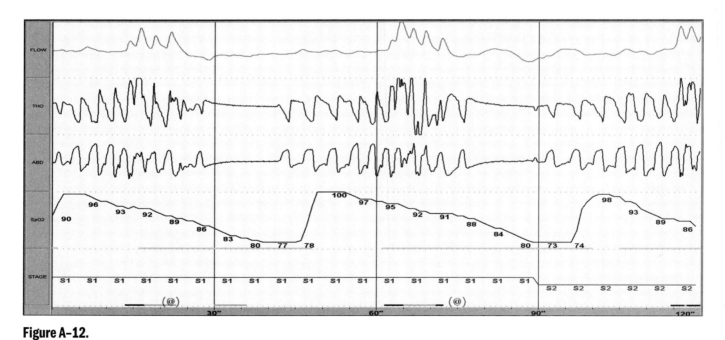

Figure A-12.

Mixed apnea. A mixed apnea is a cessation or reduction of airflow for at least 10 seconds with an initial central component and a terminal obstructive component.

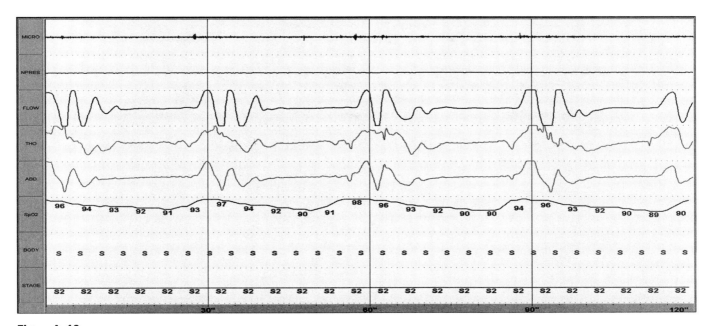

Figure A-13.
Central apnea. A central apnea is a cessation or reduction of airflow for at least 10 seconds that occurs in association with the absence of ventilatory efforts.

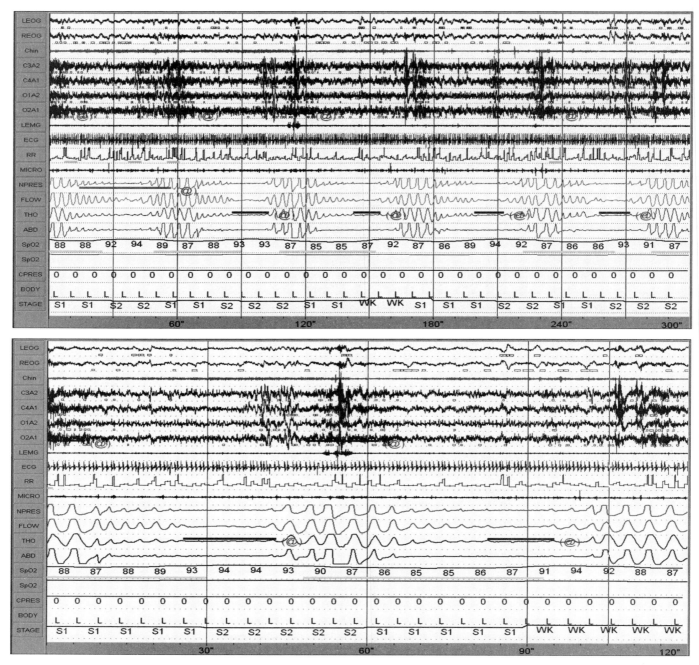

Figures A–14 and A–15.
Cheyne-Stokes respiration. Crescendo-decrescendo variability in respiratory rate and tidal volume is evident. The period of hyperpnea is longer, and the waxing and waning of ventilation is less abrupt (typically more than 45 seconds) than in other forms of central sleep apnea. Arousals and modest oxygen desaturation may accompany the respiratory events.

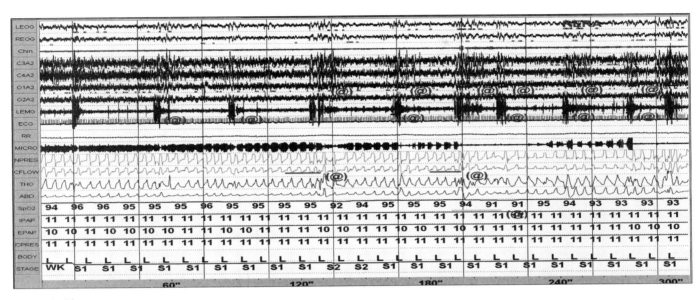

Figure A–16.

Periodic limb movements during sleep. This figure demonstrates repetitive leg electromyographic activity. Movements are counted if they occur during sleep, have a duration of 0.5 to 5 seconds, and occur in a series of four or more consecutive contractions with intervals between movements of between 5 to 90 seconds from the *onset* of one limb movement to the *onset* of the next. The amplitude of the electromyograpic activity is at least 25% greater than that of baseline during biocalibrations.

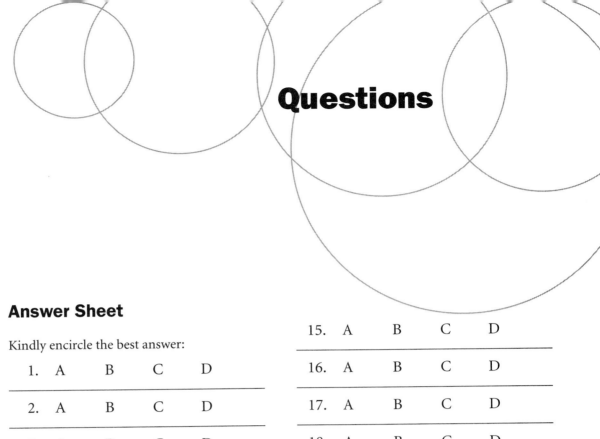

Questions

Answer Sheet

Kindly encircle the best answer:

1.	A	B	C	D
2.	A	B	C	D
3.	A	B	C	D
4.	A	B	C	D
5.	A	B	C	D
6.	A	B	C	D
7.	A	B	C	D
8.	A	B	C	D
9.	A	B	C	D
10.	A	B	C	D
11.	A	B	C	D
12.	A	B	C	D
13.	A	B	C	D
14.	A	B	C	D

15.	A	B	C	D
16.	A	B	C	D
17.	A	B	C	D
18.	A	B	C	D
19.	A	B	C	D
20.	A	B	C	D
21.	A	B	C	D
22.	A	B	C	D
23.	A	B	C	D
24.	A	B	C	D
25.	A	B	C	D
26.	A	B	C	D
27.	A	B	C	D
28.	A	B	C	D
29.	A	B	C	D

30. A	B	C	D
31. A	B	C	D
32. A	B	C	D
33. A	B	C	D
34. A	B	C	D
35. A	B	C	D
36. A	B	C	D
37. A	B	C	D
38. A	B	C	D
39. A	B	C	D
40. A	B	C	D
41. A	B	C	D
42. A	B	C	D
43. A	B	C	D
44. A	B	C	D
45. A	B	C	D
46. A	B	C	D
47. A	B	C	D
48. A	B	C	D
49. A	B	C	D
50. A	B	C	D
51. A	B	C	D
52. A	B	C	D

53. A	B	C	D
54. A	B	C	D
55. A	B	C	D
56. A	B	C	D
57. A	B	C	D
58. A	B	C	D
59. A	B	C	D
60. A	B	C	D
61. A	B	C	D
62. A	B	C	D
63. A	B	C	D
64. A	B	C	D
65. A	B	C	D
66. A	B	C	D
67. A	B	C	D
68. A	B	C	D
69. A	B	C	D
70. A	B	C	D
71. A	B	C	D
72. A	B	C	D
73. A	B	C	D
74. A	B	C	D
75. A	B	C	D

76. A   B   C   D

77. A   B   C   D

78. A   B   C   D

79. A   B   C   D

80. A   B   C   D

81. A   B   C   D

82. A   B   C   D

83. A   B   C   D

84. A   B   C   D

85. A   B   C   D

86. A   B   C   D

87. A   B   C   D

88. A   B   C   D

89. A   B   C   D

90. A   B   C   D

91. A   B   C   D

92. A   B   C   D

93. A   B   C   D

94. A   B   C   D

95. A   B   C   D

96. A   B   C   D

97. A   B   C   D

98. A   B   C   D

99. A   B   C   D

100. A   B   C   D

101. A   B   C   D

102. A   B   C   D

103. A   B   C   D

104. A   B   C   D

105. A   B   C   D

106. A   B   C   D

107. A   B   C   D

108. A   B   C   D

109. A   B   C   D

110. A   B   C   D

111. A   B   C   D

112. A   B   C   D

113. A   B   C   D

114. A   B   C   D

115. A   B   C   D

116. A   B   C   D

117. A   B   C   D

118. A   B   C   D

119. A   B   C   D

120. A   B   C   D

121. A   B   C   D

122.	A	B	C	D		145.	A	B	C	D
123.	A	B	C	D		146.	A	B	C	D
124.	A	B	C	D		147.	A	B	C	D
125.	A	B	C	D		148.	A	B	C	D
126.	A	B	C	D		149.	A	B	C	D
127.	A	B	C	D		150.	A	B	C	D
128.	A	B	C	D		151.	A	B	C	D
129.	A	B	C	D		152.	A	B	C	D
130.	A	B	C	D		153.	A	B	C	D
131.	A	B	C	D		154.	A	B	C	D
132.	A	B	C	D		155.	A	B	C	D
133.	A	B	C	D		156.	A	B	C	D
134.	A	B	C	D		157.	A	B	C	D
135.	A	B	C	D		158.	A	B	C	D
136.	A	B	C	D		159.	A	B	C	D
137.	A	B	C	D		160.	A	B	C	D
138.	A	B	C	D		161.	A	B	C	D
139.	A	B	C	D		162.	A	B	C	D
140.	A	B	C	D		163.	A	B	C	D
141.	A	B	C	D		164.	A	B	C	D
142.	A	B	C	D		165.	A	B	C	D
143.	A	B	C	D		166.	A	B	C	D
144.	A	B	C	D		167.	A	B	C	D

168. A   B   C   D

169. A   B   C   D

170. A   B   C   D

171. A   B   C   D

172. A   B   C   D

173. A   B   C   D

174. A   B   C   D

175. A   B   C   D

176. A   B   C   D

177. A   B   C   D

178. A   B   C   D

179. A   B   C   D

180. A   B   C   D

181. A   B   C   D

182. A   B   C   D

183. A   B   C   D

184. A   B   C   D

185. A   B   C   D

186. A   B   C   D

187. A   B   C   D

188. A   B   C   D

189. A   B   C   D

190. A   B   C   D

191. A   B   C   D

192. A   B   C   D

193. A   B   C   D

194. A   B   C   D

195. A   B   C   D

196. A   B   C   D

197. A   B   C   D

198. A   B   C   D

199. A   B   C   D

200. A   B   C   D

201. A   B   C   D

202. A   B   C   D

203. A   B   C   D

204. A   B   C   D

205. A   B   C   D

206. A   B   C   D

207. A   B   C   D

208. A   B   C   D

209. A   B   C   D

210. A   B   C   D

211. A   B   C   D

212. A   B   C   D

213. A   B   C   D

214.	A	B	C	D	237.	A	B	C	D
215.	A	B	C	D	238.	A	B	C	D
216.	A	B	C	D	239.	A	B	C	D
217.	A	B	C	D	240.	A	B	C	D
218.	A	B	C	D	241.	A	B	C	D
219.	A	B	C	D	242.	A	B	C	D
220.	A	B	C	D	243.	A	B	C	D
221.	A	B	C	D	244.	A	B	C	D
222.	A	B	C	D	245.	A	B	C	D
223.	A	B	C	D	246.	A	B	C	D
224.	A	B	C	D	247.	A	B	C	D
225.	A	B	C	D	248.	A	B	C	D
226.	A	B	C	D	249.	A	B	C	D
227.	A	B	C	D	250.	A	B	C	D
228.	A	B	C	D	251.	A	B	C	D
229.	A	B	C	D	252.	A	B	C	D
230.	A	B	C	D	253.	A	B	C	D
231.	A	B	C	D	254.	A	B	C	D
232.	A	B	C	D	255.	A	B	C	D
233.	A	B	C	D	256.	A	B	C	D
234.	A	B	C	D	257.	A	B	C	D
235.	A	B	C	D	258.	A	B	C	D
236.	A	B	C	D	259.	A	B	C	D

260. A   B   C   D

261. A   B   C   D

262. A   B   C   D

263. A   B   C   D

264. A   B   C   D

265. A   B   C   D

266. A   B   C   D

267. A   B   C   D

268. A   B   C   D

269. A   B   C   D

270. A   B   C   D

271. A   B   C   D

272. A   B   C   D

273. A   B   C   D

274. A   B   C   D

275. A   B   C   D

276. A   B   C   D

277. A   B   C   D

278. A   B   C   D

279. A   B   C   D

280. A   B   C   D

281. A   B   C   D

282. A   B   C   D

283. A   B   C   D

284. A   B   C   D

285. A   B   C   D

286. A   B   C   D

287. A   B   C   D

288. A   B   C   D

289. A   B   C   D

290. A   B   C   D

291. A   B   C   D

292. A   B   C   D

293. A   B   C   D

294. A   B   C   D

295. A   B   C   D

296. A   B   C   D

297. A   B   C   D

298. A   B   C   D

299. A   B   C   D

300. A   B   C   D

301. A   B   C   D

302. A   B   C   D

303. A   B   C   D

304. A   B   C   D

305. A   B   C   D

306.	A	B	C	D		329.	A	B	C	D
307.	A	B	C	D		330.	A	B	C	D
308.	A	B	C	D		331.	A	B	C	D
309.	A	B	C	D		332.	A	B	C	D
310.	A	B	C	D		333.	A	B	C	D
311.	A	B	C	D		334.	A	B	C	D
312.	A	B	C	D		335.	A	B	C	D
313.	A	B	C	D		336.	A	B	C	D
314.	A	B	C	D		337.	A	B	C	D
315.	A	B	C	D		338.	A	B	C	D
316.	A	B	C	D		339.	A	B	C	D
317.	A	B	C	D		340.	A	B	C	D
318.	A	B	C	D		341.	A	B	C	D
319.	A	B	C	D		342.	A	B	C	D
320.	A	B	C	D		343.	A	B	C	D
321.	A	B	C	D		344.	A	B	C	D
322.	A	B	C	D		345.	A	B	C	D
323.	A	B	C	D		346.	A	B	C	D
324.	A	B	C	D		347.	A	B	C	D
325.	A	B	C	D		348.	A	B	C	D
326.	A	B	C	D		349.	A	B	C	D
327.	A	B	C	D		350.	A	B	C	D
328.	A	B	C	D		351.	A	B	C	D

352. A   B   C   D
353. A   B   C   D
354. A   B   C   D
355. A   B   C   D
356. A   B   C   D
357. A   B   C   D
358. A   B   C   D
359. A   B   C   D
360. A   B   C   D
361. A   B   C   D
362. A   B   C   D
363. A   B   C   D
364. A   B   C   D
365. A   B   C   D
366. A   B   C   D
367. A   B   C   D
368. A   B   C   D
369. A   B   C   D
370. A   B   C   D
371. A   B   C   D
372. A   B   C   D
373. A   B   C   D
374. A   B   C   D

375. A   B   C   D
376. A   B   C   D
377. A   B   C   D
378. A   B   C   D
379. A   B   C   D
380. A   B   C   D
381. A   B   C   D
382. A   B   C   D
383. A   B   C   D
384. A   B   C   D
385. A   B   C   D
386. A   B   C   D
387. A   B   C   D
388. A   B   C   D
389. A   B   C   D
390. A   B   C   D
391. A   B   C   D
392. A   B   C   D
393. A   B   C   D
394. A   B   C   D
395. A   B   C   D
396. A   B   C   D
397. A   B   C   D

398.	A	B	C	D
399.	A	B	C	D
400.	A	B	C	D
401.	A	B	C	D
402.	A	B	C	D
403.	A	B	C	D
404.	A	B	C	D
405.	A	B	C	D
406.	A	B	C	D
407.	A	B	C	D
408.	A	B	C	D
409.	A	B	C	D
410.	A	B	C	D
411.	A	B	C	D
412.	A	B	C	D
413.	A	B	C	D
414.	A	B	C	D
415.	A	B	C	D
416.	A	B	C	D
417.	A	B	C	D
418.	A	B	C	D
419.	A	B	C	D
420.	A	B	C	D

421.	A	B	C	D
422.	A	B	C	D
423.	A	B	C	D
424.	A	B	C	D
425.	A	B	C	D
426.	A	B	C	D
427.	A	B	C	D
428.	A	B	C	D
429.	A	B	C	D
430.	A	B	C	D
431.	A	B	C	D
432.	A	B	C	D
433.	A	B	C	D
434.	A	B	C	D
435.	A	B	C	D
436.	A	B	C	D
437.	A	B	C	D
438.	A	B	C	D
439.	A	B	C	D
440.	A	B	C	D
441.	A	B	C	D
442.	A	B	C	D
443.	A	B	C	D

444.	A	B	C	D	467.	A	B	C	D
445.	A	B	C	D	468.	A	B	C	D
446.	A	B	C	D	469.	A	B	C	D
447.	A	B	C	D	470.	A	B	C	D
448.	A	B	C	D	471.	A	B	C	D
449.	A	B	C	D	472.	A	B	C	D
450.	A	B	C	D	473.	A	B	C	D
451.	A	B	C	D	474.	A	B	C	D
452.	A	B	C	D	475.	A	B	C	D
453.	A	B	C	D	476.	A	B	C	D
454.	A	B	C	D	477.	A	B	C	D
455.	A	B	C	D	478.	A	B	C	D
456.	A	B	C	D	479.	A	B	C	D
457.	A	B	C	D	480.	A	B	C	D
458.	A	B	C	D	481.	A	B	C	D
459.	A	B	C	D	482.	A	B	C	D
460.	A	B	C	D	483.	A	B	C	D
461.	A	B	C	D	484.	A	B	C	D
462.	A	B	C	D	485.	A	B	C	D
463.	A	B	C	D	486.	A	B	C	D
464.	A	B	C	D	487.	A	B	C	D
465.	A	B	C	D	488.	A	B	C	D
466.	A	B	C	D	489.	A	B	C	D

490.	A	B	C	D	513.	A	B	C	D
491.	A	B	C	D	514.	A	B	C	D
492.	A	B	C	D	515.	A	B	C	D
493.	A	B	C	D	516.	A	B	C	D
494.	A	B	C	D	517.	A	B	C	D
495.	A	B	C	D	518.	A	B	C	D
496.	A	B	C	D	519.	A	B	C	D
497.	A	B	C	D	520.	A	B	C	D
498.	A	B	C	D	521.	A	B	C	D
499.	A	B	C	D	522.	A	B	C	D
500.	A	B	C	D	523.	A	B	C	D
501.	A	B	C	D	524.	A	B	C	D
502.	A	B	C	D	525.	A	B	C	D
503.	A	B	C	D	526.	A	B	C	D
504.	A	B	C	D	527.	A	B	C	D
505.	A	B	C	D	528.	A	B	C	D
506.	A	B	C	D	529.	A	B	C	D
507.	A	B	C	D	530.	A	B	C	D
508.	A	B	C	D	531.	A	B	C	D
509.	A	B	C	D	532.	A	B	C	D
510.	A	B	C	D	533.	A	B	C	D
511.	A	B	C	D	534.	A	B	C	D
512.	A	B	C	D	535.	A	B	C	D

536.	A	B	C	D	559.	A	B	C	D
537.	A	B	C	D	560.	A	B	C	D
538.	A	B	C	D	561.	A	B	C	D
539.	A	B	C	D	562.	A	B	C	D
540.	A	B	C	D	563.	A	B	C	D
541.	A	B	C	D	564.	A	B	C	D
542.	A	B	C	D	565.	A	B	C	D
543.	A	B	C	D	566.	A	B	C	D
544.	A	B	C	D	567.	A	B	C	D
545.	A	B	C	D	568.	A	B	C	D
546.	A	B	C	D	569.	A	B	C	D
547.	A	B	C	D	570.	A	B	C	D
548.	A	B	C	D	571.	A	B	C	D
549.	A	B	C	D	572.	A	B	C	D
550.	A	B	C	D	573.	A	B	C	D
551.	A	B	C	D	574.	A	B	C	D
552.	A	B	C	D	575.	A	B	C	D
553.	A	B	C	D	576.	A	B	C	D
554.	A	B	C	D	577.	A	B	C	D
555.	A	B	C	D	578.	A	B	C	D
556.	A	B	C	D	579.	A	B	C	D
557.	A	B	C	D	580.	A	B	C	D
558.	A	B	C	D	581.	A	B	C	D

582. A B C D

583. A B C D

584. A B C D

585. A B C D

586. A B C D

587. A B C D

588. A B C D

589. A B C D

590. A B C D

591. A B C D

592. A B C D

593. A B C D

594. A B C D

595. A B C D

596. A B C D

597. A B C D

598. A B C D

599. A B C D

600. A B C D

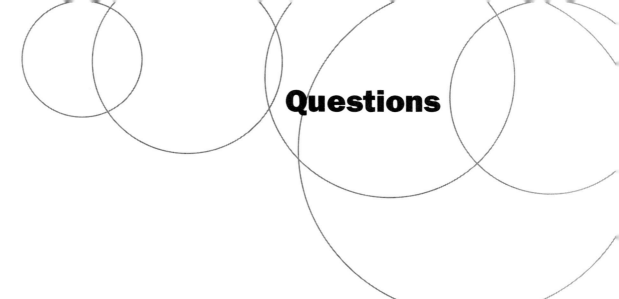

Questions

1. **Which of the following descriptions of apnea in an adult is correct?**

   a) Apnea is the absence of nasal and oral airflow for greater than 10 seconds.

   b) An apnea is classified as central if nasal and oral airflow ceases accompanied by absence of respiratory efforts.

   c) An apnea is considered obstructive if partial cessation of airflow occurs because of ineffectual respiratory efforts.

   d) A mixed apnea consists of an initial obstructive component followed by a central apnea.

2. **Persons are considered excessively sleepy if they are unable to consistently achieve and sustain wakefulness and alertness to accomplish the tasks of daily living. Which of the following statements about excessive sleepiness is correct?**

   a) Among young adults, hours of weekday sleep predict daytime sleepiness.

   b) Those who are single are less likely to develop daytime sleepiness than married individuals.

   c) Sleepiness is less prevalent among persons employed full-time than among those who are employed part-time or are unemployed.

   d) Prevalence is less among adolescents and older adults compared to middle-aged adults.

3. **The ability to initiate and maintain sleep may change in some older adults. Which of the following statements regarding sleep in older adults is true?**

   a) Older adults often have lower sleep efficiencies and more nighttime awakenings than younger adults.

   b) Older adults are less sleepy during the day than younger adults.

   c) Compared with elderly women, men are better able to maintain satisfactory sleep with aging.

   d) Older adults have increased NREM stages 3 and 4 sleep compared with younger adults.

4. **Which of the following best describes the demographic characteristics of restless legs syndrome?**

   a) Prevalence is increased with pregnancy, uremia, and anemia.

   b) Prevalence decreases with aging and is highest among young children, in whom it can be mistaken for rhythmic movement disorder.

   c) Course is chronic, and spontaneous remission does not occur.

   d) A majority of patients with periodic limb movements during sleep has concurrent restless leg syndrome.

5. **Which of the following is NOT an indication for specific therapy of parasomnias?**

   a) Associated with daytime impairment

   b) Associated with significant sleep disturbance

   c) When injurious

   d) When it persists for more than 3 months

6. **Which of the following statements describes sleep among women during the menstrual cycle?**

   a) Subjective sleepiness increases during the follicular phase.

   b) Sleep efficiency decreases during the follicular phase compared with the luteal phase.

   c) There is a decrease in sleep spindles during the luteal phase compared with the follicular phase.

   d) There is a decrease in REM sleep during the luteal phase compared with the follicular phase.

7. Which of the following disorders is characterized by recurrent, massive myoclonic jerks involving large muscle groups that occur only during sleep among infants during the first year of life?

   a) Fragmentary myoclonus

   b) Benign sleep myoclonus of infancy

   c) Propriospinal myoclonus at sleep onset

   d) Rhythmic movement disorder

8. Which of the following statements best characterizes caffeine?

   a) Adenosine receptor agonist

   b) Enhances phosphodiesterase that degrades adenosine

   c) Decrease drowsiness during sleep deprivation

   d) Increases REM sleep

9. According to the American Academy of Sleep Medicine 2005 *International Classification of Sleep Disorders*, which of the following is NOT considered a sleep-related movement disorder?

   a) Sleep-related bruxism

   b) Sleep-related leg cramps

   c) Sleep-related rhythmic movement disorder

   d) Sleepwalking

10. Which of the following statements is consistent with the American Academy of Sleep Medicine 2001 Practice Parameters for the Treatment of Narcolepsy?

    a) Failure to respond to seemingly adequate doses of stimulants should prompt rapid escalation to supranormal doses because excessive sleepiness related to narcolepsy is often refractory to conventional doses of stimulants.

    b) Methylphenidate is unsafe and should be avoided in children between the ages of 6 and 15 years.

    c) Scheduled naps are useful to combat sleepiness and are generally sufficient as primary and sole therapy for daytime sleepiness.

    d) Regular follow-up is necessary to monitor response to treatment and address adverse effects of medications.

11. The initial sleep episode is often REM sleep in young infants. At what age does the adult pattern of NREM sleep during sleep onset first develop?

    a) 1 to 2 months

    b) 3 to 4 months

    c) 9 to 12 months

    d) 12 to 15 months

12. Genetics appear to have an important role in the development of restless legs syndrome (RLS). Which of the following statements is true?

    a) A positive family history is more common in persons with secondary RLS than in those with idiopathic RLS.

    b) About one-third of cases of RLS is associated with an autosomal recessive mode of transmission.

    c) There is a low concordance rate of RLS symptoms between twins.

    d) RLS is more frequent in first- and second-degree relatives of individuals with RLS.

13. Which of the following statements regarding alcohol and its effect on sleep is correct?

    a) Alcohol has stimulatory effects at high doses and on the falling phase of alcohol levels.

    b) Alcohol's sedating effect can be additive with other agents such as benzodiazepines.

    c) Acute ingestion increases sleep latency, decreases NREM stages 3 and 4 sleep, and increases REM sleep during the first half of the sleep period.

    d) Alcohol causes a decrease in REM sleep during the second part of the night.

14. Which of the following antidepressant agents is preferable for patients with restless legs syndrome because it has no appreciable effect on the incidence or severity of this disorder?

    a) Bupropion

    b) Lithium

    c) Selective serotonin reuptake inhibitors

    d) Tricyclic antidepressants

15. Which of the following statements concerning the demographics of obstructive sleep apnea is correct?

    a) The prevalence of obstructive sleep apnea among women increases with menopause.

    b) There is a greater prevalence of obstructive sleep apnea among Caucasians than among African Americans.

c) Prevalence peaks during the fourth decade of life and remains stable with aging.

d) Because of differences in percentage and distribution of body fat, women are more likely to develop obstructive sleep apnea than men at all age groups.

16. **Which of the following statements regarding sleep disturbances in patients with Alzheimer disease is NOT correct?**

a) "Sun downing"

b) Increase in REM sleep

c) Reversal of sleep-wake rhythms

d) Sleep fragmentation with repetitive arousals and awakenings

17. **Which of the following is associated with the use of tetrahydrocannabinol (THC)?**

a) Administration at low doses results in increase in alertness

b) High doses can produce hallucinations

c) High doses increase REM sleep

d) Increase in total sleep time during THC discontinuation

18. **Which of the following medications can decrease REM sleep latency?**

a) Amphetamine

b) Barbiturates

c) Reserpine

d) Selective serotonin reuptake inhibitors

19. **Episodes of obstructive sleep apnea are commonly associated with brady-tachycardia. When does tachycardia typically occur during a period of sleep apnea?**

a) At the onset of apnea

b) During arousals following apnea termination

c) Immediately prior to apnea termination

d) At the nadir of oxygen saturation

20. **Which of the following statements regarding monoamine oxidase (MAO) inhibitors is correct?**

a) MAO inhibitors are classified as either classic agents that cause reversible enzyme inhibition (eg, phenelzine and tranylcypromine), or newer irreversible agents (eg, brofaromine).

b) MAO inhibitors increase REM sleep.

c) MAO inhibitors decrease REM sleep latency.

d) REM sleep rebound can occur during drug withdrawal.

21. **Which of the following statements concerning sleep during alcohol withdrawal is true?**

a) There is an increase in total sleep time.

b) Sleep latency decreases.

c) A decrease in wake time after sleep onset is common.

d) Delirium tremens is associated with markedly decreased total sleep time.

22. **Which of the following statements regarding confusional arousals is NOT correct?**

a) Occur following arousals from sleep, typically from NREM stages 3 and 4 sleep.

b) Usually occur in the first third of the night.

c) There is often amnesia for the event.

d) Signs of fear or autonomic hyperactivity are prominent.

23. **Compared with narcolepsy, naps in patients with idiopathic hypersomnia are generally:**

a) More likely to be associated with REM sleep

b) Shorter

c) More refreshing

d) More likely to be associated with difficulty awakening from sleep

24. **Which of the following is NOT a risk factor for REM sleep behavior disorder?**

a) Aging

b) Female gender

c) Multiple system atrophy

d) Parkinson disease

25. **One of the following statements regarding selective serotonin reuptake inhibitors (SSRIs) is correct?**

a) Excessive sleepiness has been reported following the use of citalopram or fluoxetine.

b) Fluvoxamine and paroxetine are among the most alerting SSRIs.

c) SSRIs are the preferred antidepressant agents for

patients with periodic limb movements of sleep and restless legs syndrome because they do not precipitate or aggravate these conditions.

d) SSRIs can increase eye movements during NREM sleep.

26. **When should nighttime feedings in children be discontinued?**

a) 2 months or older

b) 4 months or older

c) 6 months or older

d) 12 months or older

27. **Sudden unexplained nocturnal death syndrome (SUNDS) is characterized by sudden death that occurs during sleep without any apparent cause. Which of the following statements regarding SUNDS is correct?**

a) Victims are mostly older Southeast Asian males between the ages of 60 and 70 years with known cardiovascular disease.

b) Witnessed reports include descriptions of moaning, thrashing, screaming, violent motor activity, perspiration, and labored breathing that usually last for a few minutes prior to death.

c) All victims had evidence of atherosclerotic coronary artery disease, myocarditis, cardiomyopathy, or congenital cardiac anomalies.

d) Mutations in SCN5A, the gene known to cause Brugada syndrome, have been identified in all victims of SUNDS.

28. **Oxygen desaturation is commonly observed during sleep apnea. Which of the following factors is related to the severity of oxygen desaturation in sleep apnea?**

a) The degree of oxygen desaturation is related to the duration of apnea or hypopnea but not to the duration of ventilation between periods of apnea.

b) Oxygen desaturation is worse in persons with lower baseline awake supine SaO_2, and lower sleep SaO_2.

c) There is no significant difference in the degree of oxygen desaturation during apneas of equal duration occurring during NREM sleep compared with REM sleep.

d) Because of the absence of ventilatory efforts during central apneas, this type of apnea is

associated with more severe oxygen desaturation compared to obstructive apneas.

29. **Changes in sleep architecture can persist during abstinence from alcohol. Which of the following statements is true of sleep during alcohol abstinence?**

a) Total sleep time is increased.

b) NREM stages 3 and 4 sleep are increased.

c) There is a decrease in frequency of arousals.

d) Sleep disturbance can persist for several years following cessation of alcohol use.

30. **Which of the following agents is not effective in treating cataplexy, sleep paralysis, and sleep hallucinations?**

a) Modafinil

b) Fluoxetine

c) Protriptyline

d) Gamma-hydroxybutyrate

31. **Which of the following statements regarding upper airway resistance syndrome is correct?**

a) Repetitive sleep-related episodes of increasing upper airway resistance occur with a decrease in inspiratory airflow.

b) Respiratory effort is decreased.

c) Oxygen desaturation is present.

d) Snoring is essential for the diagnosis.

32. **Which of the following medications can increase REM sleep?**

a) Acetylcholine

b) Barbiturates

c) Selective serotonin reuptake inhibitors (fluoxetine)

d) Tricyclic antidepressants (except trimipramine)

33. **Which of the following is indicated in every patient with suspected obstructive sleep apnea?**

a) Multiple sleep latency test

b) Imaging studies, including lateral cephalometric views

c) Thyroid function tests

d) Physical examination

34. **Many factors increase the risk of developing obstructive sleep apnea (OSA). Which of the following statements regarding risk factors for OSA is correct?**

    a) The risk of developing OSA is greater among offsprings and first-degree relatives of OSA patients.

    b) Male gender is a risk factor for the occurrence of childhood OSA.

    c) OSA is relatively less common during childhood (ages 3 to 5 years) than during adolescence and early adulthood.

    d) Prevalence may be higher among Caucasians than among African Americans.

35. **Which of the following is NOT associated with the administration of opiates?**

    a) Excessive sleepiness during opiate use

    b) Development of insomnia during opiate withdrawal

    c) Exacerbation of obstructive sleep apnea

    d) Worsening symptoms of restless legs syndrome

36. **Which one of the following is an effect of hormonal agents on sleep?**

    a) Estrogen decreases REM sleep latency.

    b) Estrogen decreases REM sleep.

    c) Progesterone decreases REM sleep latency.

    d) Progesterone increases REM sleep.

37. **There are several mechanisms by which obesity may cause obstructive sleep apnea (OSA). Which one of the following mechanisms is NOT related to excess weight?**

    a) Reduction of upper airway caliber

    b) Increase in upper airway compliance

    c) Decrease in upper airway muscle tone

    d) Increase in lung residual volume

38. **Which of the following statements regarding the demographic features of central sleep apnea (CSA) is correct?**

    a) Prevalence is greater among women.

    b) The idiopathic form of CSA is more common than secondary causes of CSA.

    c) Prevalence increases in middle-aged and older adults compared with younger adults.

    d) CSA is more common than obstructive sleep apnea in the general population.

39. **One of the following statements about trazodone is correct?**

    a) It is an alerting agent.

    b) Trazodone can cause postural hypotension and priapism.

    c) It increases sleep latency and decreases sleep efficiency.

    d) Total sleep time is reduced.

40. **Which of the following statements regarding alcohol-dependent sleep disorder is correct?**

    a) Persons commonly exhibit other patterns of behavior compatible with overt alcoholism.

    b) Patients use alcohol regularly and consumption typically occurs throughout the day.

    c) Abruptly terminating alcohol use can precipitate profound insomnia with frequent awakenings.

    d) Use of alcohol a few hours prior to anticipated bedtime has no significant effects on sleep quality.

41. **At what age do children first develop the ability to postpone voiding in response to a full bladder?**

    a) By 12 to 18 months of age

    b) By 18 to 36 months of age

    c) By 36 to 48 months of age

    d) By 48 to 60 months of age

42. **Prevalence of nighttime fears peaks at what age?**

    a) Between 2 and 3 years of age

    b) Between 3 and 6 years of age

    c) Between 6 and 9 years of age

    d) Between 9 and 12 years of age

43. **Which of the following statements about sleepwalking is correct?**

    a) Adult sleepwalking is infrequent among those who had never walked in their sleep during childhood

    b) Eyes are usually closed during sleepwalking

    c) Full alertness when awakened from the episode

    d) Heightened autonomic activation

44. Which of the following antidepressants is typically alerting and can cause insomnia when taken close to bedtime?

    a) Amitriptyline

    b) Doxepin

    c) Fluoxetine

    d) Trazodone

45. Which of the following factors increases the risk of developing central sleep apnea?

    a) Low CO_2 ventilatory drive

    b) Female gender

    c) Younger age group

    d) Ascent to high altitude

46. Which of the following is an indication for autotitrating continuous positive airway pressure (APAP) devices?

    a) Comorbid congestive heart failure and obstructive sleep apnea (OSA)

    b) Respiratory failure

    c) Obesity hypoventilation syndrome

    d) To determine a single continuous positive airway pressure (CPAP) during attended polysomnography for the therapy of OSA

47. Which of the following statements best describes the association between excess body weight and the risk of developing obstructive sleep apnea (OSA)?

    a) The risk of developing OSA is not influenced by intra-abdominal fat or percentage of body fat.

    b) Excess body weight may be particularly important in persons without any apparent craniofacial or oropharyngeal features that would predispose them to developing OSA.

    c) Obesity in general (ie, body weight) appears to correlate better with OSA severity than central or nuchal obesity (increased waist-hip ratio and neck circumference).

    d) The apnea hypopnea index is not correlated with leptin levels.

48. Which of the following statements regarding bupropion is correct?

    a) It is a dopamine and norepinephrine reuptake inhibitor.

    b) It is sedating and can cause excessive daytime sleepiness.

    c) It can exacerbate or worsen periodic limb movements of sleep.

    d) It decreases REM sleep.

49. Which of the following antidepressants decreases REM sleep and increases REM sleep latency?

    a) Bupropion

    b) Mirtazapine

    c) Monoamine oxidase inhibitors

    d) Nefazodone

50. Which of the following agents can be used to improve sleep in patients with narcolepsy?

    a) Dextroamphetamine

    b) Methylphenidate

    c) Gamma-hydroxybutyrate

    d) Fluoxetine

51. Which of the following antidepressants either decreases or has no significant effect on NREM stages 3 and 4 sleep?

    a) Mirtazapine

    b) Nefazodone

    c) Selective serotonin reuptake inhibitors

    d) Trazodone

52. Which of the following statements about the effects of antihistamine agents on sleep is correct?

    a) Second-generation H_1 antagonists can induce sedation and cause excessive sleepiness.

    b) Multiple sleep latency studies following administration of second-generation H_1 antagonists reveal a decrease in daytime sleep latency.

    c) Second-generation H_1 antagonists are generally not sedating even at high doses.

    d) H_2 antagonists do not generally produce sedation.

53. Which of the following statements best describes caffeine?

    a) It acts by increasing adenosine transmission in the central nervous system.

    b) Adverse effects on sleep are dose-dependent and may last up to 8 hours after caffeine ingestion.

c) Tolerance to objective measures of alertness may develop more rapidly than subjective reports.

d) Elimination half-life is increased among smokers.

54. **Patients with asthma may present with episodic dyspnea and wheezing that can be worse at night and can give rise to repeated awakenings from sleep. Which of the following statements concerning nocturnal asthma is correct?**

a) A circadian variability in airflow exists with greatest airflow in the early morning and lowest airflow in the late afternoon.

b) Corticosteroid administration during the daytime does not diminish the circadian variability in airway tone that is observed at night.

c) Snoring and upper airway obstruction does not increase the frequency of nocturnal asthma attacks in individuals with coexisting asthma and obstructive sleep apnea.

d) Sleep, itself, is a major determinant of the variation in peak expiratory flow rate.

55. **Which of the following statements best describes the polysomnographic features of central sleep apnea?**

a) Loss of chest and abdominal movement occurs on strain gauges or respiratory inductance plethysmography.

b) Central hypopneas have a flattened profile on nasal pressure monitoring.

c) Snoring is absent.

d) Central apneas occur more frequently during REM sleep.

56. **In patients with chronic obstructive pulmonary disease (COPD), airflow limitation is usually progressive and is not fully reversible. COPD is often associated with poor sleep quality. Which of the following statements regarding sleep in patients with COPD is true?**

a) The increase in frequency of arousals seen in patients with COPD is primarily due to hypoxemia that occurs during sleep.

b) Episodes of oxygen desaturation are more frequent, of greater duration, and more severe during REM sleep than during NREM sleep.

c) Because patients with COPD who develop sleep-related hypoxemia have altered ventilatory responses to hypoxemia and hypercarbia, providing low-flow oxygen therapy frequently results in significant increases in nocturnal $PaCO_2$.

d) The severity of arterial oxygen desaturation during sleep is influenced by baseline lung function but is independent of awake PaO_2 and $PaCO_2$.

57. **Neuromuscular disorders, including muscular dystrophy, myotonic dystrophy, amyotrophic lateral sclerosis, poliomyelitis, and myasthenia gravis, are commonly associated with sleep-related breathing disorders. Which of the following statements about sleep in patients with neuromuscular disorders is true?**

a) Nocturnal respiratory impairment usually follows abnormalities during wakefulness by months to years.

b) Individuals with neuromuscular disorders often have an altered sense of dyspnea and there are generally no nighttime symptoms of dyspnea.

c) The likelihood of sleep-related oxygen desaturation is greater in patients with maximal inspiratory pressures less than 100 cm H_2O.

d) The likelihood of sleep-related oxygen desaturation is greater in patients with forced vital capacity less than 50% of predicted.

58. **Which of the following factors does NOT increase the risk of developing obstructive sleep apnea?**

a) Untreated hypothyroidism (myxedema)

b) Acromegaly

c) Strokes

d) Use of zolpidem for the therapy of insomnia

59. **Which of the following is a polysomnographic feature of lithium administration?**

a) Decrease in total sleep time

b) Decrease in NREM stage 2 sleep

c) Decrease in NREM stages 3 and 4 sleep

d) Increase in REM sleep latency

60. **When does electroencephalographic slow wave activity first appear in a child?**

a) 1 to 2 weeks of age

b) 4 to 8 weeks of age

c) 8 to 12 weeks of age

d) 12 months of age

61. **Which of the following statements about idiopathic hypersomnia is correct?**

a) Excessive sleepiness usually begins during infancy or early childhood

b) Onset is heralded by a viral illness (mononucleosis or hepatitis) in some cases.

c) There is a male predominance in prevalence.

d) A high frequency of DQ6 [DQB1*0602] has been described for some familial cases of the disorder.

62. **Which of the following polysomnographic features associated with the use of quetiapine is true?**

a) Increase in sleep latency

b) Increase in NREM stages 3 and 4 sleep

c) Decrease in REM sleep

d) Decrease in REM density

63. **Which of the following statements regarding Duchenne muscular dystrophy is NOT correct?**

a) It can present with central apneas.

b) It can present with obstructive apneas.

c) It is associated with an increase in frequency of arousals.

d) It is associated with an increase in REM sleep.

64. **Which of the following is NOT an effect of amphetamine administration?**

a) Improvements in alertness and reaction time

b) Reductions in sleepiness and fatigue

c) Sleep disturbance including insomnia and frequent awakenings

d) Pupillary constriction

65. **Which of the following statements regarding the regulation of sleep and wakefulness is correct?**

a) Sleep homeostasis is independent of the sleep-wake cycle.

b) Circadian rhythms are dependent on the sleep-wake cycle.

c) Sleep homeostasis is characterized by an increase in sleep pressure following sleep deprivation that is related to the duration of prior wakefulness followed by a decline in sleep need as sleep accumulates.

d) Electroencephalographic slow-wave activity is often used as a marker for circadian sleep-wake rhythms.

66. **Which of the following factors does NOT contribute to the development of Cheyne-Stokes respiration?**

a) Heightened hypercapnic respiratory drive

b) Long circulation time

c) Low daytime and sleep-related $PaCO_2$ levels

d) Low hypoxic respiratory drive

67. **Identify the two circadian peaks in wakefulness.**

a) Near the maximum core body temperature about 8 hours before the minimum core body temperature [Tmin] and about 4 to 8 hours after the Tmin.

b) Near the Tmin and about 9 hours after the Tmin.

c) Near the maximum core body temperature about 8 hours before the Tmin and about 9 hours after the Tmin.

d) Near the Tmin and about 4 to 8 hours after the Tmin.

68. **Methylphenidate acts by blocking the reuptake and enhancing the release of which neurotransmitter?**

a) Dopamine

b) Histamine

c) Hypocretin (orexin)

d) Serotonin

69. **Which of following best describes the changes in sleep associated with poliomyelitis?**

a) Increase in REM sleep

b) Increase in sleep efficiency

c) No change in frequency of arousals

d) Nocturnal hypoventilation

70. **Which of the following statements regarding excessive sleepiness in patients with obstructive sleep apnea (OSA) is true?**

a) Excessive daytime sleepiness (EDS) is present in all patients with OSA, and its absence excludes the diagnosis.

b) Nocturnal oxygen desaturation is the primary cause of EDS in OSA.

c) There is poor correlation between apnea indices and mean sleep latency during the Multiple Sleep Latency Test.

d) There is excellent correlation between apnea indices and subjective (Epworth Sleepiness Scale) measures of sleepiness.

71. **Which of the following is NOT true about corticosteroids and their effect on sleep?**

    a) Can cause insomnia

    b) Can cause nightmares

    c) Decrease NREM stages 3 and 4 sleep

    d) Increase REM sleep

72. **Based on criteria proposed by the American Academy of Sleep Medicine 1997 *International Classification of Sleep Disorders*, sleepiness is considered to be of moderate severity if:**

    a) Sleepiness occurs during times of rest or when little attention is required (eg, reading or watching television).

    b) Sleepiness occurs daily and during physical activities that involve mild to moderate degree of attention (eg, conversation, eating, or driving).

    c) Sleepiness occurs daily and during mild physical activities that involve some degree of attention (eg, group meetings).

    d) Sleepiness is associated with marked impairment of social or occupational functioning.

73. **Which of the following statements best describes the changes in sleep associated with myasthenia gravis?**

    a) Increased likelihood of developing central sleep apnea but not obstructive apneas and hypopneas

    b) Nocturnal oxygen desaturation predominantly during REM sleep

    c) An autoimmune disease characterized by the presence of antibodies directed against norepinephrine receptors at the neuromuscular junction

    d) Nocturnal oxygen desaturation predominantly during NREM sleep

74. **Which of the following statements concerning the regulation of sleep and wakefulness is correct?**

    a) Sleep latency and subsequent sleep duration and quality are influenced by sleep deprivation but not by circadian factors.

    b) Sleep inertia refers to the short-lived reduction in alertness that occurs immediately prior to sleep onset.

    c) Post-sleep reduction in alertness is greater following awakenings from REM sleep.

    d) The timing of sleep is determined by autonomic nervous system tone.

75. **A sleep cycle refers to the period from NREM stages 1 to 4 to REM sleep. Which of the following statements regarding sleep cycles among humans is correct?**

    a) There are commonly three to five NREM-REM sleep cycles, each occurring every 60 minutes in adults.

    b) Sleep cycles occur every 90 to 120 minutes in infants and young children.

    c) Every sleep stage (NREM stages 1 to 4 and REM sleep) is present in every sleep cycle.

    d) REM density (frequency of rapid eye movements during REM sleep) and percentage REM sleep increase during the latter portion of the night.

76. **Which of the following statements regarding sleep in animals is correct?**

    a) Mammals have cycling of quiet and paradoxical sleep.

    b) Among mammals, sleep spindles, but no delta waves, can be seen during NREM sleep.

    c) Sleep spindles are present in birds.

    d) Avian sleep is characterized by prolonged REM sleep periods.

77. **Which of the following factors does NOT influence the degree of oxygen desaturation during sleep apnea?**

    a) Baseline oxygen saturation prior to the apnea

    b) Lung volume

    c) Duration of apnea

    d) Location of oximetry probe

78. **Which of the following statements about the changes in sleep that occur in patients with diaphragm paralysis is correct?**

    a) Nocturnal hypoxemia is common

    b) Sleep-related breathing disorders occur in patients with unilateral but not bilateral diaphragmatic paralysis

    c) There is an increase in NREM stages 3 and 4 sleep

    d) An increase in REM sleep is often present.

79. **Which of the following factors related to obstructive sleep apnea has NOT been shown to increase the risk of developing hypertension?**

    a) Percent sleep time with oxygen saturation below 90%

b) Apnea index

c) Apnea hypopnea index

d) Sleep efficiency

80. **Which of the following measures is a reliable method of reducing sleepiness during night shift work?**

a) Increase in levels of physical activity or frequent changes in posture during work

b) External stimulation, such as loud music, in the workplace

c) Exposure to bright lights in the workplace

d) Administration of melatonin prior to daytime sleep

81. **Which of the following sleep stages accounts for the greatest percentage of sleep among healthy adults?**

a) NREM stage 1 sleep

b) NREM stage 2 sleep

c) NREM stages 3 and 4 sleep

d) Stage REM sleep

82. **Which of the following statements regarding the polysomnographic features of REM sleep is correct?**

a) REM sleep is composed of two components, namely, tonic (with rapid eye movements) and phasic (without rapid eye movements) sleep.

b) Saw-tooth waves may be present in the electroencephalogram and are more prominent over the vertex and frontal leads.

c) Alpha waves are 1 to 2 Hz faster than those occurring during wakefulness and NREM stage 1 sleep.

d) The amplitude of chin electromyography is similar to or higher than the lowest amplitude during NREM sleep.

83. **Which of the following neurotransmitters participates in the generation and maintenance of REM sleep?**

a) Acetylcholine

b) Dopamine

c) Histamine

d) Hypocretin

84. **Which of the following statements about stage Wake is true?**

a) Persons who are drowsy are often unable to keep their eyes open, and blinking or rapid eye movements are generally noted during this time.

b) Slow rolling eye movements are present when a person is awake and alert, a phenomenon referred to as "scanning."

c) Chin electromyographic activity is low due to muscle relaxation.

d) Electroencephalographic and electro-oculographic tracings may demonstrate muscle artifact when a person is tense.

85. **Which of the following statements about the causes of cardiac ischemia developing during sleep is NOT correct?**

a) Sleep-related hypotension is particularly prominent during REM sleep.

b) Sympathetic surges with increase in blood pressure and heart rate occur during arousals or awakenings from sleep.

c) REM sleep can be associated with instability of heart rate and blood pressure.

d) Hypoxemia develops during apneic episodes and increases in blood pressure and heart rate occur during the post-arousal period in patients with obstructive sleep apnea.

86. **Which of the following statements regarding blood pressure in patients with obstructive sleep apnea (OSA) is NOT correct?**

a) Increased risk of hypertension in OSA is associated with greater frequency of apneic episodes and but not nocturnal oxygen saturation.

b) Prevalence of OSA is increased in patients with hypertension.

c) Blood pressure increases following termination of the apneic episode.

d) Treatment of OSA may decrease blood pressure.

87. **Which of the following is associated with the administration of risperidone?**

a) Increase in frequency of awakenings

b) No change in NREM stages 3 and 4 sleep

c) No change in REM sleep latency

d) No change in REM sleep

88. **Which of the following statements best characterizes venlafaxine's effect on sleep?**

a) Decrease in wake time after sleep onset

b) Decrease in REM sleep latency

c) Increase in REM sleep

d) Can cause or exacerbate periodic limb movements of sleep

89. Cataplexy is characterized by an abrupt, transient, and bilateral loss or reduction of postural muscle tone occurring during wakefulness and precipitated by intense emotion such as laughter. Which of the following statements regarding cataplexy is correct?

a) Cataplexy may also be triggered by stress, fatigue, or medications, but it does not occur spontaneously without apparent provocation.

b) Prolonged episodes of cataplexy may give rise to REM sleep with hypnagogic hallucinations and dreaming.

c) Cataplexy last only several seconds and does not persist for more than a minute.

d) Severity is maximal at the start of the attack and improves gradually over several seconds.

90. In which of the following phases of schizophrenia is a decrease in sleep efficiency commonly noted?

a) Waning phase

b) Waxing phase

c) Postpsychotic phase

d) Remission phase

91. In which of the following patients is the development of pulmonary hypertension LEAST likely?

a) A patient with severe obstructive sleep apnea (OSA)

b) A patient with OSA and daytime hypoxemia and hypercapnia due to concurrent chronic obstructive pulmonary disease ("overlap" syndrome)

c) A patient with OSA and obesity-hypoventilation syndrome

d) A patient with mild OSA and systemic hypertension

92. Which of the following medications increases NREM stages 3 and 4 sleep?

a) Adenosine agonists

b) Barbiturates

c) Benzodiazepines

d) Selective serotonin reuptake inhibitors

93. Which of the following conditions is NOT associated with greater frequency of arousals among infants?

a) Bottle-feeding (relative to breast-feeding)

b) Colic

c) Cosleeping

d) Otitis media

94. Which of the following statements about the relationship between sleep and congestive heart failure (CHF) is NOT correct?

a) Obstructive sleep apnea and central sleep apnea can develop in patients with CHF.

b) Left ventricular systolic dysfunction is an independent risk factor for the development of sleep apnea in patients with CHF.

c) Untreated severe sleep-related breathing disorders may further impair left ventricular function.

d) A decrease in circulation time is responsible for most cases of obstructive sleep apnea in patients with CHF.

95. Which of the following neurotransmitters associated with the regulation of wakefulness has neurons located in the locus ceruleus in the dorsal pontine tegmentum?

a) Dopamine

b) Histamine

c) Hypocretin (orexin)

d) Noradrenaline

96. What do lesions of the central midbrain tegmentum produce?

a) Cortical inactivation without affecting behavioral responsiveness to sensory stimulation

b) Cortical inactivation affecting behavioral responsiveness to sensory stimulation

c) Behavioral somnolence and unresponsiveness without loss of cortical activation

d) Behavioral and cortical activation

97. Which of the following statements regarding the neurotransmitter gamma-aminobutyric acid (GABA) is correct?

a) GABA neurons are located in the ventrolateral preoptic (VLPO) area, thalamus, hypothalamus, basal forebrain, and cerebral cortex

b) GABA is the main central nervous system excitatory neurotransmitter.

c) Barbiturates, benzodiazepines, and nonbenzodiazepine benzodiazepine receptor agonists (eg, eszopiclone or zolpidem) act on the GABA-B receptor.

d) Sodium oxybate acts on the GABA-A receptor.

98. **Which of the following is the main excitatory central nervous system neurotransmitter?**

a) Glutamate

b) Histamine

c) Hypocretin

d) Serotonin

99. **In which sleep stage/s does Cheyne-Stokes respiration typically occur?**

a) NREM stages 1 and 2 sleep

b) NREM stages 3 and 4 sleep

c) REM sleep

d) Equally distributed across the different sleep stages

100. **Which of the following medications is NOT used for the therapy of cataplexy in patients with narcolepsy?**

a) Fluoxetine

b) Gamma-hydroxybutyrate

c) Modafinil

d) Protriptyline

101. **When does daytime sleepiness develop in persons with seasonal affective disorder?**

a) Major depressive episodes during fall and winter.

b) Major depressive episodes during spring and summer.

c) Hypomanic episodes during fall and winter.

d) Hypomanic episodes during spring and summer.

102. **Which neurotransmitter causes cortical electroencephalographic desynchronization during wakefulness and REM sleep?**

a) Acetylcholine

b) Hypocretin

c) Norepinephrine

d) Serotonin

103. **In contrast to patients with obstructive sleep apnea (OSA) who complain of excessive sleepiness, those who present with insomnia have which of the following characteristics?**

a) More obese

b) More severe OSA

c) Milder oxygen desaturation

d) Higher apnea hypopnea indices

104. **The methylxanthines, including caffeine and theophylline, are psychostimulants that block the action of which neurotransmitter?**

a) Adenosine

b) Gamma-aminobutyric acid

c) Histamine

d) Serotonin

105. **Which of the following is NOT a polysomnographic feature of stimulant agents?**

a) Increase in sleep latency

b) Decrease in total sleep time

c) Increase in NREM stages 3 and 4 sleep

d) Increase in REM sleep latency

106. **Which of the following is NOT a clinical feature of agrypnia excitata?**

a) Autonomic sympathetic discharge

b) Loss of NREM stages 3 and 4 sleep

c) Oneirism

d) Reduced motor activity and hypotonia

107. **Which of the following is a known physiologic consequence of obstructive sleep apnea?**

a) Decrease in pulmonary artery pressure

b) Increase in systemic blood pressure

c) Increase in right ventricular output

d) Decrease in vascular resistance

108. **Which of the following statements best describes the sleep-related changes in cardiac rhythm?**

a) Risk of ventricular arrhythmias is increased during arousals from sleep.

b) Frequency of premature ventricular beats generally increases during NREM sleep.

c) In patients with obstructive sleep apnea, heart rate increases at the onset of the apneic episode, with relative bradycardia after the termination of the event.

d) Sinus arrhythmias are rare in obstructive sleep apnea.

109. What is the frequency of an electroencephalographic (EEG) delta wave?

a) < 4 Hz

b) 4–7 Hz

c) 8–13 Hz

d) 13 Hz

110. Which of the following statements about electrocephalographic (EEG) waveforms is correct?

a) Beta waves consist of oscillations with a frequency of 4–7 Hz.

b) Delta waves are high-amplitude (peak to peak of > 75 µV), slow (< 2 Hz) EEG activity.

c) Saw-tooth waves are beta waves with a notched waveform that occurs during REM sleep.

d) Theta waves are maximal over the occipital leads.

111. Which of the following statements regarding polysomnography is correct?

a) Chin electromyography is necessary to identify sleep onset.

b) A 12-lead electrocardiogram is commonly used to monitor cardiac rate and rhythm.

c) Of the techniques used to measure airflow, only $PetCO_2$ monitoring measures airflow directly.

d) Thermal sensors provide indirect estimates of airflow.

112. Which of the following statements regarding cataplexy is correct?

a) Respiratory muscles are spared.

b) Oculomotor muscles are affected and blurring of vision may occur.

c) Memory and consciousness are impaired.

d) Frequency of cataplexy does not decrease over time.

113. Which of the following statements does NOT describe sleep in patients with peptic ulcer disease?

a) There is greater gastric acid secretion during sleep.

b) Nocturnal abdominal pain is common.

c) Onset of abdominal pain occurs within the last 4 hours of sleep.

d) Repeated arousals and awakenings are common.

114. Which of the following statements regarding surface diaphragmatic electromyography (EMG) and strain gauges during polysomnography is correct?

a) Both surface diaphragmatic EMG and strain gauges are used to measure rib cage and abdominal excursions during sleep.

b) Surface diaphragmatic EMG can measure respiratory effort directly.

c) With strain gauges, only quantitative measures of volume changes are useful during polysomnography.

d) Quantitative measurements of volume changes require calibration of the rib cage and abdominal strain gauges against another volume-measuring device.

115. Which of the following statements best describes the relationship between sleep and gastroesophageal reflux (GER)?

a) The prevalence of GER is not increased by the presence of obstructive sleep apnea.

b) The primary mechanism of GER is transient relaxation of the upper esophageal sphincter.

c) More prolonged esophageal acid clearance times are associated with sleep-related GER compared to GER occurring during wakefulness.

d) Production of saliva, which helps neutralize acid refluxate, increases during sleep.

116. When does an arousal typically occur during an apneic event in patients with obstructive sleep apnea?

a) At the termination of the apneic event

b) At the nadir of oxygen saturation

c) At the start of the apneic event

d) Sporadically during sleep

117. Which of the following statements related to sleep among women is true?

a) The prevalence of obstructive sleep apnea is greater among postmenopausal women who use hormone replacement therapy (HRT) than among those not on HRT.

b) In polycystic ovarian syndrome, there is an increased risk of developing obstructive sleep apnea.

c) Central sleep apnea is more common in premenopausal women than in men.

d) Compared with men, women tend to demonstrate greater supine position dependency in respiratory events.

118. **Which of the following statements about HLA typing in the evaluation of patients with suspected narcolepsy is correct?**

a) The prevalence of DR2 in African Americans with narcolepsy is 90%.

b) HLA DQB1*0602 is present in most patients with narcolepsy with cataplexy (90%) and in about 40% to 60% of those with narcolepsy without cataplexy.

c) HLA DRB1*1501 is common among African Americans with narcolepsy with cataplexy.

d) DQB1 *0602 is more specific among Asians and Caucasians with narcolepsy.

119. **At which of the following age groups is the proportion of NREM stages 3 and 4 sleep greatest during the night?**

a) Newborn period

b) Early childhood

c) Middle adulthood

d) Older adulthood

120. **Which of the following antidepressants increase REM sleep?**

a) Mirtazapine

b) Nefazodone

c) Trazodone

d) Venlafaxine

121. **Which of the following disorders is characterized by asynchronous, asymmetric and brief contractions of the muscles of the face, trunk, and extremities appearing at the onset of sleep and continuing throughout the night?**

a) Benign sleep myoclonus of infancy

b) Fragmentary myoclonus

c) Propriospinal myoclonus at sleep onset

d) Rhythmic movement disorder

122. **Which of the following statements best describes the changes in sleep in patients with end-stage renal disease (ESRD)?**

a) Disturbances in sleep are uncommon (less than 15%) among patients on maintenance hemodialysis for ESRD.

b) Sleep disturbance is more severe in patients on continuous peritoneal dialysis compared to those on hemodialysis.

c) Obstructive sleep apnea is not improved by hemodialysis.

d) Correction of anemia in ESRD patients can improve sleep quality.

123. **Which of the following factors does NOT contribute to the greater likelihood of developing obstructive sleep apnea in patients with untreated hypothyroidism?**

a) Deposition of mucopolysaccharides in the upper airway

b) Impaired central respiratory drive

c) Myopathy

d) Presence of myxedema

124. **Which of the following factors is important in the development of nocturnal cardiac ischemia in patients with obstructive sleep apnea?**

a) Endothelial dysfunction and accelerated atherosclerosis

b) Decreased sympathetic activity

c) Postapneic bradycardia

d) Increased left ventricular preload

125. **Changes in sleep architecture seen during menopause include which of the following?**

a) Decrease in sleep latency

b) Decrease in sleep efficiency

c) Increase in total sleep time

d) Decrease in wake time after sleep onset

126. **Which of the following factors does NOT contribute to the greater likelihood of developing obstructive sleep apnea in patients with acromegaly?**

a) Abnormalities in craniofacial dimensions, predominantly of the mandible

b) Biochemical parameters of disease activity, such as growth hormone levels

c)   Greater initial tongue volume

d)   Upper airway narrowing due to changes in pharyngeal soft tissues

127. **Which of the following factors does NOT influence the accuracy of conventional pulse oximetry used during polysomnography?**

a)   Pulse oximeter response times

b)   Use of nail polish for finger probes

c)   Reduced skin vascular perfusion

d)   Presence of dyshemoglobin species such as carboxyhemoglobin or methemoglobin

128. **Which of the following newborn electroencephalographic waveforms is not present during active sleep?**

a)   High-voltage slow pattern

b)   Low-voltage irregular pattern

c)   Trace alternant

d)   Mixed pattern

129. **How do electrode popping artifacts appear on the polysomnogram?**

a)   As sudden, sharp high-amplitude deflections

b)   As slow-frequency undulating movements

c)   As dense, almost square-shaped electroencephalogram tracing

d)   As isolated mixed frequency low-amplitude waveforms in the chin electromyogram

130. **Which of the following statements best describes the changes in sleep architecture in patients with Cushing syndrome?**

a)   Increase in sleep efficiency

b)   Increase in NREM stages 3 and 4 sleep

c)   Decrease in REM latency

d)   Decrease in REM density

131. **What level of diagnostic sleep study consists of a cardiorespiratory sleep study, or modified portable sleep apnea testing with four or more parameters (eg, airflow, SaO2, respiratory effort, electrocardiography, or body position)?**

a)   Level 1 study

b)   Level 2 study

c)   Level 3 study

d)   Level 4 study

132. **Which of the following statements about actigraphy is true?**

a)   Actigraphy is routinely indicated for the evaluation of suspected circadian rhythm sleep disorders.

b)   Data obtained from actigraphs placed on the wrists are superior to those placed on the lower extremities.

c)   Actigraphy is a reliable and valid method of detecting sleep in normal, healthy adults.

d)   Actigraphy monitoring should include at least 7 days of data collection.

133. **Which of the following statements regarding the relationship between congestive heart failure (CHF) and obstructive sleep apnea (OSA) is correct?**

a)   Compared with those with symptomatic CHF, patients with asymptomatic left ventricular dysfunction do not have an increased risk of developing OSA.

b)   The presence of isolated OSA does not increase the likelihood of developing CHF.

c)   OSA is associated with a decrease in left ventricular afterload and more positive intrathoracic pressure.

d)   OSA is associated with sympathetic nervous system activation due to hypoxemia and repeated arousals during sleep.

134. **Which of the following statements best describes the performance of the Multiple Sleep Latency Test (MSLT)?**

a)   A nocturnal polysomnography during the patient's usual major sleep period should always be performed on the evening immediately before an MSLT.

b)   MSLT can be performed after a split-night sleep study.

c)   The first nap opportunity generally starts immediately after awakening from the previous night's polysomnography.

d)   The patient is instructed to lie quietly; assume a comfortable position; close his/her eyes; and try to stay awake in a dark, quiet room.

135. **Alternating current (AC) amplifiers in a polygraph are generally used to monitor which of the following sleep-related parameters?**
    a) Continuous positive airway pressure levels
    b) Electroencephalography
    c) Esophageal pressures
    d) Oxygen saturation

136. **What is the reference standard for identifying central sleep apnea–hypopnea syndromes?**
    a) Esophageal pressure monitoring
    b) Expired carbon dioxide ($PetCO_2$) monitoring
    c) Respiratory inductance plethysmography
    d) Surface diaphragmatic electromyography

137. **Which of the following statements best describes the effect on sleep architecture of bedtime administration of hydrocortisone in patients with Addison disease?**
    a) Increase in sleep efficiency
    b) Greater wake time after sleep onset
    c) Increase in REM latency
    d) Decrease in REM sleep

138. **Which of the following statements regarding pulse transit time is correct?**
    a) It is the time it takes the arterial pulse pressure wave to travel from the aortic valve to the periphery.
    b) It decreases during obstructive sleep apnea–related inspiratory fall in blood pressure.
    c) It increases during the rise in blood pressure related to arousals.
    d) It is useful in distinguishing obstructive apneas from obstructive hypopneas.

139. **Which of the following statements best describes modafinil?**
    a) It possesses no major addiction potential.
    b) It can produce sleep rebound with drug discontinuation.
    c) There is no development of tolerance.
    d) It is indicated for excessive sleepiness regardless of etiology.

140. **Which of the following statements regarding REM sleep–related sinus arrest is correct?**
    a) It affects adults with ischemic heart disease, many of whom also have obstructive sleep apnea syndrome.

    b) Episodes are accompanied by arousals or sleep disruption.
    c) Periods of asystole last up to 9 seconds in duration.
    d) Sinus arrest is commonly present during daytime electrocardiography but are less frequent than during REM sleep.

141. **What percentage of total sleep time does REM sleep occupy in the newborn period?**
    a) 10%
    b) 25%
    c) 50%
    d) 75%

142. **Which of the following statements regarding cataplexy is correct?**
    a) Cataplexy can be considered as intrusion of REM sleep–related muscle atonia during wakefulness.
    b) During episodes of cataplexy, neurologic examination demonstrates muscle flaccidity but persistence of deep tendon and pupillary light reflexes.
    c) Cataplexy is produced by excitation of lower motor neurons as well as deep tendon and H reflexes by noradrenergic areas of the pons and basal forebrain.
    d) There is a glutamate-mediated hyperpolarization of the anterior horn cells of the spinal cord.

143. **At what age does an increase in frequency of awakenings during the night ("night wakings") develop?**
    a) Between 6 and 12 months
    b) Between 1 and 6 years
    c) Between 6 and 10 years
    d) Between 10 and 14 years

144. **Which of the following statements regarding cataplexy is correct?**
    a) Cataplexy generally first develops several months or years before the onset of excessive sleepiness.
    b) Cataplexy is required for the diagnosis of narcolepsy and all patients with this disorder have cataplexy.
    c) The absence of cataplexy excludes the diagnosis of narcolepsy.
    d) Cataplexy can also be seen in association with midbrain tumors, Niemann-Pick disease (type C) and Norrie disease.

145. What is the reference standard for identifying respiratory effort–related arousals?

    a) Measurement of esophageal pressure

    b) Measurement of nasal pressure

    c) Strain gauges

    d) Surface diaphragmatic electromyography

146. Which of the following is NOT an effect of weight reduction on upper airway and lung parameters in patients with obstructive sleep apnea?

    a) Increase upper airway caliber

    b) Decrease airway collapsibility

    c) Decrease upper airway critical closing pressure

    d) Increase functional residual capacity and residual volume

147. Which of the following types of rhythmic movement disorders is generally associated with the earliest mean age of onset?

    a) Body rocking

    b) Body rolling

    c) Head banging

    d) Head rolling

148. Which of the following medications is the most potent REM sleep inhibitor?

    a) Bupropion

    b) Monoamine oxidase inhibitors

    c) Selective serotonin reuptake inhibitors

    d) Tricyclic antidepressants

149. When may oral devices be reasonably considered for the treatment of obstructive sleep apnea in children?

    a) In young children before the rapid growth of craniofacial bones

    b) In young children with significant adenotonsillar enlargement

    c) In older adolescents when the growth of craniofacial bones and upper airway soft tissues is largely complete

    d) In children without dental braces

150. Which of the following statements is associated with sleep terrors?

    a) Full memory for the episode

    b) Generally responsive to external stimuli and are easily arousable

    c) Minimal autonomic activation

    d) Sleep terrors in adults can begin in NREM sleep stage 2

151. Which of the following is NOT a characteristic feature of Down syndrome that increases the risk of developing obstructive sleep apnea?

    a) Enlarged tongue

    b) Maxillary hyperplasia

    c) Short neck

    d) Small nose

152. Which of the following factors related to human immunodeficiency virus (HIV) infection is NOT associated with sleep disturbance in patients with acquired immunodeficiency syndrome (AIDS)?

    a) Presence of underlying encephalopathy

    b) Age of patient

    c) Severity of HIV-related symptoms

    d) Selection of antiviral therapy

153. Which of the following statements regarding sleep in patients with Lyme disease is correct?

    a) Caused by *Trypanosoma brucei*

    b) Transmission of human disease via flea bites

    c) Sleep disturbances can persist for several years in patients with previous Lyme disease

    d) No alpha wave intrusion into NREM sleep

154. What is the reference standard for identifying Cheyne-Stokes respiration?

    a) Esophageal pressure monitoring

    b) Respiratory inductance plethysmography

    c) Surface diaphragmatic electromyography

    d) Strain gauges

155. Polysomnographic features of high altitude–related periodic breathing include which of the following?

    a) Repetitive central apneas occur primarily during REM sleep

    b) Respiration is more regular during REM sleep

    c) Decrease in total sleep time

    d) No significant change in frequency of arousals

156. **Alterations in circadian rhythms that accompany aging include which of the following?**

    a) Reduction in the amplitude of the circadian sleep-wake rhythms, melatonin secretion, and core body temperature

    b) Increased nocturnal levels of melatonin

    c) Increased release of growth hormone during sleep

    d) Decrease in the circadian nadir of cortisol level

157. **Which of the following statements regarding sleep-related painful erections is correct?**

    a) Generally associated with pain during sexual erections while awake

    b) Occurs during NREM sleep

    c) Often begins during adolescence

    d) Generally, normal sexual function

158. **Which of the following statements regarding the development of obstructive sleep apnea (OSA) in patients with cleft palate is correct?**

    a) Cleft palate is often accompanied by significant narrowing of the anterior-posterior dimension of the pharynx, a lower hyoid position, and a longer uvula.

    b) OSA can develop following repair of cleft palate using flap pharyngoplasty or sphincter pharyngoplasty but not by velopharyngeal ring ligation procedure.

    c) OSA does not occur in the immediate postoperative period of cleft palate repair but several years later due to the development of strictures.

    d) OSA secondary to cleft palate repair is generally progressive and does not resolve spontaneously.

159. **Sleeping sickness is an infectious cause of excessive sleepiness. Which of the following statements regarding sleeping sickness is correct?**

    a) It is a parasitic disease caused by the protozoan *Trypanosoma brucei* or *Trypanosoma rhodesiense* transmitted by the bite of the *Anopheles* mosquito.

    b) It is endemic in certain regions of South America and Asia.

    c) The disorder consists of two stages, an initial meningoencephalitic stage and a terminal hemolymphatic stage with excessive daytime sleepiness.

    d) An important feature of trypanosomiasis is disruption of the circadian rhythm, including reversal of the sleep-wake periods and plasma levels of cortisol and prolactin.

160. **What is the reference standard for identifying sleep hypoventilation syndrome?**

    a) $PaCO_2$

    b) $PetCO_2$

    c) $PtcCO_2$

    d) SaO_2

161. **Which of the following is NOT a feature of obesity hypoventilation syndrome?**

    a) Severe obesity (defined as a body mass index > 40 kg/m^2)

    b) Hypercapnia ($PaCO_2 > 45 \text{ mmHg}$) during wakefulness

    c) Rare obstructive sleep apnea

    d) Polycythemia, pulmonary hypertension, and cor pulmonale due to chronic hypoxemia

162. **Excessive sleepiness and sleep attacks can occur in patients with narcolepsy. Which of the following statements is correct?**

    a) Excessive daytime sleepiness is typically the least disabling manifestation of narcolepsy.

    b) Excessive sleepiness is chronic and may manifest as pervasive drowsiness and subwakefulness, frequent napping, microsleep episodes, and unexpected and overpowering sleep attacks occurring almost daily for at least 3 months.

    c) Patients with narcolepsy typically describe constant sleepiness without any waxing and waning periods of alertness.

    d) Sleepiness is constant and not relieved by napping.

163. **Acute and chronic pain can give rise to sleep disruption. Which of the following statements regarding the association between pain syndromes and sleep is correct?**

    a) Polysomnographic studies of patients with acute pain may reveal sleep fragmentation, and increase in both NREM stages 3 and 4 sleep and REM sleep.

    b) Development of depression in patients with chronic pain can further disturb sleep.

    c) Polysomnographic findings in patients with chronic pain consist of an increase in sleep latency, increase in wake time after sleep onset, and increase in NREM stages 3 and 4 sleep.

d) Poor sleep has no significant effect on the daytime perception of pain intensity.

164. **Which of the following is a polysomnographic feature seen in patients with fibromyalgia?**

a) No change in total sleep time

b) Decrease in frequency of arousals

c) Decrease in NREM stages 3 and 4 sleep

d) Increase in REM sleep

165. **Which of the following statements regarding congenital central hypoventilation syndrome is true?**

a) Hypoventilation and failure of autonomic respiratory control develop during puberty.

b) It is associated with a disorder of peripheral chemoreceptor responsiveness to hypoxia and hypercapnia.

c) Death is usually due to cardiac failure.

d) Apparent life-threatening events, respiratory arrest, or pulmonary hypertension may develop during infancy.

166. **Which of the following best describes the newborn electroencephalographic trace alternant pattern?**

a) Continuous, medium- to high-amplitude (between 50 and 150 µV) waveforms; frequencies between 0.5 and 4.0 Hz

b) Low-amplitude (between 14 and 35 µV) waveforms; frequencies between 5.0 and 8.0 Hz

c) Bursts of slow (0.5 to 3 Hz), high-amplitude waves, fast low-amplitude waves, and sharp waves (2 to 4 Hz) lasting several seconds interspersed with periods of relative quiescence (mixed frequency waveforms) lasting 4 to 8 seconds

d) High- and low-voltage waveforms

167. **What is the reference standard for identifying obstructive sleep apnea–hypopneas?**

a) Pneumotachometer

b) Respiratory inductance plethysmography

c) Strain gauges

d) Thoracic impedance

168. **Polysomnographic features of a major depressive episode include which of the following?**

a) Increase in sleep efficiency

b) Increase in total sleep time

c) Increase in NREM stages 3 and 4 sleep

d) Decrease in REM sleep latency

169. **Patients with genetic syndromes characterized by maxillary hypoplasia are more likely to develop obstructive sleep apnea. Which of the following statements about these syndromes is correct?**

a) The syndromic craniosynostoses (eg, Apert syndrome, Crouzon syndrome, and Pfeiffer syndrome) arise as a result of mutations in fibroblast growth factor receptor genes that inhibit the lateral growth of the cranium.

b) Patients with maxillary hypoplasia typically possess a facial profile that is anteriorly protuberant in shape.

c) Midfacial hypoplasia displaces the palate anteriorly closer to the posterior wall of the nasopharynx.

d) Features of Antley-Bixler syndrome include craniosynostosis, frontal bossing, midfacial hypoplasia, choanal atresia or stenosis, and depression of the nasal bridge.

170. **Which of the following clinical subtypes of depression is LEAST likely to give rise to excessive daytime sleepiness?**

a) Major depression

b) Depressive phase of a bipolar disorder

c) Seasonal affective disorder

d) Atypical depression

171. **Insomnia is the most common sleep complaint among older adults. Which of the following statements best describes insomnia in older adults?**

a) Among the elderly, the prevalence of insomnia is higher in men compared to women.

b) There is a poorer correlation between subjective complaints and objective sleep parameters in older men compared to women.

c) The development of insomnia in the elderly is due most frequently to aging itself.

d) Increasing age is associated with a greater likelihood that insomnia becomes chronic.

172. **Primary or idiopathic restless legs syndrome (RLS) can be classified into two subtypes: early onset (before the age of 35 to 45 years) and late onset. Relative to the late onset type, the early onset**

type is characterized by which of the following statements?

a) More rapid progression of symptoms

b) Greater family history of RLS

c) Greater association with abnormalities in dopaminergic neurotransmitter systems

d) Less likely to respond to dopaminergic therapy

173. **Which of the following statements regarding nasal pressure is correct?**

a) Respiration produces fluctuations on the nasal pressure transducer signals that are proportional to flow.

b) The shape and amplitude of the nasal cannula signal are superior to those obtained from face mask pneumotachographs.

c) The presence of a flattening on the inspiratory flow signal is associated with central apneic events.

d) Tracings are reduced and rounded with obstructive apneic events.

174. **Pierre-Robin syndrome is characterized by the presence of a small jaw, retropositioned tongue and soft palate, displacement of the larynx, and, in some cases, a cleft palate. Which of the following statements does NOT describe the pathophysiology of obstructive sleep apnea in this syndrome?**

a) Mandibular hypoplasia in utero displaces the tongue anteriorly.

b) Posterior displacement of the tongue impairs the midline closure of the palate.

c) Breathing difficulties that develop in the early days of life improve significantly during the first 2 years with growth of the lower jaw in relation to the cranial dimensions.

d) Persistent micrognathia increases the risk of snoring and obstructive sleep apnea in later life.

175. **In which of the following clinical scenarios is obtaining cerebrospinal fluid hypocretin-1 rarely useful?**

a) In patients who are taking medications (eg, stimulants or REM sleep suppressants) that may interfere with proper interpretation of Multiple Sleep Latency Test (MSLT) results

b) In patients who are too young to undergo MSLT

c) During the early course of the disease prior to the development of cataplexy

d) In patients with suspected narcolepsy but without cataplexy

176. **Which of following is NOT a behavioral state described in young infants?**

a) Quiet sleep

b) Active sleep

c) Intermediate sleep

d) Vocalization

177. **Which of the following statements regarding the differences in sleep-related breathing disorders between men and women is correct?**

a) There is increased susceptibility to upper airway collapse during sleep among women relative to men.

b) There are significant gender differences in pharyngeal cross-sectional area, upper airway resistance, and hypoxic and hypercapnic ventilatory response during NREM sleep.

c) There are more reports of snoring and fewer reports of daytime sleepiness, fatigue, and insomnia in women than in men.

d) The risk of obstructive sleep apnea is increased in women during menopause compared with premenopause.

178. **Which one of the following statements about non-hypercapnic central sleep apnea is correct?**

a) Not associated with daytime hypoventilation

b) High waking $PaCO_2$

c) Normal to decreased ventilatory response to hypercapnia

d) Includes patients with central alveolar hypoventilation and neuromuscular disorders

179. **Which of the following is NOT associated with congenital central hypoventilation syndrome?**

a) Dysfunction of the autonomic nervous system control of the heart

b) Hirschsprung disease

c) Metabolic acidosis

d) Tumors of neural crest derivatives (ie, ganglioneuromas and neuroblastomas)

180. **Which of the following phrases about Treacher Collins syndrome is correct?**

a) Overdeveloped mandible with bony overgrowth into the oral cavity

b) Sensory hearing loss

c) Inherited as an autosomal recessive disorder

d) Caused by mutations in the TCOF1 gene coding for the Treacle protein

181. **At what age do electroencephalographic K-complexes first appear during sleep?**
    a) After 2 to 4 weeks
    b) After 1 to 3 months
    c) After 6 months
    d) After 12 months

182. **Which of the following is NOT a polysomnographic feature of idiopathic hypersomnia?**
    a) Decrease in sleep efficiency on nocturnal polysomnography
    b) Increase in frequency of arousals during nocturnal polysomnography
    c) Fewer than two sleep onset REM periods (SOREMPS) during the Multiple Sleep Latency Test
    d) Decrease in duration of sleep over 24 hours (< 7 hours) during 24-hour continuous polysomnography

183. **Which of the following antidepressant agents does not cause or aggravate restless legs syndrome?**
    a) Bupropion
    b) Lithium
    c) Selective serotonin reuptake inhibitors
    d) Tricyclic antidepressants

184. **Which of the following statements about bipolar disorders is correct?**
    a) Excessive sleepiness may occur during manic episodes of bipolar disorder.
    b) During the depressive phase, polysomnography typically demonstrates an increase in REM sleep latency.
    c) During the acute manic phase of the disorder, total sleep time is reduced and patients do not complain of excessive sleepiness despite a shortened duration of sleep.
    d) Depressive episodes can be precipitated by sleep deprivation.

185. **Status dissociatus is a disorder characterized by the presence of complex behavior and activities due to a complete dissolution of sleep state boundaries with polysomnographic features of wakefulness, NREM sleep, and REM sleep occurring**

simultaneously. **Which of the following disorders is NOT associated with status dissociatus?**
    a) Alcohol withdrawal
    b) Fatal familial insomnia
    c) Narcolepsy
    d) REM sleep behavior disorder

186. **Which of the following features does NOT characterize obstructive sleep apnea that occur during REM sleep compared with events that occur during NREM sleep?**
    a) Respiratory events are more frequent.
    b) Respiratory events last longer.
    c) Respiratory events are associated with more profound oxygen desaturation.
    c) Respiratory events are associated with more serious neurocognitive consequences.

187. **Which of the following phrases best describes hypercapnic central sleep apnea?**
    a) Normal waking $PaCO_2$
    b) Diminished response to hypercapnia
    c) Hypoventilation that is limited to the sleep period
    d) Includes patients with congestive heart failure

188. **Which of following statements regarding cataplexy is correct?**
    a) Loss of muscle tone can be regional, affecting the face, neck, and extremities, or it can involve the entire body.
    b) Status cataplecticus, or repetitive episodes of cataplexy occurring in succession, may occur following acute administration of REM sleep suppressants.
    c) Polysomnography demonstrates REM sleep attacks, regardless of the duration of cataplexy.
    d) Cataplexy is always associated with the presence of sleep-onset REM periods on multiple sleep latency testing.

189. **Which of the following genetic syndromes characterized by mandibular hypoplasia includes clinical features consisting of vertebral abnormalities, dermal cysts, auricular malformations, and abnormalities of the upper airway?**
    a) Down syndrome
    b) Goldenhar syndrome
    c) Pierre-Robin syndrome
    d) Treacher Collins syndrome

190. **Which of the following changes in sleep is associated with the administration of nicotine?**

    a) Increase in wake time after sleep onset during the first few days of smoking cessation

    b) Nicotine gum increases NREM stages 3 and 4 sleep

    c) Produces mild sedation in high blood concentrations

    d) Smoking close to bedtime decreases sleep latency

191. **Breast-feeding during the postpartum period is associated with which of the following sleep characteristics?**

    a) Decrease in subjective perception of sleep quality

    b) Increase in total sleep time

    c) Decrease in NREM stages 1 and 2 sleep

    d) Decrease in NREM stages 3 and 4 sleep (compared to bottle-feeding)

192. **Which of the following statements is NOT consistent with the diagnostic criteria for restless legs syndrome among adults based on the recommendations of the International Restless Legs Syndrome Study Group?**

    a) An urge to move the legs is usually accompanied or caused by uncomfortable and unpleasant sensations (paresthesias or dysesthesias) in the limbs.

    b) The urge to move or unpleasant sensations begin or worsen during periods of rest or inactivity (eg, lying or sitting).

    c) The urge to move or unpleasant sensations are partially or totally relieved by movement (eg, walking or stretching).

    d) The urge to move or unpleasant sensations are worse during the day or early afternoon than during the evening or night.

193. **Compared with nocturnal seizures, parasomnias are more likely to be associated with which of the following?**

    a) Complex or stereotypic activities or behavior

    b) Occurence at the transition between sleep and wakefulness

    c) Tongue biting

    d) Urinary incontinence

194. **Which of the following clinical features is NOT associated with propriospinal myoclonus at sleep onset?**

    a) Spontaneous sudden muscle jerks that occur typically during relaxed wakefulness in the transition from wakefulness to sleep

    b) Jerks starting in the proximal limb and neck muscles that spread centrally to the abdominal and truncal muscles

    c) Nonperiodic trunk flexion and extension that disappear at sleep onset or with mental activation

    d) Polysomnographic features including brief, recurring myoclonic electromyographic activity associated with alpha electroencephalographic (EEG) rhythms that disappear with EEG desynchronization and remain absent during sleep

195. **Which statement best describes the pathophysiology of congenital central hypoventilation syndrome?**

    a) Lack of ventilatory or arousal responses can give rise to significant hypoventilation (reduction in tidal volume and respiratory rate) during sleep.

    b) Hypercapnia but not hypoxemia is seen during sleep.

    c) Hypoventilation is typically most severe during REM sleep.

    d) Frank central apneas, snoring or paradoxical breathing are common.

196. **Which of the following best describes the effects of sodium oxybate on the sleep of patients with fibromyalgia?**

    a) No change in sleep latency

    b) Increase in REM sleep

    c) No change in alpha-NREM phenomena

    d) Increase in NREM stages 3 and 4 sleep

197. **Which of the following statements regarding thermal sensing devices for the measurement of airflow is correct?**

    a) They provide an indirect and semiquantitative measurement of airflow.

    b) They sense airflow by differences in the temperature between warmer inspired air and cooler exhaled air.

    c) Sensor temperature is measured as electrical resistance by a thermocouple and as change in voltage by a thermistor.

    d) They reliably detect the presence of hypopneas but not apneas.

198. Compared with continuous positive airway pressure, autotitrating continuous positive airway pressure is associated with which of the following?

    a) Greater efficacy

    b) Higher compliance

    c) Higher peak airway pressure

    d) Higher mean delivered pressure

199. Compared with the mother sleeping alone during the postpartum period, cosleeping with the newborn infant during the postpartum period is associated with which of the following maternal sleep characteristics?

    a) Increase in frequency of arousals

    b) Increase in NREM stages 3 and 4 sleep

    c) Decrease in sleep efficiency

    d) Decrease in total sleep time

200. Which of the following techniques is considered the gold standard for measuring airflow?

    a) Pneumotachography

    b) Thermistors

    c) Thermocouples

    d) End-tidal carbon dioxide ($PetCO_2$) monitoring

201. When is polysomnography indicated for patients with suspected parasomnias?

    a) REM sleep behavior disorder

    b) Sleepwalking

    c) Parasomnias in older adults

    d) Sleep enuresis during pre-adolescence

202. Which of the following is NOT classified as a nocturnal frontal lobe epilepsy?

    a) Episodic nocturnal wanderings

    b) Nocturnal paroxysmal dystonia

    c) Paroxysmal arousals

    d) Paroxysmal nocturnal automatisms

203. A 62-year-old gentleman reports that he repeatedly awakens at night with coughing, choking, or gagging. He says that he has difficulty swallowing his saliva during sleep. His wife, who has accompanied him to the sleep clinic, reports that he produces a "gurgling" sound before he starts coughing. The most likely diagnosis is:

    a) Nocturnal gastroesophageal reflux

    b) Sleep-related abnormal swallowing syndrome

    c) Sleep-related choking syndrome

    d) Sleep-related laryngospasm

204. Amphetamine use is associated with which of the following changes in sleep architecture?

    a) Decrease in sleep latency

    b) Increase in sleep efficiency

    c) Increase in total sleep time

    d) Decrease in REM sleep

205. Which of the following is an appropriate recommendation for the evaluation of patients with craniofacial syndromes?

    a) Routine screening for obstructive sleep apnea (OSA) is indicated for patients with craniofacial syndromes.

    b) Periodic reassessment following initial evaluation is not necessary.

    c) After the presence of OSA has been established by polysomnography, additional studies are unnecessary.

    d) Imaging studies to visualize both key skeletal structures and soft tissues (eg, tonsils and adenoids) and their relationships to each other are not generally indicated.

206. Which of the following best describes expired carbon dioxide monitoring of airflow?

    a) It utilizes infrared analyzers placed in front of the nose and mouth.

    b) It provides a quantitative measure of airflow.

    c) Ambient air contains a greater concentration of carbon dioxide compared to expired air from the lungs.

    d) A falling $PetCO_2$ level indicates the presence of hypoventilation.

207. Which of the following is NOT a limitation to the use of transcutaneous oxygen ($PtcO_2$) monitoring during polysomnography?

    a) Lack of correlation to cutaneous perfusion

    b) Need for periodic site changes

    c) Slow response that fails to mirror rapid changes in PaO_2

    d) Variable relationship between PaO_2 and $PtcO_2$

208. Which of the following statements is consistent with the American Academy of Sleep Medicine 2006 practice parameters for the medical therapy of obstructive sleep apnea (OSA)?

    a) Selective serotonin reuptake inhibitors are recommended for the therapy of patients with predominantly REM sleep-related OSA.

    b) Estrogen therapy with or without progesterone is recommended for postmenopausal women with mild OSA.

    c) Topical nasal corticosteroids may be a useful adjunct to primary therapies for OSA in patients with concurrent rhinitis.

    d) Modafinil is recommended for treating patients with OSA who are unable to tolerate positive airway pressure treatment.

209. One of the following features distinguishes idiopathic hypersomnia from narcolepsy. In comparison to patients with narcolepsy, those with idiopathic hypersomnia have:

    a) Less refreshing sleep

    b) More sleep onset REM periods (SOREMPs) during multiple sleep latency testing

    c) More predictable improvement to stimulant therapy

    d) Greater prevalence of HLA DQB1*0602

210. Which of the following statements regarding sleep in premature infants is NOT true?

    a) Active sleep is recognizable by 32 to 36 weeks of gestation and constitutes the majority of sleep at this age group.

    b) No clearly definable sleep states are present from 24 to 26 weeks of gestation.

    c) At the same conceptual age, premature and full-term infants attain similar electroencephalographic milestones.

    d) Development of spindles is more advanced in premature infants compared to full-term infants.

211. Which of the following is NOT a cause of multiple sleep onset REM periods (SOREMPs)?

    a) Narcolepsy

    b) Obstructive sleep apnea

    c) Normal healthy adults

    d) Acute administration of REM sleep-suppressing agents

212. Which of the following statements regarding REM sleep behavior disorder is true?

    a) Absent or partial dream recall on awakening

    b) Episode ends with a rapid awakening and full alertness

    c) Eyes are usually open during the event

    d) A history of violent or aggressive behavior during the day while awake is common

213. Which of the following is NOT a feature of Beckwith-Wiedeman syndrome?

    a) Affects only males

    b) Small noses

    c) Umbilical abnormalities

    d) Unusually large tongues

214. Which of the following disorders is classified as a nonhypercapnic form of central sleep apnea?

    a) Neuromuscular disease

    b) Congestive heart failure

    c) Central alveolar hypoventilation

    d) Neurologic disorders affecting the brainstem

215. The perimenopausal period is associated with changes in sleep. Which of the following statements related to the perimenopause is true?

    a) Hormone replacement therapy increases sleep duration and improves subjective sleep quality in women with climacteric symptoms such as hot flashes.

    b) Administration of progesterone is associated with an increase in wake time after sleep onset.

    c) Women taking estrogen report greater insomnia and sleep disturbance.

    d) Hormone replacement therapy is associated with increased prevalence of obstructive sleep apnea.

216. Which of the following is the most common cause of excessive sleepiness in the general population?

    a) Insufficient sleep

    b) Narcolepsy

    c) Obstructive sleep apnea syndrome

    d) Use of sedative-hypnotic agents

217. Differences in the clinical features of obstructive sleep apnea (OSA) in older adults compared with younger adults include which of the following?

a) Clinical symptoms associated with OSA, such as excessive daytime sleepiness, appear to be less common, and, if present, less severe in older adults than in younger adults.

b) Most of the increase in prevalence of OSA among older adults occurs after 65 years of age.

c) The increased risk of cardiopulmonary diseases appears to be greater among the elderly than among younger individuals.

d) Excess body weight, snoring, and witnessed apneas are more consistent indicators for the presence of OSA in older adults than in younger individuals.

218. Which of the following features is NOT associated with a manic episode of mood disorder?

a) Decrease in both amount of and requirement for sleep

b) Development of insomnia

c) Increase in frequency of awakenings

d) Increase in REM sleep latency

219. Which of the following features of lower airway obstruction is associated with an increased likelihood of sleep-related hypoventilation?

a) Forced expiratory volume exhaled in 1 second/forced vital capacity (FEV_1/FVC) > 60%

b) Daytime hyperventilation

c) Daytime hypocapnia

d) Comorbid obstructive sleep apnea

220. Which of the following is an effect of continuous positive airway pressure on Cheyne-Stokes respiration?

a) Decreases cardiac function

b) Lowers oxygen saturation

c) Reduces blood pressure

d) Decreases $PaCO_2$

221. Which of the following statements regarding transcutaneous carbon dioxide (PtcCO2) monitoring is true?

a) $PtcCO_2$ represents the CO_2 tension at the epidermal surface.

b) $PtcCO_2$ is generally similar to a simultaneously obtained $PaCO_2$.

c) It is regularly indicated during adult polysomnography.

d) Its rapid response time makes it suitable for monitoring blood gas tensions during adult polysomnography.

222. What are the standard electrode derivations for monitoring electroencephalography (EEG) based on Rechtschaffen and Kales criteria?

a) C3/A2 or C4/A1

b) F3/A2 or F4/A1

c) O3/A2 or O4/A1

d) T3/A2 or T4/A1

223. Which of the following statements regarding the patterns of eye movements during polysomnography is correct?

a) Slow rolling eye movements are present during drowsiness with open eyes.

b) Slow rolling eye movements disappear during stage NREM stage 1 sleep.

c) Rapid eye movements are not present during wakefulness.

d) Frequency of rapid eye movements per minute of REM sleep is less during early REM sleep episodes and progressively increases during later REM sleep periods.

224. What is the most common arrhythmia associated with obstructive sleep apnea?

a) Atrioventricular block

b) Premature ventricular contractions

c) Sinus arrhythmia

d) Sinus pauses or arrest

225. Which of the following factors is associated with a greater likelihood of developing Cheyne-Stokes respiration in patients with congestive heart failure?

a) Low ejection fraction

b) High awake $PaCO_2$

c) Age < 60 years

d) Female gender

226. Which of the following is NOT an indication for continuous positive airway pressure therapy for children with obstructive sleep apnea?

    a) When adenotonsillectomy is not indicated or contraindicated

    b) When significant symptoms persist following adenotonsillectomy

    c) During the perioperative period in children with severe disease

    d) In all children with severe obstructive sleep apnea associated with significant oxygen desaturation and daytime sleepiness

227. What medication can cause eye movements during NREM sleep?

    a) Benzodiazepines

    b) Melatonin

    c) Selective serotonin reuptake inhibitors

    d) Trazodone

228. Which of the following psychostimulants has been withdrawn from the U.S. market due to concerns regarding hepatic toxicity?

    a) Dextroamphetamine

    b) Methamphetamine

    c) Pemoline

    d) Selegiline

229. Which of the following is NOT a characteristic of patients with insomnia?

    a) Greater subjective sleep disturbance compared with changes in objective polysomnographic parameters

    b) Enhanced ability to distinguish sleep from wakefulness

    c) Greater tendency to describe, when awakened from sleep, of being awake all along, when compared with those without insomnia

    d) Often overestimate the duration of sleep latencies

230. Which of the following best describes the term "ultradian" frequency?

    a) One oscillation lasting less than 24 hours

    b) One oscillation approximately every 24 hours

    c) One oscillation lasting more than 24 hours

    d) One oscillation per year

231. Unihemispheric sleep, with electroencephalography showing wakefulness in one hemisphere and sleep in the opposite hemisphere, can be seen in which animal?

    a) Whale

    b) Alligator

    c) Manatee

    d) Penguin

232. Which of the following best describes the performance of multiple sleep latency testing (MSLT)?

    a) A nocturnal polysomnography is not routinely performed immediately before MSLT.

    b) An adequate duration of nocturnal sleep (at least 6 hours) should be present prior to MSLT.

    c) An adequate sleep duration and regular sleep-wake schedule for 2 to 3 days is sufficient before proceeding with MSLT.

    d) Discontinuing medications that can potentially influence sleep latency and REM sleep (eg, REM sleep suppressants) for 2 to 3 days is sufficient before proceeding with the study.

233. Which of the following statements regarding methylphenidate is true?

    a) It is a piperidine derivative structurally similar to modafinil.

    b) It increases total sleep time.

    c) It decreases wake time after sleep onset.

    d) It increases REM sleep latency.

234. Which one of the following statements about selegiline in the therapy of patients with narcolepsy is correct?

    a) Selegiline is a tricyclic antidepressant.

    b) It has sedating and anticataplectic actions, and it should preferably be taken at bedtime.

    c) Adverse effects include confusion, dizziness, dry mouth, and nausea.

    d) To be effective, a diet high in tyramine is required when taking this medication.

235. Which of the following statements regarding Frederick Bremmer's animal brain transection studies related to sleep is true?

    a) In cerveau isole, transection is at the C1 vertebral level in the lower part of the medulla between the brain and spinal cord.

    b) Electroencephalography (EEG) demonstrates only sleep state in cerveau isole.

    c) EEG demonstrates only wake state in cerveau isole.

    d) In encephale isole, transection is at the midcollicular level caudal to the origin of the oculomotor nerves in the midbrain, which disrupts the projections of the brainstem ascending reticular activating system.

236. What percentage of delta electroencephalographic activity defines NREM stage 3 sleep?

    a) Less than 20% of an epoch

    b) Greater than 10% but less than 50% of an epoch

    c) Between 20% and 50% of an epoch

    d) Greater than 50% of an epoch

237. Which of the following changes in sleep is generally associated with the administration of beta-adrenergic blockers?

    a) Decrease in wake time after sleep onset

    b) No change in NREM stage 1 sleep

    c) No change in REM sleep latency (except atenolol and metoprolol)

    d) Decrease in REM sleep (except atenolol and metoprolol)

238. Which of the following demographic factors is associated with a greater prevalence of insomnia?

    a) Children and young adults

    b) Individuals who belong to a high socioeconomic status

    c) Shift workers

    d) Men

239. Which of the following best describes the polysomnographic features of primary insomnia?

    a) Increase in sleep latency

    b) Normal total sleep time

    c) Increase in NREM stages 3 and 4 sleep

    d) Always abnormal sleep architecture

240. Which of the following statements about the effect of theophylline on sleep is correct?

    a) Decrease in sleep latency

    b) Decrease in wake time after sleep onset

    c) Decrease in NREM stage 1 sleep

    d) Decrease in REM sleep

241. Which of the following statements regarding the basic stages of human sleep is true?

    a) Sleep is generally staged using specific electro-encephalographic and electro-oculographic characteristics only.

    b) Sleep can be differentiated into non-rapid eye movement NREM sleep and rapid eye movement REM sleep.

    c) REM sleep can be further subdivided into stages 1, 2, 3, and 4 sleep.

    d) NREM stages 1 and 2 sleep are often collectively referred to as slow wave sleep or delta wave sleep.

242. Which of the following statements about post-traumatic hypersomnia is correct?

    a) There is generally no correlation between the degree of sleepiness and the severity of head trauma.

    b) Hypersomnia typically begins immediately after head trauma.

    c) Symptoms are usually maximal immediately after head trauma.

    d) Polysomnography reveals severe derangements in sleep architecture with increase in total sleep time and absence of NREM stages 3 and 4 sleep and REM sleep.

243. Which of the following is NOT a common polysomnographic feature of generalized anxiety disorder?

    a) Increase in sleep latency

    b) Increase in wake time after sleep onset

    c) Increase in total sleep time

    d) Decrease in NREM stages 3 and 4 as well as REM sleep

244. Which of the following statements regarding paradoxical insomnia is correct?

    a) Significant impairment of daytime function consistent with subjective reports of extreme sleep loss occurs.

b) Frequent daytime napping occurs.

c) Prevalence is higher in men than in women.

d) Despite subjective reports of little or no sleep during polysomnography, the study demonstrates a normal or near normal sleep latency, quality, and architecture.

245. **Which of the following statements about fatal familial insomnia (FFI) is true?**

a) This autosomal recessive disorder is secondary to a prion disease.

b) It is associated with autonomic dysregulation and neurologic abnormalities.

c) It typically has its onset during early childhood.

d) The course and prognosis of FFI is influenced by the type of substitution, with methionine in codon 129 on the nonmutated allele associated with a less severe and longer course.

246. **Which of the following statements regarding the use of sedating tricyclic antidepressants for patients with insomnia is correct?**

a) Low risk of abuse

b) Decrease REM sleep latency

c) Increase REM sleep

d) No effect on symptoms of restless legs and periodic limb movements during sleep

247. **What is the ideal electrode impedance for electroencephalography?**

a) Less than 5000

b) Between 5000 and 7500

c) Between 7500 and 10,000

d) Greater than 10,000

248. **Which of the following statements best describes the pattern of esophageal pressure tracing in patients with upper airway resistance syndrome (UARS)?**

a) Increasingly more negative immediately preceding an arousal, with a positive overshoot after the arousal

b) Increasingly more negative immediately preceding an arousal, after which the esophageal pressure rapidly returns to baseline levels

c) Increasingly more negative immediately after an arousal, after which the esophageal pressure rapidly returns to baseline levels

d) Increasingly more positive immediately preceding an arousal, after which the esophageal pressure rapidly returns to baseline levels

249. **Which of the following polysomnographic features is associated with stimulant-dependent sleep disorder?**

a) No change in sleep latency during stimulant use

b) No change in frequency of arousals during stimulant use

c) REM sleep rebound during stimulant withdrawal

d) No change in daytime sleep latency on multiple sleep latency test during stimulant withdrawal

250. **Which of the following is an appropriate recommendation for treating children with insomnia?**

a) Fix bedtimes of children to the parent's own bedtime to allow the family to sleep and awaken at the same time each day

b) Consistent bedtime routines (minimal stimulating activities) and sleep schedules

c) Placing the child in bed asleep beginning at 2 to 4 months of age

d) Transitioning the infant to the final sleep environment (eg, crib in infant's room) by 6 months of age

251. **Which of the following is a polysomnographic feature of pemoline use?**

a) Increase in total sleep time

b) Decrease in wake time after sleep onset

c) Increase in NREM stages 3 and 4 sleep

d) Decrease in REM sleep

252. **Which of the following statements about respiratory inductance plethysmography (RIP) and thoracic impedance (TI) during polysomnography is correct?**

a) RIP provides information regarding airflow.

b) Paradoxical motion of the chest and abdomen during RIP monitoring suggests an obstructive event rather than a central process and is most pronounced during NREM sleep compared with REM sleep.

c) With RIP, a current is applied across the thorax, which serves as an electrical conductor.

d) TI varies with the relative amount of conductive materials (body fluids and tissue) and nonconductive air between a pair of electrodes placed at opposite sides of the thoracic cage.

253. **Which of the following clinical features is true of Huntington disease?**

a) Progressive chorea

b) Normal mental status

c) Autosomal recessive disorder

d) Chorea typically occurs during REM sleep

254. **Which of the following changes in sleep is NOT generally seen following traumatic brain injury?**

a) Insomnia

b) Excessive sleepiness

c) Circadian rhythm sleep disturbances (eg, delayed sleep phase syndrome)

d) Decrease in frequency of awakenings

255. **Which of the following statements about sleep staging is NOT correct?**

a) Polysomnographic data are divided into 30-second time periods or epochs.

b) Standard sleep study paper speed is 10 millimeters per second.

c) Electroencephalographic evaluation of seizure activity usually utilizes a paper speed of 60 millimeters per second.

d) Each epoch is assigned a sleep stage according to the stage that occupies the majority of the epoch.

256. **Which one of the following statements about the effect of clonidine on sleep is correct?**

a) Excessive sleepiness

b) No significant change in sleep latency

c) No significant change in total sleep time

d) No significant change in REM sleep

257. **Which of the following polysomnographic features is NOT associated with alcohol-dependent sleep disorder?**

a) Vivid, disturbing dreams precipitated by abrupt termination of alcohol use

b) Possible persistence of sleep fragmentation

during abstinence among chronic heavy alcohol users

c) REM-sleep fragmentation during alcohol use

d) Decrease in REM sleep during alcohol withdrawal

258. **Which of the following statements regarding scheduled awakenings for children is correct?**

a) The parent wakes up the child at the same time each night approximately 2 hours after sleep onset.

b) The frequency of scheduled awakenings is progressively reduced until the child is able to sleep through the night, at which time they are discontinued.

c) Treatment time is rapid and is often shorter than that of extinction procedures.

d) An advantage is that children are taught sleep initiation skills at least twice each night, namely at sleep onset and again following scheduled awakenings.

259. **Which of the following is NOT an indication for polysomnography in the evaluation of transient or chronic insomnia?**

a) When clinical history cannot be obtained or is deemed unreliable

b) Strong evidence based on clinical history for insomnia due to periodic limb movement disorder

c) Strong evidence based on clinical history for insomnia due to sleep-related breathing disorder

d) When insomnia is severe and persists despite an adequate trial of behavioral therapy, sleep hygiene, and pharmacologic intervention

260. **Which of the following statements about decongestants and their effect on sleep is correct?**

a) Possess central nervous system sedating effects

b) Can cause hypersomnolence

c) Prolong sleep latency

d) Decrease in wake time after sleep onset

261. **Closed eyes, visible movements, vocalizations, irregular respiration, low-voltage irregular or mixed electroencephalographic pattern, positive eye movements on electro-oculography, and low electromyographic tone characterize which of the following newborn sleep stages?**

a) Active REM sleep

b) Intermediate sleep

c) Quiet sleep

d) Wake state

262. **Arousal threshold is highest (ie, the individual is most difficult to awaken) during which stage of sleep?**

   a) NREM stage 1 sleep

   b) NREM stage 2 sleep

   c) NREM stages 3 and 4 sleep

   d) REM sleep

263. **Which of the following statements about recurrent hypersomnia is true?**

   a) During periods of hypersomnia, daily sleep duration may reach 10 to 12 hours but typically does not exceed 14 to 16 hours.

   b) Sleep, alertness, behavior, and cognitive function are normal between episodes.

   c) Kleine-Levin syndrome affects mostly females.

   d) Frequency, severity, and duration of episodes generally worsen over time.

264. **Which of the following statements is consistent with the Rechtschaffen and Kales criteria for scoring NREM stage 2 sleep?**

   a) Sleep spindles and K-complexes should be present in every epoch.

   b) An epoch is scored as stage 2 sleep if the intervening period between sleep spindles or K-complexes is less than 3 minutes and would otherwise meet criteria for stage 1 sleep with low-amplitude, mixed-frequency EEG activity.

   c) An epoch is scored as stage 2 sleep if the intervening period is between sleep spindles or K-complexes, even if it is associated with an arousal.

   d) An epoch is scored as stage wake sleep if the intervening period between sleep spindles or K-complexes is equal to or greater than 3 minutes.

265. **Which of the following is NOT generally useful in the evaluation of patients with insomnia?**

   a) Multiple sleep latency test

   b) Psychologic screening tests

   c) Self-administered questionnaires

   d) Sleep logs

266. **Which of the following statements regarding the clinical features of narcolepsy is correct?**

   a) Only half of patients of narcolepsy demonstrate the full clinical tetrad of excessive sleepiness, cataplexy, sleep paralysis, and sleep hallucinations.

   b) Patients with narcolepsy often have nocturnal sleep disturbance with frequent arousals and awakenings.

   c) The prevalence of cataplexy is lower than that of sleep paralysis in patients with narcolepsy.

   d) Automatic behavior is rare in patients with narcolepsy without comorbid psychiatric disorders.

267. **Which of the following statements regarding sleep in neonates (newborn to 2 months) is true?**

   a) Sleep periods occur throughout the 24-hour day with no clear diurnal-nocturnal pattern.

   b) Aggregate hours of sleep per day are higher among full-term infants compared to premature infants.

   c) Sleep periods tend to be longer among breast-fed infants than among bottle-fed infants.

   d) Awakenings are more likely to occur from quiet rather than active sleep.

268. **The effects of oxygen therapy for the treatment of obstructive sleep apnea (OSA) include which of the following?**

   a) Increase central and mixed apneas

   b) Decrease obstructive sleep apneas (OSAs)

   c) Decrease apnea duration

   d) Decrease frequency of recorded hypopneas

269. **Which of the following is NOT a relaxation technique used for therapy of patients with insomnia?**

   a) Extinction

   b) Electromyographic biofeedback

   c) Guided imagery

   d) Progressive muscle relaxation

270. **Which of the following statements regarding NREM stage 3 sleep is correct?**

   a) Along with NREM stage 4 sleep, it has the highest arousal threshold by external stimuli among the different sleep stages.

b) Sleep spindles must not be present on electroen-cephalography.

c) It is more prominent during the second half of sleep.

d) NREM stage 3 sleep accounts for about 20% to 25% of total sleep time in adults.

271. Which of the following is NOT a major contributory factor in the pathophysiology of sleep disturbance in patients with Parkinson disease?

a) Adverse effects of medications

b) Muscle spasms

c) Nocturia

d) Reversal of sleep-wake schedules

272. Which of the following statements characterizes stage Wake?

a) Prominent alpha (8–13 Hz) electroencephalo-graphic (EEG) activity occurs when a person is alert and the eyes are open.

b) Low-voltage, high-frequency activity occurs when a person is drowsy and the eyes are closed.

c) Alpha activity is generally more prominent in the central leads than in the occipital leads.

d) Eye opening suppresses alpha EEG activity.

273. Which of the following instructions to patients is NOT part of stimulus control therapy for insomnia?

a) Use the bedroom only for sleep and sexual activity.

b) Get into bed at the same time each night even when not sleepy.

c) Refrain from engaging in activities in bed that are not compatible with sleep, such as eating or watching television.

d) Maintain a consistent arising time in the morning.

274. Paradoxical breathing is NOT present in which of the following disorders?

a) Central sleep apnea

b) Diaphragm paralysis

c) Respiratory muscle weakness

d) Upper airway obstruction

275. Which of the following statements regarding NREM stage 4 sleep is correct?

a) Delta electroencephalographic (EEG) activity occupies greater than 50% of the epoch.

b) Sleep spindles must not be present.

c) Slow rolling eye movements are present.

d) Chin muscle electromyographic activity is high and generally greater than that in stages 1 and 2 sleep.

276. Which of the following electroencephalographic (EEG) activity is present during NREM stage 1 sleep?

a) Prominent alpha (8–13 Hz) activity occupying more than 50% of the epoch

b) Presence of sleep spindles and K-complexes

c) Prominent theta activity

d) Delta activity occupying more than 20% of the epoch

277. Which of the following statements is NOT correct about temporal control therapy for insomnia?

a) It is designed to enhance sleep efficiency.

b) It promotes constancy of sleep-wake schedules.

c) Patients are instructed to get out of bed at the same time each day regardless of the quality and quantity of the preceding evening's sleep.

d) Daytime naps are allowed but should be limited to less than 30 minutes.

278. Which of the following statements regarding the clock genes of circadian rhythms is correct?

a) Cycle is required for light-related degradation of Timeless.

b) Down regulation of Period and Timeless transcription occurs due to interactions with Clock and Cycle.

c) Peak protein levels of Period and Timeless are reached by mid-morning.

d) Period and Timeless transcription starts in the early evening to midnight.

279. At what age does the polyphasic sleep pattern (occurring several times throughout the 24-hour day) seen in infancy and early childhood become monophasic (occurring only once generally at night)?

a) 6 months to 1 year

b) 1 to 2 years

c) 2 to 3 years

d) 3 to 5 years

280. **Which one of the following statements best describes the evaluation of patients with suspected narcolepsy?**

a) Narcolepsy with cataplexy cannot be diagnosed by clinical history alone.

b) Polysomnography followed by multiple sleep latency testing (MSLT) is always indicated in every patient with suspected narcolepsy even if cataplexy is present.

c) MSLT measures a person's ability to remain awake in quiet situations.

d) The Maintenance of Wakefulness Test (MWT) is useful for monitoring treatment response to stimulant medications used for the therapy of excessive sleepiness.

281. **Which of the following factors is NOT known to increase the risk of developing nocturnal leg cramps?**

a) Fluid and electrolyte imbalances (eg, hypocalcemia)

b) Pregnancy

c) Use of oral contraceptives

d) Warm ambient temperature

282. **Which of the following is NOT a known risk factor for adult nocturnal bruxism?**

a) History of childhood bruxism

b) Restless legs syndrome

c) Sleep talking

d) Smoking

283. **Which of the following best describes sleep-related groaning (catathrenia)?**

a) Occurrence of episodes predominantly or exclusively during NREM sleep

b) Inspiratory groaning during sleep

c) More common among females

d) An asymptomatic individual, generally with a normal physical examination

284. **At what age do distinct electroencephalographic features develop that allow differentiation of NREM sleep into four specific stages (ie, stages 1, 2, 3, and 4 sleep)?**

a) 1 to 2 weeks

b) 4 to 8 weeks

c) 8 to 12 weeks

d) 3 to 6 months

285. **Which of the following is a clinical feature of sub-wakefulness syndrome?**

a) It is a common and transient condition affecting mostly adolescents and young adults.

b) Subjective sensation of constant daytime sleepiness parallels abnormalities in objective measures of excessive sleepiness.

c) Frequent napping is common.

d) Nocturnal polysomnography is normal.

286. **Which of the following stages of sleep present in the first 6 months of life is the first behavioral sleep state to appear and is the predominant sleep state in the newborn?**

a) Active sleep

b) Quiet sleep

c) Intermediate sleep

d) Transitional sleep

287. **According to the American Academy of Sleep Medicine International Classification of Sleep Disorders (2nd edition), which of the following is required for the diagnosis of sleep-related bruxism?**

a) At least one episode per hour of sleep

b) At least one individual muscle burst per hour of sleep

c) At least one audible bruxism episode per polysomnographic study

d) No abnormal encephalographic activity such as seizures

288. **How many hours does a toddler (1 to 3 years of age) sleep on average per day?**

a) 8 to 11

b) 11 to 12

c) 12 to 14

d) 14 to 16

289. **Which of the following techniques is NOT used in cognitive therapy for insomnia?**

a)   Attention shifting

b)   Decatastrophizing

c)   Guided imagery

d)   Reappraisal

290. **Which of the following statements best describes cognitive-behavioral therapy for insomnia?**

a)   It is not effective unless performed as individualized one-on-one sessions with the therapist.

b)   It benefits patients with primary, but not secondary, insomnia.

c)   Beneficial effects on sleep are sustained over time after the initial treatment period.

d)   Most patients undergoing this therapy achieve complete normalization of sleep.

291. **Which of the following statements about the performance of the Maintenance of Wakefulness Test (MWT) is correct?**

a)   It consists of five nap opportunities, each 20 minutes in duration, performed at 2-hour intervals.

b)   The patient is asked to lie down in bed in a dark, quiet room.

c)   Whether sleep logs are used or if a polysomnography is to be performed prior to the test should be individualized as determined by the clinician.

d)   Measures to stay awake such as singing are allowed.

292. **Which of the following headaches occur only during sleep?**

a)   Chronic paroxysmal hemicrania

b)   Cluster headaches

c)   Hypnic headaches

d)   Migraine headaches

293. **Which of the following agents is classified as a short-acting benzodiazepine?**

a)   Clorazepate

b)   Flurazepam

c)   Temazepam

d)   Triazolam

294. **Administration of positive airway pressure (PAP) therapy is the treatment of choice for most patients with obstructive sleep apnea (OSA). Which of the following statements regarding PAP therapy is NOT correct?**

a)   Bilevel positive airway pressure provides two pressure levels during the respiratory cycle, namely a higher level during inspiration and a lower pressure during expiration.

b)   PAP increases nasal pressure above the critical closing pressure.

c)   Higher pressures are required to reverse airway occlusion during REM sleep and during sleep in a supine position.

d)   Spit-night studies always overestimate the severity of OSA.

295. **Which of the following statements about snoring among children is true?**

a)   Incidence peaks at 12 to 14 years of age during the rapid growth noted at puberty.

b)   Snoring is related to significant adenotonsillar hypertrophy in fewer than 40% of cases.

c)   Prevalence is estimated to be about 3% to 20%.

d)   Isolated snoring (ie, without obstructive sleep apnea) is not associated with behavioral and academic problems, or excessive sleepiness.

296. **A patient has inquired about the possibility of having repetitive transient ischemic attacks. He reports recurrent transient episodes of being unable to move occurring on awakening. Which of the following statements is the most appropriate response?**

a)   Sleep paralysis occurs in approximately 90% of persons with narcolepsy.

b)   Sleep paralysis does not occur in an isolated form or affect normal individuals.

c)   Sleep paralysis involves all voluntary muscles, including the ocular muscles.

d)   Sensorium is generally unaffected during episodes of sleep paralysis.

297. **Which of the following statements best describes chronic paroxysmal hemicrania?**

a)   It is most commonly associated with NREM sleep.

b)   It is often temporal, orbital, or supraorbital in location.

c)   It is generally responsive to therapy with low-dose benzodiazepines.

d)   It is characterized by severe bilateral headaches.

298. **Which of the following statements best describes NREM stage 2 sleep?**

    a) Delta electroencephalographic (EEG) activity occupies more than 20% of the epoch.

    b) Low-voltage, mixed-frequency EEG activity is present.

    c) Slow rolling eye movements occur.

    b) Sleep spindles and K-complexes are generally more prominent in the occipital leads than over the vertex.

299. **Which of the following benzodiazepines has a more delayed onset of action?**

    a) Clorazepate

    b) Diazepam

    c) Flurazepam

    d) Temazepam

300. **Which of the following is NOT an indication for the use of bilevel positive airway pressure (BPAP) therapy for patients with sleep-related breathing disorders?**

    a) An optional therapy to continuous positive airway pressure (CPAP) in selected patients who require high pressures and report difficulty exhaling against a fixed CPAP pressure

    b) Morbidly obese patients with obstructive sleep apnea with or without obesity hypoventilation syndrome

    c) Patients with coexisting hypoventilation syndrome

    d) Patients with complaints of aerophagia and gastric distention due to CPAP therapy

301. **Colic is defined as repeated sustained episodes of crying, generally over 3 hours, and irritability or fussing with no apparent reason. Which of the following statements about colic is true?**

    a) Present in more than 80% of infants

    b) Generally begins at about 3 months of age

    c) Usually resolves by 1 year of age

    d) Associated with a shorter sleep duration

302. **Which of the following statements best describes REM sleep?**

    a) The loss of postural muscle tone is due to postsynaptic hyperpolarization of the spinal motoneurons.

    b) Chin electromyographic activity is absent during phasic REM sleep.

    c) It accounts for nearly 50% of total sleep time in the adult.

    d) There is often three to five periods of REM sleep during the night, with progressively less REM sleep during the latter part of sleep.

303. **Which of the following is NOT characteristic of complex partial seizures?**

    a) Associated with localized sensorimotor manifestations

    b) Automatisms, such as lip smacking, vocalization, or sleepwalking

    c) Commonly originate from the temporal or frontal lobes

    d) No change of consciousness

304. **Which of the following neurotransmitters participates in the generation and maintenance of wakefulness?**

    a) Acetylcholine

    b) Adenosine

    c) Gamma-aminobutyric acid

    d) Glycine

305. **Which of the following benzodiazepine receptor agonists is least likely to be associated with rebound insomnia?**

    a) Eszopiclone

    b) Flurazepam

    c) Temazepam

    d) Triazolam

306. **Which of the following polysomnographic features is associated with cocaine use?**

    a) Increase in total sleep time during cocaine use

    b) Increase in REM sleep during cocaine use

    c) Increase in total sleep time during initial cocaine discontinuation

    d) Persistent decrease in REM sleep during initial cocaine discontinuation

307. **Which of the following genetic syndromes is associated with a greater likelihood of obstructive sleep apnea due to the presence of mandibular hypoplasia?**

a) Achondroplasia

b) Apert syndrome

c) Crouzon syndrome

d) Pierre-Robin sequence

308. **Which of the following sleep stages in the first 6 months of life is characterized by minimal or no body movements and by regular breathing?**

a) Active sleep

b) Quiet sleep

c) Intermediate sleep

d) Transitional sleep

309. **Which of the following changes in sleep architecture is related to oral contraceptive use?**

a) Decrease in NREM stage 2 sleep

b) No change or decrease in NREM stages 3 and 4 sleep

c) Increase in REM sleep latency

d) Decrease in REM sleep

310. **Which of the following disorders is defined by the presence of motor restlessness usually related to the use of neuroleptic agents or dopamine receptor antagonists and is not improved by movement?**

a) Akathisia

b) Myoclonus

c) Painful toes-moving legs syndrome

d) Vesper's curse

311. **What is the primary therapy for a short sleeper?**

a) Aside from reassurance, no specific therapy

b) Properly timed light therapy

c) Cognitive behavioral therapy for insomnia

d) Low-dose benzodiazepine receptor agonists

312. **Which of the following statements about continuous positive airway pressure (CPAP) adherence is NOT true?**

a) Self-report often overestimates actual CPAP use.

b) The percentage of days in which CPAP is not used correlates with decreased duration of nightly use.

c) Long-term use of CPAP is related to the level of prescribed pressure.

d) Patterns of nightly use are often discernible within the first few days or weeks of initiating treatment.

313. **Lethality with overdose of benzodiazepines increases with coingestion of which of the following agents?**

a) Alcohol

b) Cimetidine

c) Furosemide

d) Isoniazid

314. **Which of the following interventions has NOT been shown to improve continuous positive airway pressure (CPAP) adherence?**

a) Airway humidification

b) Bilevel positive airway pressure therapy

c) CPAP education and support

d) Motivational enhancement to reduce ambivalence regarding treatment

315. **Which of the following statements regarding therapy of childhood obstructive sleep apnea (OSA) is NOT correct?**

a) Adenotonsillectomy is the first-line and most common therapy for children with OSA.

b) Adenotonsillectomy is effective in most cases of uncomplicated childhood OSA (ie, without craniofacial anomalies, choanal atresia, macroglossia, or hypotonia).

c) Postoperative polysomnography following adenotonsillectomy is always required to assess the efficacy of the procedure.

d) OSA may recur during adolescence in children with initial success with adenotonsillectomy.

316. **Which of the following statements regarding sleep-related breathing disorders during pregnancy is correct?**

a) Factors responsible for the increased incidence of snoring and obstructive sleep apnea during pregnancy include weight gain and upper airway congestion (related to progesterone).

b) Estrogen may protect against worsening sleep apnea.

c) Sleep-related breathing disorders during pregnancy are related to lower rates of maternal hypertension and preeclampsia.

d) Sleep-related breathing disorders during pregnancy are related to higher rates of both intrauterine growth retardation and low birth weight.

317. **Which of the following statements regarding restless legs syndrome is correct?**

    a) A complaint of pain excludes the diagnosis.

    b) Uncomfortable sensations only involves the legs (thus its name) and does not involve the arms.

    c) An isolated urge to move may be present without any accompanying unpleasant sensations.

    d) There is always complete relief of the unpleasant sensations with movement.

318. **The characteristic movement of periodic limb movements of sleep consists of which of the following?**

    a) Partial extension of the ankle

    b) Extension of the knee

    c) Flexion of the big toe

    d) Fanning of the small toes

319. **Which of the following characteristics of the non-benzodiazepine benzodiazepine receptor agonists (eg, zolpidem, zaleplon, and eszopiclone) differentiate them from benzodiazepines?**

    a) Greater hypnosedative action

    b) No myorelaxant or antiseizure activities

    c) More lethal with overdose given their longer duration of action

    d) Greater changes in sleep architecture

320. **Which of the following statements regarding autotitrating positive airway pressure (APAP) devices is correct?**

    a) Snorers should not be titrated with APAP devices using diagnostic algorithms that rely on vibration or sound production.

    b) APAP devices are recommended for split-night positive airway pressure titration.

    c) Different devices utilize different algorithms for monitoring respiratory events and for altering delivered pressures.

    d) Proper mask fitting is not as crucial during unattended APAP use as with CPAP use.

321. **Which of the following sleep disorders is NOT present in infants (2 to 12 months of age)?**

    a) Bedtime resistance

    b) Sleep onset association disorder

    c) Rhythmic movement disorders

    d) Limit-setting sleep disorder

322. **Which of the following is a polysomnographic feature of narcolepsy?**

    a) Few awakenings

    b) Decreased in REM sleep latency of 20 minutes or less

    c) Increase in total sleep time

    d) Increase in REM sleep

323. **Which of the following polysomnographic features best describes the effect of sedating antidepressants on sleep?**

    a) Increase in sleep latency

    b) Decrease in frequency of awakenings

    c) Decrease in total sleep time

    d) Decrease in sleep efficiency

324. **Continuous spike waves during sleep are associated with which statement?**

    a) Course tends to be lifelong.

    b) Encephalographic (EEG) discharges decrease during NREM sleep.

    c) This was formerly referred to as electrical status epilepticus of sleep.

    d) Generalized continuous EEG spike and slow-wave complexes occur continuously throughout REM sleep.

325. **Which of the following neurotransmitters participates in the generation and maintenance of NREM sleep?**

    a) Acetylcholine

    b) Gamma-aminobutyric acid

    c) Histamine

    d) Hypocretin

326. **Where are dopamine-containing neurons located in the brain?**

    a) Ventral mesencephalic tegmentum and substantia nigra

    b) Locus ceruleus

c) Mesopontine neurons

d) Perifornical neurons

327. **Which of the following statements regarding multiple system atrophy is true?**

a) Onset is generally during childhood.

b) Patients can develop REM sleep behavior disorder.

c) There is an increase in sleep efficiency.

d) There is an increase in total sleep time.

328. **Which of the following statements regarding the neurotransmitter glycine is true?**

a) Neurotransmitter release occurs during NREM sleep.

b) It is the main excitatory neurotransmitter in the spinal cord.

c) It causes sleep-related paralysis.

d) Depolarization of spinal motoneurons is the mechanism responsible for REM sleep–related paralysis.

329. **Which of the following statements regarding hypocretin (orexin) is correct?**

a) Neurons are located in the locus ceruleus in the dorsal pontine tegmentum.

b) Neurons project widely to the spinal cord.

c) Narcolepsy is observed in animals with hypocretin (orexin) gene deletion.

d) Destruction of hypocretin neurons results in a marked reduction in total amount of waking.

330. **When do most seizures occur during sleep?**

a) NREM stages 1 and 2 sleep

b) NREM stages 3 and 4 sleep

c) REM sleep

d) Throughout the night

331. **Ramelteon has greatest affinity for which of the following melatonin receptors?**

a) ML1

b) ML2

c) ML3

d) ML4

332. **Bilevel positive airway pressure (BPAP) devices provide two pressure levels during the respiratory cycle, namely a higher level during inspiration and a lower pressure during expiration. Which of the following is NOT an indication for BPAP therapy in patients with sleep-related breathing disorders?**

a) Poor continuous positive airway pressure (CPAP) adherence

b) Development of aerophagia and gastric distention due to CPAP therapy

c) Concurrent chronic obstructive pulmonary disease and obstructive sleep apnea (overlap syndrome)

d) Presence of obesity hypoventilation syndrome

333. **Which of the following is associated with the administration of antiparkinsonian drugs?**

a) High-dose levodopa causes sedation and improves sleep quality.

b) Levodopa increases NREM stages 3 and 4 sleep.

c) Benztropine increases REM sleep latency.

d) Pramipexole, ropinirole, and benztropine can cause hallucinations.

334. **Based on the American Academy of Sleep Medicine (AASM) International Classification of Sleep Disorders (2nd edition), which of the following is NOT considered a parasomnia usually associated with REM sleep?**

a) Recurrent isolated sleep paralysis

b) REM sleep behavior disorder

c) Sleep-related dissociative disorder

d) Status dissociatus

335. **Which of the following statements best describes Rett disorder?**

a) It is characterized by developmental delay following a period of normal psychomotor development during the first few months after birth.

b) It is reported to occur only in males.

c) Some cases are related to mutations in MECP2 gene in chromosome Y.

d) There is a decrease in total sleep time during a 24-hour day

336. The brainstem tegmentum (laterodorsal and pedunculopontine tegmental nuclei) and basal forebrain (substantia innominata, and diagonal band of Broca and septum) contain which of the following neurotransmitters?

    a) Acetylcholine

    b) Histamine

    c) Hypocretin

    d) Norepinephrine

337. Which of the following statements regarding the use of trazodone for patients with insomnia is correct?

    a) Trazodone possesses both anxiolytic and sedative properties.

    b) It increases sleep efficiency but decreases total sleep time.

    c) The drug is associated with high potential for tolerance and dependency.

    d) Trazodone has a higher anticholinergic action than the tricyclic antidepressants.

338. Which of the following statements regarding oral devices for obstructive sleep apnea is NOT correct?

    a) The degree of anterior displacement of the tongue influences the effectiveness of these devices.

    b) A repeat sleep study for patients given oral devices for snoring or obstructive sleep apnea is recommended once the device has been optimally adjusted.

    c) Tongue-retaining devices are preferred for edentulous patients or those with compromised dentition.

    d) Oral devices should be avoided in patients unable to breathe nasally or who have a high resistance to nasal airflow.

339. What percentage of time in a 24-hour day does a newborn infant spend sleeping?

    a) 40%

    b) 50%

    c) 60%

    d) 70%

340. In the evaluation of patients presenting with excessive sleepiness, which of the following is an indication for polysomnography?

    a) Sleepiness is clearly related to insufficient sleep.

    b) Sleepiness is related to a diagnosed medical, neurologic, or psychiatric disorder.

    c) Sleepiness resolves with appropriate therapy of the underlying condition.

    d) Sleepiness is due to suspected narcolepsy.

341. To which of the following gamma-aminobutyric acid (GABA)–benzodiazepine receptors does non-benzodiazepine benzodiazepine receptor agonists selectively bind?

    a) BZ1

    b) BZ2

    c) BZ4

    d) BZ8

342. The neurotransmitter norepinephrine plays a role in the regulation of sleep and wakefulness. Which of the following statements regarding norepinephrine is correct?

    a) Its neurons are located in the laterodorsal tegmentum/pedunculopontine tegmentum.

    b) Norepinephrine is involved with maintenance of NREM sleep.

    c) Neurotransmitter release occurs during NREM sleep.

    d) It is not released during REM sleep.

343. Which of the following statements is true of temporal lobe seizures?

    a) Often occur only during sleep

    b) Generally not accompanied by impaired consciousness or postictal confusion

    c) Does not begin focally

    d) Most common during REM sleep

344. The laterodorsal tegmentum/pedunculopontine tegmentum (LDT/PPT) contain which of the following neurotransmitters?

    a) Acetylcholine

    b) Dopamine

    c) Gamma-aminobutyric acid

    d) Histamine

345. Which of the following statements regarding the factors causing and maintaining insomnia is NOT correct?

    a) Predisposing factors are present before the start of insomnia that increases the likelihood of developing insomnia.

    b) Predisposing factors cannot independently cause insomnia.

c) Precipitating factors trigger the start of insomnia.

d) Perpetuating factors sustain sleep disturbance and contribute to the persistence of insomnia independent of the precipitating causes.

346. **What percentage of chronic insomnia is due to psychophysiologic insomnia?**

a) 3%

b) 15%

c) 25%

d) 50%

347. **Which of the following statements about rapid eye movement (REM) sleep is true?**

a) There is a low arousal threshold by external stimuli.

b) Generalized skeletal muscle atonia or hypotonia spares the diaphragm and extraocular muscles but not the sphincter muscles.

c) There is a decrease in middle ear muscle activity during phasic REM sleep.

d) Penile tumescence in men and vaginal vascular engorgement and clitoral erection in women are seen.

348. **When are tics most frequently observed during sleep in patients with Tourette syndrome?**

a) NREM stages 1 and 2 sleep

b) NREM stages 3 and 4 sleep

c) REM sleep

d) Throughout the night

349. **Which of the following features is NOT present in Prader-Willi syndrome?**

a) Obesity

b) Hyperphagia

c) Short stature

d) Low-arched palate

350. **Which of the following surgical procedures for obstructive sleep apnea is designed to increase the dimensions of the retropalatal airspace?**

a) Genioglossal advancement

b) Hyoid myotomy and suspension

c) Mandibular advancement

d) Uvulopalatopharyngoplasty

351. **Which of the following statements about the clinical subtypes of narcolepsy is true?**

a) In patients with narcolepsy with cataplexy, normal hypocretin-1 levels in the cerebrospinal fluid (CSF) are present in up to 50% of cases.

b) Narcolepsy without cataplexy is always associated with normal hypocretin-1 levels in the CSF.

c) HLA DQB1*0602-negative narcolepsy without cataplexy patients generally have low CSF hypocretin-1 levels.

d) Low CSF hypocretin-1 level (< 110 pg/mL) is present in up to 20% of cases of narcolepsy with cataplexy-like or atypical episodes.

352. **Which of the following statements about the Maintenance of Wakefulness Test (MWT) is correct?**

a) It is an objective measure of an individual's ability to maintain wakefulness for a defined time.

b) The MWT and Multiple Sleep Latency Test measure the same parameters and are interchangeable.

c) It cannot assess response to treatment in patients with excessive sleepiness.

d) The 20-minute protocol is preferred over the 40-minute protocol.

353. **Which of the following statements regarding transient insomnia is NOT correct?**

a) Sleep is already abnormal prior to the start of insomnia.

b) Sleep normalizes with resolution of the inciting event.

c) Individuals have increased central nervous system arousal.

d) Individuals are more vulnerable to acute stresses.

354. **Which of the following is NOT a feature of Down syndrome?**

a) Hypertonia

b) Midfacial hypoplasia

c) Mandibular hypoplasia

d) Glossoptosis

355. **What is the only surgical procedure that is consistently effective as a sole procedure for obstructive sleep apnea?**

a) Genioglossal advancement

b) Maxillomandibular osteotomy and advancement

c) Tracheostomy

d) Uvulopalatopharyngoplasty

356. **Which of the following statements regarding the pathophysiology of central sleep apnea (CSA) is correct?**

a) A correlation exists between CSA and decreased left ventricular function due, partly, to a delay in circulatory time to respiratory control centers.

b) Carbon dioxide (CO_2) ventilatory drive is decreased in patients with idiopathic CSA, and results in a $PaCO_2$ that is high during both wakefulness and sleep.

c) At sleep onset, repetitive episodes of central apneas may occur if $PaCO_2$ (lower during sleep and higher during wakefulness) fluctuates above or below the apnea threshold.

d) CSA can develop during administration of opiate drugs due to stimulation of hypoxic and hypercapnic ventilatory drives.

357. **Which of the following statements regarding REM sleep is correct?**

a) Dreaming occurs only during REM sleep.

b) An increase in sympathetic activation occurs during tonic REM sleep.

c) Ponto-geniculo-occipital waves occur during REM sleep in the cat.

d) There is a decrease in brain metabolism and temperature relative to NREM sleep.

358. **Which of the following statements about the relationship between sleep and cerebrovascular disease is NOT correct?**

a) Patients with stroke may complain of recurrent awakenings and insomnia.

b) Subdural hematomas may give rise to excessive sleepiness.

c) Obstructive sleep apnea (OSA) increases the risk of cerebrovascular disease, but the presence of stroke does not increase the risk of developing OSA.

d) Ondine curse has been described following brainstem strokes.

359. **Which of the following factors is NOT responsible for the development of an adjustment sleep disorder?**

a) Momentous or stressful life events

b) Change in the sleeping environment

c) An acute medical disorder or physical illness

d) Childhood history of sleep disturbance

360. **Which of the following statements regarding the therapy of central sleep apnea (CSA) is correct?**

a) Supplemental oxygen therapy results in worsening hypercapnia in patients with nonhypercapnic CSA.

b) Positive airway pressure therapy can decrease left ventricular ejection fraction and increase left ventricular afterload in patients with CSA due to congestive heart failure.

c) Acetazolamide is effective in improving CSA in patients with high-altitude periodic respiration.

d) Benzodiazepines and narcotics are safe in patients with hypercapnic forms of CSA but not for those with nonhypercapnic CSA.

361. **Compared with adult obstructive sleep apnea (OSA), childhood OSA is associated with which of the following statements?**

a) Excessive sleepiness is more common.

b) There is greater prevalence among females.

c) Continuous positive airway pressure is more effective than upper airway surgery.

d) Adenotonsillar enlargement is a more important risk factor.

362. **Which of the following statements about the nocturnal eating (drinking) syndrome is true?**

a) Consumption of alcohol is common.

b) Patients are unaware or only partly conscious of the abnormal behavior.

c) There is full recall of the episode on awakening.

d) It is typically associated with daytime abnormal eating behavior.

363. **Which of the following factors does NOT influence the severity of symptoms in patients with periodic breathing related to high altitude?**

a) Altitude

b) Gender

c) Hypercapnic ventilatory chemoresponsiveness

d) Speed of ascent

364. Which of the following statements best describes juvenile myoclonic epilepsy?

a) Bilateral massive myoclonic jerks occur soon after sleep onset.

b) Episodes can be precipitated by sleep deprivation or alcohol use.

c) Onset is generally during prepuberty.

d) EEG can demonstrate asymmetric and asynchronous 4–6 Hz polyspike and wave discharges.

365. Which of the following statements regarding the control of respiration and cardiovascular function during REM sleep is correct?

a) Regular respiratory pattern

b) Increase in hypoxic and hypercapnic ventilatory responses relative to NREM sleep

c) Decrease in activity of upper airway dilator muscles

d) Decrease in systemic blood pressure accompanying skeletal muscle hypotonia

366. Which of the following statements is true of nocturnal frontal lobe epilepsy?

a) Abnormal behaviors (eg, sleep terrors or sleepwalking) can be observed.

b) Abnormal ictal or interictal electroencephalographic activity is readily apparent.

c) Onset is generally during adulthood.

d) Response to antiseizure medications, including carbamazepine, is poor.

367. Which of the following best describes the polysomnographic features of psychophysiologic insomnia?

a) Possibly normal polysomnography

b) Normal number of awakenings

c) "First-night effect" (better sleep than usual during the first night in the sleep laboratory)

d) "Reverse first-night effect" (worse sleep than usual during the first sleep laboratory night)

368. Which of the following statements regarding the difference between Cheyne-Stokes respiration and obstructive and central apneas is correct?

a) Periods of hyperpnea in Cheyne-Stokes respiration are shorter than that seen in central sleep apnea.

b) Arousals in Cheyne-Stokes respiration occur at the peak of ventilation or a few breaths after ventilation resumes, whereas arousals in obstructive sleep apnea occur at the termination of apnea.

c) Waxing and waning of ventilation is more abrupt in Cheyne-Stokes respiration than in central sleep apnea.

d) The nadir of oxygen desaturation immediately follows apneic events in Cheyne-Stokes respiration.

369. Which of the following is a characteristic feature of sleep during adolescence (14 to 18 years)?

a) Decrease in daytime sleepiness

b) Decrease in required total sleep time

c) Phase delay in circadian sleep-wake rhythms

d) Decrease in frequency of sleep-maintenance insomnia

370. Which of the following is the most effective countermeasure for excessive sleepiness secondary to sleep deprivation?

a) Increasing levels of external stimulation (eg, loud noises)

b) Napping

c) Bright ambient lights

d) Changes in posture, such as standing or stretching

371. Both primary and secondary enuresis can result from organic or functional causes. Which of the following factors suggests a functional etiology of enuresis?

a) Urinary urgency

b) Abnormality in urinary flow

c) Involuntary voiding during wakefulness

d) Presence of psychosocial stressors

372. Which of the following benzodiazepines has the shortest half-life?

a) Flurazepam

b) Temazepam

c) Estazolam

d) Triazolam

373. "Pseudo-spindles" or "drug spindles" with a frequency of about 15 Hz are associated with which of the following medications?

    a) Selective serotonin reuptake inhibitors

    b) Benzodiazepines

    c) Trazodone

    d) Dopamine agonists

374. Which of the following statements regarding melatonin is correct?

    a) Evening melatonin secretion is increased among older adults with insomnia.

    b) Minimal melatonin is secreted in infants younger than 3 months of age.

    c) Peak melatonin levels occur shortly after sleep onset in the early to mid-evening.

    d) Secretion of melatonin is stimulated by light exposure.

375. Which of the following statements regarding psychophysiologic insomnia is NOT correct?

    a) The onset of insomnia is related to a stressor, and sleep disturbance abates with resolution of the stressful event.

    b) There is heightened somatized tension, such as increased agitation and muscle tone.

    c) Conditioned arousal is limited to the person's own bed and bedroom, and he or she commonly reports sleeping better in any room other than his or her own.

    d) Its course is commonly chronic, and if left untreated, may progressively worsen.

376. Which of the following does NOT contribute to hypercapnia in obesity hypoventilation syndrome?

    a) Increased production of CO_2 due to greater work of breathing

    b) Increased chest wall compliance

    c) Decreased ventilation

    d) Decreased ventilatory responses to hypercapnia and hypoxemia

377. Which of the following is the most important risk factor for obstructive sleep apnea in children?

    a) Male gender

    b) Excess body weight

    c) Adenotonsillar enlargement

    d) Ethnicity

378. When does circadian sleep phase preference (ie, a person's "eveningness" versus "morningness") first develop?

    a) Between 3 and 6 years of age

    b) Between 6 and 12 years of age

    c) Between 12 and 15 years of age

    d) Between 15 and 18 years of age

379. Pregnancy has profound effects on sleep quality. Which of the following statements about sleep among pregnant women is correct?

    a) The frequency of napping increases during the second trimester.

    b) Sleep quality typically is best during the third trimester.

    c) Sleep is most disrupted during the second trimester of pregnancy.

    d) The direct effects of the growing fetus disrupt sleep.

380. Which of the following genetic syndromes is NOT associated with mandibular hypoplasia?

    a) Apert syndrome

    b) Cri du chat

    c) Pierre-Robin sequence

    d) Treacher-Collins syndrome

381. Which of the following statements regarding sleep during perimenopause and postmenopause is true?

    a) Compared with men, healthy older women are less likely to complain of insomnia, poor sleep quality, insufficient or nonrestorative sleep, and need for daytime naps.

    b) Older women report less use of sedative-hypnotic agents than men.

    c) There is a more pronounced decrease in NREM stages 3 and 4 sleep with aging in healthy women than in men.

    d) There is greater NREM stages 3 and 4 sleep in perimenopause than in premenopause.

382. **Panic disorders occur most commonly during which period of sleep?**

    a) Transition from drowsiness to NREM stage 1 sleep

    b) Transition from NREM stage 2 sleep to NREM stages 3 and 4 sleep

    c) NREM stages 3 and 4 sleep

    d) REM sleep

383. **Sleep starts, hypnic jerks, or hypnic myoclonia, consist of sudden muscle contractions of part or all of the body that occur at sleep onset. Which of the following statements about sleep starts is correct?**

    a) This condition commonly presents as several repetitive brief body jerks occurring in rapid succession and are accompanied by a sensation of "falling" or "dreaming."

    b) It can also present as visual (flashes of light or vivid imagery), auditory (loud bangs), or somesthetic (floating) phenomena.

    c) It is a common experience among many normal individuals during NREM stages 3 and 4 sleep.

    d) Sleep starts are spontaneous phenomena and are not triggered by external stimuli.

384. **Which of the following mutations has been described in patients with congenital central hypoventilation syndrome?**

    a) PHOX2B

    b) Hypocretin null

    c) Autosomal recessive hypoventilation gene

    d) EDN1 frameshift point mutation

385. **Which of the following changes in sleep architecture is associated with the administration of chlorpromazine?**

    a) Increase in sleep latency

    b) Decrease in sleep efficiency

    c) No consistent changes in NREM stages 3 and 4 sleep

    d) Decrease in REM sleep latency

386. **Which statement concerning sleep disorders during pregnancy is correct?**

    a) The prevalence of restless legs syndrome (RLS) peaks during the second trimester of pregnancy.

    b) The risk of developing RLS is greater among women who have experienced similar complaints

during previous pregnancies.

    c) There is no significant difference in the frequency of leg cramps in women with twin pregnancies than in those with single pregnancies.

    d) There is no significant difference in the frequency of leg cramps among the different trimesters.

387. **When does daytime napping in children usually cease?**

    a) Between 1 and 2 years of age

    b) Between 2 and 3 years of age

    c) Between 3 and 5 years of age

    d) Between 5 and 7 years of age

388. **Sleep hallucinations are common experiences in persons with narcolepsy. Which of the following statements regarding sleep hallucinations is correct?**

    a) They are not pathognomonic for narcolepsy and have been described in normal persons.

    b) Hallucinations may occur during wakefulness at sleep onset, referred to as hypnopompic, or on awakening, referred to as hypnagogic.

    c) Hallucinatory phenomena are only visual.

    d) Sleep hallucinations often begin several months to years before the onset of excessive sleepiness in patients with narcolepsy.

389. **Which of the following statements regarding benzodiazepines is NOT true?**

    a) Decrease in REM sleep can occur following sudden drug discontinuation.

    b) They can reduce upper airway muscle tone and worsen obstructive sleep apnea.

    c) They can depress respiration.

    d) They reduce severity of symptoms of restless legs syndrome.

390. **Hot flashes during the perimenopausal period affect sleep quality. Which of the following statements related to hot flashes and sleep is correct?**

    a) Hot flashes occurring at night can significantly disturb sleep, leading to a decrease in sleep efficiency and increase in frequency of awakenings.

    b) Hot flashes cause excessive sleepiness and paradoxically increase subjective sleep quality.

c) The frequency of hot flashes is not influenced by environmental temperature prior to bedtime.

d) Hot flashes generally resolve immediately after menopause once hormonal levels stabilize.

391. **Which of the following polysomnographic features associated with the use of olanzapine is true?**

    a) Increase in sleep latency

    b) Decrease in sleep efficiency

    c) Increase in total sleep time

    d) No change in REM sleep

392. **Which of the following statements about idiopathic sleep-related hypoventilation is correct?**

    a) Arterial blood gas analysis during sleep demonstrates an absolute ($PaCO_2 > 45$ mm Hg) or relative hypercapnia compared with levels during wakefulness that are not related to apneas or hypopneas.

    b) Hypoxemic and hypercapnic chemoresponsiveness are decreased, leading to decreased respiratory rate but increased tidal volume.

    c) It appears to be more common among females than among males.

    d) Hypoventilation is more severe during NREM sleep than during REM sleep.

393. **Which of the following statements regarding sleep spindles is correct?**

    a) Oscillations with a frequency of 15 to 18 Hz

    b) More prominent over the occipital leads

    c) Are seen during NREM stage 2 sleep and are absent during NREM stages 3 and 4 sleep

    d) Generated in midline thalamic nuclei

394. **Where are electroencephalographic K-complexes seen maximally?**

    a) Frontal leads

    b) Frontoparietal leads

    c) Occipital leads

    d) Vertex (central and central-parietal leads)

395. **Which of the following statements best describes idiopathic insomnia?**

    a) It is a long-standing sleep disturbance that generally starts during infancy or in early childhood.

b) Spontaneous remission is common.

c) It generally responds to low-dose benzodiazepines.

d) There is no change in total sleep time.

396. **Which of the following statements best describes Asperger disorder?**

    a) Stereotypical activities and behavior develop but without impairment in social interaction.

    b) Cognitive and language development are normal.

    c) Women are affected more commonly than men.

    d) Increase in sleep time occurs during the first part of the night with no changes in REM sleep.

397. **Which of the following statements regarding glucose and energy balance during sleep is correct?**

    a) Blood levels of glucose and insulin increase during sleep.

    b) Leptin stimulates the intake of food.

    c) Highest serum levels of leptin occur between 12:00 PM and 4:00 AM.

    d) Serum levels of ghrelin increase during wakefulness and decrease at night.

398. **Which of the following increases the likelihood of sleep-related hypoventilation in the various neuro-muscular disorders?**

    a) Daytime hyperventilation

    b) Daytime hypocapnia

    c) Increased chemosensitivity

    d) Presence of bulbar dysfunction

399. **Which of the following is associated with the administration of antipsychotic medications?**

    a) Shortened sleep latency

    b) Decrease in sleep efficiency

    c) Increase in wake time after sleep onset

    d) Decrease in total sleep time

400. **Preeclampsia, or pregnancy-induced hypertension, is associated with which of the following?**

    a) Higher frequency of snoring

    b) No change in airflow and upper airway dimensions

    c) No change in frequency of arousals

    d) No change in prevalence of periodic limb movements during sleep

401. Which of the following statements regarding benzodiazepines is NOT true?

    a) Act via the GABA receptors

    b) Increase NREM stages 3 and 4 sleep

    c) Increase spindle (12–14 cycles per second) density

    d) Increase "pseudospindles" (14–18 cycles per second)

402. Which of the following statements regarding electroencephalographic alpha waveforms is correct?

    a) Oscillations with a frequency of 8 to 13 Hz

    b) Present when a person is relaxed and drowsy and eyes are open

    c) Originates in the frontal cortex

    d) More prominent in the frontal leads compared to central leads

403. Which of the following statements is a feature of frontal lobe seizures?

    a) Consciousness is lost.

    b) Postseizure confusion is significant.

    c) "Jacksonian march" with seizure activity starting at the distal part of the extremity and moving proximally is associated with onset in the posterior frontal lobes.

    d) Abnormal interictal electroencephalographic discharges are common.

404. Which of the following changes in hormone levels occurs during the first half compared with the second half of the night?

    a) Increase in adrenocorticotropic hormone

    b) Increase in cortisol

    c) Increase in growth hormone

    d) No change in growth hormone

405. Which of the following statements regarding morning light exposure for sleep-onset insomnia is correct?

    a) Produces a phase delay in circadian sleep-wake, core body temperature, and melatonin rhythms

    b) Shortens sleep latency

    c) No change in total sleep time

    d) Causes a later final awakening time

406. Which of the following statements regarding the Multiple Sleep Latency Test (MSLT) is correct?

    a) It is an objective measure of an individual's ability or tendency to fall asleep.

    b) It is routinely indicated in the initial evaluation of patients with obstructive sleep apnea who present with complaints of sleepiness.

    c) A repeat MSLT is indicated annually following an abnormal study.

    d) A repeat MSLT testing is indicated when results fail to confirm the diagnosis of narcolepsy in patients with low cerebrospinal fluid hypocretin levels.

407. What is the standard gain for electroencephalography used for polysomnography?

    a) 1 mm for every 50 μV

    b) 1 cm for every 25 μV

    c) 1 cm for every 50 μV

    d) 1 cm for every 100 μV

408. Which of the following cytokines inhibits sleep?

    a) Interleukin-1 (IL-1)

    b) IL-2

    c) IL-4

    d) IL-8

409. Which of the following statements is true of limit-setting sleep disorder?

    a) Sleep-onset insomnia is commonly severe and resistant to behavioral therapy.

    b) Prevalence is greater among girls.

    c) The disorder is not commonly encountered until the child reaches puberty.

    d) Sleep is typically normal on polysomnography.

410. Which of the following are considered "REM-on cells" (ie, neurons that are active during REM sleep)?

    a) Cholinergic neurons

    b) Histaminergic neurons

    c) Noradrenergic neurons

    d) Serotonergic neurons

411. **Narcolepsy can occur without cataplexy. Which of the following statements regarding this subset of narcolepsy is true?**

    a) Cataplexy-like symptoms, including prolonged episodes of tiredness, or muscle weakness related to atypical triggers (exercise, stress, or sex) may be present.

    b) It accounts for less than 10% of cases of narcolepsy.

    c) Most have low levels of cerebrospinal fluid hypocretin-1.

    d) Loss of hypocretin-containing hypothalamic neurons is more pronounced than with narcolepsy with cataplexy.

412. **Which of the following statements regarding phototherapy for delayed sleep phase syndrome is correct?**

    a) Timed early morning exposure and evening avoidance of bright lights produce a phase advance in the sleep-wake circadian cycle.

    b) Light exposure is of greatest benefit if timed close before the temperature nadir (Tmin).

    c) The body temperature nadir (Tmin) is often about 1 to 2 hours before the habitual mid-sleep time.

    d) Phototherapy can be used for patients with retinopathy if commercial light boxes that provide narrow spectrum light are used.

413. **Which of the following is associated with the administration of clozapine?**

    a) Increase in sleep latency

    b) Decrease in sleep efficiency

    c) Decrease in total sleep time

    d) No change in REM sleep

414. **At what age does the prevalence of childhood obstructive sleep apnea peak?**

    a) Between 1 to 2 years

    b) Between 2 to 5 years

    c) Between 5 to 10 years

    d) Between 10 to 12 years

415. **In animal models of REM sleep, ponto-geniculo-occipital waves are generated by which of the following neural systems?**

    a) Locus ceruleus

    b) Mesopontine neurons

    c) Perifornical neurons

    d) Posterior hypothalamus

416. **Which of the following statements best describes behavioral therapy for insomnia?**

    a) Improvements in sleep parameters following behavioral therapy are sustained over time.

    b) Everyone who benefits from behavioral therapy becomes good sleepers.

    c) Improvements in nighttime sleep with behavioral therapy are always associated with positive changes in daytime symptoms.

    d) Subjective reports of improvements in sleep are less than objective measures obtained with polysomnography.

417. **Which of the following statements about the electroencephalographic alpha-NREM sleep anomaly is true?**

    a) It is specific for fibromyalgia.

    b) It is present in every patient with fibromyalgia.

    c) It can be seen in otherwise healthy individuals.

    d) It is not related to medication use.

418. **Which of the following statements about hypocretin (orexin) is correct?**

    a) Neurons are located in the tuberomammillary nucleus of the posterior hypothalamus.

    b) Neurotransmitter is released during REM sleep.

    c) It acts on other central nervous system centers related to sleep-wake regulation, including the dorsal raphe, locus ceruleus, tuberomammillary nuclei, and spinal cord.

    d) Hypocretin system dysfunction is associated with idiopathic hypersomnia.

419. **It is NOT possible to obtain which of the following sleep-related data by actigraphy?**

    a) REM sleep latency

    b) Sleep latency

    c) Total sleep time

    d) Wake time after sleep onset

420. **Serotonin is a neurotransmitter involved in the regulation of sleep and wakefulness. Which of the following statements regarding serotonin is correct?**

a) Serotonergic neurons are located in the raphe nuclei and thalamus.

b) Neurotransmitter release is highest during REM sleep.

c) Its release is lowest during wakefulness.

d) Agents that inhibit serotonin (eg, selective serotonin receptor inhibitors) increase REM sleep.

421. **When does nocturnal hypoventilation-induced oxygen desaturation occur in patients with amyotrophic lateral sclerosis?**

a) During NREM stage 2 sleep

b) During NREM stages 3 and 4 sleep

c) During REM sleep

d) Immediately preceding arousals

422. **Which of the following statements best characterizes normal adult sleep?**

a) Long sleep latency (> 15 minutes)

b) Low sleep efficiency (< 95%)

c) Sleep is entered into through NREM sleep.

d) REM sleep predominates during the first half of the night, whereas NREM sleep percentage is greatest during the second half of the night.

423. **Which of the following statements about altitude insomnia is NOT true?**

a) Sleep disturbance develops following ascent to elevations greater than 2000 to 4000 meters.

b) There is a decrease in sleep efficiency.

c) Incidence increases in persons with underlying cardiorespiratory disorders or anemia.

d) Arousals can occur during the apneic and hypopneic phase of periodic breathing.

424. **Which of the following statements regarding sleep during pregnancy, labor, and delivery is true?**

a) Decrease in sleep efficiency during pregnancy

b) Decrease in total sleep time during early pregnancy and increase in total sleep time during late pregnancy

c) Increase in REM sleep

d) Association of longer nighttime sleep duration in the period before labor and delivery with longer labor and increased likelihood of cesarean delivery

425. **Differences in polysomnographic features between childhood and adult obstructive sleep apnea (OSA) include which of the following?**

a) Sleep architecture is generally normal in childhood OSA.

b) Oxygen desaturation is less severe in adult OSA.

c) Respiratory events are more frequently associated with arousals in childhood OSA.

d) There are few respiratory event-related arousals in adult OSA.

426. **Which of the following neuronal systems is associated with the neurotransmitter histamine?**

a) Basal forebrain (substantia innominata and diagonal band of Broca and septum)

b) Brainstem tegmentum (laterodorsal and pedunculopontine tegmental nuclei)

c) Locus ceruleus in the dorsal pontine tegmentum

d) Tuberomammillary nucleus in the posterior hypothalamus

427. **Which of the following statements about sleep restriction therapy for insomnia is NOT true?**

a) It creates a state of sleep deprivation to increase sleep efficiency.

b) Time in bed is allowed to be less than 4 hours each night.

c) No change in allowable bedtime is made if sleep efficiency is between 80% and 90%.

d) Naps are not allowed.

428. **Patients in the intensive care unit (ICU) may complain of sleep disturbance. Which of the following statements describe sleep in the ICU patient?**

a) The ICU syndrome is characterized by reversible mental status changes, including delirium, among patients 3 to 7 days after admission to the ICU.

b) There is an increased tendency for patients to sleep more during the day and night.

c) Poor sleep quality is influenced by gender, age, and duration of ICU stay.

d) Because of decreased mobility of most patients in the ICU, nursing observations often underestimate sleep time compared to objective data obtained with polysomnography.

429. Which of the following is NOT an indication for polysomnography in patients with suspected parasomnias?

a) Cases with forensic implications

b) Failure to respond to therapy

c) Typical noninjurious cases

d) Unusual or atypical features

430. Which of the following polysomnographic features is associated with sleep initiated during the rising phase of the temperature rhythm?

a) Increase in sleep latency

b) Increase in total sleep time

c) Increase in NREM stages 3 and 4 sleep

d) Decrease in REM sleep

431. Which of the following statements regarding thiothixene is true?

a) Decrease in sleep latency

b) Decrease in sleep efficiency

c) Decrease in total sleep time

d) Decrease in REM sleep latency

432. Which extinction technique involves having the parent put the child in bed, leaving the child alone in his or her room, and responding to the child's inappropriate demands in a progressively decreasing fashion until parental intervention is finally stopped?

a) Fast extinction approach

b) Absolute extinction approach

c) Gradual extinction approach

d) Parental presence extinction approach

433. Which of the following statements regarding the nonbenzodiazepine benzodiazepine receptor agonists is correct?

a) They act via the gamma-aminobutyric acid receptor complex.

b) Tolerance and withdrawal symptoms are common.

c) They have significant adverse effects on respiratory status.

d) Zolpidem has a shorter half-life than zaleplon.

434. Which of the following statements about the afferent pathways of the suprachiasmatic nucleus is correct?

a) The alternate afferent photic connection involves the thalamic intergeniculate leaflet of the lateral geniculate nuclei via the geniculohypothalamic tract using neuropeptide γ and gamma-aminobutyric acid as its neurotransmitters.

b) The cholinergic photic pathway involves the tuberomammillary complex neurons in the posterior basal hypothalamus.

c) Midbrain medial raphe nuclei via serotonergic pathways is a photic afferent pathway.

d) Light entrainment is lost with disruption of either the retinohypothalamic or alternate geniculohypothalamic tracts.

435. Which of the following statements about pulse transit time (PTT) is correct?

a) PTT is represented by the interval between the electrocardiographic R-wave and the subsequent pulse shock wave at the finger.

b) PTT is typically about 500 ms.

c) PTT decreases during inspiratory falls in blood pressure and increases during arousal-induced increases in blood pressure in patients with obstructive sleep apnea.

d) PTT is directly related to blood pressure.

436. The susceptibility to sleep deprivation is best described by which statement?

a) There is no interindividual vulnerability to sleep deprivation.

b) Compared with older adults, younger individuals appear to be less susceptible to the effects of total sleep deprivation.

c) Variability among individuals in susceptibility to sleep deprivation becomes less prominent as the duration of sleep deprivation increases.

d) The adverse physiologic, neurocognitive, and behavioral consequences of acute total sleep deprivation are similar to that generally observed with chronic partial sleep deprivation (sleep restriction).

437. The "overlap syndrome" is defined by the presence of both chronic obstructive pulmonary disease and obstructive sleep apnea. Compared with patients with obstructive sleep apnea alone, those with the overlap syndrome have which of the following features?

a) Higher awake and sleep PaO_2

b) Higher sleep PaO_2 only

c) Lower sleep $PaCO_2$

d) Higher pulmonary artery mean pressures

438. **Which of the following statements about electro-oculography (EOG) is correct?**

    a) EOG records the difference in potentials (dipole) between the cornea (negative) and the retina (positive).

    b) A positive voltage (downward deflection) is recorded when the eye moves toward an electrode.

    c) EOG electrodes are placed using collodion.

    d) EOG electrodes are generally placed lateral and superior to the outer canthus of both eyes.

439. **Which of the following statements about nocturnal seizures is true?**

    a) Sleep deprivation is a recognized precipitant of seizure activity, and sleep protects against the development of seizures.

    b) There are two peaks in the occurrence of nocturnal seizures, the first immediately following sleep onset and the second immediately prior to awakening.

    c) They occur more frequently during NREM stages 1 and 2 sleep than NREM stages 3 and 4 or REM sleep.

    d) Seizure thresholds are generally greater during NREM sleep than during REM sleep.

440. **Which of the following statements regarding pupillary changes during sleep is correct?**

    a) There is no change in pupil size during sleep compared with wakefulness.

    b) Constriction of the pupils occurs during phasic REM sleep.

    c) Constriction of the pupils occurs during tonic REM sleep.

    d) Dilation of the pupils occurs during NREM sleep.

441. **Patients with cystic fibrosis may present with complaints of poor sleep quality and sleep fragmentation. Which of the following statements regarding cystic fibrosis is true?**

    a) Cystic fibrosis is an autosomal recessive disease characterized by abnormal transport of sodium and chloride across the epithelium in all exocrine and endocrine tissues.

    b) Nocturnal episodes of coughing can occur, but oxygen desaturation is rarely seen.

    c) The likelihood of sleep-related hypoxemia is greater in patients with low FEV_1 and low awake SaO_2.

    d) Sleep quality deteriorates during disease exacerbations but is otherwise independent of physiologic variables of disease severity.

442. **The parents of a child with narcolepsy have asked you about the likelihood of another child developing this disorder. What is the most appropriate reply to their inquiry?**

    a) Most cases of narcolepsy are sporadic.

    b) A clear familial tendency is present in up to two-thirds of patients.

    c) About 30% of patients have a first-degree relative with cataplexy and excessive sleepiness.

    d) The risk of developing the disorder is increased by 100 times among first-degree relatives of narcoleptic individuals.

443. **When does minimum core body temperature typically occur?**

    a) 2 to 4 hours after the end of the sleep period

    b) 2 to 4 hours prior to the end of the sleep period

    c) At sleep onset

    d) On awakening

444. **Which of the following hypnotic agents has the shortest elimination half-life?**

    a) Temazepam

    b) Triazolam

    c) Zaleplon

    d) Zolpidem

445. **Which of the following statements about expired end-tidal carbon dioxide (PetCO2) monitoring is correct?**

    a) $PetCO_2$ is generally similar to $PaCO_2$.

    b) The measured level of $PetCO_2$ at the end of a complete expiration is related to $PaCO_2$.

    c) $PetCO_2$ may overestimate $PaCO_2$ when the dead space to tidal volume ratio is increased during sleep.

    d) $PetCO_2$ remains accurate during positive airway pressure therapy but not during supplemental oxygen therapy.

446. **Which of the following statements best describes benign epilepsy of childhood with centrotemporal spikes?**

a) Perioral numbness and clonic focal twitching of the face and mouth do not occur during drowsiness, start immediately following sleep onset, and are not present during sleep.

b) Secondarily generalized tonic-clonic seizures do not occur.

c) EEG demonstrates rolandic or centrotemporal spike and sharp waves.

d) Spontaneous resolution does not occur.

447. **Which of the following hormones decrease during sleep compared to levels present during wakefulness?**

a) Aldosterone

b) Parathyroid hormone

c) Renin (during REM sleep)

d) Testosterone (adult men)

448. **Which of the following statements defines obstructive hypoventilation in children?**

a) Prolonged periods of hypoventilation, with hypercapnia and hypoxemia, due to persistent but partial upper airway obstruction that can occur with or without arousals

b) Prolonged periods of hypoventilation, without hypercapnia and hypoxemia, due to partial upper airway obstruction typically associated with arousals

c) Prolonged periods of hypoventilation, with hypercapnia and hypoxemia, due to partial upper airway obstruction that are not associated with arousals

d) Prolonged periods of hypoventilation with hypercapnia due to partial upper airway obstruction that are not associated with hypoxemia or arousals

449. **During polysomnography, what is the reference standard for detecting respiratory effort?**

a) Esophageal pressure monitoring

b) Respiratory inductance plethysmography

c) Strain gauges

d) Surface diaphragmatic electromyography

450. **Which of the following is NOT a generalized seizure?**

a) Absence seizures (petit mal)

b) Complex frontotemporal seizures

c) Generalized tonic-clonic seizures

d) Juvenile myoclonic seizures

451. **Which of the following statements best describes the relationship between sleep and thyroid-stimulating hormone (TSH)?**

a) TSH levels are highest during the daytime.

b) The nadir of TSH is at night prior to sleep onset.

c) Sleep, particularly NREM stages 3 and 4 sleep, inhibits the secretion of TSH.

d) Levels of TSH decline during sleep deprivation.

453. **Which of the following statements best describes the sleep-related changes in thermoregulation?**

a) Readjustment of the thermal set point to a higher level than that during wakefulness occurs.

b) Response to thermal challenge is lower during NREM sleep than during REM sleep.

c) Sweating and shivering are present during NREM sleep.

d) Heat production with shivering is present during REM sleep.

454. **What percentage of an epoch should be obscured by movement artifact for it to be scored as "movement time?"**

a) More than 25%

b) More than 30%

c) More than 50%

d) More than 90%

455. **When does the greatest phase delay shifting occur during light exposure?**

a) Anytime in the late afternoon or early evening

b) During the subjective day

c) Immediately after the minimum core body temperature (Tmin)

d) Immediately prior to Tmin

456. **Which of the following is NOT a known risk factor for infant sleep apnea?**

a) Family history of sudden infant death syndrome

b) Low birth weight

c) Comorbid medical disorders (eg, anemia or infection)

d) Neurologic disorders

457. Which of the following agents decreases the occurrence of cataplexy?

   a) α_1-receptor antagonists

   b) α_2-receptor agonists

   c) α_2-receptor antagonists

   d) β-antagonists

458. You have been asked to review a polysomnography that demonstrates repetitive and brief activation of the anterior tibialis electromyography of one leg followed by a similar activation of the other leg. Each activation has a duration of 0.1 to 0.5 seconds, with four or more muscle activations occurring in sequence lasting from 1 to 30 seconds. There is less than 2 seconds between activations. The most likely diagnosis is:

   a) Hypnagogic foot tremor

   b) Alternating leg muscle activation

   c) Periodic limb movement during wakefulness

   d) Rhythmic movement disorder

459. Barbiturate use is associated with which of the following changes in sleep architecture?

   a) Increase in sleep latency

   b) Increase in NREM stages 3 and 4 sleep

   c) Increase in spindle density

   d) Decrease in REM sleep latency

460. Which of the following statements about the retinohypothalamic pathway of the suprachiasmatic nucleus is NOT correct?

   a) It is the main afferent pathway for photic stimuli in the suprachiasmatic nucleus.

   b) Photosensitive retina ganglion cells contain the photopigment, melanopsin.

   c) It uses glutamate and pituitary adenylate cyclase-activating polypeptide as its neurotransmitters.

   d) Retinal photoreceptors involved with circadian processes are most sensitive to visible light of longer wavelengths (ie, yellow to orange).

461. Which of the following phrases best describes the changes in sleep architecture following the administration of benzodiazepines?

   a) Decrease in total sleep time

   b) Increase in NREM stage 2 sleep

   c) Decrease in number of sleep spindles

   d) Increase in REM sleep

462. Which of the following is NOT a feature of cluster headaches?

   a) Associated features include lacrimation and conjunctival injection.

   b) Onset is gradual with a peak in symptoms after several hours.

   c) Headaches tend to occur during sleep, particularly during REM sleep.

   d) Obstructive sleep apnea is a known trigger.

463. Which of the following mechanisms contributes to the fall in core body temperature during sleep?

   a) Greater heat loss mediated by peripheral vasoconstriction

   b) Less heat generation due to a decrease in metabolism

   c) Readjustment of the thermal set point to a higher level, leading to increased sweating

   d) Complete loss of thermoregulation during both NREM and REM sleep

464. Which of the following statements regarding the use of melatonin in the treatment of delayed sleep phase syndrome is correct?

   a) Melatonin given in the evening is effective in inducing a phase advance of the sleep period.

   b) It can increase sleep latency when given too early in the evening.

   c) Its phase shifting effect is comparable to that of bright light.

   d) Melatonin has a paradoxical alerting effect when ingested in supraphysiologic doses.

465. Which of the following is NOT a characteristic of noninvasive methods of measuring oxygenation and ventilation as compared with direct arterial blood gas measurements during sleep?

   a) Afford continuous monitoring

   b) Less intrusive of the patient's sleep

   c) Capable of monitoring carbon dioxide

   d) As accurate as direct arterial blood gas sampling

466. What is the generally accepted definition of the phenomenon of blood pressure "dipping"?

a) Nighttime systolic blood pressure is about 10% greater than that during the daytime.

b) Nighttime mean blood pressure is about 10% less than that during the daytime.

c) Nighttime systolic blood pressure is about 10% less than that during the daytime.

d) Nighttime systolic blood pressure is about 25% less than that during the daytime.

467. Which of the following phrases best describes respiratory effort–related arousals?

a) Reduction in airflow associated with reduced inspiratory effort

b) Associated with significant oxygen desaturation

c) Transient flattening of the nasal pressure signal

d) Increasing positive deflections on esophageal pressure monitoring followed by a sudden change in pressure to a less positive level and an arousal

468. Which of the following cardiovascular parameters does NOT increase during phasic REM sleep compared with NREM and tonic REM sleep?

a) Cardiac output

b) Peripheral vascular resistance

c) Stroke volume

d) Systemic blood pressure

469. What term defines the free-running endogenous circadian period?

a) Delta

b) Omega

c) Sigma

d) Tau

470. Patients with neurodegenerative disorders often complain of poor sleep quality. Which of the following statements regarding sleep in patients with neurodegenerative disorders is correct?

a) Muscular contractions and gross body movements occur during wakefulness and generally disappear during sleep with the development of muscle hypotonia.

b) There is an increased likelihood of REM sleep behavior disorder.

c) There is an increase in NREM stages 3 and 4 sleep.

d) There is an increase in REM sleep.

471. Which of the following statements best characterizes the changes in autonomic tone during REM sleep compared with NREM sleep?

a) Decrease in parasympathetic tone during tonic REM sleep

b) Increase in sympathetic tone, particularly during phasic REM sleep

c) Lower average blood pressure

d) Lower average heart rate

472. Which of the following does NOT contribute to the generation of 60-Hz interference in the polysomnogram?

a) High and unequal electrode impedance

b) Interference from 60-Hz electrical activity from power lines

c) Lead failure

d) Respiratory movements

473. Which of the following factors increase REM sleep latency?

a) Depression

b) Mirtazapine

c) Monoamine oxidase inhibitors

d) Nefazodone

474. Which of the following statements best describes the effect of melatonin on circadian rhythms?

a) It causes a phase advance when taken in the morning.

b) It causes a phase delay when given in the afternoon or early evening.

c) It is as effective in phase shifting the circadian rhythm as light exposure.

d) Melatonin alters the phase of circadian rhythms by its effect on the suprachiasmatic nucleus.

475. Which of the following statements best describes sweat artifacts that can be seen during polysomnography?

a) Slow-frequency undulating movements that are present only in the electroencephalographic (EEG) leads and often synchronous with respiration

b) Due to alterations in electrode potentials by salt in sweat

c) May resemble alpha waves and may result in overscoring of wakefulness

d) Can be prevented and minimized by using collodion for EEG leads

476. **Which of the following phrases about hypnic headaches is NOT true?**

a) Most common during NREM sleep

b) No significant autonomic manifestations

c) Occur during sleep and awaken the patient

d) Respond to therapy with lithium

477. **Which of the following phrases regarding gastrointestinal physiology during sleep is correct?**

a) Increase in salivary production

b) No change in esophageal motility

c) Delay in esophageal acid clearance following gastroesophageal reflux

d) Peak secretion of gastric acid occurs between 5:00 and 8:00 AM

478. **Which of the following factors is capable of producing a phase advance of the circadian sleep-wake rhythm?**

a) Light exposure before the core body temperature nadir

b) Light exposure near the end of the subjective night

c) Passive body heating in the evening

d) Physical exercise in the evening

479. **Which of the following statements regarding REM sleep latency is NOT true?**

a) It is the period from lights out to the first epoch of REM sleep.

b) It is the period from the first epoch of sleep to the first epoch of REM sleep.

c) It usually ranges from 60 to 120 minutes

d) Sleep-onset REM period is generally defined as the occurrence of REM sleep within 10 to 15 minutes of sleep onset

480. **What is the main REM sleep neurotransmitter?**

a) Acetylcholine

b) Histamine

c) Hypocretin

d) Norepinephrine

481. **Neurons of the locus ceruleus, midbrain reticular formation, thalamus, lateral hypothalamus, and basal forebrain have a tonic high rate of discharge during wakefulness. Which statement related to these systems is correct?**

a) Histamine is contained in neurons in the dorsal raphe.

b) The locus ceruleus in the dorsal pontine tegmentum contain norepinephrine, and discharge during both waking and REM sleep.

c) Neurons located in the substantia nigra and ventral tegmental area contain dopamine.

d) Serotonin-containing neurons are located in the locus ceruleus in the dorsal pontine tegmentum.

482. **Where are the suprachiasmatic nuclei located in mammals?**

a) Dorsal to the optic chiasm in the anterior hypothalamus

b) Ventral to the optic chiasm in the anterior hypothalamus

c) Dorsal to the optic chiasm in the posterior hypothalamus

d) Ventral to the optic chiasm in the posterior hypothalamus

483. **Which of the following is an indication for split-night polysomnography?**

a) An apnea hypopnea index (AHI) > 10 during a minimum of 2 hours of monitoring in a diagnostic polysomnography

b) An AHI of 5 to 10, and the presence of repetitive prolonged obstructions or marked oxygen desaturations

c) Duration of time available for continuous positive airway pressure (CPAP) titration of greater than 4 hours

d) CPAP titration successfully eliminates or nearly eliminates respiratory events during sleep, including REM sleep in a supine position

484. **Where are hypocretin neurons located?**

a) Laterodorsal tegmentum/pedunculopontine tegmentum

b) Perifornical region of lateral hypothalamus

c) Locus ceruleus

d) Raphe nuclei

485. What is the role of the nucleus ambiguus in the control of respiration?

    a) Generates the basic respiratory rhythm

    b) Modulates respiration by its action on laryngeal and pharyngeal muscles

    c) Regulates inspiration

    d) Regulates expiration

486. Which of the following statements best describes the use of chronotherapy for the treatment of delayed sleep phase syndrome?

    a) With progressive phase delay, bedtime is delayed by 20 to 40 minutes each day but arising time is fixed regardless of bedtime.

    b) Napping should be encouraged during progressive phase delay because it strengthens the phase altering effect of chronotherapy.

    c) Physical activities, meal times, and light exposure should be timed during both progressive phase delay and phase advance to coincide with wake times.

    d) Progressive phase advance usually utilizes greater changes in bedtimes (often by 3 to 6 hours each 24-hour day) than progressive phase delay.

487. Which of the following is a common clinical feature of narcolepsy?

    a) Automatic behavior with good recall of the event

    b) Sleep disruption with repetitive nighttime awakenings

    c) Decreased prevalence of REM sleep behavior disorder

    d) Decreased prevalence of sleep apnea

488. Which of the following must be present during polysomnography for periodic limb movements to be counted?

    a) Duration of greater than 10 seconds

    b) Occurrence in a series of at least two consecutive contractions

    c) Intervals between movements of between 5 to 90 seconds from the onset of one limb movement to the onset of the next

    d) Amplitude of the electromyogram greater than 50% than that of baseline during biocalibrations

489. Which of the following is NOT a known adverse effect from chronic use of benzodiazepines?

    a) Tolerance

    b) Dependency

    c) Increase in restless leg symptoms

    d) Rebound insomnia

490. Hurler syndrome (mucopolysaccharidosis type I) and Hunter syndrome (mucopolysaccharidosis type II) are characterized by the accumulation of glycosaminoglycans in various tissues and organs of the body. Both can present with obstructive sleep apnea due to glycosaminoglycan deposition in the upper airways. Which of the following statements is correct?

    a) Hurler syndrome is an X-linked recessive disorder.

    b) Hurler syndrome is associated with increased urinary levels of chondroitin sulfate B and heparin sulfate.

    c) Hurler syndrome is associated with skeletal abnormalities, macroglossia, tracheomalacia, and a high arched palate.

    d) Hunter syndrome is an autosomal recessive disorder.

491. Which of the following is a polysomnographic feature of obstructive sleep apnea?

    a) Increase frequency of arousals

    b) Decrease in NREM stages 1 and 2 sleep

    c) Increase in NREM stages 3 and 4 sleep

    d) No change in REM sleep

492. Which of the following neurotransmitters is associated with the retinohypothalamic pathway of the suprachiasmatic nucleus?

    a) Acetylcholine

    b) Glutamate

    c) Histamine

    d) Serotonin

493. Which of the following abrupt changes in electroencephalographic frequency does NOT accompany an arousal from NREM sleep?

    a) Alpha

    b) Beta

    c) Delta

    d) Theta

494. Which of the following phrases best describes the ascending projections of the reticular formation into the forebrain that is involved in the regulation of wakefulness?

a) A lateral pathway that projects to the cerebral cortex via the hippocampus

b) A dorsal pathway that projects to the cerebral cortex via the thalamus

c) A ventral or thalamocortical pathway that projects to the cerebral cortex via the subthalamus, posterior hypothalamus, basal forebrain, and septum

d) A midline pathway that projects directly to the cerebral cortex

495. Which of the following statements regarding the neurotransmitter glycine is NOT true?

a) It is released during REM sleep.

b) It is the main inhibitory neurotransmitter in the spinal cord

c) It causes REM sleep-related paralysis via hyperpolarization of spinal motoneurons.

d) It is released during NREM sleep.

496. What modality for positive airway pressure therapy provides variable pressures using device-specific diagnostic and therapeutic algorithms?

a) Continuous positive airway pressure

b) Bilevel positive airway pressure

c) Autotitrating positive airway pressure

d) Nocturnal noninvasive positive pressure ventilation

497. Which of the following is an efferent suprachiasmatic nucleus neurotransmitter?

a) Acetylcholine

b) Glutamate

c) Histamine

d) Transforming growth factor-α

498. Lesions involving which respiratory neuron group result in apneustic breathing?

a) Dorsal respiratory group

b) Ventrolateral reticular formation

c) Pontine respiratory group

d) Nucleus ambiguus

499. Which of the following statements regarding the relationship between growth hormone and sleep is correct?

a) Growth hormone (GH)–releasing hormone increases NREM stages 3 and 4 sleep.

b) In young healthy adults, the daily peak in growth hormone (GH) secretion occurs during the second half of the sleep period.

c) Release of GH is linked to sleep, occurring among adults during NREM stages 3 and 4 sleep and does not occur without NREM stages 3 and 4 sleep.

d) There may be several peaks in GH secretion in men throughout the day and night.

500. Which of the following factors decrease REM sleep latency?

a) Mirtazapine

b) Narcolepsy

c) Nefazodone

d) Trazodone

501. Which of the following agents can increase the percentage of REM sleep?

a) Lithium

b) Mirtazapine

c) Monoamine oxidase inhibitors

d) Reserpine

502. A patient whose obstructive sleep apnea occurred predominantly during a supine sleep position is advised to try sleep-position therapy by another sleep physician. He has consulted you for a second opinion. On reviewing his polysomnographic data, you note that his total apnea hypopnea index (AHI) is 18 events per hour. A majority of the respiratory events consist of obstructive hypopneas. Supine AHI is 42 events per hour, and nonsupine AHI is 4 events per hour. Snoring is present in both supine and nonsupine sleep positions. Which is the most appropriate statement to tell your patient?

a) Positional sleep apnea has been defined as obstructive sleep apnea in which the supine sleep-related AHI is at least twice that during sleep in a nonsupine (eg, lateral recumbency) position.

b) Patients with positional sleep apnea are more likely to be more overweight.

c) Patients with positional sleep apnea are more likely to have higher AHIs.

d) Long-term adherence to sleep-position therapy is excellent and the enduring efficacy of sleep-position therapy is well established.

503. **Which of the following does the American Academy of Sleep Medicine NOT consider an effective intervention for treating bedtime problems and night wakings in young children?**

a) Unmodified extinction and extinction of undesired behavior with parental presence

b) Graduated extinction of undesired behavior

c) Paradoxical intention

d) Delayed bedtime with removal from bed, and positive bedtime routines

504. **Which of the following dopaminergic agents used for the therapy of restless legs syndrome (RLS) is most likely to give rise to augmentation (ie, RLS symptoms develop earlier in the evening or afternoon, are more severe compared to baseline prior to therapy, or affect other body parts including the upper extremities)?**

a) Carbidopa/levodopa

b) Pergolide

c) Pramipexole

d) Ropinirole

505. **Benzodiazepines act via the gamma-aminobutyric acid-A receptor complex, which consists of several benzodiazepine receptors. Which of the following receptors is primarily related to sedation?**

a) BZ1

b) BZ2

c) BZ3

d) BZ4

506. **Which of the following statements regarding prolactin levels during sleep is correct?**

a) Peak levels occur during the first half of the evening following the onset of sleep.

b) Secretion increases during REM sleep.

c) Secretion is suppressed by sleep fragmentation.

d) Administration of benzodiazepines can decrease prolactin secretion during sleep.

507. **Which of the following statements regarding dreaming is correct?**

a) Dreaming occurs only during REM sleep.

b) Compared with REM sleep-related dreams that tend to be more complex and irrational, NREM dreams are generally simpler and more realistic.

c) According to the cognitive theory of dreaming, dreaming is produced by cortical interpretation of randomly generated intrinsic subcortical activity.

d) In the activation synthesis theory, dreaming is considered an extension of awake thought that are governed by different processes.

508. **For which of the following disorders is an overnight polysomnography routinely indicated?**

a) Circadian rhythm sleep disorders

b) Narcolepsy

c) Restless legs syndrome

d) Stable asymptomatic obstructive sleep apnea treated with continuous positive airway pressure therapy

509. **Which of the following is a consequence of sleep deprivation in animal models?**

a) Weight gain due to high amounts of food intake

b) Decrease in metabolic rate

c) Decrease in plasma norepinephrine levels

d) Decrease in body temperature

510. **Which of the following is NOT an indication for terminating a Multiple Sleep Latency Test?**

a) No sleep recorded for 20 minutes

b) After at least 15 minutes after NREM sleep is recorded

c) After three consecutive epochs of NREM sleep

d) After the first epoch of unequivocal REM sleep

511. **Which of the following is a metabolic and endocrinologic consequence of sleep deprivation in humans?**

a) Decrease in evening levels of cortisol

b) Increase in levels of ghrelin and leptin

c) Blunting of sleep-dependent secretion of growth hormone and prolactin

d) Increase in metabolic rate and levels of thyroxine

512. **Which of the following is NOT an efferent projection of the suprachiasmatic nucleus?**

a) Hypothalamus

b) Locus ceruleus

c) Pineal gland

d) Retina

513. **Which of the following mechanisms does NOT contribute to the reduction of urine volume that occurs during sleep?**

a) Decrease in glomerular filtration

b) Increase in release of rennin

c) Increase in water reabsorption

d) Decrease in renal circulation

514. **Compared with wakefulness, NREM sleep is characterized by which of the following?**

a) Increase in sympathetic tone

b) Decrease in parasympathetic tone

c) Decrease in blood pressure but no change in heart rate

d) Vasoconstriction

515. **According to the 1999 Academy of Sleep Medicine Practice parameters for the use of light therapy for the treatment of sleep disorders, light therapy appears to have potential utility for the treatment of the following disorders EXCEPT:**

a) Delayed sleep phase syndrome

b) Advanced sleep phase syndrome

c) Dementia

d) Jet lag for travelers across multiple time zones

516. **Which of the following statements best describes the phenomenon of nocturnal blood pressure "dipping?"**

a) Nighttime systolic blood pressure decreases by about 10% compared with daytime values.

b) Nighttime systolic blood pressure decreases by about 20% compared with daytime values.

c) Nighttime mean blood pressure decreases by about 20% compared with daytime values.

d) Nighttime diastolic blood pressure decreases by about 10% compared with daytime values.

517. **Which of the following patient groups is most likely to benefit from paradoxical intention therapy for insomnia?**

a) Patients with secondary insomnia

b) Patients with insomnia related to mood disorders

c) Patients with psychophysiologic insomnia

d) Specific subsets of patients with insomnia that would respond to this therapy have not been defined

518. **Which of the following statements regarding respiration during sleep is correct?**

a) There is a greater reduction in hypoxic and hypercapnic ventilatory responses during REM sleep than during NREM sleep.

b) Upper airway muscle tone is diminished during sleep.

c) There is no significant change in ventilatory response to added inspiratory resistance during sleep as compared with wakefulness.

d) A greater fall in hypoxic drive from wakefulness to sleep is present in women than in men.

519. **Which of the following statements regarding the changes in cardiovascular parameters during NREM sleep relative to wakefulness is true?**

a) Marked reduction in stroke volume

b) Marked reduction in peripheral vascular resistance

c) Increase in coronary circulation

d) No significant change in renal circulation or splanchnic circulation

520. **Which of the following statements best describes the synthesis and metabolism of melatonin?**

a) Secretion of melatonin is greatest during the daytime.

b) Melatonin secretion is suppressed at night.

c) Exposure to light inhibits melatonin secretion.

d) Production of melatonin is unchanged with aging.

521. **What is the most common cause of excessive sleepiness in children?**

a) Inadequate sleep duration

b) Obstructive sleep apnea

c) Delayed sleep phase syndrome

d) Narcolepsy

522. A 72-year-old male presents with complaints of early morning awakenings. He reports getting sleepy in the early evening, which prompts him to go to bed regularly at 8:30 PM and awakening between 3:30 and 4:00 AM. He is unable to delay his bedtime despite drinking coffee with supper. His wife, who has accompanied him, reports that he often gets out of bed at 4:00 AM each day and reads a book until she gets out of bed at 6:30 AM. You diagnose him as having an advanced sleep phase syndrome. Which of the following is an appropriate recommendation regarding therapy?

    a) Bright light therapy during the early evening (7:00 to 9:00 PM) after the body temperature nadir

    b) Restricting light exposure in the evening

    c) Gradually shifting the usual sleep time until the desired bedtime is achieved

    d) Administration of melatonin during the evening

523. According to the Rechtschaffen and Kales criteria for scoring REM sleep, which of the following statements is correct?

    a) Electroencephalography (EEG), electromyography (EMG), and electro-oculography features change simultaneously at the start and end of REM periods.

    b) Any epoch contiguous with stage REM sleep with an EEG showing a relatively low-amplitude, mixed-frequency activity is scored as REM sleep if the EMG shows atonia or hypotonia and if no intervening arousals occur, whether or not rapid eye movements are observed.

    c) If an arousal occurs at the transition between NREM and REM sleep, the epochs prior to the arousal are considered stage wake even if REM-like EEG and EMG consistent with stage REM sleep are present.

    d) If an arousal occurs at the transition between NREM and REM sleep, the epochs prior to the arousal with REM-like EEG and EMG are considered stage REM sleep even if the arousal occurred less than 3 minutes after a sleep spindle or K-complex.

524. Which of the following statements best describe melatonin?

    a) It is released by the pineal gland.

    b) Neurotransmitter release occurs during the day.

    c) Neurotransmitter release is stimulated by light.

    d) Melatonin receptors are present only in the hypothalamus.

525. Which of the following neural systems that regulate NREM sleep is responsible for generating sleep spindles?

    a) Basal forebrain

    b) Reticular nucleus of the thalamus

    c) Solitary tract nuclei

    d) Ventrolateral preoptic area

526. Which of the following medications is considered the first-line therapy for both restless legs syndrome and periodic limb movement disorder?

    a) Benzodiazepines

    b) Dopaminergic agents

    c) Iron supplementation

    d) Opioids

527. Which of the following statements about the clinical course of narcolepsy is correct?

    a) Onset is generally during adolescence and early adulthood, between of 15 and 25 years of age.

    b) Cataplexy is often the first symptom to appear.

    c) Severity and frequency of cataplexy is generally persistent and unrelenting.

    d) Excessive sleepiness waxes and wanes over time.

528. Which of the following is NOT a common polysomnographic feature of obsessive-compulsive disorder?

    a) Decrease in sleep efficiency

    b) Decrease in total sleep time

    c) Decrease in NREM stages 3 and 4 sleep

    d) Increase in REM sleep latency

529. Which of the following statements regarding the irregular sleep-wake pattern is true?

    a) Sleep and wake times are disorganized with three or more short "naps" comprising the fragmentary remnants of the major sleep episode.

    b) Although sleep is disorganized within a 24-hour day, there is consistency in sleep and wake activity from one day to the next.

    c) The aggregate sleep time over a 24-hour period is generally decreased for age.

    d) The disorder is common in the general population and is most frequently encountered during adolescence and early adulthood.

530. Which of the following is associated with tonic REM sleep?

    a) Increase in heart rate relative to NREM sleep

    b) Increase in peripheral vascular resistance relative to NREM sleep

    c) Increase in systemic blood pressure relative to NREM sleep

    d) Unchanged or slight increase in splanchnic, renal, or skeletal circulation relative to NREM sleep

531. Which of the following hormones is NOT reduced with aging?

    a) Growth hormone

    b) Melatonin

    c) Prolactin

    d) Testosterone (males)

532. Which of the following statements regarding differences in narcolepsy in between children and adults is correct?

    a) Whereas adults often present initially with excessive sleepiness, most children with narcolepsy initially manifest with problematic nightwakings.

    b) Children with narcolepsy generally require shorter naps than adults with narcolepsy.

    c) Several polysomnographic studies performed over several months to years may be required for diagnosis in children with suspected narcolepsy.

    d) Multiple sleep latency test parameters for children are similar to those for adults.

533. Which of the following muscle groups is NOT spared during episodes of sleep paralysis?

    a) Ocular muscles

    b) Postural muscles

    c) Respiratory muscles

    d) Sphincter muscles

534. Many changes in sleep develop with normal aging. Which of the following phrases regarding sleep in older adults is correct?

    a) Decreased strength of homeostatic sleep drive

    b) Lower prevalence of insomnia

    c) Increase in risk of developing delayed sleep phase syndrome

    d) Increase in arousal threshold with less sensitivity to adverse environmental factors, such as noise

535. Which of the following statements regarding tricyclic antidepressants is correct?

    a) These agents can precipitate or exacerbate periodic limb movements during sleep but not restless legs syndrome.

    b) They can cause abnormal dreams and nightmares.

    c) Protriptyline can decrease upper airway muscle tone.

    d) Sudden drug withdrawal can decrease REM sleep.

536. In free-running or non-entrained type (non–24-hour sleep-wake disorder or hypernyctohemeral syndrome), there is abnormal synchronization between the endogenous sleep-wake circadian rhythm and the 24-hour environmental light-dark cycle. Which of the following statements about this disorder is correct?

    a) Free-running internal rhythms behave with a periodicity of slightly less than 24 hours.

    b) Sleep onset and wake times occur about 1 hour or more earlier each day.

    c) The relationship between the external 24-hour world and the internal 25-hour clock then tends to vary from one extreme of total asynchrony to the other extreme of complete conformity.

    d) Because of the shortened circadian sleep-wake rhythm, sleep duration is generally decreased even if patients are allowed to sleep *ab libitum*.

537. Which of the following is NOT an oropharyngeal and palatal dilator muscle?

    a) Genioglossus

    b) Sternohyoid

    c) Levator veli palatini

    d) Sternomastoid

538. Which of the following characterizes respiration during REM sleep?

    a) Regular pattern of respiration

    b) Atonia or hypotonia of the intercostal muscles

    c) Diminished activity of the phrenic motor neurons innervating the diaphragm

    d) Decrease in $PaCO_2$ and increase in PaO_2 relative to wakefulness and NREM sleep

539. Compared with the dopamine agonists (eg, ropinirole and pramipexole), carbidopa/levodopa has which of the following characteristics?

a) Similar onset of action

b) Longer duration of action

c) Greater likelihood of giving rise to augmentation

d) More effective in controlling symptoms of restless legs syndrome

540. **Which of the following statements characterize sleep in the postpartum period?**

a) Frequency of napping is increased.

b) Nighttime sleep efficiency is increased.

c) Primiparas (first-time mothers) have less sleep disruption, greater total sleep time, and higher sleep efficiency than multiparas.

d) Sleep disruption is less severe after delivery by cesarean section than after vaginal delivery.

541. **Children with circadian rhythm disorders have sleep periods occurring at inappropriate times relative to the desired, conventional, or socially acceptable bedtimes. Which of the following statements regarding circadian rhythm disorders is NOT true?**

a) Onset of delayed sleep-phase syndrome is often during early childhood.

b) The preadolescent child often has a mild degree of phase-advancement in their sleep schedules.

c) Irregular sleep wake schedule is common among newborn infants and is not considered pathologic until after 6 months of age when consolidation of nighttime sleep develops.

d) Non–24-hour sleep wake disorder is more commonly observed in blind children.

542. **You have received an e-mail message from a woman who has been informed by her primary care physician that you have an interest in sleep medicine and that you are planning to take the Sleep Medicine Board Examination. She wants to know if she would require therapy for her nightly sleep talking. Which of the following statements is an appropriate reply to her inquiry?**

a) Sleep talking or vocalization or utterance of sounds, words, or sentences during sleep can occur in all stages of sleep but is most commonly described in REM sleep related to dream sequences.

b) It affects all age groups and is more prevalent among women.

c) There is a significant genetic influence in childhood sleep talking but not in adult cases.

d) Sleep disorders, such as obstructive sleep apnea, REM sleep behavior disorder, sleep terrors, and confusional arousals, can trigger sleep talking.

543. **Which of the following statements regarding the changes in blood pressure and heart rate during each episode of obstructive sleep apnea is correct?**

a) Respiratory efforts against an occluded upper airway can result in a increase in intrathoracic pressure, which, in turn, can give rise to reductions in blood pressure and cardiac output.

b) Systemic and pulmonary artery blood pressures falls as apnea progresses, reaching their nadir in the immediate postapneic period.

c) Relative bradycardia may develop during airway obstruction followed by tachycardia during termination of apnea.

d) Events occurring during NREM sleep tend to be longer in duration and associated with greater falls in oxygen saturation.

544. **Which of the following best describes the polysomnographic features of shift work sleep disorder compared to normal adults?**

a) No change in sleep latency

b) No change in total sleep time

c) No change in sleep efficiency

d) Increase in frequency of arousals

545. **Anatomic abnormalities of the upper airway may predispose to the development of obstructive sleep apnea. Which of the following features is NOT associated with Crouzon syndrome?**

a) Choanal stenosis

b) Maxillary hypoplasia

c) Posterior displacement of the tongue

d) Shortened soft palate

546. **Which of the following factors does NOT increase the risk of developing sleep paralysis?**

a) Irregular sleep patterns (eg, shift work)

b) Prone sleep position

c) Sleep deprivation

d) Use of anxiolytic agents

547. The prevalence of nocturia, or frequent voiding during the night, increases among older adults. The mechanisms responsible for this include which one of the following?

    a) Increase in urinary bladder capacity

    b) Lesser urine production

    c) Increase in urinary concentrating ability

    d) Detrusor overactivity

548. Which of the following dopaminergic agents used for the therapy of restless legs syndrome has been associated with the development of pleuropulmonary and cardiac valve fibrosis?

    a) Bromocriptine

    b) Pergolide

    c) Pramipexole

    d) Ropinirole

549. Which of the following phrases about nightmares is NOT correct?

    a) Difficulty returning to sleep

    b) Full alertness on awakening

    c) Occurs only during REM sleep

    d) Vivid recall of the preceding dream

550. Which of the following is a polysomnographic feature of secondary amine tricyclic antidepressants?

    a) Decrease in sleep latency

    b) No change in NREM stages 3 and 4 sleep

    c) Decrease in REM sleep latency

    d) Increase in REM sleep

551. Which of the following interventions is NOT recommended for patients on shift work schedules?

    a) Administration of psychostimulants (eg, modafinil) during evening work hours

    b) Bright lights in the nighttime workplace

    c) High ambient temperature in the workplace

    d) Scheduled napping at work

552. Which of the following is an effect of benzodiazepine receptor agonists on sleep architecture?

    a) Decrease in sleep latency

    b) Decrease in frequency of awakenings

    c) Increase in total sleep time

    d) Decrease in REM sleep (nonbenzodiazepine benzodiazepine receptor agonists such as zaleplon)

553. Interaction between the two components of the autonomic nervous system, namely the sympathetic nervous system and parasympathetic nervous system, influences the regulation of sleep and wakefulness. Which of the following statements about the autonomic nervous system is correct?

    a) The sympathetic nervous system originates in the brainstem and sacral portion of the spinal cord.

    b) An increase in sympathetic activity and a decrease in parasympathetic activity occurs during the transition from wakefulness to NREM sleep.

    c) A further decrease in parasympathetic activity and increase in sympathetic activity during REM sleep.

    d) There is a transient increase in sympathetic tone during phasic REM compared to tonic REM sleep.

554. Which of the following is NOT a consequence of sleep deprivation among humans?

    a) Sleepiness and an increase in homeostatic sleep drive

    b) Increase in polysomnographic slow wave activity and NREM stages 3 and 4 sleep

    c) Increase in morbidity and mortality

    d) Hypoactive deep tendon reflexes

555. Which of the following statements regarding the pathophysiology of obstructive sleep apnea (OSA) is correct?

    a) Severity of daytime sleepiness appears to correlate better with the apnea hypopnea index than the extent of sleep fragmentation.

    b) An obstructive apnea or hypopnea occurs when the forces that maintain upper airway patency such as activation of dilator muscles are insufficient to counteract the factors that promote upper airway closure during sleep (eg, negative intraluminal pressure).

    c) The upper airways of patients with OSA tend to be stiffer and less vulnerable to collapse compared to that among persons without this disorder.

    d) The critical closing pressure is the pressure at which collapse the upper airway occurs and is more negative among patients with OSA compared to normal persons.

556. Which of the following best describes sleep-related dissociative disorders?

    a) Abnormal behaviors tend to begin immediately with the arousal from sleep.

    b) Many patients have a history of psychiatric disorders.

    c) Men are affected more commonly then women.

    d) There is full memory of the event.

557. Loss of one of the following neuronal systems in the lateral hypothalamus is the major underlying mechanism responsible for narcolepsy?

    a) Cholinergic system

    b) Dopaminergic system

    c) Hypocretin system

    d) Monoamine system

558. At what age does sleep spindles first appear?

    a) 1 to 2 weeks

    b) 4 weeks to 3 months

    c) 3 to 6 months

    d) 12 months

559. Which of the following is NOT related to the use of benzodiazepines in patients with restless legs syndrome (RLS) and periodic limb movement disorder (PLMS)?

    a) Decrease PLMS-related complaints of insomnia and arousals

    b) Reduce frequency of leg movements

    c) Improve sleep quality in RLS

    d) Decrease RLS-related paresthesias and dysesthesias

560. Which of the following statements best describes the components of the suprachiasmatic nuclei?

    a) The core region has larger neurons compared to the shell region.

    b) The core region is located in the dorsolateral part of the suprachiasmatic nuclei.

    c) The neurotransmitter of the core region is vasoactive intestinal peptide.

    d) The shell region resets the endogenous circadian rhythms.

561. Which of the following factors is NOT important in determining the susceptibility to developing time zone change (jet lag) syndrome?

    a) Direction of travel

    b) Time (daytime versus nighttime) of departure

    c) Amounts and rates of time zone transitions

    d) Age

562. Which of the following statements regarding cortisol and its relationship to sleep is correct?

    a) Secretion of cortisol appears to be linked to the circadian rhythm rather than to sleep.

    b) Sleep is associated with a modest increase in cortisol secretion.

    c) The nadir of cortisol levels occurs at midmorning.

    d) Sleep fragmentation and awakenings give rise to decreased secretion of cortisol.

563. Changes in respiration that accompanies NREM sleep include which of the following?

    a) Breathing is irregular in amplitude and frequency during NREM stages 3 and 4 sleep.

    b) Respiration is under the sole control of centrally driven metabolic processes.

    c) Periodic breathing, with hypopneas and hyperpneas, can occur at sleep onset and may persist until NREM stages 3 and 4 sleep.

    d) Increase in minute ventilation compared to wakefulness occurs during NREM sleep.

564. Which of the following statements best describes delayed sleep phase syndrome (DSPS)?

    a) Polysomnography, along with sleep diaries, is routinely indicated for the diagnosis of DSPS.

    b) Prevalence increases with aging and is highest among older adults.

    c) There is a delayed habitual bedtime coupled with an equally delayed arising time compared to conventional or socially acceptable sleep schedules.

    d) Patients also commonly have difficulty in remaining asleep (ie, sleep maintenance insomnia) following the onset of sleep.

565. Which of the following agents can be given during prolonged middle-of-the-night awakenings as long as there is at least 4 hours remaining prior to rising time?

    a) Eszopiclone

    b) Temazepam

    c) Zaleplon

    d) Zolpidem

566. A 36-year-old male was referred to your clinic for evaluation and management of snoring, witnessed apneas, and daytime sleepiness.

Past medical history is significant for hypothyroidism, rhinosinusitis, and depression. His medications consist of fluoxetine and levothyroxine. He smokes about a pack of cigarettes daily. He denies any alcohol or caffeine consumption. Family history includes a father and a brother with diagnosed obstructive sleep apnea.

An 11:00 PM bedtime and a 7:00 AM wake time are typical. He denies restless legs symptoms, periodic limb movements during his sleep, cataplexy, sleep paralysis, sleep-related hallucinations, or parasomnias.

Polysomnographic data reveal:

Total recording time	443 mutes
Total sleep time	219 mutes
Sleep efficiency	55%
Sleep latency	6 minutes

Baseline

Total apnea hypopnea index (AHI)	54.0 events per hour
Periodic limb movement index	1.2 events per hour
Lowest oxygen desaturation	83%

Continuous positive airway pressure titration

Pressure (cm H_2O)	AHI (events per hour)
5	63.2
7	51.7
11	14.2
13	11.0
15	0.4

You recommend a trial of continuous positive airway pressure (CPAP) therapy at 15 cm H_2O. Before agreeing to your advice, the patient wants to learn more about this form of treatment.

Which of the following statements about CPAP is correct?

a) Discontinuing CPAP use for several days is acceptable because beneficial effects of CPAP therapy are sustained over time.

b) CPAP therapy is indicated for all patients with an apnea hypopnea index greater than 5 events per hour.

c) Patterns of use can often be discerned within the first few days of initiating CPAP therapy.

d) CPAP therapy is not indicated in obstructive sleep apnea patients unless complaints of excessive daytime sleepiness are present.

567. Which of the following is the dominant zeitgeber for the circadian sleep-wake pacemaker?

a) Environmental light

b) Exogenous temperature

c) Meals

d) Social cues

568. Which of the following is NOT a known risk factor for sudden infant death syndrome?

a) Prematurity

b) Supine sleeping position

c) Pre- and postnatal exposure to tobacco smoke

d) Maternal substance abuse

569. Which of the following statements about the disorders of arousal is correct?

a) They occur out of NREM sleep, particularly stages 1 and 2 sleep.

b) They occur most commonly during the last third of the night.

c) They are most commonly encountered during middle to older adulthood, and their frequency increases with advancing age.

d) There is a strong familial pattern.

570. Most childhood cases of enuresis are primary. Which of the following statements regarding contributory factors for primary enuresis is NOT correct?

a) High nighttime urine volume due to exaggerated release of vasopressin during sleep.

b) Impaired arousal response secondary to very deep sleep.

c) Inappropriate or inadequate toilet training.

d) Residence in disorganized families.

571. Which of the following is a polysomnographic feature of tertiary amine tricyclic antidepressants?

a) Decrease in total sleep time

b) Increase in NREM stages 3 and 4 sleep

c) Decrease in REM sleep latency

d) Decrease in REM sleep

572. Which of the following statements about the suprachiasmatic nuclei is NOT correct?

a) Oscillate independently of the environment

b) Fire more frequently during the daytime compared to nighttime

c) Fire more frequently during NREM sleep compared to REM sleep and wakefulness

d) Promote wakefulness during the day and enhances sleep consolidation during the night

573. Which of the following was the first hypnotic agent that received U.S. Food and Drug Administration (FDA) approval without a restriction to short-term usage for chronic insomnia?

a) Eszopiclone

b) Trazodone

c) Zaleplon

d) Zolpidem

574. What is the NREM-REM cycle length during infancy?

a) 20 minutes

b) 50 minutes

c) 60 to 70 minutes

d) 90 to 120 minutes

575. Significant changes occur in the circadian regulation of sleep and wakefulness with aging. Which of the following phrases concerning circadian rhythms with aging is correct?

a) Increase in melatonin levels

b) Sleep onset and offset occurring later relative to melatonin secretion

c) Dampening of circadian sleep-wake rhythms

d) Compared with younger adults, zone of increased alertness may occur later after the nadir of core body temperature

576. What percentage of children with obstructive sleep apnea present with complaints of excessive sleepiness?

a) 95%

b) 50%

c) 30%

d) 10%

577. Which of the following statements about obstructive sleep apnea in children is true?

a) Pauses in breathing or reduction in airflow (> 30% to 50% relative to baseline) last two normal respiratory cycles or longer.

b) Five or more scorable respiratory events per hour of sleep is considered significant.

c) Increasingly positive esophageal pressure swings are present.

d) An association with electroencephalographic arousals occurring following apneas is necessary.

578. Which of the following ferritin levels is associated with fewer symptoms of restless legs syndrome and has been used as a goal for iron supplementation therapy?

a) Any normal value of ferritin

b) Ferritin levels between 10 and 30 µg/1

c) Ferritin levels between 30 and 50 µg/1

d) Ferritin levels greater than 50 µg/1

579. Psychiatric disorders can give rise to insomnia, excessive sleepiness, or parasomnias (eg, nightmares or sleep terrors). Which of the following psychiatric disorders is more likely to be associated with excessive sleepiness rather than insomnia?

a) Atypical depression

b) Generalized anxiety disorder

c) Major depression

d) Post-traumatic stress disorder

580. Which of the following statements regarding nefazodone's effect on sleep is correct?

a) Decrease in sleep efficiency

b) Increase in NREM stages 3 and 4 sleep

c) Increase in REM sleep latency

d) Decrease in REM sleep

581. Which of the following variables peak during the sleep phase?

    a) Body temperature

    b) Forced expiratory volume

    c) Insulin levels

    d) Growth hormone

582. A 64-year old male with a history of chronic obstructive pulmonary disease (COPD) and snoring is referred for a polysomnography for evaluation of a suspected obstructive sleep apnea syndrome. He was diagnosed with emphysema 8 years ago after presenting with progressive dyspnea and coughing. His forced expiratory volume in 1 second (FEV1) was 1.5 1during a recent pulmonary function test. Arterial blood gases performed on room air during his last office visit three months ago demonstrated a pH of 7.39, PaCO2 of 44 mm Hg, and a PaO2 of 53 mm Hg.

    Aside from COPD, the patient has a past medical history significant for hypertension and depression for which he takes a calcium channel blocker and a selective serotonin reuptake inhibitor, respectively. Another physician recommended continuous low-flow oxygen therapy several years ago, but the patient had declined this, explaining that this would restrict his activities. He reports a 40-pack year smoking history and currently averages a half pack of cigarettes daily. He consumes several cans of beer on weekends and does not drink coffee, tea, or soda. Exercise is limited to walking his Maltese dog around the block twice each day.

    Examination findings are notable for moderate obesity, low-lying palate, prominent P2, diminished breath sounds with no wheezing, a slightly distended abdomen, and pedal edema.

    Polysomnographic data reveal:

Total recording time	443 minutes
Total sleep time	306 minutes
Sleep efficiency	69%
Sleep latency	38 minutes

Total AHI	37.6 events per hour
Supine AHI	51.2 events per hour
Non-supine AHI	18.0 events per hour
NREM AHI	34.1 events per hour

REM AHI	64.0 events per hour

Periodic limb movement index	3.2 events per hour
Lowest oxygen desaturation	96%

Which of the following statements about the relationship between obstructive sleep apnea (OSA) and COPD is correct?

    a) OSA has a more severe course in individuals with coexisting COPD.

    b) Sleep-related PaO_2 is similar in patients with both OSA and COPD compared to those with COPD alone.

    c) There is no significant difference in $PaCO_2$ in patients with OSA and COPD compared to those with COPD alone.

    d) Pulmonary artery mean pressure is lower in patients with OSA and COPD compared to those with COPD alone.

583. Which of the following agents enhance REM sleep?

    a) Cholinergic medications

    b) Lithium

    c) Monoaminergic medications

    d) Selective serotonin reuptake inhibitors

584. Which of the following adverse effects led to the withdrawal of pemoline from the market?

    a) Cardiac toxicity

    b) Hepatic toxicity

    c) Pulmonary toxicity

    d) Renal toxicity

585. Which of the following statements is NOT true about dim light melatonin onset?

    a) Generally occurs 2 to 3 hours after bedtime in normally entrained persons

    b) Is commonly > 3 and 10 pg/ml for salivary and plasma melatonin, respectively

    c) Is the time when melatonin levels starts to rise

    d) Is used to estimate the timing of circadian rhythms

586. **Which of the following phrases best describes the agent ecstasy?**
    a) Chemically related to modafinil
    b) Produces an increase in REM sleep
    c) No changes in sleep latency associated with use
    d) Causes a decrease in total sleep time

587. **Which of the following phrases about chloral hydrate is correct?**
    a) Acts via histamine receptors
    b) Causes a decrease in sleep latency
    c) Extremely long half-life
    d) No change in total sleep time

588. **Which of following refers to the time interval between two consecutive events in a cycle?**
    a) Acrophase
    b) Amplitude
    c) Period length
    d) Phase

589. **Which of the following is associated with the administration of haloperidol?**
    a) No consistent changes in sleep latency
    b) No consistent changes in sleep efficiency
    c) No consistent changes in total sleep time
    d) No consistent changes in NREM stages 3 and 4 sleep

590. **Which of the following levels of oxygen desaturation and hypercapnia related to respiratory events in children is considered significant?**
    a) Oxygen desaturation nadir < 92%, or change in oxygen desaturation nadir from baseline by greater than 4%
    b) Maximal end-tidal CO_2 > 45 to 50 mm Hg
    c) Increase in end-tidal CO_2 > 45 mm Hg for greater than 20% of total sleep time
    d) Increase in end-tidal CO_2 > 50 mm Hg for greater than 5% of total sleep time

591. **What is the term that describes the maximal excursion of a cycle from peak to trough?**
    a) Acrophase
    b) Amplitude
    c) Mesor
    d) Nadir

592. **Mirtazapine's effects on sleep architecture include which of the following?**
    a) Increase in sleep latency
    b) Increase in total sleep time
    c) Decrease in sleep efficiency
    d) Decrease in REM sleep latency

593. **A 35-year-old gentleman presents with complaints of daytime sleepiness if he sleeps less than 10 hours during a 24-hour period. He states that this started during his childhood. His polysomnography documents normal sleep efficiency, an increase in total sleep time (11 hours), normal amounts of NREM stages 3 and 4 sleep, and increases in NREM stage 2 and REM sleep. Mean sleep latency on the Multiple Sleep Latency Test (MSLT) is normal. The most likely diagnosis is:**
    a) Idiopathic hypersomnia
    b) Insufficient sleep syndrome
    c) Long sleeper
    d) Narcolepsy

594. **Which of the following abnormalities has NOT been described in animal models of narcolepsy?**
    a) Canine mutations of hypocretin receptor-2 gene (Hcrt2) in lateral hypothalamic neurons
    b) Hypocretin knockout rodents with null mutation of the preprohypocretin gene
    c) Autosomal dominant mode of inheritance of narcolepsy in canine models
    d) Increase in pontine cholinergic M_2 muscarinic receptors, and basal ganglia and amygdala M_1 receptors in narcoleptic dogs

595. **What is the annual spontaneous cure rate of primary sleep enuresis in children?**
    a) 5%
    b) 10%
    c) 15%
    d) 25%

596. **Which of the following parasomnias is NOT classified as a disorder of arousal?**

a)   Confusional arousals

b)   Sleep-related eating disorder

c)   Sleep terrors

d)   Sleepwalking

597. **Which of the following statements about sleep during pregnancy, labor, and delivery is true?**

a)   Increase in levels of progesterone during pregnancy can give rise to insomnia.

b)   Estrogen increases REM sleep.

c)   Significant nighttime oxygen desaturation occurs in most pregnant women.

d)   Shorter nighttime sleep duration in the period before labor and delivery is associated with longer labor and increased likelihood of cesarean delivery.

598. **Which of the following statements regarding parasomnias is correct?**

a)   They are undesirable physical phenomena or behavior that develop predominantly or exclusively during the sleep period.

b)   They are associated with abnormalities of the states of sleep and wakefulness.

c)   They are associated with major complaints of excessive sleepiness or insomnia.

d)   They occur only during the transition from wakefulness to sleep or vice versa.

599. **At what age do infants achieve nocturnal sleep consolidation (ie, ability to sleep through the night)?**

a)   6 to 9 months

b)   9 to 12 months

c)   12 to 15 months

d)   15 to 18 months

600. **Which of the following statements regarding the demographics of narcolepsy is correct?**

a)   Narcolepsy affects an estimated 0.05% of the general population in the United States.

b)   Prevalence is lower in Japan than in Israel.

c)   Onset is often during mid-adulthood in the third to fourth decades of life.

d)   Narcolepsy with cataplexy appears to affect females slightly more frequently than men.

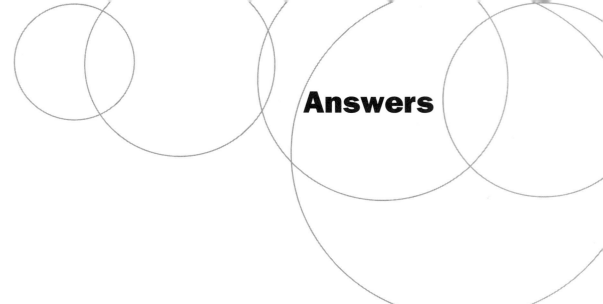

Answers

1. Answer: B

Educational objective: Distinguish the different types of apneas in adults.

Explanation: Apnea in an adult is defined as the absence of nasal and oral airflow for at least 10 seconds in duration. It is classified as central if respiratory efforts are absent, and as obstructive if cessation of airflow is noted despite the persistence of respiratory effort. A third type, mixed apnea, consists of an initial central apnea followed by an ineffectual respiratory effort consistent with obstructive apnea.

2. Answer: A

Educational objective: Describe the demographics of excessive sleepiness in the general population.

Explanation: Excessive sleepiness is estimated to affect 5% of the general population. Occasional excessive daytime sleepiness may be present in up to 33% of the general adult population. Among young adults, hours of weekday sleep predict daytime sleepiness, as does snoring, depression, marital state (those who are single are more likely to develop daytime sleepiness than married individuals) and employment status (sleepiness is more prevalent among persons employed full-time than among those who are employed part-time or are unemployed). Prevalence is greater among adolescents and older adults. Both genders appear to be affected equally.

3. Answer: A

Educational objective: Describe changes in sleep that accompany normal aging.

Explanation: Normal aging is associated with changes in sleep architecture. These include a decrease in sleep efficiency, an increase in frequency and duration of nighttime awakenings, and a decrease in NREM stages 3 and 4 and REM sleep. The decrease in daytime sleep latency on multiple sleep latency test is manifested by an increase in frequency of naps. Older men are less able to maintain satisfactory sleep compared to women.

4. Answer: A

Educational objective: Understand the demographic characteristics of restless legs syndrome.

Explanation: Restless legs syndrome can be seen in approximately 1% to 15% of individuals in the general population. Prevalence is increased with pregnancy, uremia, anemia, and rheumatoid arthritis. Women are affected more commonly than men are. Onset can occur at any age. Prevalence increases with aging, and is highest among middle-aged and elderly adults. Course is chronic but spontaneous remissions have been reported. A majority has concurrent periodic limb movements during sleep (PLMS). About 70% to 90% of patients with RLS have PLMS, but only about a third of patients with PLMS have RLS.

5. Answer: D

Educational objective: Identify the indications for specific therapy of parasomnias.

Explanation: Unless injurious or associated with significant distress, sleep disturbance or daytime impairment, parasomnias require no specific therapy. Known risk or precipitating factors should be avoided or eliminated. Instructions regarding proper sleep hygiene and safety issues are important.

6. Answer: D

Educational objective: Describe how the menstrual cycle affects sleep among women.

Explanation: The usual 28- to 30-day menstrual cycle is divided into two phases, each lasting about 14 to 15 days. The initial follicular phase starts on the first day of menses, and the second luteal phase begins at ovulation. Compared with the follicular phase, the luteal phase is associated with a longer sleep latency and lower sleep efficiency. During the luteal phase, there is an increase in sleep spindles and decrease in REM sleep.

7. Answer: B

Educational objective: Describe the clinical features of benign sleep myoclonus of infancy.

Explanation: Benign sleep myoclonus of infancy is characterized by recurrent, massive myoclonic jerks involving large muscle groups (ie, entire body, trunk or extremities) that occur only during sleep (predominantly during quiet sleep) among infants during the first year of life, usually from birth to 6 months of age. The muscle jerks are not associated with arousals or awakenings. It has a self-limited course with resolution by 6 months of age in most infants. Video-encephalographic (EEG) and electromyographic monitoring during polysomnography demonstrates muscle activity with a frequency of 4 to 5 jerks per second, occurring in clusters lasting 3 to 15 minutes. It is generally observed during quiet sleep but can sometimes occur during active sleep. No seizure activity is present on EEG tracings.

8. Answer: C

Educational objective: Describe caffeine's effect on sleep and wakefulness.

Explanation: Caffeine is the most commonly used psychostimulant worldwide, being ingested as coffee, tea, caffeinated beverages, or caffeine tablets. Chemically classified as a methylxanthine, caffeine acts by antagonizing central nervous system adenosine receptors located on the basal forebrain neurons. Adenosine is a sleep-promoting neurotransmitter. Caffeine may also increase cortical release of acetylcholine and affect the GABAergic neurons located in the posterior hypothalamus. Caffeine can increase wakefulness and alertness as well as decrease drowsiness during sleep deprivation. Insomnia can occur following ingestion of large quantities of caffeine. Excessive sleepiness can develop during withdrawal following chronic large-quantity caffeine use. Polysomnographic features during caffeine ingestion include an increase in sleep latency, a decrease in total sleep time, an increase in frequency of arousals, an increase in NREM stage 1 sleep, a decrease in NREM stages 3 and 4 sleep, and a decrease in REM sleep.

9. Answer: D

Educational objective: Identify the different sleep-related movement disorders.

Explanation: Sleep-related movement disorders are simple, often stereotypical, movements that can give rise to sleep disturbance. In contrast, parasomnias consist of relatively complex, apparently purposeful, behavior or movements, The American Academy of Sleep Medicine 2005 International Classification of Sleep Disorders Diagnostic and Coding Manual classifies the following disorders as sleep-related movement disorders, namely restless legs syndrome, periodic limb movement disorder, sleep-related leg cramps, sleep-related bruxism, and sleep-related rhythmic movement disorder. Sleepwalking is considered a NREM parasomnia.

10. Answer: D

Educational objective: Know the American Academy of Sleep Medicine Practice Parameters for the Treatment of Narcolepsy.

Explanation: The American Academy of Sleep Medicine (AASM) recommendations for the treatment of narcolepsy include:

1.   A diagnosis of narcolepsy must be established.
2.   Goals of therapy should be established for each patient.
3.   Regular follow-up is necessary to monitor response to treatment and address adverse effects of medications.
    a.   A health care provider should evaluate a patient stabilized on stimulant medication at least annually (preferably once every 6 months) to determine any adverse effects to the medication.
    b.   Follow-up is necessary to assess treatment adherence, efficacy, and safety, and to assist the patient with occupational and social difficulties.
    c.   Until sleepiness is appropriately controlled by stimulants, patients should be advised to avoid potentially dangerous activities, including operating a motor vehicle.
    d.   Amphetamines, especially at high doses, are the most likely of the stimulants used for narcolepsy to lead to tolerance.
    e.   Failure to respond to adequate doses of stimulants should prompt assessment for other sleep disorders that may contribute to excessive sleepiness.
    f.   Clinicians are advised to refer to appropriate sources for up-to-date information on drugs useful for narcolepsy including their adverse effects, dosage ranges, and use during pregnancy and nursing.
    g.   Methylphenidate appears relatively safe for treatment of narcolepsy in children between the ages of 6 and15 years. Caution must be exercised regarding the use of other medications for narcolepsy in this age group.
    h.   Patients should be provided assistance for specific narcolepsy-related disabilities.
    i.   Repeat polysomnography is indicated if there is a significant increase in sleepiness, or if new or worsening sleep abnormalities (eg, obstructive sleep apnea or periodic limb movement disorder) are suspected.
4.   Scheduled naps are useful to combat sleepiness but are seldom sufficient as primary therapy.
5.   The following medications are effective treatments for patients with narcolepsy:
    a.   Modafinil for daytime sleepiness
    b.   Amphetamine, methamphetamine, dextroamphetamine, and methylphenidate for daytime sleepiness
    c.   Selegiline for all narcoleptic symptoms

d. Tricyclic antidepressants and fluoxetine for cataplexy, sleep paralysis, and hypnagogic hallucinations

e. Combinations of long- and short-acting stimulants may be effective for some patients.

f. Pemoline for daytime sleepiness (Note: Pemoline has been withdrawn from the market due to concerns regarding hepatotoxicity.)

(From Littner, et al. Practice parameters for the treatment of narcolepsy: an update for 2000. Sleep. 2001;24(4).

11. Answer: B

Educational objective: *Identify when the adult pattern of NREM sleep during sleep onset first develops.*

Explanation: *In infants less than 3 months of age, the initial sleep episode is REM sleep. NREM sleep generally becomes the initial sleep episode by 3 to 4 months of age.*

12. Answer: D

Educational objective: *Understand the possible genetic mechanisms associated with restless legs syndrome.*

Explanation: *A positive family history can be elicited in up to 92% of persons with idiopathic restless legs syndrome (RLS) and in about 13% of persons with secondary RLS. An estimated one-third of cases of RLS is associated with an autosomal dominant mode of transmission. There is a high concordance rate of RLS symptoms between twins. RLS is more frequent in first- and second-degree relatives of individuals with RLS.*

13. Answer: B

Educational objective: *Understand the biphasic effect of alcohol ingestion on nighttime sleep.*

Explanation: *Alcohol has both stimulatory effects (at low doses and on the rising phase of alcohol levels) and sedative effects (at high doses and on the falling phase of alcohol levels). Alcohol's sedating effect can be additive with other agents such as benzodiazepines. Acute ingestion decreases sleep latency, increases NREM stages 3 and 4 sleep, and reduces REM sleep during the first half of the sleep period. Alcohol causes a rebound increase in the frequency of arousals and awakenings, and increase in REM sleep during the second part of the night.*

14. Answer: A

Educational objective: *Know which antidepressant agents can cause restless legs syndrome or aggravate an existing restless legs disorder.*

Explanation: *Selective serotonin reuptake inhibitors, tricyclic antidepressants, and lithium may precipitate or exacerbate restless legs syndrome or periodic limb movements during sleep. Bupropion, on the other hand, has no significant effect on these two disorders.*

15. Answer: A

Educational objective: *Describe the demographic characteristics of obstructive sleep apnea.*

Explanation: *Obstructive sleep apnea (OSA) is most prevalent between the fifth and seventh decades. It is more common in men than in women with a ratio of 2–10:1. Prevalence in women increases with menopause. Greater prevalence of OSA has also been reported among African Americans, Pacific Islanders, and Mexican Americans compared with Caucasians. Prevalence increases with age.*

16. Answer: B

Educational objective: *Describe the clinical features of Alzheimer disease.*

Explanation: *Alzheimer disease is the most common degenerative disorder of the central nervous system that causes dementia. Fragmentation and repetitive arousals/awakenings characterize the sleep of persons with dementia. Confusion, agitation, and wandering can occur at night ("sun downing"), further contributing to sleep disruption. Reversal of the sleep-wake rhythms can be seen with patients complaining of nocturnal insomnia and excessive daytime sleepiness. Polysomnography may demonstrate decreases in REM sleep time and REM density. Sleep efficiency is often reduced.*

17. Answer: B

Educational objective: *Describe the pharmacologic features of tetrahydrocannabinol.*

Explanation: *Tetrahydrocannabinol (THC) is one of the active constituents found in marijuana. Administration of THC at low doses results in mild sedation. Higher doses can produce hallucinations. During administration at low doses, there is an increase in total sleep time, increase in NREM stages 3 and 4 sleep, and a mild decrease in REM sleep. At high doses (hallucinatory action), there is a reduction of both NREM stages 3 and 4 sleep and REM sleep. THC discontinuation is often associated with a decrease in total sleep time, increase in sleep latency, and increase in REM sleep.*

18. Answer: C

Educational objective: *Identify the medications that can increase or decrease REM sleep latency.*

Explanation: *Medications that can increase REM sleep latency include alcohol (acute ingestion), amphetamine, barbiturates, benzodiazepines, chlorpromazine, clonidine, doxepin, haloperidol, levodopa, lithium, loxapine, methylphenidate, mirtazapine, phenelzine, progesterone, scopolamine, selective serotonin reuptake inhibitors, trazodone, tricyclic antidepressants, and trifluoperazine. Medications that can decrease REM sleep latency include estrogen and reserpine.*

19. Answer: B

Educational objective: Describe the types of cardiac arrhythmias related to obstructive sleep apnea.

Explanation: Bradytachycardia generally occurs during episodes of obstructive sleep apnea, with relative bradycardia at the onset of apnea and relative tachycardia during arousals following apnea termination. Heart rate remains between 60 and 100 beats per minute in many patients. Some may develop heart blocks (second- or third-degree) or premature ventricular complexes.

20. Answer: D

Educational objective: Understand the effects of monoamine oxidase inhibitors on sleep.

Explanation: Monoamine oxidase (MAO) inhibitors act via inhibition of enzymes involved in the metabolism of norepinephrine, dopamine and serotonin. They are classified as either classic agents that cause irreversible enzyme inhibition (eg, phenelzine and tranylcypromine), or newer reversible agents (eg, brofaromine). MAO inhibitors are the most potent REM inhibitors. Polysomnographic features include decrease in total sleep time, increase in wake time after sleep onset, no change in NREM stages 3 and 4 sleep, and increase in REM sleep latency. REM sleep rebound can occur during drug withdrawal.

21. Answer: D

Educational objective: Describe the changes in sleep that develop during alcohol withdrawal.

Explanation: During alcohol withdrawal, there is a decrease in total sleep time, and increase in sleep latency, wake time after sleep onset, and REM sleep. REM sleep latency is decreased. NREM stages 3 and 4 sleep are reduced. Delirium tremens is associated with markedly decreased total sleep time.

22. Answer: D

Educational objective: Describe the clinical features of confusional arousals.

Explanation: Confusional arousals are characterized by episodes of confusion following spontaneous or forced arousals from sleep, typically from NREM stages 3 and 4 sleep. They usually occur in the first third of the night. Disorientation, confusion, inappropriate behavior (moving around in bed, thrashing, crying or sleep talking), amnesia for the event, and inconsolability are common. Other features include diminished vigilance and blunted response to s or external stimuli. Behavior may, at times, become violent. However, signs of fear or autonomic hyperactivity are minimal or absent. Episodes may last from several minutes to hours, with most spontaneously resolving within 5 to 15 minutes.

23. Answer: D

Educational objective: Differentiate the characteristics of napping in patients with narcolepsy and idiopathic hypersomnia.

Explanation: In idiopathic hypersomnia, unintended naps are longer and are typically less refreshing than in narcolepsy. Affected individuals often report difficulty awakening from sleep. Sleep onset REM periods (SOREMP) are more frequent in patients with narcolepsy.

24. Answer: B

Educational objective: Identify the risk factors for REM sleep behavior disorder.

Explanation: Male gender, aging and an underlying neurologic condition (Parkinson disease or multiple system atrophy) are important predisposing factors for REM sleep behavior disorder. REM sleep behavior disorder may be quite prevalent in Parkinson disease and parkinsonian disorders. Indeed, a substantial number of cases of REM sleep behavior disorder considered to be idiopathic may merely be an early manifestation of a parkinsonian disorder.

25. Answer: D

Educational objective: Understand the effects of selective serotonin reuptake inhibitors on sleep.

Explanation: Selective serotonin reuptake inhibitors (SSRIs) include citalopram, fluoxetine, fluvoxamine, paroxetine, and sertraline. Polysomnographic features include an increase in sleep latency, increase in frequency of awakenings, increase in wake time after sleep onset, decrease in sleep efficiency and decrease in total sleep time. There is an increase in REM sleep latency, decrease in REM sleep and increase in REM density. Fluvoxamine and paroxetine are among the most sedating SSRIs. Insomnia can develop during citalopram or fluoxetine administration. SSRIs can precipitate or worsen periodic limb movements of sleep and restless legs syndrome. SSRIs can also cause REM sleep behavior disorder. An increase in eye movements during NREM sleep (so called "Prozac eyes") has been described.

26. Answer: C

Educational objective: Identify when nighttime feedings can be discontinued in children.

Explanation: Nighttime feedings can be discontinued for most children 6 months of age or older.

27. Answer: B

Educational objective: Describe the clinical features of sudden unexplained nocturnal death syndrome.

Explanation: Sudden unexplained nocturnal death syndrome (SUNDS) is characterized by sudden death that occurs during sleep without any apparent cause. Victims are mostly healthy adult Southeast Asian males between the ages of 25 and 44 years. Witnessed reports include descriptions of moaning, thrashing, screaming, violent motor activity, perspiration, and labored breathing that usually last for a few minutes prior to death. Resuscitated victims have reported sensations of airway obstruction, chest discomfort or pressure, and numb or weak limbs. They are unresponsive and difficult to arouse during the event. Ventricular fibrillation has been described in cases of successful resuscitation or monitored death. However, some victims had no evidence of atherosclerotic coronary artery disease, myocarditis, cardiomyopathy, or congenital cardiac anomalies. Mutations in SCN5A, the gene known to cause Brugada syndrome, have been identified in some, but not all, families with SUNDS.

28. Answer: B

Educational objective: Enumerate the different factors that determine the severity of oxygen desaturation during sleep apnea.

Explanation: The following factors are associated with greater oxygen desaturation in sleep apnea: (1) lower baseline awake supine and sleep SaO_2, (2) longer duration of apnea or hypopnea, and shorter duration of ventilation between periods of apnea, (3) increase in percentage of sleep time with apneas or hypopneas, (4) lower functional residual capacity and expiratory reserve volume, and (5) presence of comorbid lung disorders such as chronic obstructive pulmonary disease. Oxygen desaturation is also more severe with apneas occurring during REM sleep than during NREM sleep and with obstructive apneas compared to central apneas.

29. Answer: D

Educational objective: Understand the changes in sleep that occur during abstinence from alcohol.

Explanation: Sleep disturbance, including insomnia, can persist during abstinence from alcohol. Total sleep time and NREM stages 3 and 4 sleep are reduced, and frequency of arousals is increased. Sleep disturbance can persist for several years following cessation of alcohol use.

30. Answer: A

Educational objective: Enumerate the medications that are effective in treating cataplexy, sleep paralysis, and sleep hallucinations.

Explanation: Medications capable of suppressing REM sleep (eg, selective serotonin reuptake inhibitors [SSRIs], non–tricyclic serotonin-norepinephrine reuptake inhibitors [venlafaxine], and tricyclic antidepressants [TCAs]) are generally used to treat cataplexy, sleep paralysis, and sleep hallucinations. Other medications that can be tried for persistent cases of cataplexy include carbamazepine, clonidine, gamma-hydroxybutyrate, monoamine oxidase

inhibitors, and viloxazine. SSRIs inhibit the processes that generate REM sleep. TCAs inhibit adrenergic uptake and the descending cholinergic pathways responsible for the production of cataplexy. Sudden discontinuation of medications used to treat cataplexy can give rise to status cataplecticus (continuous attack of cataplexy). Modafinil, a wakefulness promoting agent, has no effect on cataplexy, sleep paralysis or sleep hallucinations.

31. Answer: A

Educational objective: Describe the clinical features of upper airway resistance syndrome.

Explanation: Upper airway resistance syndrome describes a pattern of repetitive sleep-related episodes of increasing resistance in the upper airways with decreased inspiratory airflow, increased or constant respiratory effort, and arousals from sleep (respiratory effort related arousals). The apnea hypopnea index is less than five events per hour, and there is no accompanying oxygen desaturation. Snoring may or may not be present.

32. Answer: A

Educational objective: Identify the medications that can increase or decrease REM sleep.

Explanation: Medications that can increase REM sleep include acetylcholine, bupropion, carbachol, estrogen, methyldopa, nefazodone, physostigmine, reserpine and yohimbine. Medications that can decrease REM sleep include alcohol (acute ingestion), amphetamines, antihistamines, atropine, barbiturates, benzodiazepines, benztropine, beta-blockers, caffeine, carbamazepine, chlorpromazine, clonidine, corticosteroids, ethosuximide, haloperidol, lithium, loxapine, maprotiline, metoclopramide, narcotic agents (morphine), nicotine, phenelzine, phenytoin, progesterone, scopolamine, selective serotonin reuptake inhibitors (fluoxetine), selegiline, stimulants, tricyclic antidepressants (except trimipramine), trifluoperazine, trihexyphenidyl, and venlafaxine.

33. Answer: A

Educational objective: Understand which factors increase the risk of developing obstructive sleep apnea.

Explanation: The Multiple Sleep Latency Test may be indicated in patients with obstructive sleep apnea (OSA) whose sleepiness persists despite optimal continuous positive airway pressure therapy. Imaging studies, including lateral cephalometric views, computed tomography, or magnetic resonance imaging of the upper airways, may be required in patients with craniofacial syndromes or in whom surgical therapy is being considered. Thyroid function tests may be helpful in patients with a clinical history suggestive of hypothyroidism. None of these tests are routinely indicated in the evaluation of patients suspected of having OSA. A thorough physical examination should always be performed in patients with this disorder.

34. Answer: A

Educational objective: *Understand which factors increase the risk of developing obstructive sleep apnea.*

Explanation: *Patients with obstructive sleep apnea (OSA) often have a positive family history of the disorder. The risk of developing OSA is greater among offsprings and first-degree relatives of OSA patients. Male gender is a risk factor for the occurrence of adult OSA. Among women, menopause increases the predisposition for developing OSA. In contrast, there appears to be no gender difference in OSA prevalence among children. OSA is relatively more common during childhood (ages 3 to 5 years) than during adolescence and early adulthood. Prevalence progressively increases in middle-aged individuals until the sixth and seventh decade of life. Finally, prevalence may be higher among African Americans, Mexican Americans, and Pacific Islanders than among Caucasians.*

35. Answer: D

Educational objective: *Describe the pharmacologic features of opiates.*

Explanation: *Opiates, including codeine, heroin, methadone, morphine, oxycodone, and propoxyphene, are used primarily for analgesia. They can cause excessive sleepiness, and may exacerbate obstructive sleep apnea. They improve symptoms of restless legs syndrome. Polysomnographic features during opioid use include a decrease in sleep efficiency, increase in sleep fragmentation, decrease in total sleep time, decrease in NREM stages 3 and 4 sleep, and decrease in REM sleep. Opioid discontinuation can give rise to sleep disturbance, insomnia, and nightmares.*

36. Answer: A

Educational objective: *Identify the effects of hormonal agents on sleep.*

Explanation: *Hormonal agents, including estrogen and progesterone, can have profound effects on sleep. Polysomnographic features of estrogen administration include a decrease in sleep latency, increase in total sleep time, decrease in REM sleep latency and increase REM sleep. Polysomnographic features of progesterone use include an increase in REM sleep latency and decrease in REM sleep.*

37. Answer: D

Educational objective: *Describe the mechanisms by which obesity may cause obstructive sleep apnea.*

Explanation: *Excess weight can reduce upper airway caliber due to fat deposition, increase upper airway compliance (increase in collapsibility) due to a reduction in*

muscle tone, and decrease lung residual volume. All of these factors can increase the likelihood of developing obstructive sleep apnea.

38. Answer: C

Educational objective: *Describe the demographic characteristics of central sleep apnea.*

Explanation: *Central sleep apnea (CSA) can either result from failure of ventilatory drive (idiopathic form) or may be due to secondary causes, such as congestive heart failure or neurologic disorders. The true incidence of idiopathic CSA is not known but appears to be rare and is less common than secondary causes of CSA. Central apneas can also occur during sleep onset in otherwise healthy individuals and during sleep at high altitude. CSA is estimated to represent about 5% to 10 % of patients with sleep-related breathing disorders. Prevalence of CSA is greater among men and increases in middle-aged and older adults.*

39. Answer: B

Educational objective: *Describe the effects of trazodone on sleep.*

Explanation: *Trazodone blocks serotonin, alpha 1, and histamine receptors. It is also a serotonin reuptake inhibitor and serotonin-2 antagonist. Polysomnographic features include a decrease in sleep latency, increase in sleep efficiency, increase in total sleep time, and decrease in wake time after sleep onset. Trazodone is a sedating antidepressant that has been used to treat insomnia. Adverse effects include postural hypotension and priapism.*

40. Answer: C

Educational objective: *Understand the differences in patterns of alcohol use between alcohol-dependent sleep disorder and alcoholism.*

Explanation: *Persons with alcohol-dependent sleep disorder do not exhibit other patterns of behavior compatible with overt alcoholism, and appear to use alcohol only for its sedative effects. However, habitual use of alcohol a few hours prior to anticipated bedtime in an attempt to enhance sleep onset could paradoxically lead to insomnia. Attempts to abruptly terminate alcohol use can precipitate profound insomnia with frequent awakenings.*

41. Answer: B

Educational objective: *Identify at what age children first develop the ability to postpone voiding in response to a full bladder.*

Explanation: *By 18 months to 3 years of age, children develop the ability to postpone voiding in response to a full bladder, initially during wakefulness and eventually during sleep as well.*

42. Answer: B

Educational objective: *Describe the clinical features of nighttime fears among children.*

Explanation: *Nighttime fears of the dark or being left alone can result in significant bedtime resistance and problematic night wakings. Prevalence peaks between 3 and 6 years of age. Many of these fears are benign age-appropriate behaviors. They respond to reassurance and resolve spontaneously by 5 to 6 years of age. Parents should be instructed to avoid reacting excessively because this may reinforce their child's fears.*

43. Answer: A

Educational objective: *Describe the clinical features of sleepwalking.*

Explanation: *Sleepwalking or somnambulism refers to ambulation that occurs during sleep. It is considered a disorder of arousal. Sleepwalking is associated with an altered state of consciousness, diminished arousability, impaired judgment and inappropriate behavior (eg, climbing out of a window). It can either be calm, or agitated and violent. Autonomic activation is generally minimal. The sleepwalker's eyes are usually open (described as a blank stare) but attempts to communicate with the sleepwalker are generally unsuccessful. Some activities are highly elaborate, such as driving a car. The individual is typically confused when awakened from the episode, with partial or complete amnesia for the event. Sleepwalking is most commonly seen during the first third or first half of the night and typically originates from NREM stages 3 and 4 sleep. It can, however, occur throughout the entire sleep period in adults. A positive history of sleepwalking during childhood is present in most adult sleepwalkers. Conversely, adult sleepwalking is infrequent among those who had never walked in their sleep during childhood.*

44. Answer: C

Educational objective: *Distinguish antidepressant agents that are sedating from those that can potentially cause insomnia.*

Explanation: *Some antidepressants can disrupt sleep and cause insomnia (fluoxetine). Others are sedating and improve sleep (amitriptyline, doxepin, and trazodone).*

45. Answer: D

Educational objective: *Identify the factors that increase the risk of developing central sleep apnea.*

Explanation: *Factors that increase the risk of developing central sleep apnea (CSA) include a high CO_2 ventilatory drive; increased frequency of sleep-wake transitions; male gender (men are more likely to have central apneas due to a higher hypocapnic apneic threshold during NREM sleep); age (more common in older adults); and ascent to high altitude.*

46. Answer: D

Educational objective: *Enumerate the indications for autotitrating continuous positive airway pressure devices.*

Explanation: *Autotitrating continuous positive airway pressure (APAP) titration or treatment is not indicated for patients with congestive heart failure, significant respiratory diseases such as chronic obstructive pulmonary disease or daytime hypoxemia and respiratory failure from any cause, and nocturnal arterial oxygen desaturation secondary to disorders other than obstructive sleep apnea (eg, obesity hypoventilation syndrome). APAP may be used to determine a single continuous positive airway pressure (CPAP) during attended polysomnography for the therapy of OSA (APAP titration) or may be used in a self-adjusting mode for the therapy of OSA after an initial successful attended polysomnography-guided CPAP or APAP titration (APAP treatment).*

47. Answer: B

Educational objective: *Understand the relationship between excess body weight and the likelihood of developing obstructive sleep apnea.*

Explanation: *Excess body weight (overweight defined as a body mass index [BMI] $\geq$ 25 kg/m² and obese defined as BMI $\geq$ 30–40 kg/m²) is a major risk factor for OSA. The prevalence of OSA increases with greater excess body weight, and is especially high among morbidly obese persons. Other factors influencing the risk of OSA include fat skin fold thickness, intra-abdominal fat, and percentage of body fat. Excess body weight may be particularly important in persons without any apparent craniofacial or oropharyngeal features that would predispose them to developing OSA.*

Distribution of fat is important because central or nuchal obesity (increased waist-hip ratio and neck circumference) appears to correlate better with OSA severity than obesity in general (ie, body weight). The apnea hypopnea index is correlated with leptin levels. Excess body weight can contribute to the development of OSA either by fatty deposition in the upper airways leading to reduced airway size and decreased muscle tone, or by reducing lung volumes, which, in turn, decreases upper airway size.

48. Answer: A

Educational objective: *Describe the effects of bupropion on sleep.*

Explanation: *Bupropion, a dopamine and norepinephrine reuptake inhibitor, is alerting and can cause insomnia. Polysomnographic features include a decrease in NREM stage 2 sleep, increase in NREM stages 3 and 4 sleep, decrease in REM sleep latency, and increase in REM sleep. It has no significant effect on periodic leg movements of sleep.*

49. Answer: C

Educational objective: Describe the effects of antidepressant agents on REM sleep.

Explanation: Antidepressants (except nefazodone, bupropion, and mirtazapine) decrease REM sleep and increase REM sleep latency. Bupropion and nefazodone increase REM sleep. Sudden discontinuation of REM-suppressant antidepressants can lead to a rebound in REM sleep.

50. Answer: C

Educational objective: Know which agents can improve nocturnal sleep in patients with narcolepsy.

Explanation: Gamma-hydroxybutyrate or a hypnotic agent can be used to treat nocturnal sleep disturbance and consolidate nocturnal sleep in patients with narcolepsy. Gamma-hydroxybutyrate (sodium oxybate), a gamma aminobutyric (GABA) precursor, increases sleep continuity and decreases the frequency of cataplexy in persons with narcolepsy. Gradual and mild improvement in daytime sleepiness has also been reported with chronic use. Adverse effects include headaches, dizziness, and nausea. Overdosage can result in respiratory depression, seizures, coma, or death. Gamma-hydroxybutyrate has a U.S. Food and Drug Administration (FDA) schedule III rating and is associated with potential for abuse. It has a short half-life and has to be administered at bedtime and again several hours later.

51. Answer: C

Educational objective: Enumerate which antidepressant agents are capable of altering NREM sleep stages.

Explanation: Mirtazapine, nefazodone, tricyclic antidepressants, trazodone, and lithium increase NREM stages 3 and 4 sleep, whereas selective serotonin reuptake inhibitors either decrease or have no significant effect on NREM stages 3 and 4 sleep.

52. Answer: D

Educational objective: Describe the pharmacologic features of the antihistamine agents.

Explanation: There are two types of histamine receptor antagonists, namely histamine 1 (H_1) and histamine 2 (H_2) antagonists. H_1 antagonists are commonly used for allergies. First-generation H_1 antagonists (eg, chlorpheniramine, clemastine, diphenhydramine, and hydroxyzine) are lipophilic and easily cross the blood-brain barrier. First-generation H_1 antagonists can induce sedation and cause excessive sleepiness, and multiple sleep latency testing reveals a decrease in daytime sleep latency. Second-generation H_1 antagonists (eg, cetirizine, fexofenadine, loratadine, and terfenadine) are hydrophilic and do not readily cross the blood-brain barrier. Second-generation H_1 antagonists are generally not sedating and do not impair performance; however, they may produce sedation at high doses. H_2 antagonists (eg, cimetidine, famotidine, and ranitidine) are used for peptic ulcer disease. They do not readily cross the blood-brain barrier, and they do not generally produce sedation except in the elderly and in patients with renal impairment in whom excessive sleepiness has been reported.

53. Answer: B

Educational objective: Understand the pharmacology of caffeine.

Explanation: Caffeine, a stimulant, acts by decreasing adenosine transmission from both central nervous system A_1 and A_{2A} receptors. Caffeine increases objective measures of wakefulness as well as subjective alertness. When ingested close to bedtime, caffeine can result in sleep disturbance. Adverse effects on sleep may last up to 8 hours after caffeine ingestion. Habitual use of caffeine can give rise to tolerance and withdrawal symptoms with a decrease in performance. Tolerance to subjective reports of alertness may develop more rapidly than objective measures. Elimination half-life, which is usually 3 to 6 hours, is decreased among smokers.

54. Answer: D

Educational objective: Understand the pathophysiology of nocturnal asthma and the circadian variability of airway tone.

Explanation: Patients with nocturnal asthma often present with poor sleep quality and frequent arousals. Several mechanisms are responsible for the overnight bronchoconstriction noted in nocturnal asthma. There is a circadian variability in airflow, which is greatest in the late afternoon and lowest in the early morning. Sleep, itself, is also a major determinant of the variation in peak expiratory flow rate. Finally, decreases in functional residual capacity, minute ventilation and tidal volume that occur during sleep may be exaggerated in individuals with nocturnal asthma. Corticosteroid administration can diminished the circadian variability in airway tone. Both snoring and upper airway obstruction can increase the frequency of nocturnal asthma attacks in those with both asthma and obstructive sleep apnea.

55. Answer: A

Educational objective: Describe the polysomnographic features of central sleep apnea.

Explanation: Polysomnography is necessary for the diagnosis of central sleep apnea. Central apneas tend to occur more frequently at sleep onset and during NREM stages 1 and 2 sleep. Events are less frequent during NREM stages 3 and 4 sleep, and REM sleep. Pauses in respiration and absent ventilatory effort last 10 seconds or longer. There is loss of chest and abdominal movement (strain gauges or respiratory inductance plethysmography), and no electromyographic activity of the respiratory muscles, including the diaphragm. No change in intrathoracic pressures (esophageal balloon) is noted. Central hypopneas have a rounded profile on nasal pressure monitoring. Events are associated with oxygen desaturation (generally mild) and, occasionally, arousals. Snoring may occur but is less prominent than in obstructive sleep apnea.

56. Answer: B

Educational objective: Explain the characteristics of nocturnal hypoxemia seen in patients with chronic obstructive pulmonary disease.

Explanation: Chronic obstructive pulmonary disease (COPD) is characterized by airflow limitation that is usually progressive and is not fully reversible. Dyspnea and/or chronic cough are the chief complaints. In patients with moderate to severe COPD, significant oxygen desaturation may develop during sleep. Episodes of oxygen desaturation are more frequent, of greater duration, and more severe during REM sleep compared with NREM sleep. The severity of arterial oxygen desaturation during sleep is influenced by baseline lung function as well as awake PaO_2 and $PaCO_2$. Arousals appear to be unrelated to hypoxemia. Low-flow oxygen therapy seldom leads to a significant increase in nocturnal $PaCO_2$; nonetheless, caution and close monitoring are indicated in patients with comorbid obstructive sleep apnea in whom apnea duration may lengthen and nocturnal hypercapnia may worsen with oxygen therapy.

57. Answer: D

Educational objective: Describe the clinical features of the various neuromuscular disorders.

Explanation: Individuals with neuromuscular disorders can present with complaints of insomnia, sleep disturbance, excessive sleepiness, fatigue, morning headaches, and nighttime symptoms of dyspnea and intermittent snoring. Nocturnal respiratory impairment, including alveolar hypoventilation, can precede abnormalities during wakefulness by months to years. The likelihood of sleep-related oxygen desaturation is greater in patients with maximal inspiratory pressures < 60 cm H_2O and forced vital capacity $< 50\%$ of predicted.

58. Answer: D

Educational objective: Understand which factors increase the risk of developing obstructive sleep apnea.

Explanation: Risk factors for obstructive sleep apnea (OSA) include:
1. Untreated hypothyroidism—myxedema can precipitate, or exacerbate existing, OSA, possibly secondary to upper airway narrowing, macroglossia (due to deposits of mucoproteins), upper airway myopathy, or impairment of ventilatory control systems
2. Acromegaly
3. Strokes
4. Neuromuscular conditions, such as Duchenne muscular dystrophy, myotonic dystrophy, post-polio syndrome, neuropathies, and myopathies
5. Smoking and alcohol use
6. Medications, including muscle relaxants, sedative-hypnotics (benzodiazepines and barbiturates), narcotics, and anesthetics, can induce OSA by reducing upper airway dilator muscle tone. Neither zolpidem nor eszopiclone, both nonbenzodiazepine benzodiazepine receptor agonist hypnotic agents used for the treatment of insomnia, appear to significantly affect the apnea hypopnea index
7. Nasal congestion, due to allergic or nonallergic chronic rhinitis

59. Answer: D

Educational objective: Describe the polysomnographic changes following administration of lithium.

Explanation: Lithium can cause excessive sleepiness and impairment of cognitive and psychomotor functions. Polysomnographic features include an increase in total sleep time, decrease in NREM stage 1 sleep, increase in NREM stages 2, 3 and 4 sleep, increase in REM sleep latency and a variable decrease in REM sleep. Abrupt withdrawal of lithium administration may cause REM sleep rebound.

60. Answer: C

Educational objective: Describe the characteristic features of sleep during infancy and childhood.

Explanation: Electroencephalographic slow wave activity can be first discerned by 8 to 12 weeks of age.

61. Answer: B

Educational objective: Describe the distinguishing features of idiopathic hypersomnia.

Explanation: Idiopathic hypersomnia has a prevalence of approximately 0.002% to 0.005% and accounts for about 1% to 10% of patients referred to sleep clinics for excessive sleepiness. Excessive sleepiness usually begins insidiously during adolescence or early adulthood (onset often before 25 years of age). In some cases, onset may be heralded by a viral illness (mononucleosis or hepatitis). It affects males and females equally. After an initial period of progressive worsening of sleepiness, the latter may either become stable or continue to worsen throughout life. Some cases may be familial with an autosomal dominant inheritance pattern. Although there is no obvious association with specific HLAs, a high frequency of HLA-Cw2 has been described for some familial cases of the disorder.

62. Answer: C

Educational objective: Describe the pharmacologic features of quetiapine.

Explanation: Quetiapine is an atypical antipsychotic agent that causes a decrease in sleep latency, decrease in wake time after sleep onset, increase in sleep efficiency, increase in total sleep time, increase in NREM stage 2 sleep, and decrease in REM sleep. There are no changes in NREM stages 3 and 4 sleep, REM sleep latency, and REM density. It can cause or increase periodic leg movements of sleep.

63. Answer: D

Educational objective: Describe the clinical features of Duchenne muscular dystrophy.

Explanation: Patients with Duchenne muscular dystrophy can present with both central and obstructive apneas. Polysomnography may reveal an increase in the frequency of arousals and a decrease in REM sleep.

64. Answer: D

Educational objective: Describe the physiologic effects of amphetamine administration.

Explanation: Amphetamine is a stimulant agent that can cause dose-related improvements in alertness, mood, performance, and reaction time, as well as reductions in sleepiness and fatigue. Sleep disturbance may develop with insomnia, frequent awakenings, and decrease in sleep quality. The incidence of physiologic effects (tachycardia, and increase in body temperature and blood pressure) and adverse effects (headaches, nervousness, anxiety, tremulousness, restlessness, agitation, and ventricular arrhythmias) is also dose-dependent. Euphoria and pupillary dilation are commonly noted.

65. Answer: C

Educational objective: Identify the factors that regulate sleep and wakefulness.

Explanation: Two basic intrinsic components, namely circadian rhythm and sleep homeostasis, interact to regulate the timing and consolidation of sleep and waking. Sleep homeostasis is dependent on the sleep-wake cycle, whereas circadian rhythms are independent of it. Sleep homeostasis is characterized by an increase in sleep pressure following sleep deprivation, and electroencephalographic slow-wave activity is often used as a marker for it.

66. Answer: D

Educational objective: Understand the factors contributing to the genesis of Cheyne-Stokes respiration.

Explanation: The mechanism responsible for Cheyne-Stokes respiration (CSR) is believed to be instability of the control of ventilation due to a long circulation time, lower daytime and sleep-related $PaCO_2$ levels (< 45 mm Hg), and greater hypercaphic respiratory drive compared with patients with congestive heart failure but without CSR.

67. Answer: A

Educational objective: Identify the circadian peaks in wakefulness and sleep propensity.

Explanation: Circadian process promotes wakefulness during the day. There are two circadian peaks in wakefulness (wake-maintenance zones): one occurring near the maximum core temperature about 8 hours before the minimum core body temperature [Tmin] (early evening), and a second peak about 4 to 8 hours after the Tmin (late morning). Greatest sleep propensity occurs during periods of circadian troughs in arousal (overnight between 3:00 and 5:00 AM, and early-mid afternoon between 3:00 and 5:00 PM), or near the Tmin (early morning), and about 9 hours after the Tmin (early-mid afternoon), respectively.

68. Answer: A

Educational objective: Identify the neurotransmitter affected by the administration of methylphenidate.

Explanation: Methylphenidate, a piperidine derivative, acts by blocking dopamine reuptake and enhancing release of dopamine and norepinephrine. Methylphenidate has been shown to improve alertness and psychomotor performance. It produces an increase in sleep latency during multiple sleep latency and maintenance of wakefulness tests. It is indicated for the treatment of attention deficit hyperactivity disorder and excessive sleepiness related to narcolepsy.

69. Answer: D

Educational objective: Describe the clinical features of poliomyelitis.

Explanation: Poliomyelitis is a lower motor neuron disease that can involve the respiratory motor nuclei. It can give rise to dysfunction of respiratory muscles, including the diaphragm. Sleep-disordered breathing (eg, nocturnal hypoventilation and obstructive apneic and hypopneic events) can develop. Hypersomnolence is a common complaint. Polysomnographic features consist of a decrease in sleep efficiency and increase in frequency of arousals. There is often an increase in NREM stage 1 sleep and a decrease in REM sleep.

70. Answer: C

Educational objective: Describe the features of excessive sleepiness associated with obstructive sleep apnea.

Explanation: Excessive daytime sleepiness is present in a majority of patients with obstructive sleep apnea (OSA), and is secondary to sleep fragmentation. There is poor correlation between apnea indices and objective (Multiple Sleep Latency Test) and subjective (Epworth Sleepiness Scale) measures of sleepiness. Sleepiness improves with therapy of OSA.

71. Answer: D

Educational objective: Describe corticosteroids' effects on sleep.

Explanation: Corticosteroids, such as dexamethasone and hydrocortisone, can cause insomnia and nightmares. Polysomnographic features of corticosteroid administration include an increase in NREM stage 2 sleep as well as a decrease in NREM stages 3 and 4 sleep and REM sleep.

72. Answer: C

Educational objective: Classify excessive sleepiness based on clinical severity.

Explanation: According to the American Academy of Sleep Medicine 1997 International Classification of Sleep Disorders (revised) Diagnostic and Coding Manual, excessive sleepiness is considered mild if sleepiness occurs during times of rest or when little attention is required (eg, reading or watching television) and is associated with minor impairment of social and occupational functioning; moderate if sleepiness occurs daily and during mild physical activities that involve some degree of attention (eg, group meetings) and is associated with moderate impairment of social or occupational functioning; and severe if sleepiness occurs daily and during physical activities that involve mild to moderate degree of attention (eg, conversation, eating, or driving) and is associated with marked impairment of social or occupational functioning.

73. Answer: B

Educational objective: Describe the clinical features of myasthenia gravis.

Explanation: Myasthenia gravis is an autoimmune disease characterized by the presence of antibodies directed against acetylcholine receptors that result in impairment of transmission at the neuromuscular junction. There is a higher incidence of both central and obstructive apneas and hypopneas in patients with myasthenia gravis. Significant oxygen desaturation can develop and is seen predominantly during REM sleep.

74. Answer: D

Educational objective: Identify the factors that influence the propensity for sleep and wakefulness.

Explanation: Sleep latency and subsequent sleep duration and quality are influenced by both sleep deprivation and circadian factors. Sleep inertia refers to the short-lived reduction of alertness that occurs immediately following awakening from sleep, disappears within 2 to 4 hours, and is more pronounced following awakenings from NREM stages 3 and 4 sleep. Timing of sleep is also determined by autonomic nervous system tone (ie, a decrease in sympathetic activation and an increase in parasympathetic discharge facilitate the onset of sleep).

75. Answer: D

Educational objective: Describe the characteristics of human sleep architecture.

Explanation: There are commonly three to five NREM-REM sleep cycles, each occurring every 90 to 120 minutes in adults (every 60 minutes in infants and young children) during the night. Each sleep stage is not necessarily present in every sleep cycle. The percentage of NREM stages 3 and 4 sleep is greater during the initial part of sleep, whereas REM sleep is relatively more common during the latter part of sleep. REM density (frequency of rapid eye movements during REM sleep) also increases during the latter portion of the night.

76. Answer: A

Educational objective: Characterize the unique features of sleep in animals.

Explanation: Mammals have cycling of NREM (quiet) and REM (paradoxical) sleep. Sleep spindles and delta waves can be seen during NREM sleep among mammals. Avian sleep is characterized by the absence of spindles during NREM sleep and brief REM sleep periods.

77. Answer: D

Educational objective: Identify the determinants of oxygen desaturation during episodes of sleep apnea.

Explanation: The severity of oxygen desaturation during episodes of sleep apnea is dependent on baseline oxygen saturation prior to the apnea, lung volume, and duration of apnea; thus, oxygen desaturation is more severe with lower baseline oxygen levels, lesser lung volumes, and long apneic episodes.

78. Answer: A

Educational objective: Describe the clinical features of diaphragm paralysis.

Explanation: Unilateral diaphragmatic paralysis leads to significant nocturnal hypoxemia but in the absence of systemic lung disease, it does not generally result in chronic respiratory failure or cor pulmonale. Bilateral diaphragmatic paralysis can lead to the development of sleep apnea. The most common causes of bilateral diaphragmatic paralysis include high spinal cord injury, thoracic trauma, multiple sclerosis, anterior horn disease, and muscular dystrophy. Unilateral paralysis of the diaphragm is much more common than bilateral paralysis, the most frequent cause of which is nerve invasion from malignancy (usually a bronchogenic carcinoma). Polysomnography in patients with diaphragmatic paralysis can demonstrate decreases in NREM stages 3 and 4 sleep and REM sleep.

79. Answer: D

Educational objective: Describe the relationship between sleep and hypertension.

Explanation: Sleep-related breathing disorder is a risk factor for hypertension independent of other known confounding factors. In the Sleep Heart Health Study, mean systolic and diastolic blood pressures as well as the prevalence of hypertension increased significantly with increasing measures of sleep-related breathing disorder (eg, apnea hypopnea index [AHI] and percent sleep time with oxygen saturation below 90%). The odds of hypertension were observed to increase by about 1% for each additional apneic event per hour of sleep and to increase by 13% for each 10% decrease in nocturnal oxygen saturation. In the Wisconsin Sleep Cohort Study, subjects with an AHI of at least 15 events per hour had an odds ratio for the presence of hypertension of 2.89 compared with those with an AHI of 0 events per hour over 4 years of follow-up. A nocturnal fall in blood pressure can usually be observed in hypertensive patients without obstructive sleep apnea ("dippers"). Some patients with obstructive sleep apnea (OSA) fail to demonstrate this sleep-related nighttime fall in blood pressure ("non-dippers"). The risk of cardiovascular disease may be greater among "non-dippers" than among "dippers."

Some, but not all, investigators observed a reduction in blood pressure during administration of therapeutic continuous positive airway pressure (CPAP) but not subtherapeutic CPAP in patients with coexisting OSA.

80. Answer: C

Educational objective: Describe effective countermeasures for sleepiness during shift work.

Explanation: Intermittent exposure to bright lights in the workplace, administration of wake-promoting agents (e.g., caffeine, methamphetamine or modafinil) during evening work hours, use of hypnotic agents to improve daytime sleep, and scheduled napping might enhance alertness and reduce sleepiness. The effectiveness of behavioral countermeasures (e.g., increasing levels of activity or changes in posture) or external stimulation (e.g., loud noises) in reducing sleepiness during night work is unpredictable but appears limited. Melatonin given to night workers prior to their daytime sleep period has been shown to improve daytime sleep quality and duration, but has no effect on subsequent nighttime alertness.

81. Answer: B

Educational objective: Identify the percentages of sleep stages in healthy adults.

Explanation: Percentages of sleep stages in healthy adults are typically as follows: stage 1 sleep (2–5%), stage 2 sleep (45–55%), stages 3 and 4 sleep (20–25%), and REM sleep (5–20%).

82. Answer: B

Educational objective: Describe the polysomnographic features of REM sleep.

Explanation: REM sleep is composed of two components, namely, tonic (without rapid eye movements) and phasic (with rapid eye movements) sleep. Electroencephalography demonstrates low-voltage, mixed-frequency activity (theta and beta rhythms). Saw-tooth waves may be present and are more prominent over the vertex and frontal leads. Alpha waves are generally 1 to 2 Hz slower than those occurring during wakefulness and NREM stage 1 sleep. Vertex sharp waves are not prominent. Electro-oculography may show either no movements (tonic REM sleep) or bursts of conjugate (out-of-phase) rapid eye movements (phasic REM sleep). The amplitude of chin electromyography is reduced or absent (ie, at least equal to or, more commonly, lower than the lowest amplitude during NREM sleep).

83. Answer: A

Educational objective: Know the various neurotransmitters that play a role in the regulation of wakefulness, NREM sleep, and REM sleep.

Explanation: The main REM sleep neurotransmitter is acetylcholine. Other neurotransmitters include gamma-aminobutyric acid and glycine.

84. Answer: D

Educational objective: Describe the polysomnographic features of stage Wake.

Explanation: There are two types of eye movements that occur during stage Wake, namely (1) blinking or rapid eye movements when a person is awake and alert, and (2) slow rolling eye movements when a person is drowsy and eyes are closed. Stage Wake is also associated with high chin electromyographic tone. Electroencephalographic and electro-oculographic tracings may demonstrate muscle artifacts when a person is tense.

85. Answer: A

Educational objective: Describe the relationship between sleep and coronary artery disease.

Explanation: Pathogenetic mechanisms responsible for cardiac ischemia developing during sleep include marked sleep-related hypotension as well as sympathetic surges with increases in blood pressure and heart rate occurring during arousals or awakenings from sleep. Hypotension may be particularly prominent during NREM stages 3 and 4 sleep. REM sleep can be associated with instability of heart rate and blood pressure. The risk of sleep-related cardiac events is increased in patients with obstructive sleep apnea due, in part, to the hypoxemia that develops during the apneic episodes and the post-arousal increase in blood pressure and heart rate. The risk of developing cardiovascular disease is increased in middle-aged patients with obstructive sleep apnea. This elevated risk is independent of age, body mass index, blood pressure, and smoking.

The increased risk of cardiovascular disease, including myocardial infarction, angina, coronary revascularization procedure, heart failure, and stroke, is present even in patients with obstructive sleep apnea whose apnea-hypopnea indices are considered only mildly elevated.

Risk is reduced by reversal of obstructive sleep apnea. Mechanisms responsible for the increased risk of cardiovascular events in patients with obstructive sleep apnea include increase in sympathetic activity during sleep, inflammation, hypercoagulability, endothelial dysfunction, oxidative stress, and insulin resistance.

86. Answer: A

Educational objective: *Describe the association between obstructive sleep apnea and hypertension.*

Explanation: *Systemic blood pressure normally falls during NREM sleep ("dipping"). Many patients with obstructive sleep apnea (OSA) may fail to demonstrate this sleep-related fall in blood pressure ("non-dipping"). Blood pressure increases following termination of the apneic episode. The risk of hypertension is increased, and is associated with greater frequency of apneic episodes and severity of nocturnal oxygen desaturation. Conversely, the prevalence of OSA is increased in patients with hypertension. Treatment of OSA may result in a decrease in blood pressure and improved hypertension control.*

87. Answer: C

Educational objective: *Describe the pharmacologic features of risperidone.*

Explanation: *Polysomnographic features of risperidone, an atypical antipsychotic, consist of a decrease in frequency of awakenings, an increase in NREM stages 3 and 4 sleep, and a decrease in REM sleep. There is generally no change in REM sleep latency. Risperidone can cause or exacerbate periodic limb movements of sleep.*

88. Answer: D

Educational objective: *Describe the changes in sleep related to the use of venlafaxine.*

Explanation: *Venlafaxine is a serotonin and norepinephrine reuptake inhibitor. It can cause either insomnia or excessive sleepiness. Polysomnographic features include a decrease in sleep efficiency, an increase in wake time after sleep onset, an increase in REM sleep latency, and a decrease in REM sleep. It can cause or exacerbate periodic limb movements of sleep.*

89. Answer: B

Educational objective: *Describe the clinical features of cataplexy.*

Explanation: *Cataplexy may also be triggered by stress or fatigue, medications (alpha-1 adrenergic blockers, or during the switch to modafinil from amphetamines), or may occur spontaneously without apparent provocation. Although recovery is generally immediate and complete, prolonged episodes of cataplexy may give rise to REM sleep with hypnagogic hallucinations and dreaming. Episodes of muscular atonia or hypotonia may last from a few seconds to several minutes (generally <2 minutes in duration), and they can either be maximal at the start of the attack or worsen over several seconds or minutes.*

90. Answer: B

Educational objective: *Describe the disturbances in sleep associated with schizophrenia.*

Explanation: *There is often a reduction in both total sleep time and duration of REM sleep during the waxing phase of schizophrenia, which normalizes during the waning, postpsychotic, and remission phases of the disorder. Rebound sleepiness with an increase in sleep efficiency can occur during the waning phase of schizophrenia or during residual schizophrenia.*

91. Answer: D

Educational objective: *Identify the risk factors for pulmonary hypertension in patients with obstructive sleep apnea.*

Explanation: *Pulmonary hypertension and cor pulmonale are more likely to develop in patients with severe obstructive sleep apnea, especially in patients with daytime hypoxemia and hypercapnia due to concurrent chronic obstructive pulmonary disease ("overlap" syndrome) or morbid obesity (obesity-hypoventilation syndrome).*

92. Answer: A

Educational objective: *Identify the medications that can increase or decrease NREM stages 3 and 4 sleep.*

Explanation: *Medications that increase NREM stages 3 and 4 sleep include adenosine agonists, alcohol (acute ingestion), antihistamines, apomorphine, benztropine, carbamazepine, clonidine, interleukin-1, lithium, 1-tryptophan, maprotiline, mirtazapine, phenytoin, ritanserin, trazodone, tricyclic antidepressants, and trihexyphenidyl. Medications that decrease NREM stages 3 and 4 sleep include adenosine antagonists, alcohol (withdrawal), barbiturates, benzodiazepines, beta-adrenergic blockers, caffeine (during first half of the sleep period), corticosteroids, levodopa, methyldopa, prostaglandin E_2, selective serotonin reuptake inhibitors, selegiline, and stimulants.*

93. Answer: A

Educational objective: *Identify the factors associated with greater frequency of arousals among infants.*

Explanation: *Most infants are capable of sleeping through the night by 6 months of age. However, arousals occur normally four to six times each night. Certain conditions, such as cosleeping, colic, otitis media, and breast-feeding, may increase the frequency of arousals.*

94. Answer: D

Educational objective: *Describe the relationship between sleep and congestive heart failure.*

Explanation: *Obstructive sleep apnea (OSA), central sleep apnea (CSA), or both, can develop in patients with congestive heart failure (CHF). Left ventricular systolic dysfunction is an independent risk factor for the development of sleep apnea in patients with CHF. Moreover, untreated severe sleep-related breathing disorders may further impair left ventricular function. Why CSA develops in certain patients with CHF and not in others remains incompletely understood. There are several possible mechanisms responsible for the occurrence of CSA in patients with CHF, including the presence of pulmonary congestion, changes in end-tidal carbon dioxide pressures, and a decrease in circulation time.*

95. Answer: D

Educational objective: *Locate the neurons associated with specific neurotransmitters that regulate wakefulness.*

Explanation: *The following table matches the neurons that regulate wakefulness and their corresponding neurotransmitters:*

Location of neurons	Neurotransmitter
Locus ceruleus in the dorsal pontine tegmentum	Noradrenaline
Substantia nigra and ventral tegmental area	Dopamine
Tuberomammillary nucleus in the posterior hypothalamus	Histamine
Perifornical neurons in the lateral hypothalamus	Hypocretin (orexin)
Brainstem tegmentum (laterodorsal and pedunculopontine tegmental nuclei)	Acetylcholine
Basal forebrain (substantia innominata and diagonal band of Broca and septum)	Acetylcholine
Dorsal raphe	Serotonin

96. Answer: A

Educational objective: *Describe the effects of lesions of the central midbrain or ventral tegmentum.*

Explanation: *Lesions of the central midbrain tegmentum produce cortical inactivation without affecting behavioral responsiveness to sensory stimulation, whereas lesions of the ventral tegmentum produce behavioral somnolence and unresponsiveness without loss of cortical activation.*

97. Answer: A

Educational objective: *Understand the role of gamma-aminobutyric acid in the regulation of sleep and wakefulness.*

Explanation: *Gamma-aminobutyric acid (GABA) is the main central nervous system inhibitory neurotransmitter. This neurotransmitter is released primarily during sleep. Neurons are located in the ventrolateral preoptic (VLPO) area, thalamus, hypothalamus, basal forebrain, and cerebral cortex. Alcohol, barbiturates, benzodiazepines, and nonbenzodiazepine benzodiazepine receptor agonists (eg, eszopiclone or zolpidem) act on the GABA-A receptor, whereas sodium oxybate acts on the GABA-B receptor.*

98. Answer: A

Educational objective: *Identify the roles of the different neurotransmitters in the regulation of sleep and wakefulness.*

Explanation: *Glutamic acid is the main excitatory central nervous system neurotransmitter. Histamine is released by the tuberomammillary nucleus of the posterior hypothalamus during wakefulness. Histamine H-1 receptor blockers increase sleepiness.*

99. Answer: A

Educational objective: *Describe the features of Cheyne-Stokes respiration.*

Explanation: *Cheyne-Stokes respiration (CSR) is characterized by periodic crescendo/decrescendo breathing with apneas or hypopneas. It can be encountered in patients with congestive heart failure. Sleep disruption secondary to arousals associated with the hyperpneic phase of CSR as well as hypoxemia can develop in these patients. CSR occurs predominantly during NREM stages 1 and 2 sleep, and it occurs less frequently during NREM stages 3 and 4 sleep and REM sleep.*

100. Answer: C

Educational objective: *Identify the medications that are useful for treating cataplexy in patients with narcolepsy.*

Explanation: *The following agents are effective for treating cataplexy in patients with narcolepsy: carbamazepine, clomipramine, clonidine, desipramine, fluoxetine,* gamma-hydroxybutyrate, imipramine, nortriptyline, paroxetine, protriptyline, sertraline, venlafaxine, and viloxazine. Modafinil is a wake-promoting agent and does not prevent the occurrence of cataplexy.

101. Answer: A

Educational objective: Describe the sleep disturbances that can develop in persons with seasonal affective disorder.

Explanation: In seasonal affective disorder, the appearance of mood disorders (eg, depressive, manic, and hypomanic episodes) is closely associated with certain seasons of the year. Individuals commonly have major depressive episodes during the fall and winter; daytime sleepiness and fatigue can occur and may be accompanied by an increase in total sleep time. Depression is absent during spring and summer, during which times some patients may experience hypomanic symptoms, including increases in activity levels.

102. Answer: A

Educational objective: Describe the role of acetylcholine in the regulation of sleep and wakefulness.

Explanation: Acetylcholine causes cortical electroencephalographic (EEG) desynchronization during wakefulness and REM sleep. Its neurons are located in the basal forebrain and laterodorsal tegmentum/pedunculopontine tegmentum (LDT/PPT). Neurotransmitter release increases during wakefulness and REM sleep and decreases during NREM sleep.

103. Answer: C

Educational objective: Identify the factors that are associated with insomnia in patients with obstructive sleep apnea.

Explanation: Both obstructive sleep apnea (OSA) and central sleep apnea can result in either insomnia or excessive somnolence. In contrast to obese persons with severe OSA who typically present with excessive sleepiness, those with complaints of insomnia generally have less severe sleep-disordered breathing and are less likely to be obese. Apnea frequency and duration tend to be lower, and oxygen desaturation is milder in persons with insomnia compared to hypersomnolent individuals with OSA.

104. Answer: A

Educational objective: Identify the agents that block the action of the neurotransmitter adenosine.

Explanation: Levels of adenosine increase during prolonged wakefulness (ie, sleep deprivation) and decrease during sleep recovery. The methylxanthines, including caffeine and theophylline, are psychostimulants that block the action of adenosine.

105. Answer: C

Educational objective: Describe the changes in sleep architecture associated with the use of stimulant agents.

Explanation: Following the administration of stimulants, polysomnography typically demonstrates an increase in sleep latency, a decrease total sleep time, an increase in NREM stage 1 sleep, a decrease in NREM stages 3 and 4 sleep, an increase in REM sleep latency, and a decrease in REM sleep. Hypersomnia accompanied by a decrease in sleep latency, an increase in total sleep time, a decrese in REM sleep latency, and REM sleep rebound can develop during drug withdrawal.

106. Answer: D

Educational objective: Describe the clinical features of agrypnia excitata.

Explanation: Agrypnia excitata is a clinical syndrome that consists of oneirism (REM sleep-related dream enactment), enhanced motor activity, autonomic sympathetic discharge, and sleep disturbances (eg, sleeplessness and loss of NREM stages 3 and 4 sleep). It can be present in familial fatal insomnia, delirium tremens, and Morvan fibrillary chorea.

107. Answer: B

Educational objective: Enumerate the consequences of obstructive sleep apnea.

Explanation: Obstructive sleep apnea is associated with a decrease in SaO_2 and PaO_2, an increase in $PaCO_2$, an increase in systemic and pulmonary artery pressures, a decrease in left and right ventricular output, and an increase in vascular resistance secondary to heightened sympathetic nervous system activity.

108. Answer: A

Educational objective: Describe the relationship between sleep and cardiac arrhythmias.

Explanation: The risk of ventricular arrhythmias appears to be increased during arousals from sleep due to the associated surge in sympathetic activity. In contrast, the frequency of premature ventricular beats may diminish during sleep because of a greater parasympathetic tone. In individuals with obstructive sleep apnea (OSA), the heart rate typically slows at the onset of the apneic episode and increases after the termination of the event. Other rhythm disturbances have been described in patients with OSA and include ventricular tachycardia or fibrillation, complex ventricular ectopy, supraventricular tachycardia, sinus pauses, and second- or third-degree heart block. The severity of arrhythmias appears to be correlated with the degree of OSA.

109. Answer: A

Educational objective: Identify the frequencies of the different electroencephalographic waveforms.

Explanation: The frequencies in Hz or cycles per second of the electroencephalographic waveforms are delta waves (< 4), theta waves (4–7), alpha waves (8–13), and beta waves (> 13).

110. Answer: B

Educational objective: Describe the features of the different electroencephalographic waveforms.

Explanation: Beta waves are electroencephalographic (EEG) oscillations with frequencies of 13–35 Hz and amplitudes that is usually < 30 μV. They are present during alert wakefulness. Delta waves are high-amplitude (peak to peak of > 75 μV), slow (< 2 Hz) EEG waves that are predominant during NREM stages 3 and 4 sleep. Saw-tooth waves are theta waves with a notched waveform and are more prominent over the vertex and frontal leads. Saw-tooth waves occur during REM sleep. Theta waves are EEG oscillations with a frequency of 4–7 Hz and are maximal over the central and temporal leads.

111. Answer: D

Educational objective: Describe the features of the different electrodes used during polysomnography.

Explanation: Chin electromyography (EMG) leads are placed in the mental and submental areas to identify REM sleep. An additional EMG electrode can be placed over the masseter muscle to detect bruxism. Electrocardiography usually consists of a single channel, with one electrode placed near the sternum at the area of the right clavicle and another over the lateral chest wall near the seventh rib, and is used to monitor cardiac rate and rhythm. Techniques to measure airflow include nasal pressure, pneumotachography, thermistors, thermocouples, and end-tidal carbon dioxide ($PetCO_2$) monitoring. Only pneumotachography measures airflow directly. Thermal sensors and $PetCO_2$ monitoring provide indirect estimates of airflow based on the changing thermal and chemical characteristics of inspired ambient air and expired air originating from the lungs and airways.

112. Answer: A

Educational objective: Describe the clinical features of cataplexy.

Explanation: Memory and consciousness are unaffected. Although respiratory and oculomotor muscles are spared, blurring of vision may occur. Frequency of cataplexy may decrease over time.

113. Answer: C

Educational objective: Describe the relationship between sleep and gastrointestinal disorders.

Explanation: There is increased gastric acid secretion during sleep in patients with peptic ulcer disease compared with normal individuals. Persons may present with repeated arousals and awakenings from their sleep due to peptic ulcer disease. The abdominal pain is commonly described as dull, steady, or intermittent and is localized to the epigastric area. Onset of abdominal pain is commonly within the first 4 hours of sleep.

114. Answer: D

Educational objective: Describe the features of surface diaphragmatic electromyography and strain gauges during polysomnography.

Explanation: Surface diaphragmatic electromyography (EMG) and strain gauges are used to measure respiratory effort during polysomnography. With surface diaphragmatic EMG, signal tracings derived from electrodes placed on the chest wall may infer respiratory effort indirectly. Strain gauges, which are length-sensitive, can be positioned below the axilla and at the level of the umbilicus to measure rib cage and abdominal excursions, respectively. A single uncalibrated abdominal or chest gauge can be used to detect respiratory movements. Quantitative measurements of volume changes require calibration of the rib cage and abdominal gauges against another volume-measuring device.

115. Answer: C

Educational objective: Describe the relationship between sleep and gastroesophageal reflux.

Explanation: Gastroesophageal reflux (GER) is caused by backflow of gastric acid and other gastric contents into the esophagus due to incompetent barriers at the gastroesophageal junction. This leads to irritation and damage to the esophageal mucosa, and produces heartburn, pain or discomfort in the retrosternal area, and a sour or bitter taste. Prevalence increases with aging, and its course is generally chronic. Nocturnal GER appears to be common in patients with obstructive sleep apnea. The primary mechanism for GER is transient relaxation of the lower esophageal sphincter, the main deterrent against GER. The pressure of the upper esophageal sphincter, which acts as a further barrier to nocturnal regurgitation, also diminishes during sleep. Other factors contributing to the pathogenesis of GER include hiatal hernia, poor esophageal clearance, delayed gastric emptying, and impaired mucosal defense factors. GER during sleep is associated with a more prolonged acid contact time. Sleep prolongs esophageal acid clearance times. Furthermore, the production of saliva, which helps neutralize acid refluxate, ceases during sleep. Patients with nocturnal GER may complain of recurrent awakenings with a sensation of substernal burning or discomfort, indigestion, sour or bitter taste, or water brash. Dyspnea, coughing, and choking may be reported. Insomnia or sleep fragmentation due to frequent arousals may develop.

Continuous positive airway pressure (CPAP) therapy decreases the frequency of nocturnal GER symptoms, not only in patients with obstructive sleep apnea, but also in those without sleep-related breathing disorders. This anti-reflux activity may be due to elevation of intraesophageal pressure as well as lower esophageal sphincter constriction. Higher CPAP pressures produce greater improvements in GER.

116. Answer: A

Educational objective: Identify when arousals occur during obstructive sleep apnea.

Explanation: Arousals generally occur at the termination of the apneic-hypopneic event in patients with obstructive sleep apnea.

117. Answer: B

Educational objective: Describe the features of sleep in women.

Explanation: The prevalence of obstructive sleep apnea is less among postmenopausal women who use hormone replacement therapy (HRT) than among those not on HRT. In polycystic ovarian syndrome, there is an increased risk of developing obstructive sleep apnea. Central sleep apnea is less common in premenopausal women than in men. Compared with men, women tend to demonstrate less supine position dependency in respiratory events.

118. Answer: B

Educational objective: Determine the utility of HLA typing in the evaluation of patients with suspected narcolepsy.

Explanation: Narcolepsy is associated with certain human leukocyte antigens, namely DR2 (particularly the subtype DR15) and DQ1 (in particular DQ6 [DQB1*0602]). Most multiplex family cases (multiple members of the family with narcolepsy) are HLA DQB1*0602 positive. The prevalence of DR2 in subjects with narcolepsy is about 100% in Japanese subjects, 90% to 95% in Caucasians, and 60% in African Americans. However, HLA typing has limited diagnostic utility. HLA DQB1*0602 is present in most patients with narcolepsy with cataplexy (90%) and in about 40% to 60% of those with narcolepsy without cataplexy. HLA DRB1*1501 is also common among Asians and Caucasians with narcolepsy with cataplexy, whereas DQB1 *0602 is more specific among African Americans with narcolepsy.

119. Answer: B

Educational objective: Describe the characteristic features of sleep during infancy and childhood.

Explanation: The proportion of NREM and REM sleep are equal during early infancy. NREM stages 3 and 4 sleep are greatest during early childhood and progressively decline with aging.

120. Answer: B

Educational objective: Describe the changes in REM sleep associated with the use of antidepressant agents.

Explanation: Except for bupropion and nefazodone, antidepressants generally increase REM sleep latency and decrease REM sleep. MAOIs are the most potent REM sleep inhibitors. Bupropion and nefazodone increase REM sleep.

121. Answer: B

Educational objective: Describe the clinical features of fragmentary myoclonus.

Explanation: Fragmentary myoclonus is characterized by asynchronous, asymmetric and brief contractions of the muscles of the face, trunk and extremities appearing at the onset of sleep and continuing throughout the night. They may also be present during wakefulness. Episodes last from 10 minutes to over an hour. Affected individuals are typically unaware of these movements, with the fragmentary myoclonus being merely an incidental electromyographic (EMG) finding during polysomnography. Excessive fragmentary myoclonus may be seen in association with obstructive and central sleep apnea, hypoventilation syndromes, narcolepsy, insomnia, periodic limb movement disorder, restless legs syndrome and Niemann-Pick disease (type C) disease. Fragmentary myoclonus can be exacerbated by excessive sleepiness. Polysomnography demonstrates brief EMG potentials in various muscle groups, with more than five potentials per minute for at least 20 minutes of NREM stages 2, 3, or 4 sleep. Although muscle twitches may accompany EMG discharges, no movements may be evident. No accompanying electroencephalographic changes are present.

122. Answer: D

Educational objective: Describe the relationship between sleep and renal disorders.

Explanation: Disturbances in sleep can be encountered in 60% to 80% of patients on maintenance hemodialysis for end-stage renal disease (ESRD). Common sleep complaints include insomnia, prolonged awakenings, early morning awakenings, excessive sleepiness, reversal of day-night sleep patterns, and disturbed nocturnal sleep. There appear to be no differences in sleep characteristics between patients on hemodialysis versus continuous peritoneal dialysis. Excessive daytime sleepiness is a major problem in some patients with ESRD, and can be due to metabolic disturbances (eg, uremia); dialysis treatments (with its accompany changes in serum electrolytes, osmolarity, and acid-base balance); parathyroid hormone excess; changes in levels of neurotransmitters; and the production of somnogenic substances, such as interleukin-1 and tumor necrosis factor-alpha during dialysis. There is also a high prevalence of obstructive sleep apnea, restless legs syndrome, and periodic limb movement disorder in this patient population. Sleep apnea is improved by hemodialysis. Polysomnographic features of renal failure include an increase in sleep latency, a decrease in sleep efficiency, an increase in sleep fragmentation, an increase in frequency of awakenings, a decrease in total sleep time, an increase in NREM stages 1 and 2 sleep, a decrease in NREM stages 3 and 4 sleep, and a decrease in REM sleep. In one study, sleep quality in ESRD patients with anemia improved following therapy with recombinant human erythropoietin.

123. Answer: B

Educational objective: Describe the relationship between sleep and hypothyroidism.

Explanation: Patients with hypothyroidism may present with excessive sleepiness and fatigue. Polysomnography may reveal a decrease in NREM stages 3 and 4 sleep, which normalizes with thyroid hormone replacement. A high incidence of obstructive sleep apnea has been reported in patients with untreated hypothyroidism, especially when myxedema is present. Pathogenesis appears to involve obesity, myopathy, upper airway edema, and deposition of mucopolysaccharides in the upper airway. Central sleep apnea secondary to an impaired central respiratory drive may also be present. Indices of sleep apnea severity do not diminish significantly in all patients following attainment of a euthyroid state.

124. Answer: A

Educational objective: Identify the factors that contribute to nocturnal cardiac ischemia in patients with obstructive sleep apnea.

Explanation: Increased risk of coronary artery disease (CAD) in patients with obstructive sleep apnea (OSA) may be related to endothelial dysfunction, accelerated atherosclerosis, hypertension, and comorbid obesity. Nocturnal ischemia in patients with CAD and OSA may be due to increased sympathetic activity, arousal-related tachycardia, and increased left ventricular afterload. This ischemia may improve with therapy of OSA.

125. Answer: B

Educational objective: Describe the changes in sleep associated with menopause.

Explanation: Menopause is associated with hot flashes, insomnia, an increase in sleep latency, a decrease in sleep efficiency, a decrease in total sleep time, an increase in wake time after sleep onset, and possibly a decrease in REM sleep.

126. Answer: B

Educational objective: Describe the relationship between sleep and acromegaly.

Explanation: Acromegaly is a condition resulting from excessive levels of growth hormone (GH). Obstructive sleep apnea is common in patients with acromegaly. The risk of developing obstructive sleep apnea is increased with greater age, larger neck circumference, greater initial tongue volume, presence of abnormalities in craniofacial dimensions (predominantly of the mandible) and upper airway narrowing due to changes in pharyngeal soft tissues. Other factors that might contribute to the development of obstructive sleep apnea are facial bone deformities, mucosal edema, hypertrophy of the pharyngeal and laryngeal cartilages, and presence of nasal polyps. There appears to be no correlation between obstructive sleep apnea and biochemical parameters of disease activity (eg, GH and insulin-like growth factor 1 [IGF-1] levels). Improvements in indices of sleep apnea severity have been reported following therapy of acromegaly with bromocriptine, octreotide (a long-acting somatostatin analog), and pituitary surgery (adenomectomy or hypophysectomy). Nonetheless, sleep apnea may persist despite normalization of GH levels during therapy. Central sleep apnea is also common in patients with acromegaly. Possible mechanisms for the development of central apneas include reflex inhibition of the respiratory center due to narrowing of the upper airways, or increase in ventilatory response to carbon dioxide. Central sleep apnea is associated with higher levels of GH and IGF-1 than obstructive apnea.

127. Answer: B

Educational objective: Describe the features of pulse oximetry used during polysomnography.

Explanation: Pulse oximeters, using either spectrophotometric technique or photoelectric plethysmography, are routinely utilized during overnight polysomnography to monitor SaO_2. A pulsating vascular bed (eg, earlobe or fingertip) is placed between a two-wavelength light source and a sensor. A pulse oximeter responds rapidly to changes in SaO_2 and permits continuous monitoring of SaO_2. Altering the pulse oximeter response time influences the accuracy of pulse oximeters in measuring changes in SaO_2. For instance, SaO_2 recordings may be inaccurate if the oximeter response time approximates the duration of oxygen desaturation events. Sensitivity is greater with shorter sampling intervals, and the least filtering to achieve the most rapid response is recommended. Signal amplitude is affected by reduced skin perfusion due to hypothermia, hypotension or vasoconstriction and by poor sensor attachment. In addition, oximetry readings may overestimate low oxygen saturation values. Lastly, due to its reliance on only two light wavelengths, the presence of dyshemoglobin species such as carboxyhemoglobin or methemoglobin produces errors in measurement

128. Answer: C

Educational objective: Describe the features of the different newborn electroencephalographic waveforms.

Explanation: High-voltage slow pattern is present in both quiet and active REM sleep, low-voltage irregular pattern is present in active REM sleep, trace alternant is present in quiet sleep, and mixed pattern is present in both quiet and active REM sleep.

129. Answer: A

Educational objective: *Describe the different artifacts that might be encountered during polysomnography.*

Explanation: *Electrode popping consists of sudden, sharp high-amplitude, "spike-like" deflections due to electrode leads being pulled away from the skin (change in impedance) brought about by body or respiratory movements, or when the patient lies on the electrode itself. Popping may also be due to drying out of the electrode gel or faulty electrodes. Fixing electrode placement, changing to an alternate lead, or applying more electrode gel can correct electrode popping.*

130. Answer: C

Educational objective: *Describe the relationship between sleep and Cushing disease.*

Explanation: *Patients with Cushing syndrome or Cushing disease have an excess of adrenocorticosteroid hormones. Sleep complaints, including insomnia, are common. There is an increased incidence of obstructive sleep apnea. Changes in sleep architecture, including a decrease in sleep efficiency, an increase in sleep fragmentation, poorer sleep continuity, a decrease in NREM stages 3 and 4 sleep, a decrease in REM latency, and an increase in REM density, have been described.*

131. Answer: C

Educational objective: *Describe the different levels of diagnostic sleep studies.*

Explanation: *Several levels of diagnostic sleep studies, both in attended and unattended settings, have been described. A level 1 study consists of an attended in-laboratory full polysomnography, typically including electroencephalography (EEG), electro-oculography (EOG), chin electromyography (EMG), airflow, respiratory effort, oxygen saturation (SaO_2), electrocardiography (EKG), leg EMG, and body position. A level 1 study is the gold standard for the diagnosis of obstructive sleep apnea (OSA). A level 2 study is a comprehensive portable polysomnography or an unattended full polysomnography. It monitors the same parameters as a level 1 study, including EEG, EOG, chin EMG, airflow, respiratory effort, SaO_2, EKG, leg EMG, and body position. A level 3 cardiorespiratory sleep study, or modified portable sleep apnea test, consists of four or more parameters (eg, airflow, SaO_2, respiratory effort, EKG, or body position). It is may be useful when there is a high pretest likelihood of OSA, levels 1 or 2 studies are not readily available, and a delay in testing is unacceptable; it may also be useful for follow-up evaluation following therapy of patients previously diagnosed with OSA. A level 4 study involves a continuous single or dual bioparameter recording (eg, SaO_2,*

airflow, or snoring) and has a poor specificity and sensitivity. It is not recommended for the diagnosis of OSA.

132. Answer: C

Educational objective: *Describe the use of actigraphs for patients with sleep complaints.*

Explanation: *Actigraphy is a reliable and valid method of detecting sleep in normal, healthy adults. Actigraphy monitoring should include at least three consecutive 24-hour periods. Superiority of one actigraphy placement over others on different parts of the body is not established.*

(Standards of Practice Committee of the American Academy of Sleep Medicine (AASM). Practice parameters for the role of actigraphy in the study of sleep and circadian rhythms: an update for 2002. Sleep. 2003;26(3):337–41.)

133. Answer: D

Educational objective: *Describe the relationship between obstructive sleep apnea and congestive heart failure.*

Explanation: *The prevalence of obstructive sleep apnea is increased in patients with moderate to severe congestive heart failure (CHF) or in asymptomatic patients with left ventricular dysfunction. Possible mechanisms for the development of CHF in patients with OSA include an increase in left ventricular afterload due to greater peripheral resistance (hypertension) and more negative intrathoracic pressure (inspiration against a closed airway) as well as sympathetic nervous system activation by hypoxemia and repeated arousals during sleep.*

134. Answer: A

Educational objective: *Describe the features of the Multiple Sleep Latency Test.*

Explanation: *The Multiple Sleep Latency Test (MSLT) measures a person's physiologic propensity to fall asleep in quiet situations. A nocturnal polysomnography during the patient's usual major sleep period should be performed on the evening immediately before an MSLT to exclude the presence of other sleep disorders and to ensure an adequate duration of nocturnal sleep (at least 6 hours). An MSLT should not be performed after a split-night sleep study. It consists of four or five nap opportunities, each 20 minutes in duration, performed every 2 hours. It is usually scheduled between 8:00 to 9:00 AM and 5:00 to 6:00 PM, with the first nap opportunity starting about 1.5 to 3 hours after awakening from the previous night's polysomnography. Breakfast is provided at least 1 hour before the first nap, and lunch is given immediately after the second nap study. Smoking should be stopped 30 minutes before the start of every test. Bathroom trips, if needed, are scheduled prior to each trial. Caffeinated beverages, unusual bright light exposure, and vigorous physical activity should be avoided during the day of the study. Stimulating activities should be stopped 15 minutes prior to each nap trial.*

Electrodes should be connected and calibrated 5 minutes before lights out. Standard biocalibrations are performed before each trial. During the test, electroencephalography (central C3-A2, C4-A1, and occipital O1-A2, O2-A1), electro-oculography, chin electromyography, and electrocardiography are monitored to determine sleep latency (time from lights out to the onset of sleep) and the occurrence of REM sleep for each nap. The patient is instructed to lie quietly, assume a comfortable position, close his/her eyes and try to fall asleep in a dark, quiet room. Room temperature should be adjusted based on the patient's level of comfort. Lights are then turned off ("lights out") and monitoring is started. Between nap opportunities, the patient is asked to get out of bed and to remain awake until the next test.

Sleep onset for clinical MSLTs is defined as the first epoch of any stage of sleep. Sleep latencies (from lights out to the first epoch of sleep [sleep onset]), and the number of sleep-onset REM periods (SOREMPs), defined as greater than 15 s of REM sleep in a 30-s epoch, are determined for each nap. REM latency is the duration from the first epoch of sleep to the beginning of the first epoch of REM sleep. An adequate sleep duration and regular sleep-wake schedule, as documented by sleep diaries or actigraphy, must have been maintained for at least 1 to 2 weeks preceding MSLT. Furthermore, medications that can potentially influence sleep latency and REM sleep, such as stimulants, opiates, benzodiazepines, narcotics, and REM suppressants, should be discontinued for at least 2 weeks before the study. A urine drug screen during the study is required to rule out the recent use of opiates, sedatives, hypnotics, and stimulants. Obstructive sleep apnea, if present, should be appropriately treated before performing an MSLT. In patients using continuous positive airway pressure (CPAP) for obstructive sleep apnea, both polysomnography and MSLT are performed at the usual prescribed CPAP pressure. MSLT parameters are not as well established for children younger than 8 years of age.

135. Answer: B

Educational objective: *Describe the use of amplifiers during polysomnography.*

Explanation: *A polygraph is used to monitor and record several physiologic variables during sleep. It consists of a series of alternating current (AC) and direct current (DC) amplifiers as well as filters.*

AC amplifiers are used to record high-frequency parameters, such as electroencephalographs, electro-oculographs, electromyographs, and electrocardiographs. Filters are commonly incorporated into AC amplifier systems. High-frequency filters attenuate fast, presumably nonphysiologic, potentials, and low-frequency filters reduce slow potentials that might interfere with proper recording of physiologic parameters.

DC amplifiers, on the other hand, are used to record low-frequency physiologic variables, including oxygen saturation,

esophageal pressures, or continuous positive airway pressure levels. DC amplifiers are not equipped with low-frequency filters. Either AC or DC amplifiers can be used to record airflow and respiratory effort.

136. Answer: A

Educational objective: *Describe the methods of monitoring central sleep apnea–hypopneas.*

Explanation: *Central sleep apnea–hypopnea syndrome is defined by the presence of repetitive episodes of apnea during sleep that are not accompanied by upper airway obstruction. A central apnea–hypopnea event consists of a cessation or reduction of airflow lasting 10 seconds or longer along with a reduction in esophageal pressure excursion compared to baseline. Respiratory events are often associated with oxygen desaturation and arousals. Esophageal pressure monitoring is the reference standard measurement for central apnea-hypopneas. Respiratory inductance plethysmography, surface diaphragmatic electromyography, thermal sensors, expired carbon dioxide (PetCO$_2$), piezo sensors, and strain gauges are relatively insensitive in identifying central apnea-hypopneas.*

137. Answer: B

Educational objective: *Describe the relationship between sleep and Addison disease.*

Explanation: *Patients with Addison disease (primary adrenal insufficiency) may present with complaints of weakness, fatigue, anorexia, gastrointestinal symptoms, weight loss, hyperpigmentation, and hypotension. Sleep disturbances in patients with Addison disease include sleep-onset insomnia, repeated awakenings, and early morning awakenings. Polysomnographic features include a decrease in NREM stages 3 and 4 sleep. Administration of hydrocortisone at bedtime in patients with Addison disease can lead to a decrease in REM latency, an increase in REM sleep, and a greater wake time after sleep onset.*

138. Answer: A

Educational objective: *Describe the characteristics of pulse transit time.*

Explanation: *Pulse transit time is defined as the time it takes for the arterial pulse pressure wave to travel from the aortic valve to the periphery. It increases during obstructive sleep apnea–related inspiratory fall in blood pressure and decreases during arousal-related rise in blood pressure, and it is useful in distinguishing obstructive from central respiratory events.*

139. Answer: A

Educational objective: *Describe the pharmacologic features of modafinil.*

Explanation: *Modafinil is an atypical psychostimulant whose precise mechanism of action remains incompletely understood. Compared with the other stimulating compounds, modafinil appears to possess no major addiction potential. It does not produce sleep rebound with drug discontinuation. Development of tolerance has been described. Polysomnographic features include a decrease in total sleep time. It is indicated for excessive sleepiness secondary to narcolepsy and shift work sleep disorders. It is also used for residual sleepiness in patients with obstructive sleep apnea who are being treated with CPAP therapy.*

140. Answer: C

Educational objective: *Describe the clinical features of REM sleep–related sinus arrest.*

Explanation: *REM sleep–related sinus arrest is a cardiac rhythm disorder characterized by sinus arrest, often in clusters, with periods of asystole lasting up to 9 seconds that usually recur frequently during REM sleep. It is a rare condition affecting apparently healthy young adults without any identified cardiac pathology. Episodes of nocturnal sinus arrest are not accompanied by arousals or sleep disruption, and are not associated with obstructive sleep apnea. Most patients are asymptomatic, although palpitations or vague chest discomfort may occasionally be present. Daytime electrocardiography and angiography are usually unremarkable.*

141. Answer: C

Educational objective: *Describe the characteristic features of sleep during infancy and childhood.*

Explanation: *The percentage of REM sleep decreases with aging, from 50% of total sleep time in the newborn period to 20% to 25% of total sleep time by adulthood. A marked reduction of REM sleep occurs during the first 6 months of life.*

142. Answer: A

Educational objective: *Describe the clinical features of cataplexy.*

Explanation: *Cataplexy can be considered as intrusion of REM sleep–related muscle atonia during wakefulness. Cataplexy is produced by inhibition of lower motor neurons, and deep tendon and H reflexes by cholinergic areas of the pons and basal forebrain. There is a glycine-mediated hyperpolarization of the anterior horn cells of the spinal cord. During episodes of cataplexy, neurologic examination demonstrates muscle flaccidity, reduction or absence of deep tendon reflexes, loss of pupillary light response and, occasionally, a positive Babinski sign.*

143. Answer: B

Educational objective: *Identify at which age an increase in night wakings occurs among children.*

Explanation: *An increase in frequency of awakenings during the night ("night wakings") is usually noted between 12 and 72 months of age.*

144. Answer: D

Educational objective: *Describe the clinical features of cataplexy.*

Explanation: *Up to 70% to 80% of narcoleptics have cataplexy but the absence of cataplexy does not exclude a diagnosis of narcolepsy. Cataplexy can also be seen in association with midbrain tumors, Niemann-Pick disease (type C), and Norrie disease. Cataplexy generally first develops several months or years after the onset of excessive sleepiness.*

145. Answer: A

Educational objective: *Describe the methods of monitoring respiratory effort–related arousals.*

Explanation: *Respiratory effort–related arousals (RERAs) consist of increasing respiratory efforts (progressively more negative esophageal pressures) lasting 10 seconds or longer, culminating in arousal (or a change in esophageal pressure to a less negative level). These events do not fulfill the criteria for either apnea or hypopnea. The reference standard for identifying a RERA is the measurement of esophageal pressure. RERAs can also be detected using measurements of nasal pressure and surface diaphragmatic electromyography.*

146. Answer: C

Educational objective: *Describe the effects of weight reduction in patients with obstructive sleep apnea.*

Explanation: *Significant weight reduction in patients with obstructive sleep apnea can result in a reduction in the amount of adipose tissue in the upper airways; an increase in upper airway caliber; a decrease in airway collapsibility; an increase in upper airway critical closing pressure; an increase in oxygen saturation; an increase in vital capacity, functional residual capacity, and residual volume; and a decrease in the respiratory work of breathing.*

147. Answer: A

Educational objective: *Describe the clinical features of rhythmic movement disorders.*

Explanation: *Rhythmic movement disorder defines a syndrome consisting of repetitive, rhythmic, and stereotypic motions of the head, trunk, or extremities, which usually occurs during drowsiness in the transition from wakefulness to sleep or arises during sustained sleep. It is referred to as head banging (jactatio capitis nocturna) if it involves forceful anterior-posterior motions of the head and neck (ie, repeatedly lifting and banging the head back onto the bed). In addition, individuals may display head rolling (lateral movements of the head), body rolling (side-to-side* motions of the body), body rocking (entire body is rocked while positioned on hands and knees), leg rolling or banging, and rhythmic vocalizations or humming. Age of onset is typically before the first year of age (mean age of onset of 6 months for body rocking, 9 months for head banging, and 10 months for head rolling). Spontaneous resolution before 4 years of age is characteristic.

148. Answer: B

Educational objective: *Identify the medications that can suppress REM sleep.*

Explanation: *Antidepressants, including selective serotonin reuptake inhibitors, tricyclic antidepressants, and monoamine oxidase inhibitors generally increase REM sleep latency and decrease REM sleep. Monoamine oxidase inhibitors are the most potent REM sleep inhibitors.*

149. Answer: C

Educational objective: *Define the indications for oral devices in children with obstructive sleep apnea.*

Explanation: *Oral appliances may be considered in older adolescents when the growth of craniofacial bones and upper airway soft tissues is largely complete.*

150. Answer: D

Educational objective: *Describe the clinical features of sleep terrors.*

Explanation: *Sleep terrors (pavor nocturnus) consist of abrupt awakenings with profound fear usually from NREM stages 3 and 4 sleep, often in the first part of the night. Sleep terrors can cause distress and functional impairment. Individuals may suddenly bolt upright from their beds with a loud yell, cry, or scream, and this is followed, in rare instances, with sleepwalking or running. Associated clinical features include inconsolability, misperception of the environment, confusion, amnesia for the episode, autonomic and behavioral manifestations of intense fear (tachycardia, elevated blood pressure, tachypnea, dilated pupils, and profuse sweating), vocalizations, or urinary incontinence. Individuals are usually unresponsive to external stimuli and are difficult to arouse. Although usually benign, these behaviors can become violent and potentially dangerous, and injuries can be sustained during the event. Patients then spontaneously calm down and return rapidly to sleep. Sleep terrors in adults can begin in NREM sleep stage 2 and during the second half of the night.*

151. Answer: B

Educational objective: *Describe the clinical features of Down syndrome that contribute to the increased risk of obstructive sleep apnea.*

Explanation: *Patients with Down syndrome (trisomy 21) may develop apneas, hypoventilation and hypoxemia. Characteristic craniofacial features include a small head,* maxillary hypoplasia, small nose, an enlarged tongue, and a short neck, all of which increase the risk of developing obstructive sleep apnea. Down syndrome is caused in most cases by an extra chromosome at the 21 position. Incidence increases with advanced maternal age. Both genders can be affected.

152. Answer: B

Educational objective: *Describe the relationship between sleep and human immunodeficiency virus infection.*

Explanation: *Patients with human immunodeficiency virus (HIV) disease (acquired immunodeficiency syndrome [AIDS]) may present with complaints of insomnia, recurrent nighttime arousals, excessive sleepiness, and an increased tendency to nap. An estimated 35% of HIV-infected subjects have alterations in their sleep-wake patterns. Sleep disturbance may be a manifestation of an underlying encephalopathy. Increase in wake time after sleep onset, increase in frequency and longer duration of awakenings, and more frequent napping have been observed. Sleep quality is related to duration of HIV disease and the severity of HIV-related symptoms. Sleep quality is also influenced by immune status as lower T-cytotoxic/suppressor (CD3+/CD8+) cell counts are associated with greater sleep disturbances. Antiviral therapy for HIV infection can also lead to sleep disturbance. Efavirenz therapy is associated with an increase in sleep latency and decrease in NREM stages 3 and 4 sleep. It can also give rise to a number of neuropsychiatric adverse reactions (eg, vivid dreams, nocturnal awakenings, and insomnia). Zidovudine can give rise to insomnia.*

153. Answer: C

Educational objective: *Describe the relationship between sleep and Lyme infection.*

Explanation: *Lyme disease is a multisystem disorder with rheumatologic, neurologic, and dermatologic features. It is caused by Borrelia burgdorferi. Human disease is transmitted via tick bites. Sleep-related complaints are common in patients with Lyme disease and include sleep-onset insomnia, frequent awakenings, excessive daytime sleepiness, restless legs syndrome, and nocturnal leg jerking. Sleep disturbances can persist for several years in patients with previous Lyme disease, especially those who either had facial palsy or did not receive antibiotics for acute neuroborreliosis. Polysomnography may demonstrate increased sleep latency, decreased sleep efficiency, increased arousals, and greater sleep fragmentation. Some patients may have alpha wave intrusion into NREM sleep. Mean sleep onset latency during multiple sleep latency testing is typically normal.*

154. Answer: A

Educational objective: *Describe the methods of monitoring Cheyne-Stokes breathing syndrome.*

Explanation: *Cheyne-Stokes breathing syndrome consists of cyclical waxing and waning of respiration with central apneas or hypopneas alternating with periods of hyperpnea. Transient arousals often occur at the crest of hyperpnea leading to sleep fragmentation and excessive somnolence. Measurements of airflow using a pneumotachometer and esophageal pressure monitoring are the reference standards of measuring airflow and respiratory effort, respectively. Other techniques for detecting Cheyne-Stokes breathing include respiratory inductance plethysmography, surface diaphragmatic electromyography, oronasal airflow monitoring, and oximetry.*

155. Answer: B

Educational objective: *Describe the polysomnographic features of high altitude periodic breathing.*

Explanation: *Polysomnography in persons with high altitude periodic breathing can demonstrate repetitive central apneas, 10 seconds or longer in duration, occurring about every 12 to 34 seconds primarily during NREM sleep. These central apneas can be associated with oxygen desaturation and can result in arousals. Respiration is more regular during REM sleep. Finally, there can be an increase in the frequency of arousals, an increase in NREM stages 1 and 2 sleep, and a decrease in NREM stages 3 and 4 sleep. There is generally no change in total sleep time or REM sleep.*

156. Answer: A

Educational objective: *Understand the changes in circadian rhythms that occur with normal aging.*

Explanation: *There is an age-related reduction in the amplitude of the circadian sleep-wake rhythms, melatonin secretion, and core body temperature. Nocturnal levels of melatonin are reduced. There is also a diminished release of growth hormone during sleep and an increase in the circadian nadir of cortisol level.*

157. Answer: D

Educational objective: *Describe the clinical features of sleep-related painful erections.*

Explanation: *Sleep-related painful erections are not associated with any physical abnormality or any penile disorder or pain during sexual erections while awake. Sexual function while awake is generally normal. Painful penile erections occurring during REM sleep can give rise to repetitive awakenings and, in some cases, insomnia and/ or excessive daytime sleepiness. This is a rare condition that often begins after the fourth decade of life and progressively worsens with advancing age.*

158. Answer: A

Educational objective: *Understand how obstructive sleep apnea may develop following surgical repair of cleft palates.*

Explanation: *A cleft palate is often accompanied by significant narrowing of the anterior-posterior dimension of the pharynx, a lower hyoid position, and a longer uvula. Clinically significant obstructive sleep apnea (OSA) can develop following repair of cleft palates using flap pharyngoplasty, sphincter pharyngoplasty or velopharyngeal ring ligation procedure. OSA can occur in the immediate postoperative period and may, in some cases, resolve spontaneously within several months.*

159. Answer: D

Educational objective: *Describe the clinical features of sleeping sickness.*

Explanation: *Sleeping sickness, or human African trypanosomiasis, is a parasitic disease caused by the protozoan Trypanosoma brucei or Trypanosoma rhodesiense. It is endemic in certain regions of intertropical Africa.*

Following the bite of a tsetse fly, human disease evolves through two stages. The first hemolymphatic stage is characterized by fever and cervical adenopathy, followed by increasing neurologic symptoms and excessive daytime sleepiness in the meningoencephalitic stage.. An important feature of trypanosomiasis is disruption of the circadian rhythm (eg, reversal of the sleep-wake periods and plasma levels of cortisol and prolactin). If untreated, the infection culminates in altered consciousness, cachexia, coma, and eventually death.

160. Answer: A

Educational objective: *Describe the methods of monitoring sleep hypoventilation syndrome.*

Explanation: *In sleep hypoventilation syndrome, both oxygen desaturation and hypercapnia (increase in $PaCO_2$ during sleep by greater than 10 mm Hg compared with levels during wakefulness), unrelated to distinct periods of apnea-hypopnea, are present during sleep. Periods of central hypoventilation are more frequent and severe during REM sleep than during NREM sleep. Diurnal hypercapnia is frequently present. $PaCO_2$ is the reference standard measurement. Other techniques that have been utilized to monitor sleep hypoventilation include continuous oximetry (decline in SaO_2 without accompanying respiratory events), $PtcCO_2$ monitoring, calibrated respiratory inductance plethysmography (reduced tidal volume and minute ventilation), and $PetCO_2$ measurements.*

161. Answer: C

Educational objective: *Describe the clinical features of obesity hypoventilation syndrome*

Explanation: *The two key features of obesity hypoventilation syndrome (OHS) are the presence of severe obesity (defined as a body mass index > 40 kg/m^2) and hypercapnia ($PaCO_2$ > 45 mmHg) during wakefulness. Hypoventilation is not due to another respiratory or neuromuscular* *disorder. Chronic hypoxemia can result in polycythemia, pulmonary hypertension, and cor pulmonale. Most patients with OHS also have obstructive sleep apnea. Clinical manifestations include excessive sleepiness, insomnia, sleep fragmentation with frequent arousals, decreased attention or concentration, peripheral edema, and cyanosis.*

162. Answer: B

Educational objective: *Describe the features of excessive sleepiness in patients with narcolepsy.*

Explanation: *Excessive daytime sleepiness is typically the first, primary, and most disabling manifestation of narcolepsy. Excessive sleepiness is chronic and may manifest as pervasive drowsiness and subwakefulness, frequent napping, microsleep episodes, and unexpected and overpowering sleep attacks occurring almost daily for at least 3 months. Patients with narcolepsy may describe waxing and waning periods of alertness. Although lapses into sleep are more likely to occur during periods of inactivity, abrupt and unexpected sleep attacks can befall the individual at any time. Brief naps, lasting 10 to 20 minutes and seldom more than 1 hour, occur repeatedly from one to eight times throughout the day. Sleepiness is transiently relieved after awakening from a short nap, only to gradually increase again within 2 to 3 hours. Excessive sleepiness increases the risk of accidental injuries and impairs social functioning as well as school and work performance.*

163. Answer: B

Educational objective: *Describe the association between pain syndromes and sleep.*

Explanation: *Acute pain can give rise to sleep disruption, and poor sleep can magnify the perception of pain intensity. Polysomnographic studies of patients with acute pain may reveal sleep fragmentation, and decrease in both NREM stages 3 and 4 sleep and REM sleep. Development of depression in patients with chronic pain can further disturb sleep. Polysomnographic findings in patients with chronic pain consists of an increase in sleep latency, an increase in wake time after sleep onset, and a decrease in NREM stages 3 and 4 sleep.*

164. Answer: C

Educational objective: *Describe the changes in sleep architecture associated with fibromyalgia.*

Explanation: *Fibromyalgia (FM) is a syndrome characterized by chronic diffuse musculoskeletal pain and tenderness, physical discomfort, and fatigue. FM is often associated with nonrestorative sleep, insomnia, and early morning awakenings. Polysomnographic features typically include an increase in sleep latency, a decrease in sleep efficiency, a decrease in total sleep time, an increase in frequency of arousals, an increase in wake time after*

sleep onset, an increase in NREM stage 1 sleep, a decrease in sleep spindles during NREM stage 2 sleep, a decrease in NREM stages 3 and 4 sleep, and a decrease in REM sleep. An alpha-NREM sleep anomaly has been described.

165. Answer: D

Educational objective: *Describe the clinical course of congenital central hypoventilation syndrome.*

Explanation: *In patients with congenital central hypoventilation syndrome (Ondine curse or primary alveolar hypoventilation syndrome), hypoventilation and failure of autonomic respiratory control is present from birth. A disorder of central chemoreceptor responsiveness, rather than respiratory or neuromuscular disorders, gives rise to impaired ventilatory responses to hypoxia and hypercapnia. Onset of this rare disorder is typically during the newborn period. Clinical manifestations vary depending on disease severity and can include shallow breathing, episodic apnea, cyanosis, feeding difficulties, bradycardia-tachycardia, and diaphoresis. Apparent life-threatening events, respiratory arrest, or pulmonary hypertension may develop during infancy. Course is chronic, with death usually due to respiratory failure or cor pulmonale.*

166. Answer: C

Educational objective: *Describe the features of the different newborn electroencephalographic waveforms.*

Explanation: *Newborn electroencephalography waveforms are classified as:*

1. High-voltage slow pattern (continuous, medium- to high-amplitude [between 50 and 150 mV] waveforms; frequencies between 0.5 and 4.0 Hz);
2. Low-voltage irregular pattern (low-amplitude [between 14 and 35 mV] waveforms; frequencies between 5.0 and 8.0 Hz);
3. Trace alternant pattern (bursts of slow [0.5 to 3 Hz], high-amplitude waves, fast low-amplitude waves, and sharp waves [2 to 4 Hz] lasting several seconds interspersed with periods of relative quiescence [mixed frequency waveforms] lasting 4 to 8 seconds); and
4. Mixed pattern (high- and low-voltage waveforms).

167. Answer: A

Educational objective: *Describe the methods for monitoring obstructive sleep apnea–hypopneas.*

Explanation: *Obstructive sleep apnea–hypopnea syndrome is defined by the repetitive reduction or cessation of airflow despite the presence of respiratory efforts due to partial or complete upper airway occlusion during sleep. Episodes are accompanied by oxygen desaturation, arousals, and sleep disruption. This syndrome includes mixed apneas, in which an initial period of apnea secondary to an absence of respiratory effort precedes the upper airway obstruction.*

In routine clinical care, it is not necessary to distinguish apneas from hypopneas, and often the two respiratory events are scored and reported together. Measurement techniques that identify hypopneas are able to detect apneas as well; in contrast, methods that measure apneas may not necessarily be adequate in identifying hypopneic events. A reduction in total oronasal airflow detected by a pneumotachometer placed in a well-fitted face mask is the reference standard for measuring obstructive apnea-hypopneas. Other methods that can be utilized to identify obstructive apnea-hypopneas include measurement of nasal pressure, respiratory inductance plethysmography (RIP), piezo sensors, strain gauges, thoracic impedance, thermal sensors, and expired carbon dioxide (PetCO$_2$).

168. Answer: D

Educational objective: Enumerate the polysomnographic features of a major depressive episode.

Explanation: Polysomnographic features of a major depressive episode include a decrease in sleep efficiency, an increase in sleep latency, a decrease in total sleep time, an increase in wake time after sleep onset, an increase in NREM stage 1 sleep, a decrease in NREM stages 3 and 4 sleep, a decrease in REM sleep latency, and an increase in REM density. The duration of REM sleep is increased early during sleep. There is also often a delay in NREM stages 3 and 4 sleep from the first NREM cycle to the second. Changes in sleep architecture may both precede or persist after remission of major depressive episodes.

169. Answer: D

Educational objective: Describe the clinical features of the different genetic syndromes characterized by maxillary hypoplasia.

Explanation: The syndromic craniosynostoses (eg, Apert syndrome, Crouzon syndrome, and Pfeiffer syndrome) arise as a result of mutations in fibroblast growth factor receptor genes that inhibit the anterior-posterior growth of the cranium. Patients typically possess a facial profile that is either flattened or scaphoid in shape. Midfacial hypoplasia displaces the palate posteriorly closer to the posterior wall of the nasopharynx. Features of Antley-Bixler syndrome include craniosynostosis, frontal bossing, midfacial hypoplasia, choanal atresia or stenosis, and depression of the nasal bridge. Periods of apnea may occur. Most cases are sporadic, but some present as an autosomal recessive disorder.

170. Answer: A

Educational objective: Describe the disturbances in sleep associated with mood disorders.

Explanation: Insomnia is common among persons suffering from major depression. Daytime sleepiness along with an increase in total sleep time may develop during the depressive phase of a bipolar disorder, seasonal affective disorder, or atypical depression.

171. Answer: D

Educational objective: Describe the characteristics of insomnia among older adults.

Explanation: Increasing age is associated with a higher prevalence of insomnia and a greater likelihood that insomnia becomes chronic. Among the elderly, prevalence of insomnia is higher in women. There is a poorer correlation between subjective complaints and objective sleep parameters in older women than in men. Causes of insomnia in older adults include changes in circadian sleep-wake rhythms, sleep disorders, and medical, neurologic, and psychiatric disorders. Rarely is insomnia in the elderly due exclusively to aging itself.

172. Answer: B

Educational objective: Distinguish between the two clinical types of primary restless legs syndrome.

Explanation: Restless legs syndrome (RLS) can be either idiopathic (ie, primary) or secondary. Primary RLS, in turn, can be classified into two subtypes: early onset (before 35 to 45 years of age) and late onset. An earlier onset and more gradual progression of symptoms, as well as a greater family history of RLS, characterize the early onset type. Both types appear to be associated with abnormalities of the dopaminergic neurotransmitter system and respond to therapy with dopaminergic agents.

173. Answer: A

Educational objective: Describe the features of nasal pressure monitoring of airflow.

Explanation: The presence of airflow can be inferred by changes in nasal pressure during respiration. Nasal airflow can be measured quantitatively and directly with a pneumotachograph consisting of a standard oxygen nasal cannula connected to a pressure transducer and placed in the nares. Respiration produces fluctuations on the nasal pressure transducer signals (decreasing during inspiration and increasing during expiration) that are proportional to flow. The shape and amplitude of the nasal cannula signal are comparable to those obtained from face mask pneumotachographs. The presence of a plateau (flattening) on the inspiratory flow signal is associated with increased upper airway resistance and airflow limitation (obstructive event). In contrast, the signal is reduced but rounded in central events.

174. Answer: A

Educational objective: Understand how Pierre-Robin syndrome predisposes to the development of obstructive sleep apnea.

Explanation: In Pierre-Robin syndrome, mandibular hypoplasia in utero displaces the tongue posteriorly, which, in *turn, impairs the midline closure of the palate. Breathing difficulties that develop in the early days of life improve significantly during the first 2 years with growth of the lower jaw in relation to the cranial dimensions. Persistent micrognathia can increase the risk of snoring and obstructive sleep apnea in later life, and serial polysomnography is recommended.*

175. Answer: D

Educational objective: *Understand when measurement of cerebrospinal fluid hypocretin-1 is useful in the diagnosis of narcolepsy.*

Explanation: *A cerebrospinal fluid (CSF) hypocretin-1 level < or equal to 110 pg/ml (or less than one-third of mean normal control values) is highly specific and sensitive for narcolepsy with cataplexy but is rarely present in cases without cataplexy. Measuring CSF hypocretin-1 levels may be useful if patients are taking medications (stimulants or REM sleep suppressants) that may interfere with proper interpretation of Multiple Sleep Latency Test (MSLT) results, if patients are too young to undergo MSLT, or during the early course of the disease prior to the development of cataplexy.*

176. Answer: C

Educational objective: *Enumerate the behavioral states that have been described in young infants.*

Explanation: *Five behavioral states have been described in young infants, namely quiet sleep, active sleep, quiet alertness, active alertness, and vocalization.*

177. Answer: D

Educational objective: *Enumerate the differences in clinical features of sleep-related breathing disorders between men and women.*

Explanation: *There is a decreased susceptibility to upper airway collapse during sleep among women relative to men. There are no gender differences in pharyngeal cross-sectional area, upper airway resistance, and hypoxic and hypercapnic ventilatory response during NREM sleep. Women have fewer reports of snoring but more frequent reports of daytime sleepiness, fatigue, and insomnia than in men. The risk of obstructive sleep apnea is increased in women during menopause compared with premenopause.*

178. Answer: A

Educational objective: *Describe the clinical features of the different nonhypercapnic central sleep apnea syndromes.*

Explanation: *Nonhypercapnic central sleep apnea (CSA) is not associated with daytime hypoventilation (waking $PaCO_2$ is either normal or low). There is an increased ventilatory response to hypercapnia. Brief arousals are accompanied by a hyperventilatory "overshoot" that decreases $PaCO_2$ levels below the apneic threshold and*

leads to central apneas. This group includes patients with idiopathic CSA, postarousal CSA, congestive heart failure, sleep at high altitude, or during continuous positive airway pressure titration.

179. Answer: C

Educational objective: *Enumerate the clinical features of congenital central hypoventilation syndrome.*

Explanation: *Clinical features of congenital central hypoventilation syndrome include dysfunction of the autonomic nervous system control of the heart with decreased heart rate variability, hypotension, and arrhythmias (eg, heart block and sick sinus syndrome); esophageal dysmotility and swallowing difficulty; growth impairment with hypotonia or motor delay; heat intolerance; Hirschsprung disease; impaired mental processing; metabolic alkalosis; ophthalmologic abnormalities (strabismus); polycythemia; seizures; syncope; and tumors of neural crest derivatives (ie, ganglioneuromas and neuroblastomas).*

180. Answer: D

Educational objective: *Describe the characteristics of Treacher Collins syndrome.*

Explanation: *Treacher Collins syndrome is characterized by an underdeveloped mandible, receding chin, malar hypoplasia, and cleft palate. Other features include an antimongoloid palpebral fissure slant, eyelid coloboma, ear deformities, and conductive hearing loss. It is inherited as an autosomal dominant disorder and is caused by mutations in the TCOF1 gene coding for the Treacle protein. Obstructive sleep apnea has been described in patients with this syndrome.*

181. Answer: C

Educational objective: *Describe the characteristic features of sleep during infancy and childhood.*

Explanation: *K-complexes first appear after 6 months of age.*

182. Answer: C

Educational objective: *Describe the polysomnographic features of idiopathic hypersomnia.*

Explanation: *Nocturnal polysomnographic features include a decrease in sleep latency (often < 10 minutes), an increase in sleep efficiency (> 85%), an increase or normal total sleep time, a decrease in frequency of arousals, an increase in NREM stages 3 and 4 sleep (in some), and no change in REM sleep latency. Multiple sleep latency testing often reveals a decrease in mean sleep latency (< 8 minutes) and fewer than two sleep onset REM periods (SOREMPS). An increase in the duration of sleep over 24 hours (> 11 to 12 hours) is present during 24-hour continuous polysomnography.*

183. Answer: A

Educational objective: *Identify the medications that can cause or aggravate restless legs syndrome.*

Explanation: *Drugs that can potentially precipitate or worsen restless legs syndrome (RLS) include selective serotonin reuptake inhibitors, tricyclic antidepressants, sedating antihistamines, neuroleptics, lithium, and dopamine antagonists (eg, metoclopramide). Bupropion, unlike other antidepressants, increases dopamine and does not cause or exacerbate RLS.*

184. Answer: C

Educational objective: *Describe the changes in sleep associated with bipolar disorders.*

Explanation: *Excessive sleepiness may occur during depressive episodes of bipolar disorder. During this phase, polysomnography may demonstrate an increase in total sleep time and decrease in REM sleep latency. During the acute manic phase of the disorder, total sleep time is reduced and patients commonly report increased levels of energy. Manic episodes can be precipitated by sleep deprivation.*

185. Answer: D

Educational objective: *Identify the disorders that are associated with status dissociatus.*

Explanation: *Status dissociatus can be encountered in fatal familial insomnia, alcohol withdrawal, and in some patients with narcolepsy.*

186. Answer: D

Educational objective: *Differentiate obstructive sleep apneic events occurring during NREM sleep from those during REM sleep.*

Explanation: *Obstructive sleep apnea is generally more frequent, lasts longer, and is associated with more profound oxygen desaturation during REM sleep than during NREM sleep.*

187. Answer: B

Educational objective: *Describe the clinical features of hypercapnic central sleep apnea.*

Explanation: *Hypercapnic central sleep apnea (CSA) is generally associated with daytime hypoventilation (high waking $PaCO_2$), and diminished response to hypercapnia. Hypoventilation continues during sleep. It includes patients with central alveolar hypoventilation, neuromuscular disorders, or neurologic disorders affecting the brainstem. Congestive heart failure is considered a nonhypercapnic form of CSA.*

188. Answer: A

Educational objective: *Describe the clinical features of cataplexy.*

Explanation: *Severity ranges from mild weakness, such as drooping of the eyelids or sagging of the jaw, to complete lack of postural tone with a collapse to a chair or the ground. It can occur from once or twice yearly to as often as several times each day. Loss of muscle tone can be regional, affecting the face, neck, and extremities, or it can involve the entire body. Status cataplecticus (repetitive episodes of cataplexy occurring in succession) may occur following abrupt withdrawal of REM sleep suppressants. Cataplexy may present up to a year before the development of sleep-onset REM periods on multiple sleep latency testing. Polysomnography demonstrates wakefulness during brief attacks, and REM sleep during more prolonged attacks.*

189. Answer: B

Educational objective: *Differentiate among the different genetic syndromes with mandibular hypoplasia that can increase the risk of obstructive sleep apnea.*

Explanation: *In patients with mandibular hypoplasia, obstructive sleep apnea can develop as a result of posterior displacement of the base of the tongue closer to the posterior pharynx. Vertebral abnormalities, dermal cysts, and auricular malformations characterize Goldenhar syndrome. Abnormalities of the upper airway can lead to upper airway obstruction. It can either be inherited as an autosomal dominant or recessive disorder, or may occur sporadically. Males are affected more commonly than women. Features of Pierre-Robin syndrome include a small jaw, retropositioned tongue and soft palate, displacement of the larynx, and, in some cases, a cleft palate. An underdeveloped mandible, receding chin, malar hypoplasia, cleft palate, antimongoloid palpebral fissure slant, eyelid coloboma, ear deformities, and conductive hearing loss characterize Treacher Collins syndrome.*

190. Answer: A

Educational objective: *Describe the pharmacologic features of nicotine.*

Explanation: *Nicotine, present in cigarettes and other tobacco products, increases alertness and decreases sleepiness. It enhances cortical cholinergic neurotransmission. Administration close to bedtime can cause disrupted nonrestorative sleep. Low blood concentrations of nicotine produce mild sedation. Drowsiness can occur during withdrawal from nicotine. Polysomnographic features of smoking close to bedtime include an increase in sleep latency, a decrease in sleep efficiency, a decrease in total sleep time, an increase in wake time after sleep onset, and a decrease in REM sleep. Nicotine can increase restless legs symptoms, and smoking increases the risk of sleep-related breathing disorders.*

Withdrawal may result in disrupted sleep and daytime somnolence. There is an increase in wake time after sleep onset during the first few days of smoking cessation. Bupropion, an agent used to aid smoking cessation, can give rise to insomnia. Nicotine gum reduces NREM stages 3 and 4 sleep. Nicotine patch reduces sleep efficiency and prolongs sleep onset latency.

191. Answer: C

Educational objective: *Understand the effects of breast-feeding on maternal sleep.*

Explanation: *Changes in sleep associated with breast-feeding include a reduction in NREM stages 1 and 2 sleep and increase in NREM stages 3 and 4 sleep compared to bottle-feeding. There is either a decrease or no change in total sleep time. There is generally no significant change in subjective perception of sleep quality.*

192. Answer: D

Educational objective: *Enumerate the diagnostic criteria for restless legs syndrome among adults based on the recommendations of the International Restless Legs Syndrome Study Group.*

Explanation: *The International Restless Legs Syndrome Study Group has recommended the following diagnostic criteria for restless leg syndrome (RLS) in adults:*

1. An urge to move the legs, usually accompanied or caused by uncomfortable and unpleasant sensations (paresthesias or dysesthesias) in the limbs. The arms or other body parts may be involved as well. Occasionally, the urge to move is unaccompanied by uncomfortable sensations and
2. The urge to move or unpleasant sensations:
   a. Begin or worsen during periods of rest or inactivity (eg, lying or sitting)
   b. Are partially or totally relieved by movement (eg, walking or stretching), at least during the time of the activity
   c. Are worse in the evening or night than during the day or occur only in the evening or night

193. Answer: B

Educational objective: *Differentiate parasomnias and nocturnal seizures.*

Explanation: *Seizures should be considered in the differential diagnosis of any parasomnia-like behavior that is accompanied by atypical features or stereotypic activities. Seizures can occur at any time during sleep but appears to start more frequently during NREM sleep. Seizures of frontal and temporal origins may be associated with complex activities or behavior. This disorder should be highly suspected in patients who report accompanying urinary incontinence or tongue biting.*

194. Answer: B

Educational objective: *Describe the clinical and polysomnographic features of propriospinal myoclonus at sleep onset.*

Explanation: *Patients with propriospinal myoclonus at sleep onset exhibit spontaneous sudden muscle jerks that occur typically during relaxed wakefulness in the transition from wakefulness to sleep. The jerks start in the abdominal and truncal muscles and then spread slowly rostrally and caudally to the proximal limb and neck muscles. Nonperiodic trunk flexion (more common) and extension disappear at sleep onset or with mental activation. This is likely a rare disorder with a higher prevalence among adult men. Onset is generally during adulthood. Course is generally chronic. Sleep-onset insomnia may develop. Polysomnographic features include brief, recurring myoclonic electromyographic activity associated with alpha electroencephalographic (EEG) rhythms that disappear with EEG desynchronization and remain absent during sleep.*

195. Answer: A

Educational objective: *Describe the pathophysiology of congenital central hypoventilation syndrome.*

Explanation: *The lack of ventilatory or arousal responses in patients with congenital central hypoventilation syndrome can give rise to significant hypoventilation (reduction in tidal volume and respiratory rate), hypoxemia and hypercapnia during sleep. Hypoventilation is typically most severe during NREM sleep. Frank central apneas, snoring, or paradoxical breathing are uncommon. Affected patients have no subjective sensation of dyspnea. Increasing respiratory frequency rather than an augmentation of tidal volume is responsible for the increase in minute ventilation during exercise.*

196. Answer: D

Educational objective: *Identify the effects of sodium oxybate on the sleep of patients with fibromyalgia.*

Explanation: *Studies have demonstrated that sodium oxybate reduces pain and fatigue symptoms, and improves sleep quality in patients with fibromyalgia. Therapy also significantly decreases sleep latency, duration of REM sleep and the amount of alpha-NREM, and increases NREM stages 3 and 4 sleep.*

197. Answer: A

Educational objective: *Describe the features of thermal sensors used to measure airflow during polysomnography.*

Explanation: *Thermal sensing devices provide an indirect and semiquantitative measurement of airflow. Thermal sensors, placed over the nose and mouth, sense airflow by differences in the temperature between warmer expired air and cooler inhaled ambient air. The flow signal generated is related directly to the sensor temperature (measured as electrical resistance by a thermistor and as change in voltage by a thermocouple) and indirectly to airflow. It is also dependent on the pattern of airflow, and the placement of the sensor in relation to the nostril.*

Signals obtained from thermal sensors provide only qualitative data regarding airflow..

198. Answer: C

Educational objective: Enumerate the differences between continuous positive airway pressure and autotitrating continuous positive airway pressure.

Explanation: Autotitrating positive airway pressure (APAP) devices automatically and continuously adjust the delivered pressure, as required, to maintain airway patency. Pressure is increased to achieve and maintain airway patency or is gradually reduced in the absence of detectable respiratory events over a predetermined period of time. Compared with continuous positive airway pressure (CPAP), mean delivered pressure is generally lower during APAP, but peak airway pressure may be higher. APAP has not been consistently shown to result in higher compliance compared to CPAP. Studies have shown no significant differences between conventional in-laboratory CPAP titration and APAP titration in reductions in apnea-hypopnea and arousal indices, changes in sleep architecture, or oxygenation.

199. Answer: A

Educational objective: Describe the effects of infant cosleeping on maternal sleep during the postpartum period.

Explanation: Changes in maternal sleep architecture associated with infant cosleeping include an increase in frequency of arousals, a decrease in NREM stages 3 and 4 sleep, and no significant change in sleep efficiency or total sleep time compared with sleeping alone during the postpartum period.

200. Answer: A

Educational objective: Describe the methods for measuring airflow during sleep.

Explanation: A pneumotachometer is the reference standard for detecting obstructive apnea–hypopnea. Placed in a well-fitted face mask, it can measure total oronasal airflow by detecting changes in pressure between inspiration and expiration.

201. Answer: A

Educational objective: Enumerate the indications for polysomnography in patients with suspected parasomnias.

Explanation: Diagnosis of most parasomnias is based on its clinical presentation, and except for REM sleep behavior disorder, they seldom require polysomnographic documentation. A formal polysomnographic study is recommended for possible parasomnias associated with very frequent episodes, complaints of excessive sleepiness, unusual presentation, or significant sleep disturbance to the sleeper or bed partner. Polysomnography is also indicated if an underlying seizure activity is suspected

or in cases that have medicolegal implications with injury to the individual or bed partner. A single normal polysomnogram does not exclude the presence of parasomnias. Multiple studies, preferably with time-synchronized video recording (ie, simultaneous video and sleep monitoring), performed over several nights may be required. Additional electroencephalographic (EEG) electrodes are required for patients in whom a seizure disorder is being excluded.

202. Answer: D

Educational objective: Identify the disorders classified as nocturnal frontal lobe epilepsies.

Explanation: Nocturnal paroxysmal dystonia is classified as a nocturnal frontal lobe epilepsy along with two other disorders, paroxysmal arousals and episodic nocturnal wanderings. These three conditions often coexist. Nocturnal paroxysmal dystonia is characterized by an abrupt complex behavior, with dystonic-dyskinetic, choreoathetoid, or ballistic posturing, and semipurposeful activity, arising repeatedly from NREM sleep. Events may occur several times nightly, often in clusters, and can be either short (lasting 15 to 60 seconds) or more prolonged (lasting 2 minutes to less than 1 hour).

Paroxysmal arousals are brief, sudden awakenings during NREM sleep associated with transient stereotyped dystonic-dyskinetic posturing. Episodic nocturnal wanderings consist of prolonged episodes of agitated ambulation, with unintelligible speech, screaming, complex motor behavior and dystonic postures involving the head, trunk, and limbs.

203. Answer: B

Educational objective: Describe the clinical features of sleep-related abnormal swallowing syndrome, sleep-related choking syndrome, and sleep-related laryngospasm.

Explanation: Persons with sleep-related abnormal swallowing syndrome have difficulty swallowing their own saliva during sleep and have repeated transient arousals from sleep due to coughing, choking, or gagging. Abnormal swallowing mechanisms during sleep result in accumulation of saliva in the upper airway with subsequent aspiration into the trachea, leading to an arousal with coughing and a sensation of choking. A characteristic "gurgling" sound due to pooling of secretions in the oral cavity can be heard preceding each coughing spell. Transient hoarseness following awakenings can occur. With sleep-related choking syndrome, persons may complain of frequent, almost nightly, episodes of abrupt awakenings accompanied by a sensation of choking or being unable to breathe, fear, intense anxiety, sensation of dying, and tachycardia. These attacks are not accompanied by stridor, nightmares, or sleep terrors. Sleep-related laryngospasm is characterized by severe breathlessness with an initial total or near-total cessation of airflow while asleep followed by a sudden *awakening with inspiratory stridor. Events may be accompanied by temporary hoarseness, tachycardia, cyanosis, anxiety, panic, or a sensation of dying.*

204. Answer: D

Educational objective: *Describe the polysomnographic changes related to the use of amphetamines.*

Explanation: *Amphetamines increase the availability of the monoamine neurotransmitters norepinephrine, dopamine, and serotonin at the neural synapse, either by increasing their presynaptic release or by blocking their reuptake. They enhance wakefulness and alertness, and they can produce insomnia. During amphetamine use, there is a decrease in sleepiness, an increase in sleep latency, a decrease in sleep efficiency, an increase in wake time after sleep onset, a decrease in total sleep time, an increase in sleep fragmentation, a decrease in NREM stages 3 and 4 sleep, an increase in REM sleep latency, and a decrease in REM sleep. There is an increase in sleepiness, an increase in NREM stages 3 and 4 sleep, and an increase in REM sleep during amphetamine discontinuation. Amphetamines are indicated for the therapy of narcolepsy and attention deficit hyperactivity disorder. They have a high abuse potential, and both dependency and tolerance can develop.*

205. Answer: A

Educational objective: *Describe the proper evaluation of patients with craniofacial syndromes.*

Explanation: *Routine screening for obstructive sleep apnea (OSA) is recommended for patients with craniofacial syndromes. Periodic reassessment is important, because growth-related alterations in craniofacial structures may significantly affect upper airway anatomy and function. Patients with craniofacial syndromes may require more extensive evaluation. After the presence of OSA has been established by polysomnography, additional studies may be required to assess the anatomic sites of upper airway obstruction. Imaging studies include lateral cephalometric views, computed tomography, or magnetic resonance imaging to visualize both key skeletal structures and soft tissues (eg, tonsils and adenoids) along with their relationships to each other. Nasendoscopy enables visualization of the sites of upper airway obstruction.*

206. Answer: A

Educational objective: *Describe the features of expired carbon dioxide used to measure airflow during polysomnography.*

Explanation: *Expired carbon dioxide (CO_2) monitoring using infrared analyzers placed in front of the nose and mouth can provide a qualitative measure of airflow because ambient air contains negligible amounts of CO_2 compared to expired air from the lungs, which have a higher concentration*

of CO_2. One can also infer the occurrence of hypoventilation by a rising PetCO$_2$ level.

207. Answer: A

Educational objective: *Describe the use of transcutaneous oxygen (PtcO$_2$) monitoring during polysomnography.*

Explanation: *A modified Clark electrode can be used to measure oxygen tension at the skin surface (PtcO$_2$). Cutaneous perfusion, temperature, and metabolism influence the surface oxygen tension. Blood flow to the skin can be increased by local application of heat (43°C) with periodic site changes every 4 to 6 hours to prevent cutaneous thermal injury. Several factors limit the application of PtcO$_2$ monitoring during adult sleep studies, including the variable relationship between PaO$_2$ and PtcO$_2$, a slow response that fails to mirror the rapid changes in PaO$_2$, and the need for periodic site changes.*

208. Answer: C

Educational objective: *Understand the American Academy of Sleep Medicine practice parameters for the medical therapy of obstructive sleep apnea.*

Explanation: *The following are the American Academy of Sleep Medicine practice parameters for the medical therapy of obstructive sleep apnea (OSA).*

1. Dietary weight reduction may improve the apnea hypopnea index (AHI) in obese patients with OSA.
2. Dietary weight reduction should be used in conjunction with a primary treatment for OSA.
3. In obese patients, bariatric surgery may be considered as an adjunct in the treatment of OSA.
4. Selective serotonin reuptake inhibitors; protriptyline; methylxanthine derivatives, including aminophylline and theophylline; estrogen therapy with or without progesterone; and short-acting nasal decongestants are not recommended for the therapy of OSA.
5. Topical nasal corticosteroids may be a useful adjunct to primary therapies for OSA in patients with concurrent rhinitis.
6. Modafinil is recommended for treating residual daytime sleepiness in patients with OSA on effective positive airway pressure treatment and with no other known causes for sleepiness.
7. There are no or insufficient data in the literature to formulate any recommendations regarding androgen blockade, bromocriptine (for acromegaly), medroxyprogesterone (for men with OSA), mirtazapine, nicotine, and thyroid hormones (for hypothyroidism).
8. Supplemental oxygen is not recommended as a primary therapy for OSA.
9. Methods to permit sleep only in a nonsupine position are effective either as secondary therapy or as a supplement to primary therapies for OSA in patients with a low AHI in the nonsupine versus the supine position.

(From Morgenthaler TI, Kapen S, Lee-Chiong T, et al. Practice parameters for the medical therapy of obstructive sleep apnea. Sleep. 2006;29(8):1031–1035.)

209. Answer: A

Educational objective: Distinguish between narcolepsy and idiopathic hypersomnia.

Explanation: Although both narcolepsy and idiopathic hypersomnia are associated with excessive daytime sleepiness, there are distinct differences in clinical presentation between the two disorders. Cataplexy, which may be present in narcolepsy, is characteristically absent in idiopathic hypersomnia. Sleep paralysis and hypnagogic hallucinations may be present in both conditions. Although daytime naps are refreshing and can transiently improve daytime sleepiness in patients with narcolepsy, naps are generally not refreshing in idiopathic hypersomnia. Both narcolepsy and idiopathic hypersomnia are associated with short sleep latencies on multiple sleep latency testing, but only narcolepsy is associated with sleep onset REM periods. HLA typing demonstrates a greater prevalence of DQB1*0602 in narcolepsy and CW2 in idiopathic hypersomnia. Patients with narcolepsy have a more predictable response to stimulant medications.

210. Answer: A

Educational objective: Characterize sleep among premature infants.

Explanation: Among premature infants, no clearly definable sleep states are present from 24 to 26 weeks of gestation. Active sleep (presence of eye movements, body movements and irregular respiration) can be identified by 28 to 30 weeks of gestation and constitutes the majority of sleep at this age group. Quiet sleep (electroencephalographic [EEG] pattern of trace discontineau or trace alternant) can be noted by 32 weeks and 36 weeks of gestation, respectively. At the same conceptual age, premature and full-term infants attain similar EEG milestones. However, development of spindles is more advanced in premature infants compared to full-term infants.

211. Answer: D

Educational objective: Identify the causes of multiple sleep onset REM periods (SOREMPs).

Explanation: Multiple sleep onset REM periods (SOREMPs) are more specific for narcolepsy than a short sleep latency, but they can also be present in patients with significant sleep disruption such as obstructive sleep apnea (up to 5%), circadian sleep disorders, insufficient sleep, abrupt withdrawal from REM sleep-suppressing agents, and in about 1% to 3% of normal healthy adults.

212. Answer: B

Educational objective: Describe the clinical features of REM sleep behavior disorder.

Explanation: In REM sleep behavior disorder, abnormal behavior develops during REM sleep accompanied by loss of REM-related muscle atonia or hypotonia. These dream-enacting behaviors can result in sleep disruption, or injury to the sleeper or bed partner. There is often no history of violent or aggressive behavior during the day while awake. The eyes are usually closed, in contrast to the sleepwalker whose eyes are open during the episode. The episode ends with a rapid awakening and full alertness. Associated features include good dream recall on awakening. Episodes are more common during the second half of the night (eg, early morning hours) when REM sleep is most common.

213. Answer: A

Educational objective: Describe the clinical features of Beckwith-Wiedeman syndrome.

Explanation: Features of Beckwith-Wiedeman syndrome include unusually large tongues, small noses, umbilical abnormalities (eg, hernia or omphalocele), and renal/adrenal tumors. It can affect both genders.

214. Answer: B

Educational objective: Distinguish between hypercapnic and nonhypercapnic forms of central sleep apnea.

Explanation: Hypercapnic central sleep apnea (CSA) is seen in persons with ventilatory impairment due to neuromuscular diseases affecting the respiratory apparatus or due to diminished chemoresponsiveness. On the other hand, nonhypercapnic CSA consists of idiopathic CSA and central apnea in patients with congestive heart failure.

215. Answer: A

Educational objective: Explain the effects of hormone replacement therapy on sleep in perimenopausal women.

Explanation: Hormone replacement therapy (eg, oral synthetic estrogens and medroxyprogesterone) increases sleep duration and improves subjective sleep quality in both asymptomatic women during perimenopause as well as those with climacteric symptoms such as hot flashes. Administration of progesterone is associated with a decrease in wake time after sleep onset. Women receiving estrogen therapy report less insomnia and less sleep disturbance. Hormone replacement therapy is also associated with decreased prevalence of obstructive sleep apnea and hot flashes.

216. Answer: A

Educational objective: Describe the clinical features of insufficient sleep syndrome.

Explanation: Insufficient sleep is the most common cause of excessive sleepiness. It is defined as a chronic voluntary but unintentional failure to obtain nighttime sleep that is sufficient in duration to achieve and maintain normal alertness while awake. If desired, individuals have no difficulty sleeping longer. This sleep pattern is present almost daily for at least 3 months. Duration of sleep is commonly extended during weekends or vacations as compared to weekdays.

Resolution of excessive sleepiness generally occurs during a trial of nighttime sleep extension. Polysomnography demonstrates features consistent with inadequate sleep, including a reduced sleep latency and increased sleep efficiency and duration.

217. Answer: A

Educational objective: *Describe the differences in the clinical features of obstructive sleep apnea between younger and older adults.*

Explanation: *The presence of clinical symptoms associated with obstructive sleep apnea (OSA), such as excessive daytime sleepiness, appears to be less common, and, if present, less severe among older adults than in younger adults. Most of the increase in prevalence of OSA among older adults occurs prior to the age of 65 years, with the prevalence remaining relatively stable thereafter. There is a male predominance in prevalence. The risk of developing OSA among women increases after menopause. The increased risk of cardiopulmonary diseases appears to be less prominent among the elderly than among younger individuals. Unlike in younger individuals, excess body weight, snoring and witnessed apneas are less consistent indicators for the presence of OSA in older adults. Therapy for OSA is similar in both age groups.*

218. Answer: D

Educational objective: *Describe the clinical and polysomnographic features of a manic episode of mood disorder.*

Explanation: *A manic episode is associated with a decrease in both amount of and requirement for sleep, and patients often complain of insomnia, which can be severe. Polysomnographic features include an increase in awakenings, an increase in REM density, a decrease in NREM stages 3 and 4 sleep, and a decrease in REM sleep latency.*

219. Answer: D

Educational objective: *Identify the factors that increase the likelihood of developing sleep-related hypoventilation in patients with lower airway obstruction.*

Explanation: *Sleep-related hypoventilation may develop in patients with lower airway obstruction. The likelihood of sleep-related hypoventilation is greater in patients with forced expiratory volume exhaled in 1 second/forced vital capacity (FEV_1/FVC) < 60%, with daytime hypoxemia or hypercapnia, or with comorbid obstructive sleep apnea. Causes of lower airway obstruction include alpha-1* antitrypsin deficiency, bronchiectasis, cystic fibrosis, and chronic obstructive pulmonary disease (chronic bronchitis and emphysema).

220. Answer: C

Educational objective: *Describe the effects of continuous positive airway pressure on Cheyne-Stokes respiration.*

Explanation: *In Cheyne-Stokes respiration, continuous positive airway pressure (CPAP) increases $PaCO_2$, enhances cardiac function, and improves oxygen saturation. CPAP therapy generally improves blood pressure control.*

221. Answer: A

Educational objective: *Describe the features of transcutaneous carbon dioxide ($PtcCO_2$) monitoring.*

Explanation: *Transcutaneous carbon dioxide ($PtcCO_2$), the CO_2 tension at the epidermal surface, can be monitored non-invasively using a silver chloride electrode or an infrared capnometer. Although $PtcCO_2$ affords continuous monitoring during sleep, $PtcCO_2$ often differs significantly from a simultaneously obtained $PaCO_2$.*

$PtcCO_2$ monitoring is most commonly used during neonatal or pediatric polysomnography. It has less clinical utility among adults because its slow response time makes it unsuitable for monitoring blood gas tensions during sleep when rapid and short-lasting changes can occur. $PtcCO_2$ monitoring may be of some use in patients with waking hypercapnia and in those with suspected sleep-related alveolar hypoventilation.

222. Answer: A

Educational objective: *Describe the standard electrode derivations for monitoring electroencephalography.*

Explanation: *With electroencephalography (EEG), the voltage recorded from scalp electrodes originates from the summed potential activity of neuronal somas and dendrites within the cortex. Wakefulness is associated with EEG frequencies from 14 to 45 Hz, whereas sleep EEG frequencies are generally restricted to 0.5 to 14 Hz. Electrode placement is based on the International 10–20 System. In this system, electrodes are placed at 10% or 20% of the distance between specific landmarks (eg, bridge of nose [nasion], occipital prominence [inion], vertex, and preauricular location). Each electrode is provided with a letter that represents the corresponding region of the brain (F = frontal, Fp = frontopolar, O = occipital,; P = parietal, and T = temporal) and a numerical subscript (left-sided electrodes = odd numbers, right-sided electrodes = even numbers). Reference electrodes are placed over the mastoid process (A). A derivation is the difference in voltage between two electrodes. Standard electrode derivations for monitoring EEG are C3/A2 or C4/A1 (based on Rechtschaffen and Kales criteria), or 01/A2 or 02/A1. Additional EEG electrodes are necessary* to evaluate nocturnal seizure activity. A montage or set of derivations can either be bipolar (two standard electrodes are matched to each other), or referential (a standard electrode is compared to a reference electrode, such as a mastoid electrode).

223. Answer: D

Educational objective: Describe the patterns of eye movements in an electro-oculogram during polysomnography.

Explanation: There are two general patterns of eye movements, namely slow rolling and rapid eye movements. Slow rolling eye movements consist of slow undulating deflections that are present during drowsiness with closed eyes, NREM stage 1 sleep, or brief awakenings; they disappear during stage NREM stage 2 sleep. Rapid eye movements are composed of sharper deflections that can occur during wakefulness with open eyes (eye blinks) or REM sleep. Rapid eye movement density (frequency of rapid eye movements per minute of REM sleep) is less during early REM sleep episodes and progressively increases during later REM sleep periods. Conjugate eye movements create out-of-phase deflections in the two electro-oculography channels, whereas high-voltage EEG artifacts produce in-phase deflections.

224. Answer: C

Educational objective: Enumerate the types of cardiac arrhythmias associated with obstructive sleep apnea.

Explanation: The most common cardiac arrhythmia associated with obstructive sleep apnea (OSA) is sinus arrhythmia. Other arrhythmias include bradycardia, sinus pauses, sinus arrest, premature ventricular contractions, ventricular tachycardia, and atrioventricular block. There is also a higher recurrence rate of atrial fibrillation after successful cardioversion in patients with OSA.

225. Answer: A

Educational objective: Understand the factors that increase the likelihood of Cheyne-Stokes respiration in patients with congestive heart failure.

Explanation: In patients with congestive heart failure, greater risk of developing Cheyne-Stokes respiration is associated with a lower ejection fraction, the presence of atrial fibrillation, lower awake $PaCO_2$, age > 60 years, and male gender.

226. Answer: D

Educational objective: Enumerate the indications for continuous positive airway pressure for children with obstructive sleep apnea.

Explanation: Continuous positive airway pressure (CPAP) is indicated for children with obstructive sleep apnea when adenotonsillectomy is not indicated or contraindicated, when significant symptoms persist following adenotonsillectomy,

or during the perioperative period in children with severe disease. CPAP titration should be repeated periodically to account for the age-related changes in upper airway and craniofacial dimensions.

227. Answer: C

Educational objective: Identify the medications that can produce eye movements during NREM sleep.

Explanation: Administration of selective serotonin reuptake inhibitors (eg, fluoxetine) and tricyclic antidepressants may result in eye movements during NREM stages 2, 3, and 4 sleep (so-called "Prozac eyes").

228. Answer: C

Educational objective: Distinguish the pharmacologic profiles of the different psychostimulants.

Explanation: Because of the risk of hepatotoxicity, pemoline has been withdrawn from the U.S. market. Pemoline is an oxazolidine psychostimulant that acts by increasing the release, and inhibiting the reuptake, of dopamine. Improvements in performance and alertness have been described following its administration. It has an elimination half-life of approximately 12 hours.

229. Answer: B

Educational objective: Describe the clinical features of patients with insomnia.

Explanation: Patients with insomnia often report greater subjective sleep disturbance compared to changes in objective polysomnographic parameters. The discrepancy between subjective estimates and objective measures of sleep is believed to be due to persistent sensory processing during NREM sleep, which decreases the ability of patients with insomnia to distinguish sleep from wakefulness. Perception of sleep appears to be altered. Persons with insomnia may have a greater tendency to describe, when awakened from sleep, of being awake all along, compared to those without insomnia. In addition, they may overestimate the duration of their sleep latencies.

230. Answer: A

Educational objective: Define the different frequencies of rhythms.

Explanation: The frequency, or the number of oscillations per unit time, of rhythms can be classified as ultradian (one oscillation lasting less than 24 hours), circadian (one oscillation approximately every 24 hours), infradian (one oscillation lasting more than 24 hours), or circannual (one oscillation per year).

231. Answer: C

Educational objective: Characterize the unique features of sleep in animals.

Explanation: Among mammals, unihemispheric sleep can be seen in dolphins, eared seals, and manatees. Unihemispheric sleep has also been described in birds.

232. Answer: B

Educational objective: Describe how to perform multiple sleep latency testing.

Explanation: A nocturnal polysomnography should be performed immediately before MSLT to exclude the presence of other sleep disorders and to ensure an adequate duration of nocturnal sleep (at least 6 hours). Obstructive sleep apnea, if present, should be appropriately treated before performing MSLT. MSLT is usually performed between 8:00 to 9:00 AM and 5:00 to 6:00 PM, with the first nap opportunity performed about 2 hours after awakening from the previous night's polysomnography. An adequate sleep duration and regular sleep-wake schedule, as documented by sleep diaries or actigraphy, must have been maintained for at least 1 to 2 weeks preceding MSLT. Furthermore, medications that can potentially influence sleep latency and REM sleep, such as opiates, benzodiazepines, narcotics and REM sleep suppressants, should be discontinued for at least 15 days before the study.

233. Answer: D

Educational objective: Describe the changes in sleep following the administration of methylphenidate.

Explanation: Methylphenidate is a piperidine derivative structurally similar to amphetamine. It also has polysomnographic features similar to amphetamine. These include a decrease in sleep efficiency, a decrease in total sleep time, an increase in wake time after sleep onset, a decrease in NREM stages 3 and 4 sleep, an increase in REM sleep latency, and a decrease in REM sleep. It is indicated for the therapy of narcolepsy and attention deficit hyperactivity disorder.

234. Answer: C

Educational objective: Understand the role of selegiline in the treatment of narcolepsy.

Explanation: Selegiline is a monoamine oxidase (MAO) inhibitor with stimulating and anticataplectic actions. Adverse effects include confusion, dizziness, dry mouth, and nausea. Like other MAO inhibitors, a diet low in tyramine is recommended when taking this medication.

235. Answer: B

Educational objective: Describe the differences between the two cat brain sections performed by Frederick Bremmer.

Explanation: Encephale isole, in which transection is at the C1 vertebral level in the lower part of the medulla between the brain and spinal cord, is associated with electroencephalography (EEG) demonstrating alternating wake and sleep states. With cerveau isole, transection at

the midcollicular level caudal to the origin of the oculomotor nerves in the midbrain, disrupting the projections of the brainstem ascending reticular activating system, produces an EEG that demonstrates sleep state.

236. Answer: C

Educational objective: Describe the polysomnographic features of NREM stage 3 sleep.

Explanation: An epoch is scored as NREM stage 3 sleep if delta electroencephalographic activity occupies between 20% and 50% of the epoch, and it is scored as NREM stage 4 sleep if delta activity occupies greater than 50% of the epoch.

237. Answer: D

Educational objective: Describe the pharmacologic features of the beta-adrenergic blockers.

Explanation: Beta-adrenergic blockers can either be lipid soluble (eg, labetalol, oxprenolol, propranolol, and timolol) or nonlipid soluble (eg, atenolol, nadolol, and sotalol). These agents can give rise to excessive sleepiness, daytime fatigue, insomnia, nightmares, sleep terrors, and hallucinations. Polysomnographic features are drug specific; these commonly consist of an increase in wake time after sleep onset, an increase in NREM stage 1 sleep, an increase in REM sleep latency, and a decrease in REM sleep (except atenolol and metoprolol).

238. Answer: C

Educational objective: Identify the population groups that have a higher likelihood of developing insomnia.

Explanation: Insomnia is the most common sleep disorder, with about a third of adults reporting occasional insomnia and approximately 10% with chronic insomnia. The prevalence of insomnia is greater among the elderly; in individuals who belong to a low socioeconomic status; in shift workers; and in those who are widowed, divorced, or separated. Women are more likely to be affected than men. There appears to be a strong correlation between insomnia and psychiatric disorders. Many patients with insomnia have either an underlying psychiatric pathology or an increased risk of developing a new-onset psychiatric illness. A recent stressor increases the risk of developing insomnia. Finally, the prevalence of insomnia may be greater in substance and alcohol users, in hospitalized or institutionalized persons, and in individuals with an underlying medical or neurologic disorder.

239. Answer: A

Educational objective: Describe the polysomnographic features of primary insomnia.

Explanation: Insomnia is considered primary if it is not due exclusively to another sleep, medical, neurologic, or psychiatric disorder, or to the effects of substance use, abuse, or withdrawal. Three subgroups of insomnia are included in the category of primary insomnia, namely idiopathic insomnia, paradoxical insomnia (sleep state misperception), and psychophysiologic insomnia.

Polysomnographic features of primary insomnia include an increase in sleep latency, a decrease in total sleep time, a decrease in NREM stages 3 and 4 sleep, and an increase in wake time after sleep onset compared with good sleepers. Polysomnography may be normal.

240. Answer: D

Educational objective: Describe the polysomnographic features of theophylline administration.

Explanation: Theophylline is a respiratory stimulant and bronchodilator that is chemically related to caffeine. It produces sleep disruption and may result in complaints of insomnia. Polysomnographic features include an increase in sleep latency, an increase in wake time after sleep onset, an increase in NREM stage 1 sleep, and a decrease in REM sleep.

241. Answer: B

Educational objective: Describe the general divisions of human sleep.

Explanation: Sleep architecture is a term used to describe the division of sleep among the different sleep stages using specific electroencephalographic, electro-oculographic, and chin electromyographic criteria, as well as the relationship of the individual sleep stages to each other. Sleep can be differentiated into non-rapid eye movement NREM sleep and rapid eye movement REM sleep. NREM sleep can be further subdivided into stages 1, 2, 3, and 4 sleep. NREM stages 3 and 4 sleep are often collectively referred to as slow wave sleep or delta wave sleep.

242. Answer: B

Educational objective: Describe the features of post-traumatic hypersomnia.

Explanation: Central nervous system trauma, especially involving the lateral and posterior hypothalamus, basal forebrain, third ventricle, posterior fossa, midbrain, and pons, can lead to excessive sleepiness. The degree of sleepiness usually correlates with the severity of head trauma. Hypersomnia typically begins immediately after head trauma and may be accompanied by fatigue, headaches, and cognitive impairment (memory and concentration). Symptoms may transiently worsen before gradually resolving over several weeks to months. In some, lingering sleep disturbances and sleepiness may be evident. Polysomnography reveals normal sleep duration and quality.

243. Answer: C

Educational objective: Describe the changes in sleep architecture associated with generalized anxiety disorder.

Explanation: Anxiety disorders can give rise to complaints of insomnia, frequent nighttime awakenings, recurring anxiety dreams, or excessive daytime sleepiness. Some may report early morning awakenings. Polysomnographic features consist of an increase in sleep latency, a decrease in sleep efficiency, an increase in wake time after sleep onset, and a decrease in total sleep time. There is an increase in NREM stages 1 and 2 sleep, a decrease in NREM stages 3 and 4, and a decrease in REM sleep. REM sleep latency can either be normal or prolonged.

244. Answer: D

Educational objective: Describe the clinical features of paradoxical insomnia.

Explanation: In paradoxical insomnia, patients, while complaining of chronic severe insomnia, have no polysomnographic evidence of significant sleep disturbance and no impairment of daytime function consistent with subjective reports of extreme sleep loss. Patients may report having very little or no sleep during most nights and no daytime napping. This is associated with "consciousness" of the environment or ongoing thought processes during most of the night. Affected individuals often overestimate sleep latency and underestimate sleep duration compared with objective measures of sleep. Paradoxical insomnia is seen in less than 5% of chronic insomniacs. Onset is generally during early to mid-adulthood. It is less common during childhood and adolescence. Prevalence is higher among women than men. Course tends to be chronic. Despite subjective reports of little or no sleep during polysomnography, the study demonstrates a normal or near normal sleep latency, quality and architecture. Total sleep duration typically exceeds 6.5 hours.

245. Answer: B

Educational objective: Describe the clinical features of familial fatal insomnia.

Explanation: Familial fatal insomnia (FFI) is an autosomal dominant disorder secondary to a prion disease (an amino acid substitution in the prion protein related to a point mutation at codon 178 of the prion protein gene, with coding for methionine by codon 129 on the mutated allele). It is a rare disorder characterized by sleep disturbances, including relentlessly progressive insomnia, autonomic dysregulation, and neurologic abnormalities. Sleep loss eventually becomes total, terminating in stupor, coma, and death generally within 12 months to a few years after its onset. FFI typically has its onset in adulthood, often during the fifth or sixth decade. Both genders are affected equally. Similar to other human prion diseases, it is caused by a misfolded variation of a prion, an intracellular protein structure. The hereditary form results from a point (GAC to AAC) mutation (substitution of aspartic acid with asparagine) at codon 178 of the prion gene PRNP located on chromosome 20. (Interestingly, the familial form *of Creutzfeldt-Jakob disease, another prion disease, results from a similar mutation at codon 178 with coding for valine by codon 129 on the mutated allele.) The point mutation at codon 178 cosegregates with a methionine polymorphism at codon 129. A shorter disease course with a survival generally less than 12 months is seen in patients who are methionine homozygous at codon 129, whereas those who are methionine-valine heterozygous at codon 129 have a longer disease course of 1 to 6 years.*

246. Answer: A

Educational objective: *Describe the pharmacologic properties of the sedating tricyclic antidepressants.*

Explanation: *Sedating tricyclic antidepressants include amitriptyline, doxepin, nortriptyline, and trimipramine. As a group, they have low risk of abuse. It increases REM sleep latency and decreases REM sleep. Adverse effects include anticholinergic actions (eg, constipation or dry mouth), abnormalities in cardiac conduction, orthostatic hypotension, and exacerbation of symptoms of restless legs and periodic limb movements during sleep.*

247. Answer: A

Educational objective: *Identify the ideal electrode impedance for electroencephalography.*

Explanation: *Electroencephalography is commonly recorded using either gold cup or silver silver-chloride electrodes. Electrode impedance should ideally be less than 5000 Ω.*

248. Answer: B

Educational objective: *Describe the pattern of esophageal pressures seen in upper airway resistance syndrome.*

Explanation: *During episodes of respiratory event–related arousals in patients with upper airway resistance syndrome (UARS), esophageal pressures become increasingly more negative immediately preceding an arousal, after which the pressure rapidly returns to baseline levels.*

249. Answer: C

Educational objective: *Describe the clinical features of stimulant-dependent sleep.*

Explanation: *In stimulant-dependent sleep disorder, insomnia may develop whenever stimulant therapy is begun, especially when the medication is taken close to bedtime, or its dosage is increased. Sleep improves following the development of tolerance to the stimulant drugs. Polysomnographic features during stimulant use include an increase in sleep latency, an increase in frequency of arousals, a decrease in total sleep time, an increase in REM sleep latency, and a decrease in REM sleep. During stimulant withdrawal, there is a decrease in sleep latency, an increase in total sleep time, REM sleep rebound, and a decrease in daytime sleep latency on multiple sleep latency test.*

250. Answer: B

Educational objective: *Describe behavioral therapies for childhood insomnia.*

Explanation: *General recommendations for children with insomnia include selection of age-appropriate bedtimes; consistent bedtime routines (minimal stimulating activities) and sleep schedules; teaching a child to fall asleep independently by placing the child in bed sleepy but still awake, both at bedtime and during nighttime awakenings beginning at 2 to 4 months of age; transitioning the infant to the final sleep environment (eg, crib in infant's room) by 3 months of age; and proper use of transitional objects (eg, blanket or stuffed animal) at bedtime.*

251. Answer: D

Educational objective: *Describe the pharmacologic features of pemoline.*

Explanation: *Pemoline, a dopamine agonist, increases alertness and can cause insomnia. Polysomnographic features include a decrease in total sleep time, an increase in wake time after sleep onset, a decrease in NREM stages 3 and 4 sleep, and a decrease in REM sleep. Pemoline has been withdrawn from the U.S. market due to concerns regarding fatal liver failure.*

252. Answer: D

Educational objective: *Describe the features of respiratory inductance plethysmography and thoracic impedance for measuring respiratory effort during polysomnography.*

Explanation: *Changes in chest and abdominal volume during respiration can be measured semiquantitatively using respiratory inductance plethysmography (RIP). Transducers placed around the chest (at the level of the nipples) and abdomen (at the level of the umbilicus) monitor changes in the cross-sectional area of the respective body compartments as reflected in changes in inductance (resistance to change in flow of current) of the transducers. The sum of the signals from calibrated chest and abdominal sensors can afford an estimate of tidal volume and respiratory patterns during sleep. Although RIP provides data on movements of the rib cage and abdomen, it does not offer information regarding airflow.*

Paradoxical motion of the chest and abdomen suggests an obstructive event rather than a central process, and it is most pronounced during REM sleep due to chest wall muscle hypotonia. With impedance pneumography, a current is applied across the thorax, which serves as an electrical conductor. Impedance varies with the relative amount of conductive materials (body fluids and tissue) and nonconductive air between a pair of electrodes placed at opposite sides of the thoracic cage. Total impedance decreases as the volume of conductive material increases in proportion to air and vice versa, affording a qualitative measure of respiratory effort.

253. Answer: A

Educational objective: Describe the clinical features of Huntington disease.

Explanation: Huntington disease is characterized by relentlessly progressive chorea and dementia. Chorea can persist during NREM stages 1 and 2 sleep. The disease is transmitted as an autosomal dominant disorder, with the affected gene linked to the short arm of chromosome 4. Insomnia and sleep fragmentation are common in patients with advanced disease.

254. Answer: D

Educational objective: Describe the clinical features of traumatic brain injury.

Explanation: Insomnia or excessive sleepiness can complicate traumatic brain injuries. Sleep apnea syndromes and circadian rhythm sleep disturbances (eg, delayed sleep phase syndrome) can also occur. Polysomnography can reveal a decrease in total sleep time and increase in frequency of awakenings.

255. Answer: C

Educational objective: Describe the method of scoring sleep stages.

Explanation: Polysomnographic data is divided into 30-second time periods or epochs. The standard sleep study paper speed is 10 millimeters per second (ie, 30 centimeters per epoch page). In contrast, electroencephalographic (EEG) evaluation of seizure activity usually utilizes 10-second time periods (30 millimeters per second). Each epoch is assigned a sleep stage according to the stage that occupies the majority of the epoch.

256. Answer: A

Educational objective: Describe the pharmacologic features of clonidine.

Explanation: Clonidine is an alpha 2-agonist antihypertensive agent. It can cause excessive sleepiness and nightmares. Administration of clonidine can lead to changes in sleep architecture such as a decrease in sleep latency, an increase in total sleep time, a decrease in wake time after sleep onset, an increase in NREM stage 2 sleep, an increase in NREM stages 3 and 4 sleep, an increase in REM sleep latency, and a decrease in REM sleep.

257. Answer: D

Educational objective: Describe the clinical features of alcohol-dependent sleep disorder.

Explanation: Alcohol-dependent sleep disorder is defined as the habitual prebedtime self-prescribed use of alcohol in an effort to ensure sleep onset and maintain sleep continuity. This can, however, paradoxically give rise to insomnia. Alcohol consumed prior to anticipated bedtime can produce drowsiness; however, as serum levels of alcohol decline in the latter half of the night, persons may awaken repeatedly with headaches and diaphoresis. Frequent sleep-stage transitions are often seen. Abrupt termination of alcohol use can precipitate profound insomnia with frequent awakenings and vivid, disturbing dreams. Sleep fragmentation may persist during abstinence among chronic heavy alcohol users. Polysomnographic features during alcohol use include a decrease in NREM stages 3 and 4 sleep, a decrease in REM sleep, and REM-sleep fragmentation. REM sleep rebound occurs during alcohol withdrawal.

258. Answer: B

Educational objective: Describe how to perform scheduled awakenings for children.

Explanation: With scheduled awakenings, the parent wakes up the child slightly before the usual time of awakening, reassures the child, then permits the child to return to sleep. The frequency of scheduled awakenings is then progressively reduced until the awakenings are discontinued completely when the child is able to sleep through the night. Treatment time is often longer than that of extinction procedures, occasionally requiring several weeks. Children are not taught sleep initiation skills with scheduled awakenings.

259. Answer: A

Educational objective: Describe the role of polysomnography in the evaluation of transient or chronic insomnia.

Explanation: Polysomnography is not routinely indicated in the evaluation of transient or chronic insomnia and should not be used as a substitute for a careful clinical history. Polysomnography may be employed when there is strong evidence based on clinical history for insomnia to be due to periodic limb movement disorder or sleep-related breathing disorder. It may also be useful if insomnia is severe and persists despite an adequate trial of behavioral therapy, sleep hygiene, and pharmacologic intervention. Finally, polysomnography is indicated when the diagnosis is uncertain or when it is associated with violent or injurious behavior. Polysomnography is not indicated for routine evaluation of transient or chronic insomnia, evaluation of insomnia due to psychiatric disorders, distinguishing insomnia associated with dementia, or diagnosing insomnia in patients with fibromyalgia or chronic fatigue syndrome.

(From Standards of Practice Committee of the American Academy of Sleep Medicine. Practice parameters for using polysomnography to evaluate insomnia: an update for 2002. Sleep. 2003;26(6):754–60.)

260. Answer: C

Educational objective: Describe the pharmacologic features of the decongestants.

Explanation: *Decongestants, including phenylpropanolamine and pseudoephedrine, possess central nervous system stimulating effects and can cause insomnia. Polysomnographic features following their use include an increase in sleep latency and increase in wake time after sleep onset.*

261. Answer: A

Educational objective: *Describe how sleep in newborns is scored.*

Explanation: *Sleep scoring in newborns follows an "epoch" approach using behavior, respiration, electroencephalography (EEG), electro-oculography (EOG), and electromyography (EMG) data to classify sleep into active REM sleep or quiet sleep. The term "intermediate sleep" is used when epochs do not fully meet criteria for active or quiet sleep. During wakefulness, eyes are open, and visible movements and vocalizations are present. Respiration is variable. EEG demonstrates a mixed slow-wave (theta) pattern with occasional beta and delta waveforms. There are waking eye movements on the EOG, and sustained tone with burst of phasic activity on the EMG. Active REM sleep is characterized by closed eyes, visible movements (facial grimaces, smiles, movements of body and limbs), vocalizations, irregular respiration, low-voltage irregular or mixed EEG pattern, positive eye movements on the EOG and low EMG tone. Features of quiet sleep, on the other hand, include closed eyes, no body movements, regular respiration, high-voltage slow or trace alternant EEG pattern, no eye movements on the EOG, and high EMG tone.*

262. Answer: C

Educational objective: *Identify the arousal thresholds of the various sleep stages.*

Explanation: *Arousal threshold is lowest during NREM stage 1 sleep (easiest to awaken) and highest during NREM stages 3 and 4 sleep (most difficult to awaken).*

263. Answer: B

Educational objective: *Describe the clinical features of recurrent hypersomnia.*

Explanation: *Recurrent hypersomnia can manifest in two forms: hypersomnia only (monosymptomatic type) or accompanied by binge eating and hypersexuality (Kleine-Levin syndrome). Periods of hypersomnia, during which daily sleep duration may exceed 16 to 18 hours, last from a few days to several weeks (typically 2 days to 4 weeks), and recur one or more times annually. It may be associated with impaired cognition, disinhibited behavior, and weight gain (Kleine-Levin type). The episodes terminate with transient insomnia, excitement, hyperactivity, and amnesia. Between episodes, sleep, alertness, behavior, and cognitive function are normal. Recurrent episodes of somnolence begin during early adolescence. Episodes*

can be triggered by acute febrile illness (eg, viral infections). Kleine-Levin syndrome is rare and mostly affects males. Frequency, severity, and duration of episodes may decrease over time.

264. Answer: B

Educational objective: *Describe the polysomnographic features of NREM stage 2 sleep.*

Explanation: *The 3-minute NREM stage 2 sleep rule is a key element for scoring this sleep stage because sleep spindles and K-complexes are episodic and may not be present in every epoch. An epoch is scored as stage 2 sleep if the intervening period between sleep spindles or K-complexes is less than 3 minutes, would otherwise meet criteria for stage 1 sleep (low-amplitude, mixed-frequency electroencephalogram), and is not associated with an arousal. An epoch is scored as stage 1 sleep if the intervening period is equal to or greater than 3 minutes.*

265. Answer: A

Educational objective: *Describe the evaluation of transient or chronic insomnia.*

Explanation: *Self-administered questionnaires, sleep logs, bed partner interviews, and psychologic screening tests are helpful in evaluating insomnia. Multiple sleep latency testing is not routinely indicated for evaluating insomnia.*

266. Answer: B

Educational objective: *Describe the clinical features of narcolepsy.*

Explanation: *The classic clinical tetrad of narcolepsy consists of excessive sleepiness, cataplexy, sleep paralysis, and sleep hallucinations. However, only approximately 10% to 15% of patients demonstrate this full tetrad (Table). Other manifestations of narcolepsy include sleep attacks, automatic behavior, nocturnal sleep disturbance, visual changes (blurred vision, diplopia, ptosis), and lapses in memory.*

Prevalence of clinical features associated with narcolepsy

Clinical feature	Prevalence
Excessive sleepiness	≈ 100%
Cataplexy	≈ 70% to 80%
Hypnagogic/ hypnopompic hallucinations	≈ 8% to 70%
Sleep paralysis	≈ 5% to 65%

267. Answer: A

Educational objective: Describe the characteristic features of sleep among neonates.

Explanation: Neonates (newborn to 2 months) generally have aggregate hours of sleep per day of about 16 to 18 hours (higher among premature infants). Sleep periods, occurring throughout the 24-hour day with no clear diurnal-nocturnal pattern, range from 2 to 3 hours among breast-fed infants to 3 to 5 hours among bottle-fed infants; these sleep periods are separated by periods of wakefulness of 1 to 3 hours. There are frequent awakenings from sleep, with neonates more likely to awaken from active rather than quiet sleep.

268. Answer: D

Educational objective: Understand the role of oxygen therapy for obstructive sleep apnea.

Explanation: The role of oxygen therapy for the treatment of obstructive sleep apnea (OSA) is not clearly established. Although oxygen supplementation can decrease central and mixed apneas, it does not control OSA. Oxygen supplementation can potentially improve nocturnal oxygen saturation but at the risk of possibly increasing apnea duration. In addition, because the definition of a hypopnea often includes a measured reduction of oxygen saturation, administration of oxygen during polysomnography can minimize oxygen desaturation related to respiratory events and, thus, might decrease the frequency of recorded hypopneas. Oxygen supplementation may be considered for patients with marked nocturnal oxygen desaturation that is not controlled by continuous positive airway pressure (CPAP) therapy alone. However, there is no general consensus regarding the level of nocturnal oxygen desaturation that would benefit from oxygen therapy.

269. Answer: A

Educational objective: Describe the features of relaxation techniques used in the treatment of insomnia.

Explanation: Relaxation techniques include progressive muscle relaxation, electromyographic biofeedback, meditation, and guided imagery. Relaxation targets the somatic and psychic-cognitive stressors that perpetuate insomnia. Relaxation techniques are often used for patients with insomnia who are considered to have heightened cognitive and somatic arousal. Patients are taught how to use progressive muscle relaxation or biofeedback to reduce somatic arousal. Psychic-cognitive stressors may be minimized by meditation or guided imagery in which thoughts are redirected toward pleasant or neutral subjects. Sensory motor rhythm biofeedback uses electroencephalographic recordings to instruct patients on how to enhance their ability to generate sleep spindles. Thought blocking (ie, stopping racing thoughts) to decrease cognitive arousal is also used.

270. Answer: A

Educational objective: Describe the polysomnographic features of NREM stage 3 sleep.

Explanation: NREM stage 3 sleep accounts for about 10% of total sleep time in the adult. The amount of NREM stages 3 and 4, and electroencephalographic (EEG) amplitude of delta waves are increased among adolescents and reduced in older adults. Along with NREM stage 4 sleep, it has the highest arousal threshold by external stimuli among the different sleep stages. It is more prominent during the first half of sleep. Sleep spindles may be present on the EEG.

271. Answer: C

Educational objective: Identify the factors that are responsible for sleep disruption in patients with Parkinson disease.

Explanation: Poor sleep is a major complaint of persons with Parkinson disease, especially those with advanced disease, and patients may complain of either excessive sleepiness due to sleep fragmentation or insomnia. Sleep disturbance in Parkinson disease is multifactorial. Muscle spasms, decreased spontaneous body movements, painful leg cramps, repetitive body movements such as tremors, and difficulty with turning in bed secondary to rigidity can contribute to poor sleep quality. Circadian rhythm disorders, including reversal of sleep-wake schedules, have been described. Akathisia, myoclonus, frightening dreams, and dyskinesias (dystonic or choreiform) related to the use of antiparkinsonian medications can give rise to sleep fragmentation. Finally, sleep disturbance in patients with Parkinson disease may be associated with concurrent dementia, mood disorder, or other sleep disorders (eg, periodic limb movements of sleep, restless legs syndrome, and parasomnias such as REM sleep behavior disorder). Respiratory abnormalities such as obstructive and central apneas and hypopneas may develop, particularly in patients with autonomic dysfunction.

272. Answer: D

Educational objective: Describe the polysomnographic features of stage Wake.

Explanation: During stage Wake sleep, low-voltage, high-frequency electroencephalographic (EEG) activity is seen when a person is alert and the eyes are open, and prominent alpha (8–13 Hz) activity (> 50% of the epoch) when a person is drowsy and the eyes are closed. Alpha activity, which is generally more prominent in the occipital leads compared to central leads, is suppressed by eye opening.

273. Answer: B

Educational objective: Describe the features of stimulus control therapy in the treatment of insomnia.

Explanation: Stimulus control therapy aims to strengthen the association of the bedroom and bedtime to a conditioned response for sleep rather than with insomnia, arousal, and anxiety. Patients are encouraged to use the bedroom only for sleep and sexual activity. They are instructed to get into bed intending to sleep only when sleepy and to refrain from engaging in activities in bed that are not compatible with sleep, such as eating, watching television, or working. If unable to sleep or return to sleep within a reasonable time (eg, after 15 to 20 minutes in bed), patients are taught to leave the bedroom and return only when drowsy. In the interim, they are allowed to engage in restful, nonstimulating and sleep-promoting activities such as reading using a dim light. Maintaining a consistent arising time in the morning and avoiding daytime napping are important.

274. Answer: A

Educational objective: *Describe the disorders that are associated with paradoxical breathing.*

Explanation: *Paradoxical breathing or "out-of-phase" motion of the ribcage and abdomen suggesting the presence of increased upper airway resistance can be observed during obstructive apneic and hypocapneic episodes. It can also be observed in persons with neuromuscular weakness involving the respiratory muscles or diaphragm paralysis. This phenomenon is due to downward displacement of the diaphragm occurring simultaneously with occlusion of the upper airway that (1) creates negative intrapleural pressure causing retraction of the thoracic cage and (2) positive intra-abdominal pressure pushing the abdominal wall outward.*

275. Answer: A

Educational objective: *Describe the polysomnographic features of NREM stage 4 sleep.*

Explanation: *Polysomnographic features of NREM stage 4 sleep include:*

1. Electroencephalography: Delta activity occupies greater than 50% of the epoch. Sleep spindles may be present.
2. Electro-oculography: No movements are present
3. Electromyography: Chin muscle activity is low (generally less than that in stages 1 and 2 sleep)

276. Answer: C

Educational objective: *Describe the polysomnographic features of NREM stage 1 sleep.*

Explanation: *Electroencephalographic features of NREM stage 1 sleep include low-voltage, mixed-frequency activity, and prominent theta activity. Beta rhythms may be present. Alpha activity occupies less than 50% of the epoch. Vertex sharp waves (high-amplitude brief negative deflections) may be present and are more prominent in the central leads. There are no sleep spindles or K-complexes.*

277. Answer: D

Educational objective: *Describe the features of temporal control therapy in the treatment of insomnia.*

Explanation: *Temporal control therapy is designed to enhance sleep efficiency. The constancy of the sleep-wake schedule is promoted by having the patient get out of bed at the same time each day regardless of the quality and quantity of the preceding evening's sleep. Daytime naps are not allowed.*

278. Answer: B

Educational objective: *Describe the characteristics of the clock genes of circadian rhythms.*

Explanation: *Circadian rhythms are controlled by transcription-translation positive and negative feedback loops involving the clock genes and regulatory factors. Period and Timeless transcription starts in the early morning to midday, with peak protein levels of Period and Timeless by mid-evening. Levels then decrease due to phosphorylation. Down regulation of Period and Timeless transcription occurs due to interactions with Clock and Cycle. Cryptochrome is required for light-related degradation of Timeless.*

279. Answer: D

Educational objective: *Understand how the number of sleep phases that occur each day changes in difference age groups.*

Explanation: *Sleep among newborns is polyphasic (occurring several times throughout the 24-hour day). In early childhood, typically between the ages of 3 to 5 years, sleep becomes monophasic (occurring only once generally at night). Some adults continue to prefer a biphasic sleep pattern with an afternoon nap and a major nocturnal sleep period.*

280. Answer: D

Educational objective: *Understand the different tests that are available for evaluating patients with narcolepsy.*

Explanation: *Narcolepsy with cataplexy can be diagnosed by clinical history alone. A thorough evaluation of medication and substance use as well as sleep, medical, neurologic, and psychiatric history is mandatory. Polysomnography followed by multiple sleep latency testing (MSLT) is indicated when cataplexy is absent, atypical, or equivocal. MSLT measures a person's physiologic propensity to fall asleep in quiet situations. The Maintenance of Wakefulness Test (MWT) measures a person's ability to remain awake in quiet situations. The MWT may be used to monitor treatment response to stimulant medications used for the therapy of excessive sleepiness.*

281. Answer: D

Educational objective: *Identify the risk factors for nocturnal leg cramps.*

Explanation: *Nocturnal leg cramping is an almost universal experience and most individuals complain of having had these symptoms during their lifetime. Its prevalence may be increased among the elderly, in women during pregnancy, with the use of oral contraceptives, and after vigorous exercise. It also occurs in persons with diabetes mellitus and other endocrine disorders, fluid and electrolyte imbalances (eg, dehydration, hypocalcemia), peripheral vascular disease, neuromuscular disorders, Parkinson disease, and musculoskeletal disorders. A significant number of cases are idiopathic.*

282. Answer: C

Educational objective: *Identify the risk factors for adult nocturnal bruxism.*

Explanation: *A history of childhood bruxism appears to predict its presence in adulthood. The risk of developing bruxism is increased among smokers compared to nonsmokers as well as in persons with restless legs syndrome. Some cases may be related to anxiety, stress, dental disease (eg, malocclusion or mandibular malformation), caffeine ingestion, alcohol consumption, primary sleep disorders (eg, obstructive sleep apnea or REM sleep behavior disorder), neurologic conditions (eg, mental retardation, cerebral palsy, coma, tremors, dystonia, or dyskinesia), personality subtypes (eg, vigilant and highly motivated), and medication use (eg, levodopa or selective serotonin reuptake inhibitors [SSRI]).*

283. Answer: D

Educational objective: *Describe the clinical features of catathrenia.*

Explanation: *Catathrenia consists of expiratory groaning during sleep. Episodes occur predominantly or exclusively during REM sleep during the second half of the night. It appears to be a rare condition that is more common among males.*

The course tends to be chronic with a nightly occurrence. The individual is asymptomatic with no evident distress and is unaware of the events. Physical examination is generally normal.

284. Answer: D

Educational objective: *Describe the characteristic features of sleep during infancy and childhood.*

Explanation: *By 3 to 6 months of age, the development of distinct electroencephalographic features allows differentiation of NREM sleep into four specific stages.*

285. Answer: D

Educational objective: *Describe the clinical features of subwakefulness syndrome.*

Explanation: *Subwakefulness syndrome is a rare and chronic condition in which the subjective sensation of constant daytime sleepiness occurs in the absence of any objective evidence of excessive sleepiness. There is no history of frequent napping. Nocturnal polysomnography is normal; however, continuous daytime polysomnography may demonstrate intermittent episodes of NREM stage 1 sleep.*

286. Answer: A

Educational objective: *Differentiate among the four stages of sleep in the first 6 months of life.*

Explanation: *Active sleep is the first behavioral sleep state to appear and is the predominant sleep state in the newborn (accounts for 60% of sleep in the newborn, 30% of sleep in the 3 month-old infant, and 20% of sleep in the 2- to 6-year-old child).*

287. Answer: D

Educational objective: *Diagnose the diagnostic features of sleep-related bruxism.*

Explanation: *According to the American Academy of Sleep Medicine International Classification of Sleep Disorders, sleep-related bruxism is diagnosed by the presence of $\geq$ 4 episodes per hour of sleep, or $\geq$ 25 individual muscle bursts per hour of sleep, and $\geq$ 2 audible bruxism episodes per polysomnographic study, and no abnormal encephalographic activity such as seizures.*

288. Answer: B

Educational objective: *Identify the average hours of sleep per day in a toddler.*

Explanation: *The aggregate hours of sleep per day in a toddler is approximately 11 to 12 hours. There is a progressive decrease in duration of nocturnal sleep and frequency of daytime napping as a child gets older. Naps decrease to once per day by 18 months of age.*

289. Answer: C

Educational objective: *Describe the features of cognitive therapy in the treatment of insomnia.*

Explanation: *Cognitive therapy addresses unrealistic expectations about sleep and the consequences of insomnia, and it aims to reverse these dysfunctional attitudes and beliefs about sleep. Techniques may include attention shifting, decatastrophizing, and reappraisal. Guided imagery, in contrast, is a relaxation technique.*

290. Answer: C

Educational objective: *Describe the features of cognitive-behavioral therapy for insomnia.*

Explanation: *Cognitive-behavioral therapy (CBT) is a multimodality therapy often including sleep hygiene education, relaxation techniques, stimulus control therapy, sleep* *restriction therapy, and cognitive therapy. It focuses on reversing unrealistic beliefs and attitudes, unreasonable fears, and maladaptive behavior about sleep and sleep loss. Patients are also instructed about proper sleep habits. Improvements in wake time after sleep onset have been described following CBT. CBT may be utilized as a single treatment modality or combined with pharmacologic therapy (indications for combined therapy are not established). Alternative approaches to individualized therapy include group sessions, brief office encounters, phone consultations, and self-help programs. It may benefit patients with either primary or secondary insomnia. Short-term benefits are generally comparable to pharmacologic therapy, and beneficial effects are sustained over time after the initial treatment period. Treatment response is noted in an estimated 70% to 80% of patients with insomnia; however, treatment responsiveness does not necessarily result in complete normalization of sleep.*

291. Answer: C

Educational objective: *Describe the features of the Maintenance of Wakefulness Test.*

Explanation: *The Maintenance of Wakefulness Test (MWT) measures a person's ability to remain awake in quiet situations. It consists of four nap opportunities, each 40 minutes in duration, performed at 2-hour intervals. The patient is asked to sit in bed in a semireclined position with the back and head supported by a bed rest and in a dark, quiet room. Room temperature should be adjusted based on the patient's level of comfort. The first nap trial is started about 1.5 to 3 hours after the patient's customary wake time. Whether sleep logs are used or if a polysomnograph is to be performed prior to the test should be individualized as determined by the clinician. The use of tobacco, caffeine, and stimulant agents should be avoided. Drug screening may be considered. A light breakfast is provided 1 hour before the first trial, and lunch is given immediately after the second trial. Bathroom trips, if needed, are scheduled prior to each trial. Standard biocalibrations are performed before each trial. Patients are instructed to sit still, look directly while avoiding the light, and try to stay awake during the test. Measures to stay awake such as singing are not allowed. Electroencepha-lography (central and occipital leads), electro-oculography, and chin electromyography are used to determine the duration of sleep latencies (from lights out to the first epoch of sleep [sleep onset]) for each nap. The test is terminated once unequivocal sleep (defined as three consecutive epochs of stage 1 sleep, or one epoch of any other sleep stage) occurs, or after 40 minutes if no sleep is recorded.*

Mean sleep latency of less than 8 minutes on the 40-minute MWT is considered abnormal. Staying awake on all trials may provide an appropriate expectation for individuals who require the highest level of alertness for safety. Values greater than 8 minutes but less than 40 minutes are of

uncertain significance. The MWT is less sensitive than the Multiple Sleep Latency Test in measuring sleepiness but may be useful in monitoring treatment response to stimulant medications that are used for excessive sleepiness in narcolepsy or to continuous positive airway pressure (CPAP) therapy for obstructive sleep apnea.

292. Answer: B

Educational objective: *Identify the temporal association of headaches with sleep.*

Explanation: *Whereas some headaches occur during both sleep and wakefulness (eg, migraine, cluster headache, and chronic paroxysmal hemicrania), others occur only during sleep (eg, hypnic headaches). Migraines, cluster headaches, and chronic paroxysmal hemicrania commonly have their onset during sleep.*

293. Answer: D

Educational objective: *Describe the pharmacologic properties of the different benzodiazepines.*

Explanation: *Based on duration of action, benzodiazepines can be classified into short-acting (half-life of less than 3–4 hours), intermediate-acting (half-life of 8–24 hours), and long-acting (half-life of greater than 24 hours) agents. Short-acting agents include alprazolam, oxazepam, and triazolam. Intermediate-acting agents include estazolam and temazepam. Long-acting agents include clorazepate, diazepam, flurazepam, and quazepam.*

294. Answer: D

Educational objective: *Describe the features of positive airway pressure therapy for patients with obstructive sleep apnea.*

Explanation: *Positive airway pressure therapy is generally recommended for all patients with an apnea hypopnea index (AHI) $\geq$ 15/hour, and symptomatic patients (eg, excessive daytime sleepiness, insomnia, impaired cognition, mood disorder, insomnia, hypertension, ischemic heart disease, or stroke) with an AHI between 5/hour and 30/hour. Whereas continuous positive airway pressure (CPAP) provides a constant pressure through the respiratory cycle, bilevel positive airway pressure provides a higher level during inspiration and a lower pressure during expiration. Positive airway pressure is believed to function as a pneumatic splint that maintains the patency of the vulnerable portions of the nasopharyngeal airway, and increases nasal pressure above the critical closing pressure. It is generally accepted that higher pressures are required to reverse airway occlusion during REM sleep and during sleep in a supine position. A split-night study, consisting of an initial diagnostic portion followed by CPAP titration on the same night, can potentially underestimate the severity of OSA because respiratory events tend to be more common during REM sleep, which predominates during the second half of the night.*

295. Answer: C

Educational objective: Describe the significance of snoring among children.

Explanation: The prevalence of snoring among children is estimated to be about 3% to 20%. Isolated snoring in children, unaccompanied by obstructive sleep apnea, is associated with behavioral and academic problems, as well as excessive sleepiness. Such snoring is believed to be related to significant adenotonsillar hypertrophy in about 60% of cases, and incidence peaks at 2 to 8 years of age, coinciding with the peak enlargement of the tonsils and adenoids.

296. Answer: D

Educational objective: Describe the clinical features of sleep paralysis.

Explanation: Sleep paralysis involves a transient loss of the ability to move occurring at sleep onset (hypnagogic) or on awakening (hypnopompic). It occurs in approximately 25% to 80% of persons with narcolepsy. Less frequently, it can be seen either in an isolated form or in normal persons during sleep deprivation. It involves all voluntary muscles with sparing of the respiratory and ocular muscles. Sensorium is generally unaffected. Recovery, either spontaneously or following external stimulation, is immediate and complete. Differential diagnosis includes both isolated and familial (transmitted as an X-linked dominant trait) sleep paralysis and transient (hyperkalemic or hypokalemic) paralysis. Recurrent sleep paralysis can affect about 4% of the normal population.

297. Answer: B

Educational objective: Describe the clinical features of chronic paroxysmal hemicrania.

Explanation: Chronic paroxysmal hemicrania typically presents as a severe unilateral headache located in the temporal, orbital, or supraorbital region. It is most commonly associated with REM sleep and is responsive to therapy with indomethacin.

298. Answer: B

Educational objective: Describe the polysomnographic features of NREM stage 2 sleep.

Explanation: NREM stage 2 sleep accounts for the greatest proportion (45% to 55%) of total sleep time in adults. It is defined by the presence of low-voltage, mixed-frequency electroencephalographic (EEG) activity. Sleep spindles and K-complexes are present and are generally maximal over the vertex. Delta EEG activity occupies less than 20% of the epoch. Typically, there are no eye movements and chin muscle activity is low.

299. Answer: D

Educational objective: Describe the pharmacologic properties of the different benzodiazepines.

Explanation: The timing of drug administration is determined chiefly by its onset of action. Agents that are rapidly absorbed from the gastrointestinal tract have a quick onset of action and can be given at bedtime. These drugs include clorazepate, diazepam, flurazepam, and quazepam. On the other hand, benzodiazepines such as temazepam, whose action is delayed following ingestion, may need to be taken slightly earlier than the desired bedtime.

300. Answer: B

Educational objective: Provide the indications for bilevel positive airway pressure (BPAP) therapy for patients with sleep-related breathing disorders.

Explanation: Bilevel positive airway pressure (BPAP) therapy can be considered as an optional therapy to continuous positive airway pressure (CPAP) in selected patients who require high pressures, who report difficulty exhaling against a fixed CPAP pressure, or who have coexisting central hypoventilation. BPAP may also be beneficial in patients with some forms of restrictive lung disease or hypoventilation syndromes and daytime hypercapnia.

(From Kushida CA, Littner MR, Hirshkowitz M, et al. Practice parameters for the use of continuous and bilevel positive airway pressure devices to treat adult patients with sleep-related breathing disorders. Sleep. 2006;29(3):375–380.)

301. Answer: D

Educational objective: Describe the clinical features of colic.

Explanation: Colic is defined as repeated sustained episodes of crying (> 3 hours) and irritability or fussing, with no apparent reason. It has been reported in up to 20% of infants, beginning generally at about 3 weeks of age. Colic usually resolves by 3 to 4 months of age. Colic can give rise to insomnia. Infants with colic often have shorter reported sleep durations and a slightly greater prevalence of REM sleep-related obstructive apneas on polysomnography than infants without colic.

302. Answer: A

Educational objective: Describe the clinical features of REM sleep.

Explanation: The loss of postural muscle tone during REM sleep is due to postsynaptic hyperpolarization of the spinal motoneurons; however, "bursts" of chin electromyographic (EMG) activity may be present during phasic REM sleep. It accounts for about 25% of total sleep time in the adult, with three to five periods of REM sleep during the night, and progressively greater REM sleep during the latter part of sleep.

303. Answer: D

Educational objective: Describe the clinical features of complex partial seizures.

Explanation: Partial seizures (eg, frontal and temporal lobe epilepsies) are often evident during NREM sleep. They can be further subdivided into simple partial or complex partial seizures. Simple partial seizures occur without a change of consciousness. Complex partial seizures occur with a change in content, or loss, of consciousness. They commonly originate from the temporal or frontal lobes and can be associated with localized sensorimotor manifestations, wanderings, and automatisms (such as lip smacking, vocalization, or sleepwalking).

304. Answer: A

Educational objective: *Know the various neurotransmitters that play a role in the regulation of wakefulness, NREM sleep, and REM sleep.*

Explanation: Neurotransmitters involved with the regulation of wakefulness include acetylcholine, dopamine, glutamate, histamine, hypocretin (orexin), norepinephrine, and serotonin. Peptides that are important in enhancing the effect of these neurotransmitters include adrenocorticotropic hormone, corticotropin-releasing factor, neurotensin, substance P, thyroid-stimulating hormone, thyrotropin-releasing factor, and vasoactive intestinal peptide.

305. Answer: A

Educational objective: *Describe the pharmacologic properties of the different benzodiazepine receptor agonsists.*

Explanation: Benzodiazepines are associated with several adverse effects. Short-acting agents may cause rebound daytime anxiety, and greater amnesia and withdrawal symptoms (including rebound insomnia) following cessation of their use. The effect of agents with long elimination half-lives may persist into the following day, producing daytime sleepiness, poor motor coordination, delayed reaction times, and cognitive impairment. Other adverse consequences of benzodiazepines include amnesia, confusion, rebound insomnia, development of tolerance and withdrawal symptoms, and the risk of dependence and abuse. Rebound insomnia refers to the subjective and objective worsening of sleep (relative to baseline pretreatment levels) and daytime well-being that can develop for several days after drug discontinuation. It is more likely to occur with short-acting and intermediate-acting agents. The duration of sleep deterioration can be protracted. Although rebound insomnia can develop following short-term therapy with benzodiazepines, it is particularly prominent after chronic treatment.

306. Answer: C

Educational objective: *Describe the pharmacologic features of cocaine.*

Explanation: Cocaine potentiates the effects of epinephrine and norepinephrine, and it increases alertness. Polysomnographic features are similar to amphetamines.

There is a decrease in total sleep time and decrease in REM sleep during cocaine use as well as an increase in arousal and improvement in reaction time in sleep-deprived persons. During initial cocaine discontinuation, changes in polysomnographic parameters include an increase in total sleep time and increase in REM sleep. Multiple sleep latency testing during acute cocaine discontinuation demonstrates a decrease in sleep latency and an increased likelihood of sleep onset REM periods. Persistent insomnia and disturbance in REM sleep is common during chronic cocaine abstinence. Cocaine is associated with a high abuse liability.

307. Answer: D

Educational objective: *Identify the genetic syndromes associated with midfacial and mandibular hypoplasia.*

Explanation: Midfacial hypoplasia is a key feature of achondroplasia, Apert syndrome, Crouzon syndrome, and Down syndrome. Pierre-Robin sequence is associated with mandibular hypoplasia. Patients with either midfacial or mandibular hypoplasia possess an increased risk of developing obstructive sleep apnea.

308. Answer: B

Educational objective: *Differentiate among the four stages of sleep in the first 6 months of life.*

Explanation: Active sleep is characterized by the presence of frequent body and facial twitches and jerks (including limb movements, sucking movements, grimaces, vocalizations and tremors), rapid eye movements, and irregular breathing. In contrast, quiet sleep is characterized by minimal or no body movements and by regular breathing. Sleep that does not fully meet criteria for either active or quiet sleep is referred to as intermediate sleep, whereas transitional sleep occurs in the transition period between active, quiet, and intermediate sleep.

309. Answer: B

Educational objective: *Enumerate the changes in sleep architecture related to oral contraceptive use.*

Explanation: The changes in sleep architecture related to oral contraceptive use include an increase in NREM stage 2 sleep, no change or decrease in NREM stages 3 and 4 sleep, a decrease in REM sleep latency, and no change in REM sleep.

310. Answer: A

Educational objective: *Provide a differential diagnosis for restless legs syndrome.*

Explanation: Many disorders may be mistaken for restless legs syndrome. With akathisia, motor restlessness is usually related to the use of neuroleptic agents or dopamine receptor antagonists and is not improved by movement. Painful toes-moving legs syndrome is characterized by painful sensation not relieved by movement that is secondary to lumbosacral radiculopathy and is accompanied by persistent toe movements. Patients with Vesper's curse have transient lumbar stenosis due to supine-related venous plexus engorgement that gives rise to lower extremity paresthesias and lumbosacral pain.

311. Answer: A

Educational objective: Describe the clinical characteristics of a short sleeper.

Explanation: The habitual sleep duration in a short sleeper is, as the name aptly describes, less than is customary for a similarly aged person, often averaging 5 hours or less daily in an adult younger than 60 years of age. Sleep is otherwise unremarkable with normal sleep initiation, quality, continuity, and consolidation. Sleep is restorative despite its brevity. It is not associated with daytime symptoms. Short sleepers may seek medical evaluation because of concerns about their inability to sleep longer. Aside from reassurance, no specific therapy is required.

312. Answer: C

Educational objective: Describe adherence to continuous positive airway pressure therapy for obstructive sleep apnea.

Explanation: Less than optimal continuous positive airway pressure (CPAP) utilization is a significant problem in clinical practice. Self-report often overestimates actual CPAP use. Therapeutic adherence among the different studies have varied from 46% to 80% of patients that use CPAP for 4 or more hours nightly on 70% or more of monitored nights. Average nightly use is between 4 to 5 hours each night among CPAP users. The percentage of days in which CPAP is not used correlates with decreased duration of nightly use. Long-term use of CPAP does not appear to be related to the prescribed pressure. Patterns of nightly use are often discernible within the first few days or weeks of initiating treatment.

313. Answer: A

Educational objective: Describe the pharmacologic properties of the benzodiazepine agents.

Explanation: Lethality with overdose of benzodiazepines, when ingested alone, is low but rises with coingestion of other compounds such as alcohol and other central nervous system depressants.

314. Answer: B

Educational objective: Enumerate the techniques that may increase continuous positive airway pressure utilization.

Explanation: Continuous positive airway pressure (CPAP) support programs, including motivational enhancement to reduce ambivalence regarding treatment, have been shown to improve CPAP utilization. Nasal dryness, rhinorrhea, nasal congestion, sneezing, or epistaxis are common problems in patients using CPAP therapy and can adversely affect optimal CPAP utilization. Humidification can help alleviate these problems and improve CPAP use. Bilevel positive airway pressure has not been noted to consistently alter patient acceptance and CPAP adherence.

315. Answer: C

Educational objective: Identify the indications for adenotonsillectomy in children with obstructive sleep apnea.

Explanation: Adenotonsillectomy is the first-line and most common therapy for children with obstructive sleep apnea because a majority of childhood OSA is due to significant adenotonsillar enlargement. It is effective in most cases of uncomplicated childhood OSA (ie, without craniofacial anomalies, choanal atresia, macroglossia, or hypotonia). In patients with complicated cases of OSA, a postoperative polysomnogram following adenotonsillectomy is recommended to assess the efficacy of the procedure. Nevertheless, OSA may recur during adolescence in children with initial success with adenotonsillectomy.

316. Answer: D

Educational objective: Understand how sleep-disordered breathing is affected by pregnancy.

Explanation: Pregnancy increases the risk of snoring and obstructive sleep apnea. Snoring and obstructive sleep apnea can develop in women with risk factors for sleep-related breathing disorders prior to pregnancy or can worsen in pregnant women with preexisting disorders.

Factors responsible for the increased incidence of snoring and obstructive sleep apnea during pregnancy include weight gain and upper airway congestion (related to estrogen). Conversely, progesterone, a respiratory stimulant, may protect against worsening sleep apnea. Sleep-related breathing disorders during pregnancy are related to higher rates of maternal hypertension, preeclampsia, intrauterine growth retardation, and low birth weight.

317. Answer: C

Educational objective: Describe the clinical features of restless legs syndrome.

Explanation: Restless legs syndrome (RLS) or Ekbom syndrome is characterized by abnormal and unpleasant sensations (paresthesias or dysesthesias) involving the lower extremities that become apparent or worsen at rest, especially in the evening at bedtime, and are relieved, at least transiently, with movement. Although symptoms are typically not described as painful, a complaint of pain does not exclude the diagnosis. These uncomfortable sensations extend from the feet and ankle proximally to the legs and, occasionally, thighs. Similar sensations have also been described in the arms. There is often an accompanying irresistible urge to move the limbs (motor restlessness) to relieve the uncomfortable sensation. Less frequently, an isolated urge to move is present without any accompanying unpleasant sensations. Movements or walking result in temporary relief of symptoms. Relief of the unpleasant sensations is typically immediate and can be either partial or complete. However, with advanced disease, movements may be associated with minimal improvement. Symptoms tend to recur following cessation of leg motion.

318. Answer: D

Educational objective: *Describe the movement of periodic limb movement disorder.*

Explanation: *Periodic limb movements of sleep or nocturnal myoclonus consist of stereotypical, intermittent, and repetitive movements of the limbs that occur during sleep. It usually involves the lower extremities but can affect the arms as well. The characteristic movement consists of partial flexion of the ankle, knee, and hip with extension of the big toe and fanning of the small toes. Involvement of the upper extremity consists of flexion at the elbow.*

319. Answer: B

Educational objective: *Describe the pharmacologic properties of the nonbenzodiazepine benzodiazepine receptor agonists.*

Explanation: *The hypnosedative action of the nonbenzodiazepine benzodiazepine receptor agonists is comparable to that of benzodiazepines. Compared with conventional benzodiazepines, these agents do not possess myorelaxant or antiseizure activity, are less likely to cause significant rebound insomnia or tolerance, and are associated with minimal abuse liability. However, risk of abuse remains a concern, particularly in patients with a history of abuse or dependence on alcohol or other drugs and in those with psychiatric diseases.*

In addition, most of these agents are less likely than benzodiazepines to impair daytime performance and memory due to their relatively short duration of action and their low potential for residual effect. They are relatively safe and are seldom lethal even with overdosage. They are less likely to disrupt normal sleep architecture than benzodiazepines.

320. Answer: C

Educational objective: *Describe the use of autotitrating positive airway pressure devices for the therapy of obstructive sleep apnea.*

Explanation: *Not all autotitrating positive airway pressure (APAP) devices are comparable in efficacy. Different devices utilize different algorithms for monitoring respiratory events and for altering delivered pressures. Nonsnorers should not be titrated with APAP devices using diagnostic algorithms that rely on vibration or sound production alone. They are not recommended for split-night positive*

airway pressure titration. Its use can be limited by the development of significant mask/mouth leaks or central apneas, and proper mask fitting is crucial prior to unattended APAP use.

321. Answer: D

Educational objective: *Describe the sleep disorders commonly present in infants.*

Explanation: *Between the ages of 2 to 12 months, infants may develop difficulties with sleep onset, bedtime resistance, sleep onset association disorder, rhythmic movement disorders, and problematic night wakings. Limit-setting sleep disorder develops as a toddler (1 to 3 years of age) gains increasing mobility and independence.*

322. Answer: B

Educational objective: *Describe the polysomnographic features of narcolepsy.*

Explanation: *Polysomnographic features of narcolepsy include sleep fragmentation and repetitive awakenings. A short sleep latency (< 10 minutes) and sleep-onset REM period (SOREMP; decreased REM sleep latency of 20 minutes or less) may be present. SOREMPs during nocturnal polysomnography have been described in up to 25% to 50% of patients. NREM stage 1 sleep is increased. Total sleep time and percent REM sleep are often normal. Obstructive sleep apnea and periodic limb movements of sleep may be observed.*

323. Answer: B

Educational objective: *Describe the pharmacologic properties of sedating antidepressants.*

Explanation: *Sedating antidepressants have been increasingly prescribed as off-label agents for the treatment of insomnia over the past several years. However, the therapeutic efficacy and safety of sedating antidepressants used as hypnotics for patients with insomnia are incompletely understood. In general, serotonin specific antidepressants have fewer adverse effects than the older tertiary tricyclic antidepressants. Effects of sedating antidepressants on sleep architecture include a decrease in sleep latency, a decrease in frequency of awakenings, an increase in total sleep time, and an increase in sleep efficiency.*

324. Answer: C

Educational objective: *Describe the clinical features of continuous spike waves during sleep.*

Explanation: *Continuous spike waves during sleep were formerly referred to as electrical status epilepticus of sleep. Generalized continuous electroencephalographic (EEG) spike and slow-wave complexes occur continuously throughout NREM sleep with or without any apparent movements or clinical complaints. EEG discharges decrease during REM sleep and disappear with awakening. This is seen in children,* many of whom have an underlying seizure disorder. The disorder lasts for several months to years and tends to resolve within 3 years of presentation with increasing age.

325. Answer: B

Educational objective: *Know the various neurotransmitters that play a role in the regulation of wakefulness, NREM sleep, and REM sleep.*

Explanation: The main NREM neurotransmitters are serotonin and gamma-aminobutyric acid. Other neurotransmitters include adenosine and peptides (alpha melanocyte-stimulating hormone, cholecystokinin, cortistatin, growth hormone–releasing hormone, interleukins, muramyl peptides, opiates, and somatostatin).

326. Answer: A

Educational objective: *Identify the location of dopamine-containing neurons in the brain.*

Explanation: Neurons containing dopamine are located in the ventral mesencephalic tegmentum and substantia nigra. Dopamine release occurs during both wake and REM sleep and is increased by amphetamines. A decrease in arousal follows lesions involving dopamine neurons.

327. Answer: B

Educational objective: *Describe the clinical features of multiple system atrophy.*

Explanation: Multiple system atrophy, previously referred to as Shy Drager syndrome, is a multisystemic neurodegenerative disorder characterized by progressive autonomic dysfunction or failure as well as cerebellar and extrapyramidal (eg, parkinsonism) symptoms. Onset is during adulthood. Sleep disorders include sleep-related respiratory abnormalities (obstructive and central apneas and hypopneas), insomnia, and REM sleep behavior disorder. Common polysomnographic features include a decrease in sleep efficiency, an increase in frequency of awakenings, a decrease in total sleep time, a decrease in NREM stages 3 and 4 sleep, and a decrease in REM sleep.

328. Answer: C

Educational objective: *Describe the characteristics of the neurotransmitter glycine.*

Explanation: Glycine is the main inhibitory neurotransmitter in the spinal cord. By causing hyperpolarization of spinal motoneurons, it causes REM sleep-related paralysis. Glycine is released during REM sleep.

329. Answer: C

Educational objective: *Understand the role of hypocretin in the regulation of wakefulness.*

Explanation: Perifornical neurons in the lateral hypothalamus that contain hypocretin (orexin) project widely to the

cerebral cortex. Destruction of hypocretin neurons results in no significant change in the total amount of waking. Narcolepsy develops in animal models with deletion of the hypocretin (orexin) gene.

330. Answer: A

Educational objective: *Describe the clinical features of seizure disorders.*

Explanation: Polysomnography may demonstrate both ictal and interictal electroencephalographic (EEG) epileptiform activity. Nonetheless, a normal EEG does not exclude a diagnosis of seizures. A majority of seizures occur during NREM sleep, especially stages 1 and 2 sleep, and less commonly during REM sleep. Changes in sleep architecture associated with seizures include increases in sleep latency, wake time after sleep onset, and NREM stages 1 and 2 sleep, and decreases in both NREM stages 3 and 4 sleep and REM sleep.

331. Answer: A

Educational objective: *Describe the pharmacologic properties of ramelteon.*

Explanation: Ramelteon is a melatonin receptor agonist that is highly selective for ML1 receptors, which are located mainly in the cells of the suprachiasmatic nucleus, and it has less affinity for other ML receptor subtypes, including ML2. It has clinically relevant sleep-promoting effects, including a decrease in sleep latency, an increase in sleep efficiency, and an increase in total sleep time.

332. Answer: A

Educational objective: *Describe the indications for bilevel positive airway pressure therapy.*

Explanation: Patients with obstructive sleep apnea (OSA) who have persistent oxygen desaturation due to hypoventilation despite continuous positive airway pressure (CPAP) therapy may benefit from bilevel positive airway pressure (BPAP). BPAP is indicated for patients with concurrent chronic obstructive pulmonary disease (overlap syndrome), or in patients in whom hypoventilation (eg, obesity hypoventilation syndrome or neuromuscular weakness) is suspected. Although studies have not shown consistent advantages of BPAP over CPAP in patient preference and device utilization, BPAP may also be considered for patients with OSA who are unable to tolerate CPAP because of complaints of being unable to breathe out against high CPAP pressures or because of mouth leaks or aerophagia.

333. Answer: D

Educational objective: *Describe the pharmacologic features of the antiparkinsonian drugs.*

Explanation: Antiparkinsonian drugs include dopamine agonists (bromocriptine, pergolide, pramipexole and ropinirole); dopamine precursors (levodopa); anticholinergics *(benztropine); and selegiline. Amantadine, benztropine, bromocriptine, levodopa, pergolide, pramipexole, and selegiline can cause insomnia. Pramipexole and ropinirole can cause excessive sleepiness. High-dose levodopa can cause sleep disruption. Polysomnographic features of levodopa include a decrease in NREM stages 3 and 4 sleep and an increase in REM sleep latency. Polysomnographic features of benztropine consist of an increase in NREM stages 3 and 4 sleep and a decrease in REM sleep latency. Benztropine, pramipexole and ropinirole can cause hallucinations. Amantadine and levodopa can cause nightmares.*

334. Answer: C

Educational objective: *Classify the various parasomnias according to the American Academy of Sleep Medicine's International Classification of Sleep Disorders: Diagnostic and Coding Manual (2nd edition).*

Explanation: *Parasomnias can be classified into three groups based on the American Academy of Sleep Medicine International Classification of Sleep Disorders (2nd edition). Disorders of arousal from NREM sleep include confusional arousals, sleepwalking, and sleep terrors. Parasomnias usually associated with REM sleep include REM sleep behavior disorder (and parasomnia overlap disorder and status dissociatus), recurrent isolated sleep paralysis, and nightmare disorder. Other parasomnias include sleep-related dissociative disorders, sleep enuresis, sleep-related groaning (catathrenia), exploding head syndrome, sleep-related hallucinations, and sleep-related eating disorder.*

335. Answer: A

Educational objective: *Describe the clinical features of Rett disorder.*

Explanation: *Rett disorder is characterized by sleep disturbance, developmental delay, seizures, cognitive dysfunction, bruxism, hyperventilation and breath holding while awake, and speech impairment that starts within the first 18 months of age. Individuals with Rett syndrome develop a variety of deficits (eg, gait incoordination, psychomotor retardation, head growth deceleration, impairment of language development, and stereotypical hand motions) following a period of normal psychomotor development during the first few months after birth. Rett disorder has been reported only in females. Some cases are related to mutations in MECP2 gene in chromosome X. Associated sleep disturbances include an increase in total sleep time, with an increase in daytime sleep and decrease in nighttime sleep.*

336. Answer: A

Educational objective: *Locate the location of acetylcholine-containing neurons in the brain.*

Explanation: *Neurons of the brainstem tegmentum (laterodorsal and pedunculopontine tegmental nuclei) and* basal forebrain (substantia innominata and diagonal band of Broca and septum) both contain acetylcholine. The brainstem tegmentum projects to the thalamus, posterior hypothalamus, and basal forebrain. Neurons in the basal forebrain project to the cerebral cortex and hippocampus. Neuronal discharge rates increase during both waking and REM sleep.*

337. Answer: A

Educational objective: *Describe the pharmacologic properties of trazodone.*

Explanation: *Trazodone is a 5-HT (2) and alpha (1) receptor antagonist that possesses both anxiolytic and sedative properties. Although widely prescribed for chronic primary insomnia, minimal published data support its use. Its effectiveness for this indication has not been conclusively established. Trazodone increases sleep efficiency, total sleep time, and NREM stages 3 and 4 sleep, and it decreases NREM stage 2 sleep. It may or may not increase REM sleep latency and decrease REM sleep. Trazodone does not appear to possess any significant tolerance or dependence potential. It has a lower anticholinergic action and a shorter half-life compared to the tricyclic antidepressants such as amitriptyline. Side effects include cardiac arrhythmias, orthostatic hypotension, priapism (painful erection) in males, and painful clitoral engorgement in females. Concurrent administration with other serotonin-specific agents can give rise to the serotonin syndrome.*

338. Answer: B

Educational objective: *Describe the role of dental devices in the therapy of obstructive sleep apnea.*

Explanation: *Oral devices worn during sleep may be considered for snorers and individuals with mild to moderate obstructive sleep apnea (OSA) who are intolerant of positive airway pressure therapy, or whose OSA persists following upper airway surgery. The degree of anterior displacement of the tongue is considered the primary factor in influencing the effectiveness of these devices. Two types of oral devices are currently available for the therapy of OSA, namely tongue-retaining devices and mandibular repositioners. Mandibular repositioners advance the mandible (and tongue) forward, and are the most commonly used oral devices; they are contraindicated in patients with inadequate dentition to adequately support the oral device, compromised dentition (ie, loose, broken, or diseased teeth), or significant temporomandibular joint dysfunction. Tongue-retaining devices hold the tongue in an anterior (forward) position by securing the tip of the tongue in a soft bulb located anterior to the teeth; they are preferred for edentulous patients or those with compromised dentition. Oral devices should be avoided in patients who are unable to breathe nasally or have high resistances to nasal airflow, or those whose sleep apnea* is primarily central in nature. Because response rates are unpredictable, a repeat sleep study is recommended to assess its therapeutic efficacy for patients with obstructive sleep apnea once the device has been optimally adjusted. Follow-up sleep testing is not required for patients using oral devices for primary snoring.

339. Answer: D

Educational objective: *Identify the percentage of time newborn infants spend sleeping in a 24-hour day.*

Explanation: *Newborn infants spend approximately 70% of their time in a 24-hour day asleep, whereas adults sleep about 25% to 35% of the 24-hour day sleeping.*

340. Answer: D

Educational objective: *Determine when polysomnography is indicated in patients with excessive sleepiness.*

Explanation: *Polysomnography is indicated in the routine evaluation of excessive sleepiness unless the latter is clearly related to insufficient sleep, or a medical, neurologic, or psychiatric disorder, and when sleepiness resolves with appropriate therapy of the underlying condition.*

341. Answer: A

Educational objective: *Describe the pharmacologic properties of the nonbenzodiazepine benzodiazepine receptor agonists.*

Explanation: *The nonbenzodiazepine benzodiazepine receptor agonists (eg, zolpidem, zaleplon, and eszopiclone) selectively bind to the GABA-benzodiazepine-1 receptor subunit (BZ1).*

342. Answer: D

Educational objective: *Understand the role of norepinephrine in the regulation of sleep and wakefulness.*

Explanation: *Norepinephrine is involved with the maintenance of wakefulness. Neurotransmitter release occurs during wakefulness, decreases during NREM sleep, and is absent during REM sleep. Its neurons are located in the locus ceruleus.*

343. Answer: A

Educational objective: *Describe the clinical features of seizure disorders.*

Explanation: *Temporal lobe seizures occur often only during sleep and is generally accompanied by impaired consciousness and postictal confusion. They begin focally. Automatisms, including lip smacking and other facial, body, and extremity movements, are typical. Seizures are most common during NREM sleep; some can be observed at the NREM-REM sleep transition. Interictal discharges, consisting of spikes, can be present.*

344. Answer: A

Educational objective: *Match the neurotransmitters with the location of their neurons.*

Explanation: *Cholinergic neurons are located in the basal forebrain and laterodorsal tegmentum/pedunculopontine tegmentum (LDT/PPT). The locations for the other neurotransmitters are ventral mesencephalic tegmentum and substantia nigra (dopamine), ventrolateral preoptic area (VLPO), thalamus, hypothalamus, basal forebrain, and cerebral cortex (gamma-aminobutyric acid), and tuberomammillary nucleus of the posterior hypothalamus (histamine).*

345. Answer: B

Educational objective: *Describe the factors that cause and maintain insomnia.*

Explanation: *In a model proposed for the genesis and maintenance of insomnia, factors related to insomnia are classified into those that predispose a person to developing insomnia, those that trigger the start of insomnia, and those that sustain the sleep disturbance (often long after the precipitating events have resolved). Predisposing factors are present before the start of insomnia that increases the likelihood of developing insomnia. They may, if sufficiently severe, independently cause insomnia. Predisposing factors include genetic predisposition, personality traits, physiological hyperarousal (eg, increased muscle tension, body temperature, metabolic rate, and heart rate, as well as a shift in electroencephalogram to faster frequencies at sleep onset and during NREM sleep), psychologic arousal (eg, tendency to ruminate, agitation, anxiety, or heightened vigilance), and time of day sleep-wake preference. Precipitating factors trigger the start of insomnia and include stressful events; change of usual habits; abrupt alterations in sleep-wake schedules; environmental disturbances; medication use or withdrawal; substance use; or medical, neurologic, psychiatric, or sleep disorders. Perpetuating factors sustain sleep disturbance and contribute to the persistence of insomnia independent of the precipitating causes, and include poor sleep hygiene, irregular sleep-wake schedules, caffeine or alcohol consumption, ongoing worries, anxiety, unrealistic expectations about sleep, and maladaptive sleep-wake behaviors.*

(Adapted from Spielman AJ, Caruso LS, Glovinski PB. A behavioral perspective on insomnia treatment. Psychiatr Clin North Am. 1987;10:541–553.)

346. Answer: B

Educational objective: *Identify the different causes of insomnia.*

Explanation: *It is estimated that psychophysiologic insomnia is responsible for 15% of cases of chronic insomnia. Other specific causes of chronic insomnia include restless legs syndrome (about 12% of cases) and alcohol or drug use and abuse (about 12% of cases).*

347. Answer: D

Educational objective: *Describe the clinical features of rapid eye movement (REM) sleep.*

Explanation: *Rapid eye movement (REM) sleep is characterized by a high arousal threshold by external stimuli, generalized skeletal muscle atonia or hypotonia (with sparing of the diaphragm, extraocular muscles and sphincter muscles), increase in middle ear muscle activity (phasic REM sleep), presence of periorbital integrated potentials, and occurrence of penile tumescence in men and vaginal vascular engorgement and clitoral erection in women.*

348. Answer: A

Educational objective: *Describe the clinical features of Tourette syndrome.*

Explanation: *Tourette syndrome is characterized by repetitive motor and verbal tics. It may be associated with parasomnias such as disorders of arousal (eg, confusional arousals, sleepwalking, and sleep terrors). Onset of the disorder is often during childhood. During polysomnography, tics may be observed during sleep, particularly NREM stages 1 and 2 sleep.*

349. Answer: D

Educational objective: *Describe the clinical features of Prader-Willi syndrome.*

Explanation: *There is an increased likelihood of obstructive sleep apnea in patients with Prader-Willi syndrome because of obesity and hypotonia. Other features of this disorder include hyperphagia, short stature, short extremities, upsloping palpebral fissures, high-arched palate, mental retardation, hypogonadism, and abnormal ventilatory responses to hypercapnia and hypoxemia.*

350. Answer: D

Educational objective: *Describe the different surgical therapies for obstructive sleep apnea.*

Explanation: *Surgical procedures for obstructive sleep apnea are designed to increase the dimensions of the retropalatal airspace, retrolingual airway, or both. Radiofrequency palatal submucosal tissue volume reduction, laser-assisted uvulopalatoplasty, uvulopalatopharyngoplasty, and transpalatal advancement pharyngoplasty are designed to increase the dimensions of the retropalatal airspace. In contrast, radiofrequency tongue base ablation, laser midline glossectomy and lingualplasty, tongue base reduction with hyoepiglottoplasty, genioglossal advancement, hyoid myotomy and suspension, and mandibular advancement increase the dimensions of the retrolingual airway. Uvulopalatopharyngoglossoplasty and maxillomandibular advancement increase the dimensions of the retrolingual and retropalatal airway. Tracheostomy uses a percutaneous tracheal opening to bypass the area of upper airway collapse.*

351. Answer: D

Educational objective: *Differentiate among the different clinical subtypes of narcolepsy.*

Explanation: *Cerebrospinal fluid (CSF) hypocretin-1 levels are normal in up to 10% of cases of narcolepsy with cataplexy. Low CSF hypocretin-1 level (< 110 pg/mL) is present in up to 10% to 20% of cases of HLA DQB1*0602-positive narcolepsy without cataplexy.*

Patients who are HLA DQB1*0602-negative and have narcolepsy without cataplexy generally have normal CSF hypocretin-1 levels. Low CSF hypocretin-1 level (< 110 pg/mL) is present in up to 20% of cases of narcolepsy with cataplexy-like or atypical episodes.

352. Answer: A

Educational objective: *Describe the features of the Maintenance of Wakefulness Test.*

Explanation: *The Maintenance of Wakefulness Test (MWT) is an objective measure of an individual's ability to maintain wakefulness for a defined time. It may be indicated to assess response to treatment in patients with excessive sleepiness. The 40-minute protocol is recommended and is preferred over the 20-minute protocol.*

353. Answer: A

Educational objective: *Describe the features of transient insomnia.*

Explanation: *Sleep is typically normal prior to the start of sleep disturbance in individuals with transient insomnia. Sleep normalizes with resolution of the inciting event. These individuals appear to have increased central nervous system arousal, and they are more vulnerable to acute stresses (eg, changes in familiar routines or sleep schedules, significant social events, and drug ingestion or withdrawal).*

354. Answer: A

Educational objective: *Describe the clinical features of Down syndrome.*

Explanation: *Patients with Down syndrome possess a higher risk of developing obstructive sleep apnea due to hypotonia, midfacial and mandibular hypoplasia, glossoptosis, and associated obesity or hypothyroidism.*

355. Answer: C

Educational objective: *Describe the different surgical therapies for obstructive sleep apnea.*

Explanation: *Tracheostomy is the only surgical procedure that is consistently effective as a sole procedure for obstructive sleep apnea and may be considered when other therapeutic options are absent, are refused, or have failed.*

356. Answer: A

Educational objective: Identify the mechanisms underlying the development of central sleep apnea.

Explanation: Central sleep apnea (CSA) has diverse causes. Carbon dioxide (CO_2) ventilatory drive is increased in patients with idiopathic CSA and results in a $PaCO_2$ that is low during wakefulness and sleep. Both central and obstructive apneas can develop in persons with congestive heart failure, and the predominant type of respiratory event appears to depend on the size and collapsibility of the individual's upper airway. A correlation between CSA and decreased left ventricular function (due to a delay in circulatory time to respiratory control centers) and lower awake arterial $PaCO_2$ has been described. CSA is more common in persons with increased hypercapnic chemoresponsiveness during wakefulness than in those with a normal $PaCO_2$.

Several neurologic and neuromuscular disorders can decrease central ventilatory drive and can give rise to CSA. As sleep states oscillate between sleep and wake-drowsiness at sleep onset, repetitive episodes of central apneas may occur if $PaCO_2$ (higher during sleep and lower during wakefulness) fluctuates above or below the apneic threshold. Sleep-onset central apneas are generally transient, disappearing once stable sleep is attained (when $PaCO_2$ is maintained continuously at higher levels). Finally, central apneas can develop during administration of opiate drugs due to depression of the hypercapnic ventilatory drive and increase in hypoxic ventilatory drive.

357. Answer: C

Educational objective: Describe the clinical features of REM sleep.

Explanation: Dreaming has been reported during both REM and NREM sleep, but it is more frequent and more complex during REM sleep than during NREM sleep. There is an increase in sympathetic activation during phasic REM sleep. Increases in brain metabolism and temperature occur. Ponto-geniculo-occipital waves are seen during REM sleep in the cat.

358. Answer: C

Educational objective: Describe the clinical features of cerebrovascular disease.

Explanation: Patients with stroke may complain of recurrent awakenings and insomnia. Subdural hematomas may give rise to excessive sleepiness. The presence of obstructive sleep apnea (OSA) increases the risk of cerebrovascular disease. Conversely, strokes may increase the risk of developing OSA. Ondine curse has been described following brainstem strokes.

359. Answer: D

Educational objective: Identify the factors that can contribute to the development of adjustment sleep disorder.

Explanation: In adjustment sleep disorder, an identifiable acute stressor can elicit a sudden heightened state of arousal that may significantly diminish sleep propensity. Insomnia may also be precipitated by momentous or stressful life events, change in the sleeping environment, or an acute medical disorder or physical illness. Prevalence may be greater among women, older adults, and individuals with a previous history of insomnia. Course is acute and generally brief, and sleep tends to normalize once the acute stressor decreases or resolves, or if there is an increase in the individual's level of adaptation to the stressor. It is typically not associated with any major long-term complications. Polysomnographic features may include increases in sleep latency and frequency of awakenings as well as decreases in sleep efficiency and total sleep time. NREM stages 1 and 2 sleep may be increased along with decreases in NREM stages 3 and 4 and REM sleep.

360. Answer: C

Educational objective: Describe the therapy of central sleep apnea.

Explanation: By stabilizing respiratory control centers, supplemental oxygen therapy may reduce nonhypercapnic central sleep apneas (CSAs) in some but not all patients. Close monitoring of arterial blood gas parameters is crucial, because oxygen therapy in some patients (particularly those with hypercapnic CSA) can result in worsening hypercapnia. Positive airway pressure therapy can improve cardiac function (increase in left ventricular ejection fraction and reduction in left ventricular afterload) in patients with CSA due to congestive heart failure (CHF), particularly in those with elevated pulmonary capillary wedge pressures. Patients with severe CSA can be mechanically ventilated during sleep. Several pharmacologic agents, including acetazolamide, theophylline, and hypnotic agents, have been used to treat CSA. Acetazolamide, a carbonic anhydrase inhibitor, is effective in improving respiration in patients with high-altitude periodic breathing. Theophylline, a respiratory stimulant and positive inotropic agent, has been used primarily in CSA or Cheyne-Stokes respiration related to CHF. Medroxy-progesterone can stimulate ventilation and has been used in patients with obesity hypoventilation syndrome. Benzodiazepines, narcotics, and other sedatives that may suppress respiratory drive should be avoided in patients with hypercapnic forms of CSA.

361. Answer: D

Educational objective: Describe the differences between adult and childhood obstructive sleep apnea.

Explanation: Childhood obstructive sleep apnea (OSA) differs from the disorder involving adults in several ways. Excessive sleepiness, which is common among adult patients, is encountered less frequently in children. Rather, children may demonstrate behavioral problems, including hyperactivity and restlessness. There are no gender differences in prevalence among children, whereas adult OSA is more often seen among men. Finally, adenotonsillar enlargement is the most important risk factor for childhood OSA, and adenotonsillectomy is the most common therapy for this age group.

362. Answer: B

Educational objective: Describe the clinical features of nocturnal eating (drinking) syndrome.

Explanation: Nocturnal eating (drinking) syndrome consists of repetitive arousals from sleep with involuntary eating or drinking. Affected individuals are unaware or only partly conscious of the abnormal behavior. Characteristic features include partial recall or total amnesia for the episodes, and consumption of high-caloric foodstuff or inappropriate substances. Alcohol is not typically ingested. There is typically no associated daytime abnormal eating behavior, such as binge eating, anorexia, bulimia, or purging. Episodes can be observed any time during sleep, often many times each night. Women are affected more frequently than men. In many instances, the awakenings appear to be triggered by learned behavior and not by real hunger or thirst.

363. Answer: C

Educational objective: Determine the factors influencing the severity of symptoms related to periodic breathing due to high altitude.

Explanation: Severity of symptoms in patients with periodic breathing related to high altitude is influenced by altitude, speed of ascent, and individual predisposition. Persons with increased hypoxic ventilatory chemoresponsiveness appear to have a greater risk of developing high altitude–related periodic breathing. Rapid ascent and extreme elevations also increase the risk and severity of high-altitude periodic breathing. Men may be affected more commonly than women.

364. Answer: B

Educational objective: Describe the clinical features of juvenile myoclonic epilepsy.

Explanation: Juvenile myoclonic epilepsy presents as bilateral massive myoclonic jerks occurring soon after awakening. Episodes can be precipitated by sleep deprivation or alcohol use. It generally develops during adolescence. Myoclonic jerks may precede seizures by 1 to 4 years. Electroencephalography can demonstrate symmetric and synchronous 4–6 Hz polyspike and wave discharges.

365. Answer: C

Educational objective: Understand the changes in the control of respiration and cardiovascular function associated with REM sleep.

Explanation: REM sleep is associated with irregular respiratory pattern with a decrease in tidal volume accompanying rapid eye movements, a decrease in hypoxic and hypercapnic ventilatory responses, a decrease in activity of the upper airway dilator muscles, variable heart rate and blood pressure, and an increase in systemic blood pressure due to peripheral vasoconstriction.

366. Answer: A

Educational objective: Describe the clinical features of seizure disorders.

Explanation: Nocturnal frontal lobe epilepsy is characterized by abnormal behaviors (eg, sleep terrors or sleepwalking), arousals, or nocturnal paroxysmal dystonia. Because it may originate in deeper brain structures, there is typically no evident abnormal ictal or interictal electroencephalographic activity. Onset is generally during childhood. They can result in sleep disturbance and daytime sleepiness. A majority of patients respond favorably to antiseizure medications, including carbamazepine.

367. Answer: A

Educational objective: Describe the polysomnographic features of psychophysiologic insomnia.

Explanation: The diagnosis of psychophysiologic insomnia relies mainly on clinical history. Polysomnography is not routinely indicated. Polysomnography can be entirely normal or may show an increase in sleep latency, a decrease in sleep efficiency, frequent awakenings, and an increase in wake time after sleep onset. Total sleep time may be reduced. An increase in NREM stage 1 sleep and a decrease in NREM stages 3 and 4 sleep may also be observed. Both "first-night effect" (worse sleep than usual during the first night in the sleep laboratory) as well as "reverse first-night effect" (better sleep than usual during the first sleep laboratory night) can influence sleep architecture. Subjective reports of sleep time are often less than objective total sleep time determined by polysomnography. Multiple sleep latency testing demonstrates normal daytime alertness. Actigraphy is less reliable in measuring sleep in this patient group, commonly underestimating wake time and overestimating sleep time.

368. Answer: B

Educational objective: Describe the clinical features of Cheyne-Stokes respiration.

Explanation: Cheyne-Stokes respiration–related arousals occur at the peak of ventilation or a few breaths after ventilation resumes unlike that of obstructive sleep apnea in which arousals occur at the termination of apnea. In addition, the period of hyperpnea is longer and the waxing and waning of ventilation is less abrupt compared to other forms of central sleep apnea. Cycle length is related *inversely to cardiac output and directly to circulation time. There is typically a delay in the nadir of oxygen desaturation following the apneic events.*

369. Answer: C

Educational objective: *Identify the changes in sleep that accompany adolescence.*

Explanation: *An increase in daytime sleepiness and a phase delay in circadian sleep-wake rhythms occur in some individuals during puberty. There is a corresponding increase in requirements for sleep.*

370. Answer: C

Educational objective: *Identify effective countermeasures for sleepiness secondary to sleep deprivation.*

Explanation: *Sleep is the most effective countermeasure for sleep deprivation. Scheduled naps throughout the day may help alleviate sleepiness. Naps (eg, 45 minutes or longer) scheduled prior to planned prolonged wakefulness and sleep deprivation have beneficial effects on alertness and vigilance. Provision of bright ambient lights during the night augments alertness among shift work workers. Physical activity, changes in posture (such as standing), and environmental stimulation (eg, noise, cold air) do not enhance alertness or vigilance.*

371. Answer: D

Educational objective: *Describe the factors that suggest an organic cause of sleep enuresis.*

Explanation: *An organic etiology for sleep enuresis should be suspected if urinary urgency or an abnormality in urinary flow is present or involuntary voiding occurs during wakefulness as well.*

372. Answer: D

Educational objective: *Know the differences between the benzodiazepines in terms of their half-lives.*

Explanation: *Benzodiazepines differ in their half-lives. Triazolam has a shorter half-life compared to flurazepam, temazepam and estazolam (Table).*

Half-lives of benzodiazepines

Agent	Elimination half-life (hours)
Triazolam	1.5 to 5.5
Estazolam	10 to 24
Temazepam	8 to 20
Flurazepam	70 to 90

373. Answer: B

Educational objective: *Identify the medications associated with "pseudo-spindles."*

Explanation: *"Pseudo-spindles" or "drug spindles" are associated with the use of benzodiazepines and have frequencies that are faster than that of true sleep spindles.*

374. Answer: B

Educational objective: *Describe the factors that influence the secretion of melatonin.*

Explanation: *The synthesis and secretion of melatonin are suppressed by light exposure. Minimal melatonin is secreted in infants younger than 3 months of age; levels increase gradually, peak at 1 to 3 years of age, and decline thereafter. Levels of melatonin rise in the evening, peak in the early morning (between 3:00 and 5:00 AM), and decline thereafter. This pattern persists even if no sleep occurs during the night. Evening melatonin secretion is decreased among older adults with insomnia.*

375. Answer: A

Educational objective: *Describe the clinical features of psychophysiologic insomnia.*

Explanation: *In psychophysiologic insomnia, maladaptive sleep-preventing behavior develops and eventually progresses to become the predominant factor perpetuating sleep disturbances. Although the onset of insomnia is related to a stressor, sleep disturbance persists long after the stressor abates. There is heightened somatized tension, such as increased agitation and muscle tone, and mental arousal with persistent intrusive thoughts during bedtime. A vicious cycle is thus created in which patients try too hard to sleep and, in so doing, become tense and more aroused and anxious. This, in turn, diminishes further their propensity to sleep. Interestingly, sleep commences readily when they are not trying too hard to do so or when they are distracted. Conditioned arousal is limited to the person's own bed and bedroom, and they commonly report sleeping better in any room other than their own (including the sleep laboratory [reverse first-night effect]). Many patients with psychophysiologic insomnia have a lifelong history of episodic poor or light sleep, and they often demonstrate a preoccupation with their sleep duration and quality as well as the potential consequences of sleep disturbances. The course of this condition is commonly chronic, and if left untreated, it may progressively worsen.*

376. Answer: B

Educational objective: *Understand the pathophysiology of hypercapnia in patients with obesity hypoventilation syndrome.*

Explanation: *The etiology of hypercapnia in obesity hypoventilation syndrome is associated with one or more of the following, including increased production of CO_2*

due to greater work of breathing, decreased chest wall compliance, decreased ventilation, decreased expiratory reserve volume, decreased tidal volume, increased resistive load, increased dead space, and decreased ventilatory responses to hypercapnia and hypoxemia.

377. Answer: C

Educational objective: *Identify the risk factors for obstructive sleep apnea in children.*

Explanation: *Adenotonsillar enlargement is the most important risk factor for obstructive sleep apnea (OSA) in children. Whereas there is no gender difference prior to puberty, an increase in prevalence among boys after puberty has been described. Excess body weight is a risk factor, but most children with OSA are not overweight. Finally, prevalence of OSA is higher among African-American children than Caucasian children.*

378. Answer: B

Educational objective: *Describe when circadian sleep phase preference first develops.*

Explanation: *Circadian sleep phase preference ("eveningness" versus "morningness") first develops between 6 and 12 years of age.*

379. Answer: D

Educational objective: *Describe the changes in sleep among pregnant women.*

Explanation: *Pregnant women may complain of sleep disturbance as early as the first trimester. These include frequent awakenings, increase in wake time after sleep onset, and decrease in sleep duration. The frequency of napping increases during the first trimester. Sleep quality typically improves during the second trimester. Sleep is most disrupted during the third trimester of pregnancy, which is also associated with more frequent napping. Sleep can be disrupted by the direct effects of the growing fetus as well as by changes in anatomic and physiologic variables related to pregnancy. Changes in sleep architecture that develop during pregnancy include a decrease in sleep efficiency, an increase in total sleep time, an increase in frequency of awakenings and an increase in wake time after sleep onset. Whereas NREM stages 1 and 2 sleep may increase, there is often either a reduction or no change in NREM stages 3 and 4 sleep. There is no change in REM sleep, except perhaps for a decrease during late pregnancy..*

380. Answer: A

Educational objective: *Identify the genetic syndromes associated with mandibular hypoplasia.*

Explanation: *Certain genetic syndromes predispose to the development of obstructive sleep apnea due to the presence of mandibular hypoplasia. These include Cornelia de Lange syndrome, cri du chat, Down syndrome, Pierre-Robin sequence, and Treacher-Collins syndrome. Patients with Apert syndrome have midfacial hypoplasia.*

381. Answer: D

Educational objective: *Describe the changes in sleep among women during perimenopause and postmenopause.*

Explanation: *Compared with men, healthy older women are more likely to complain of insomnia (difficulty with sleep initiation or maintenance, or early morning awakening), poor sleep quality, insufficient or nonrestorative sleep, and need for daytime naps. Older women also report that their sleep is more easily disrupted and that they use sedative-hypnotic agents more often. There appears to be an increase in NREM stage 1 sleep during perimenopause and postmenopause. Unlike men, no significant decrease in NREM stages 3 and 4 sleep with aging has been described in healthy women. There is greater NREM stages 3 and 4 sleep during the perimenopausal period than during the premenopausal period.*

382. Answer: B

Educational objective: *Describe the polysomnographic features of panic disorder.*

Explanation: *Panic attacks can occur during sleep, often during the transition from NREM stage 2 sleep to NREM stages 3 and 4 sleep. Occasionally, panic attacks may arise from REM sleep. Awakenings can be accompanied by sympathetic activation (eg, tachycardia, chest discomfort, dyspnea, and diaphoresis). Patients can often recall the preceding panic attack during awakenings. Return to sleep can be delayed.*

383. Answer: B

Educational objective: *Describe the clinical features of sleep starts or hypnic jerks.*

Explanation: *Sleep starts (hypnic jerks or hypnic myoclonia) consist of sudden muscle contractions of part or all of the body that occur at sleep onset. The individual may be startled out of sleep by a single, brief body jerk accompanied by a sensation of "falling" or "dreaming." It can also present as visual (flashes of light or vivid imagery), auditory (loud bangs), or somesthetic (floating) phenomena. It is a common experience among many normal individuals during the transition between wakefulness and sleep and is a normal physiologic phenomenon. Sleep starts are believed to be due to a sudden loss of muscle tone at sleep onset and the subsequent reflex muscle contraction that develops to restore muscle tone. Although they are frequently spontaneous, sleep starts can also be triggered by external stimuli. Episodes may be precipitated by sleep deprivation, stress, excessive caffeine ingestion, stimulant use, or intense physical activity performed close to bedtime.*

Its course is generally benign, and sleep starts typically require no specific therapy.

384. Answer: A

Educational objective: *Identify the genetic mutation that is associated with the congenital central hypoventilation syndrome.*

Explanation: *Heterozygous de novo mutations in PHOX2B gene (autosomal dominant with incomplete penetrance) have been described in patients with congenital central hypoventilation syndrome (CCHS) and associated autonomic dysfunction. Most mutations consist of five to nine alanine expansions within a 20-residue polyalanine tract (exon 3). Repeat mutation length correlates with the severity of the CCHS phenotype. Less commonly, patients may have an EDN3 frameshift point mutation.*

385. Answer: C

Educational objective: *Describe the pharmacologic features of chlorpromazine.*

Explanation: *Chlorpromazine is a typical antipsychotic. Polysomnographic features associated with the use of chlorpromazine include a decrease in sleep latency, an increase in sleep efficiency, an increase in total sleep time, and an increase in REM sleep latency. There are no consistent changes in NREM stages 3 and 4 sleep.*

386. Answer: B

Educational objective: *Understand the sleep disorders that can develop or worsen during pregnancy and the postpartum period.*

Explanation: *Pregnancy can precipitate or aggravate an existing periodic limb movement disorder or restless legs syndrome (RLS). The prevalence of RLS peaks during the third trimester. RLS improves following delivery. The risk of developing RLS is greater among women who have experienced similar complaints during previous pregnancies. The prevalence of leg cramps causing awakenings from sleep is greater during pregnancy than before or after conception. The risk of developing leg cramps is increased among women with twin pregnancies than in those with single pregnancies. Frequency of leg cramps progressively increases from the first to the second to the third trimester.*

387. Answer: C

Educational objective: *Identify when daytime napping ceases among children.*

Explanation: *Cessation of daytime napping in children generally occurs between 3 and 5 years of age.*

388. Answer: A

Educational objective: *Describe the clinical features of sleep hallucinations.*

Explanation: *Sleep hallucinations are common experiences in persons with narcolepsy and are present in about 30% of cases. They are not pathognomonic for narcolepsy and have been described in normal persons as well. Hallucinations may occur during wakefulness at sleep onset (hypnagogic) or on awakening (hypnopompic). Hallucinatory phenomena often last a few seconds or minutes and can be visual, auditory, tactile, or kinetic (a sensation of movement). They often begin several months to years after the onset of excessive sleepiness.*

389. Answer: A

Educational objective: *Describe benzodiazepines' effects on sleep.*

Explanation: *Benzodiazepines can reduce upper airway muscle tone and worsen obstructive sleep apnea. They can depress respiration and should be used cautiously in patients with chronic obstructive pulmonary disease. Benzodiazepines reduce the severity of symptoms of restless legs syndrome. With shorter-acting agents, sleep improves in the first part of the night, and sleep disruption and fragmentation occur in the second part of the night due to drug withdrawal. Excessive sleepiness is more pronounced with long-acting agents. Insomnia and REM sleep rebound can occur following sudden drug discontinuation.*

390. Answer: A

Educational objective: *Understand how hot flashes occurring during the perimenopausal period can affect sleep.*

Explanation: *Hot flashes occurring at night can significantly disturb sleep, leading to a decrease in sleep efficiency, an increase in frequency of awakenings, and a decrease in subjective sleep quality. Environmental temperature prior to bedtime influences the frequency of hot flashes. Hot flashes may persist for several years after menopause.*

391. Answer: C

Educational objective: *Describe the pharmacologic features of olanzapine.*

Explanation: *An atypical antipsychotic, olanzapine causes a decrease in sleep latency, a decrease in wake time after sleep onset, an increase in sleep efficiency, an increase in total sleep time, a decrease in NREM stage 1 sleep, an increase in NREM stages 2, 3 and 4 sleep, an increase in REM sleep latency, a decrease in REM sleep, and an increase in REM sleep density.*

392. Answer: A

Educational objective: *Describe the characteristics of idiopathic sleep-related hypoventilation.*

Explanation: *In idiopathic sleep-related hypoventilation, hypoxemic and hypercapnic chemoresponsiveness are decreased leading to reduced tidal volumes and ventilation. It is not associated with lower airway, chest* *wall, diaphragm, pulmonary, or other medical or neuromuscular disorders. The disorder appears to be more common in males than in females, and it often presents during adolescence or early adulthood. Hypoventilation is more severe during REM sleep compared to NREM sleep. Arterial blood gas analysis during sleep demonstrates an absolute ($PaCO_2$ > 45 mm Hg) or relative hypercapnia compared to levels during wakefulness, with SaO_2 < 90% (nadir ≤ 85%) for greater than 5 minutes, and SaO_2 < 90% present in greater than 30% of total sleep time, that are not related to apneas or hypopneas.*

393. Answer: D

Educational objective: *Describe the features of electroencephalographic sleep spindles.*

Explanation: *Sleep spindles are brief oscillations with frequencies of 12 to 14 Hz that last from 0.5 to 1.5 seconds. Amplitude is generally less than 50 μV. Sleep spindles are more prominent and have highest voltage over the central leads. They may be seen during NREM stages 2, 3, and 4 sleep but not during NREM stage 1 sleep. Sleep spindles are generated in the midline thalamic nuclei.*

394. Answer: D

Educational objective: *Describe the features of electroencephalographic K-complexes.*

Explanation: *A K-complex is a high-amplitude, biphasic wave with an initial sharp negative deflection followed by a positive high-voltage slow wave. It has a duration of at least 0.5 seconds. K-complexes are seen maximally over the vertex (central and central-parietal leads) and are believed to represent evoked responses to internal and external stimuli.*

395. Answer: A

Educational objective: *Describe the clinical features of idiopathic insomnia.*

Explanation: *Idiopathic insomnia is characterized by long-standing sleep disturbance that generally starts during infancy or in early childhood and is not associated with any identifiable etiology. The course is chronic and relentless, and the condition persists life-long without periods of remission. Insomnia is typically refractory to therapy. Typical polysomnographic features include a significantly diminished sleep efficiency, prolonged sleep latency, a decrease in total sleep time, an increase in wake time after sleep onset, an increase in NREM stages 1 and 2 sleep, and a decrease in NREM stages 3 and 4 sleep.*

396. Answer: B

Educational objective: *Describe the clinical features of Asperger syndrome.*

Explanation: *Asperger disorder is characterized by stereotypical activities and behavior associated with significant*

impairment in daytime functioning and social interaction. Cognitive and language development are normal. Men are affected more commonly than women. Insomnia is common. Changes in sleep architecture consist of a decrease in sleep time during the first part of the night and REM sleep disruption.

397. Answer: C

Educational objective: *Describe the effects of sleep on glucose and energy balance.*

Explanation: *Blood levels of glucose and insulin may decline during sleep. Insulin resistance may develop and levels of insulin may decrease during sleep deprivation. Leptin, a product of the obese (ob) gene, is involved with the regulation of energy balance by reducing the intake of food. It is released from peripheral adipocytes, with highest serum levels between 12:00 PM and 4:00 AM. Ghrelin, like leptin, also regulates energy balance; its serum levels increase at night. Ghrelin promotes NREM sleep.*

398. Answer: D

Educational objective: *Understand the relationship between neuromuscular disorders and sleep-related hypoventilation.*

Explanation: *Neuromuscular disorders, including amyotrophic lateral sclerosis, muscular dystrophies, myopathies, postpolio syndrome, and spinal cord trauma or injury, can give rise to sleep-related hypoventilation, especially in patients with daytime hypoxemia and hypercapnia, reduced chemosensitivity, or neurologic disorders with bulbar dysfunction.*

399. Answer: A

Educational objective: *Describe the pharmacologic features of the antipsychotic agents.*

Explanation: *Antipsychotics (neuroleptics) are indicated for the treatment of schizophrenia. Typical polysomnographic features during antipsychotic administration include a shortened sleep latency, increase in sleep efficiency, decrease in wake time after sleep onset, increase in total sleep time, and decrease in REM sleep (higher doses).*

400. Answer: A

Educational objective: *Understand how preeclampsia during pregnancy affects sleep.*

Explanation: *Preeclampsia, or pregnancy-induced hypertension, is characterized by the presence of high blood pressure, proteinuria, pedal edema, and headaches. Women who develop preeclampsia have been observed to have a higher frequency of snoring, greater neck circumference, more restricted airflow secondary to narrower upper airways, increase frequency of arousals, and a higher prevalence of periodic limb movements during sleep than healthy pregnant women.*

401. Answer: B

Educational objective: Describe benzodiazepines' effects on sleep.

Explanation: Benzodiazepines act via the gamma-amino-butyric acid receptors. Polysomnographic features include a decrease in sleep latency, an increase in total sleep time, a decrease in frequency of arousals, a decrease in wake time after sleep onset, an increase in NREM stage 2 sleep, a decrease in NREM stages 3 and 4 sleep, an increase in REM sleep latency, and a decrease in REM sleep. There is an increase in spindle [12–14 cycles per second] density as well as "pseudospindles" (14–18 cycles per second).

402. Answer: A

Educational objective: Describe the features of alpha electroencephalographic waves.

Explanation: Alpha electroencephalographic waves are defined as oscillations with a frequency of 8 to 13 Hz. Frequencies are slower among children and elderly adults than among younger adults. Amplitude is variable and is generally less than 50 μV among adults. These are present when a person is relaxed and drowsy and eyes are closed but are also present during arousals from sleep. Alpha waves originate in the occipital cortex and are, therefore, more prominent in the occipital leads compared to central leads. Eye opening suppresses alpha activity.

403. Answer: C

Educational objective: Describe the clinical features of seizure disorders.

Explanation: With frontal lobe seizures, consciousness is maintained and postseizure confusion is minimal. There are often no abnormal interictal electroencephalographic discharges. They usually occur only during sleep. Clinical features vary depending on the location of the seizure focus. "Jacksonian march," with seizure activity starting at the distal part of the extremity and moving proximally, is associated with onset in the posterior frontal lobes. Onset from midline regions can give rise to complex motor activity, such as vocalizations and dystonic posturing. Seizures starting from the cingulated gyrus can present with automatisms, staring, and autonomic features (eg, tachycardia and tachypnea).

404. Answer: C

Educational objective: Describe the changes in hormone levels during sleep.

Explanation: During the first half of the night, there is an increase in growth hormone and decrease in both cortisol and adrenocorticotropic hormone (ACTH). The converse is true of the second half of the night when there is a decrease in growth hormone and increase in cortisol and ACTH.

405. Answer: B

Educational objective: Describe the role of light therapy in the treatment of transient or chronic insomnia.

Explanation: Morning light exposure for sleep-onset insomnia produces a phase advance in circadian sleep-wake, core body temperature and melatonin rhythms. This shortens sleep latency, increases total sleep time, and causes an earlier final awakening time. Evening light exposure for early morning awakenings produces a phase delay in circadian sleep-wake, core body temperature, and melatonin rhythms; it prolongs sleep efficiency, increases total sleep time, and causes a later final awakening time.

406. Answer: A

Educational objective: Describe the features of the Multiple Sleep Latency Test.

Explanation: The Multiple Sleep Latency Test (MSLT) is an objective measure of an individual's ability or tendency to fall asleep. The test is indicated for patients suspected of having narcolepsy and to distinguish between idiopathic hypersomnia and narcolepsy in patients presenting with sleepiness. The MSLT is not routinely indicated in the initial evaluation, or follow-up during continuous positive airway pressure therapy, of patients with obstructive sleep apnea, or for the evaluation of sleepiness secondary to insomnia, circadian rhythm disorders, and medical or neurologic disorders (except narcolepsy). A repeat MSLT test is indicated if appropriate study conditions are not met or if extraneous factors that might affect the results during the initial testing were present; when results are uninterpretable, vague, or uncertain; and with failure of the initial test to confirm the diagnosis of narcolepsy in patients with a high clinical suspicion of narcolepsy.

(Standards of Practice Committee of the American Academy of Sleep Medicine. Practice parameters for clinical use of the multiple sleep latency test and the maintenance of wakefulness test. Sleep. 2005;28(1):113–121.)

407. Answer: C

Educational objective: Identify the standard gain for electroencephalography electrodes.

Explanation: Standard gain for electroencephalography electrodes used for polysomnography is a deflection of 1 cm for every 50 μV. Excessively high low-frequency filter settings can decrease wave amplitude.

408. Answer: C

Educational objective: Describe the effects of cytokines on sleep.

Explanation: Interleukin-4 (IL-4), IL-10, IL-13, and insulin-like growth factor inhibit sleep. On the other hand, sleep is enhanced by fibroblast growth factor; IL-1, IL-2, IL-6, IL-8, IL-15, and IL-18; nerve growth factor; and tumor necrosis factor-α.

409. Answer: D

Educational objective: *Describe the clinical features of limit-setting sleep disorder.*

Explanation: *Limit-setting sleep disorder is seen in children who repetitively refuse to go to sleep when requested to do so and often stall going to bed. If the caregiver recognizes the child's attempts to delay his or her bedtime and limits to further activities are strictly enforced, sleep comes naturally and quickly. This disorder affects an estimated 5% to 10% of children with a greater prevalence among boys. It is not commonly encountered until children reach the age of 2 years or older when they start to develop their verbal communications skills. Sleep is normal on polysomnography.*

410. Answer: A

Educational objective: *Distinguish between "REM-on" and "REM-off" cells.*

Explanation: *REM sleep is associated with activation of "REM-on" cholinergic neurons and inhibition of "REM-off" noradrenergic neurons (locus ceruleus), serotonergic neurons (dorsal raphe), and histaminergic neurons (posterior hypothalamus).*

411. Answer: A

Educational objective: *Describe the features of narcolepsy without cataplexy.*

Explanation: *Patients with narcolepsy without cataplexy can have cataplexy-like symptoms, including prolonged episodes of tiredness, or muscle weakness related to atypical triggers (exercise, stress, or sex). It accounts for about 10% to 50% of cases of narcolepsy. Most patients have normal levels of cerebrospinal fluid hypocretin-1. Some cases of narcolepsy with cataplexy are associated with loss of hypocretin-containing hypothalamic neurons (but to a lesser degree than that seen in narcolepsy with cataplexy).*

412. Answer: A

Educational objective: *Describe the use of phototherapy for delayed sleep phase syndrome.*

Explanation: *Phototherapy, or light treatment, utilizes timed early morning exposure and evening avoidance of bright light to produce a phase advance in the sleep-wake circadian cycle for patients with delayed sleep phase syndrome. The intensity and duration of light exposure should be individualized with adjustments made as necessary depending on the person's response to therapy. The optimal timing of light exposure is important. Exposure might be of greatest benefit if timed close after the temperature nadir (Tmin). Light administered prior to the temperature nadir could further phase delay circadian rhythms. The body temperature nadir is often about 1 to 2 hours after the habitual midsleep time. Neither optimum nor minimum length of therapy has been standardized and, again, should be individualized.*

Maintenance dosing may be useful to help prevent relapse. Phototherapy should not be used in patients with retinopathy, photosensitivity, mania, and possibly migraines. An ophthalmologic examination is recommended in patients with significant retinal and ocular disorders prior to initiating bright light therapy. Adverse effects of light therapy include headaches, eye irritation, nausea, dryness of the eyes and skin, skin erythema, and precipitation of a hypomanic state in patients with bipolar disorder.

413. Answer: D

Educational objective: *Describe the pharmacologic features of clozapine.*

Explanation: *Clozapine, an atypical antipsychotic, is sedating. Polysomnographic features include a decrease in sleep latency, a decrease in wake time after sleep onset, an increase in sleep efficiency, an increase in total sleep time, an increase in NREM stage 2 sleep, and a decrease in NREM stages 3 and 4 sleep. There is generally no change in REM sleep.*

414. Answer: B

Educational objective: *Identify the peak age of prevalence of childhood obstructive sleep apnea.*

Explanation: *Childhood OSA peaks between 2 and 5 years of age, which coincides with the peak ages of adenotonsillar enlargement. A second peak in prevalence may be seen during adolescence.*

415. Answer: B

Educational objective: *Describe the neural systems that are responsible for the generation of ponto-geniculo-occipital waves.*

Explanation: *In animal models, ponto-geniculo-occipital (PGO) waves are generated by the mesopontine neurons, accompanied by activation of the lateral geniculate and occipital cortex (ie, P = pons, G = geniculate, and O = occipital).*

416. Answer: A

Educational objective: *Describe the role of behavioral therapy in the treatment of insomnia.*

Explanation: *A majority of patients (between 50% and 80%) with insomnia benefit from behavioral therapy with improvements in sleep quality and duration. Compared to hypnotic medications that can improve sleep shortly after administration, gains in sleep quality and duration with behavioral therapy for insomnia are often not immediately apparent and it might take several weeks for therapy to produce meaningful benefits. Therapeutic benefits between pharmacologic and behavioral therapy are comparable at 1 to 2 months. Improvements in sleep parameters following behavioral therapy appear to be sustained over time (ie, at least 6 months), unlike pharmacotherapy,* which does not retain any significant benefits on its discontinuation. Nonetheless, the magnitude of treatment response varies among patients, and not everyone who benefits from therapy becomes a good sleeper. Furthermore, improvements in nighttime sleep with behavioral therapy may not give rise to corresponding positive changes in daytime symptoms. Subjective reports of improvements in sleep may be greater than objective measures obtained with polysomnography.

417. Answer: C

Educational objective: Discuss the significance of the electroencephalographic alpha-NREM sleep anomaly.

Explanation: The alpha-NREM sleep anomaly is not specific for fibromyalgia and has been observed in patients with chronic pain syndromes (eg, chronic fatigue syndrome or rheumatoid arthritis), depression, psychophysiologic insomnia, febrile illness, and even in healthy individuals. In one study, fewer than 40% of subjects with this anomaly had pain syndromes, and the majority of subjects exhibiting this anomaly had a nonpainful medical or psychiatric condition. Alpha-rhythm intrusion into NREM sleep can also be seen in some individuals taking sedative-hypnotic agents. Furthermore, the alpha-NREM sleep anomaly is not universally present in patients with fibromyalgia.

418. Answer: C

Educational objective: Describe the characteristics of hypocretin (orexin).

Explanation: Neurons containing hypocretin (orexin) are located in the perifornical region of the lateral hypothalamus. Hypocretin (orexin) is released during wakefulness. It acts on other central nervous system centers related to sleep-wake regulation, including the dorsal raphe, locus ceruleus, tuberomammillary nuclei, and spinal cord. Dysfunction of the hypocretin system is associated with narcolepsy-cataplexy.

419. Answer: A

Educational objective: Describe the features of actigraphy.

Explanation: Periods of rest/sleep or activity can be discerned using actigraphs, which produce a signal whenever movement is detected. Each epoch is scored as wake or sleep based on predetermined amplitude or time thresholds for activity counts. Actigraphy permits the following data to be obtained: total wake time, total sleep time, sleep latency (if used along with an event monitor to mark the time when the patient desires to fall asleep), frequency of awakenings, and wake time after sleep onset. Actigraphy appears to be better at measuring sleep duration rather than identifying sleep initiation. There is a higher degree of correlation between polysomnography and actigraphy for total sleep time, total wake time, and sleep continuity among normal sleepers than in patients

with insomnia or sleep disturbances. Polysomnography tends to detect more sleep time compared to actigraphy in both normal sleepers and in patients with insomnia. Accuracy of recordings is decreased in persons with periodic limb movements during sleep or other sleep-related movement disorders as well as in those who habitually remain inactive in bed or in a chair while awake.

420. Answer: A

Educational objective: Identify the pattern of serotonin secretion during wakefulness, NREM sleep, and REM sleep.

Explanation: Release of serotonin is highest during wakefulness, decreases during NREM sleep, and is lowest during REM sleep. Medications that inhibit serotonin reduce REM sleep. Serotonergic neurons are located in the raphe nuclei and thalamus.

421. Answer: C

Educational objective: Describe the clinical features of amyotrophic lateral sclerosis.

Explanation: Obstructive apneic and hypopneic events in patients with amyotrophic lateral sclerosis (ALS) are seen predominantly during REM sleep. The overall index is often only mildly elevated. The development of diaphragmatic dysfunction in patients with ALS can adversely affect survival. Significant nocturnal oxygen desaturation secondary to hypoventilation can occur. Compared with those with preserved diaphragm function, these patients can have reduced REM sleep.

422. Answer: C

Educational objective: Describe the polysomnographic features of normal adult sleep.

Explanation: Normal sleep in an adult is characterized by a short sleep latency (< 15 minutes), high sleep efficiency (> 95%), and few and relatively brief awakenings. Sleep is typically entered into through NREM sleep. NREM sleep predominates during the first half of the night, whereas REM sleep percentage is greatest during the second half of the night. REM sleep occurs in three to five episodes during the night that alternate with NREM sleep every 90 to 120 minutes.

423. Answer: D

Educational objective: Describe the clinical features of altitude insomnia.

Explanation: Sleep disturbance, including insomnia, can develop following ascent to elevations greater than 2000 to 4000 meters. Sleep fragmentation, decrease in sleep efficiency, shortened total sleep time, and reduction of REM sleep can occur. Other symptoms consist of easy fatigability, headaches, and anorexia. Severity is magnified with greater altitudes. Incidence increases in persons with underlying cardiorespiratory disorders or anemia. The primary cause of sleep disruption is periodic breathing with periods of central apneas during sleep as a result of hypoxia and respiratory alkalosis. Arousals can occur during the hyperpneic phase of periodic breathing. Adverse environmental conditions may also contribute to the complaint of insomnia. Symptoms resolve with acclimatization or after descent to lower altitudes. Oxygen therapy may decrease periodic breathing but does not improve sleep quality. Acetazolamide, a carbonic anhydrase inhibitor, stimulates respiration via production of metabolic acidosis; it improves sleep quality, hypoxemia, and periodic breathing. Benzodiazepines can blunt the respiratory response to hypercapnia and should be avoided.

424. Answer: A

Educational objective: Characterize sleep during pregnancy, labor, and delivery.

Explanation: Pregnancy is associated with changes in sleep architecture that include a decrease in sleep efficiency, an increase in frequency of awakenings, an increase in wake time after sleep onset, and an increase in NREM stages 1 and 2 sleep. Total sleep time increases during early pregnancy and decreases during late pregnancy. NREM stages 3 and 4 sleep can either decrease or remain unchanged. There is no significant change in REM sleep except perhaps for a decrease during late pregnancy. With labor and delivery, shorter nighttime sleep duration in the period before labor and delivery is associated with longer labor and increased likelihood of cesarean delivery.

425. Answer: A

Educational objective: Describe the differences in polysomnographic features between childhood and adult obstructive sleep apnea.

Explanation: Childhood obstructive sleep apnea (OSA) is usually associated with normal sleep architecture, fewer respiratory event-related arousals, and less oxygen desaturation than adult OSA. There is often a decrease in NREM stages 3 and 4 as well as REM sleep in adult OSA.

426. Answer: D

Educational objective: Understand the role of the neurotransmitter histamine in the regulation of wakefulness.

Explanation: The tuberomammillary nucleus in the posterior hypothalamus has neurons that contain histamine. They project to the forebrain. Discharge rates increase during waking and are absent during REM sleep. Lesions in this area result in a decrease in arousal without a decrease in waking amount.

427. Answer: B

Educational objective: Describe the features of sleep restriction in the treatment of insomnia.

Explanation: Sleep restriction consists of limiting the amount of time a patient with insomnia spends in bed, matching the latter with the actual total sleep time. By creating a state of sleep deprivation, this method is designed to decrease sleep latency, increase sleep efficiency, and decrease wake time after sleep onset. Percentage of NREM stages 3 and 4 sleep may increase. This approach is particularly helpful in persons who spend considerable time in bed awake, frustrated and agitated. Time spent in bed is limited to actual sleeping only. For instance, in an individual with a subjective report of 6 hours of sleep duration but who spends 9 hours in bed, the initial recommended time in bed would be 6 hours from bedtime to arising time by delaying bedtime. Wake up time is kept constant. Time allowed in bed should be at least 4.5 to 5 hours per night and is adjusted periodically depending on the calculated sleep efficiency (the percentage of time in bed spent sleeping [total sleep time/time in bed] 100%) until the desired sleep duration is attained. Time in bed is increased or decreased by 15 to 30 minutes at the start of each evening's sleep when sleep efficiency is greater than 90% or lower than 80%, respectively. No change in allowable bedtime is made if sleep efficiency is between 80% and 90%. Naps are not allowed.

428. Answer: A

Educational objective: Describe the features of the intensive care unit syndrome.

Explanation: Patients in the intensive care unit (ICU) often report poorer sleep quality. Poor sleep quality does not appear to be related to gender, age or duration of ICU stay. There is also an increased tendency for patients to sleep more during the day and less at night. A variety of factors related to the patient, to therapeutic and/or diagnostic interventions, and to the ICU environment itself contribute to the genesis of sleep disruption in the ICU. The ICU syndrome is characterized by reversible mental status changes, including delirium, among patients 3 to 7 days after admission to the ICU. Other features include fear, anxiety, depression, disorientation, and hallucinations. Sleep deprivation is one of the major causes of the ICU syndrome. The ICU syndrome usually resolves within 48 hours of ICU discharge. Daily sleep assessments and charting by nurses are commonly employed to subjectively measure sleep in the ICU. However, in one study, nursing observations overestimated sleep time compared to objective data obtained with polysomnography.

429. Answer: C

Educational objective: Describe the indications for polysomnography in patients with suspected parasomnias.

Explanation: Polysomnographic evaluation, with additional electroencephalography (EEG) derivations, and video recording, is indicated for arousals and sleep disturbances that are presumed to be related to seizures when clinical evaluation and standard EEG are inconclusive; for sleep-related behaviors that are violent or potentially injurious; for presumed parasomnias with unusual or atypical features; for cases with forensic implications, either with onset following trauma, or those associated with injurious behavior; and presumed parasomnia or seizure disorder that fails to respond to therapy. Polysomnography is not routinely indicated for typical, uncomplicated, and noninjurious parasomnias, as well as for seizure disorders with no signs and symptoms consistent with a sleep disorder.

(From Kushida CA; Littner MR; Morgenthaler T, et al. Practice parameters for the indications for polysomnography and related procedures: an update for 2005. Sleep. 2005;28(4):499–521.)

430. Answer: A

Educational objective: Describe the effects of changes in body temperature on sleep.

Explanation: The onset of the major sleep period typically occurs during the declining phase of the temperature rhythm, with acceleration in the rate of fall in body temperature, following a temperature peak. The degree of heat loss at sleep onset also influences the quantity of sleep that follows. Initiating sleep during the falling phase of the temperature rhythm (increase heat loss and decrease heat production) is associated with a decrease in sleep latency, increase in total sleep time, and increase in NREM stages 3 and 4 sleep. In contrast, initiating sleep during the rising phase of the temperature rhythm (decrease heat loss and increase heat production) causes an increase in sleep latency, decrease in total sleep time, decrease in NREM stages 3 and 4 sleep, and increase in REM sleep. Awakening occurs during the rising phase of the temperature rhythm following the temperature nadir.

431. Answer: A

Educational objective: Describe the pharmacologic features of thiothixene.

Explanation: Polysomnographic features of thiothixene, a typical antipsychotic, include a decrease in sleep latency, an increase in sleep efficiency, an increase in total sleep time, and an increase in REM sleep latency. There is no consistent change in NREM stages 3 and 4 sleep.

432. Answer: C

Educational objective: Describe the different types of extinction techniques for children with sleep disorders.

Explanation: There are three general types of extinction techniques, namely the fast approach, gradual approach, and the parental presence approach. The fast approach (absolute extinction) involves having the parent put the child in bed, leaving the child alone in his or her room, and ignoring inappropriate behavior until the next morning. In extinction with parental presence, parents are allowed to sleep in a separate bed in the child's bedroom for about a

week, but are instructed to ignore any inappropriate behavior by the child. The gradual approach (graduated extinction) as described in this question involves gradually decreasing parental response to the demands of the child with progressively longer duration between interventions, shorter periods of intervention, or lesser physical contact with the child until parental intervention is finally stopped.

433. Answer: A

Educational objective: Describe the effects of the non-benzodiazepine benzodiazepine receptor agonists on sleep.

Explanation: Nonbenzodiazepine benzodiazepine receptor agonists include zaleplon, zolpidem and eszopiclone. They act via the gamma-aminobutyric acid receptor complex at a different site than the benzodiazepines. Development of tolerance and withdrawal symptoms is rare, and there is no significant effect on respiratory status. Zaleplon has a shorter half-life than zolpidem.

434. Answer: A

Educational objective: Describe the different afferent pathways of the suprachiasmatic nucleus.

Explanation: In addition to the retinohypothalamic pathway, other afferent suprachiasmatic nuclear pathways from photic stimuli include (1) thalamic intergeniculate leaflet of the lateral geniculate nuclei via the geniculohypothalamic tract using neuropeptide γ and gamma-aminobutyric acid as its neurotransmitters (alternate afferent connection); (2) tuberomammillary complex neurons in the posterior basal hypothalamus via histaminergic pathways; and (3) basal forebrain (eg, septum, diagonal band of Broca and substantia innominata) and brainstem (eg, pedunculopontine tegmentum and parabigeminal nucleus) neurons via cholinergic pathways. Afferent pathways from nonphotic stimuli include the midbrain medial raphe nuclei via serotonergic pathways. Whereas light entrainment is lost following disruption of the retinohypothalamic tract, this is unaffected by interruption of the alternate geniculohypothalamic tract.

435. Answer: A

Educational objective: Describe the features of pulse transit time.

Explanation: Pulse transit time (PTT), the transmission time for the arterial pulse pressure wave to travel from the aortic valve to the periphery (interval between the electrocardiographic R-wave and the subsequent pulse shock wave at the finger), is typically about 250 ms. The speed of the shock wave is affected by the stiffness of the arterial walls and blood pressure. PTT is inversely related to blood pressure. Therefore, PTT increases during inspiratory falls in blood pressure and decreases during arousal-induced increases in blood pressure in persons with obstructive sleep apnea. PTT has been reported to be useful in distinguishing between central and obstructive apnea-hypopneas and in differentiating those requiring nasal continuous positive airway pressure from those who do not.

436. Answer: C

Educational objective: *Understand the factors that influence susceptibility to sleep deprivation.*

Explanation: *There is significant interindividual vulnerability to sleep deprivation, with some individuals demonstrating more adverse neurocognitive effects to sleep loss than others. Compared with the elderly, younger individuals appear to be more susceptible to the effects of total sleep deprivation, with greater negative impact on alertness and cognitive performance. However, this variability among individuals becomes less prominent as the duration of sleep deprivation increases. The adverse physiologic, neurocognitive, and behavioral consequences of acute total sleep deprivation differ from those generally observed with chronic partial sleep deprivation.*

437. Answer: D

Educational objective: *Explain the characteristics of nocturnal hypoxemia seen in patients with chronic obstructive pulmonary disease.*

Explanation: *Patients with both chronic obstructive pulmonary disease (COPD) and obstructive sleep apnea ("overlap syndrome") have a more severe course compared to individuals with obstructive sleep apnea alone, and have a lower PaO_2, higher $PaCO_2$, and higher pulmonary artery mean pressures. The overlap syndrome should be suspected in patients with mild COPD presenting with daytime hypercapnia.*

438. Answer: B

Educational objective: *Describe the features of electro-oculography.*

Explanation: *Electro-oculography records the difference in potentials (dipole) between the cornea (positive) and the retina (negative). A positive voltage (downward deflection) is recorded when the eye moves toward an electrode, and a negative voltage (upward deflection) accompanies an eye movement away from an electrode. Electrodes are placed (using adhesive and not collodion) lateral and superior to the outer canthus of one eye (right outer canthus) and lateral and inferior to the outer canthus of the other eye (left outer canthus). Electrodes are connected either to the opposite or same mastoid process of the temporal bone.*

439. Answer: C

Educational objective: *Describe the clinical features of nocturnal seizures.*

Explanation: *Sleep is a recognized precipitant of seizure activity. It is estimated that about 25% of persons with* epilepsy have their seizures mostly restricted to sleep. There are two peaks in the occurrence of nocturnal seizures, the first about 2 hours after bedtime, and the second from 4:00 to 5:00 AM. Generally, sleep-related seizures occur more frequently during NREM sleep (most commonly in stages 1 and 2 sleep, and occasionally in stages 3 and 4) than REM sleep. Seizure thresholds are greater during REM sleep compared to NREM sleep.

440. Answer: C

Educational objective: *Describe pupillary changes during sleep.*

Explanation: *Constriction of the pupils secondary to parasympathetic stimulation occurs during NREM and tonic REM sleep. Dilation of the pupils due to parasympathetic inhibition is present during phasic REM sleep.*

441. Answer: C

Educational objective: *Appreciate the sleep disturbances that can occur in patients with cystic fibrosis.*

Explanation: *Cystic fibrosis is a disease characterized by abnormal transport of sodium and chloride across the epithelium in all exocrine tissues. It is an autosomal recessive disorder. Patients with cystic fibrosis can present with bronchiectasis and bronchiolectasis, exocrine pancreatic insufficiency, intestinal dysfunction, abnormal sweat gland unction, and urogenital dysfunction. Nocturnal episodes of coughing and oxygen desaturation can also occur. The likelihood of sleep-related hypoxemia is greater in patients low FEV_1 and low awake SaO_2. Sleep quality is correlated with physiological variables of disease severity and can worsen significantly during disease exacerbations. Despite poor subjective sleep quality, sleep latency, and sleep efficiency are usually normal.*

442. Answer: A

Educational objective: *Understand the risk of developing narcolepsy among relatives of patients with the disorder.*

Explanation: *Although most cases of narcolepsy are sporadic, there is a clear familial tendency in up to one-third of patients. About 3% of patients have a first-degree relative with cataplexy and excessive sleepiness. The risk of developing the disorder is increased by 10 to 40 times in first-degree relatives of narcoleptic individuals. Twin studies have described discordance in most monozygotic pairs; only about 25% to 30% of monozygotic twins are concordant.*

443. Answer: B

Educational objective: *Identify the typical timing of minimum core body temperature.*

Explanation: *The minimum of the core body temperature rhythm (Tmin) is commonly used as a biological marker to estimate the timing of circadian rhythm. Tmin typically occurs 2 to 4 hours prior to the end of the sleep period.*

444. Answer: C

Educational objective: Describe the pharmacologic properties of the benzodiazepine receptor agonists.

Explanation: *The elimination half-lives of the different hypnotic agents are zaleplon (1–1.5 hours), zolpidem (1.5–2 hours), triazolam (2–5 hours), temazepam (4–18 hours), estazolam (14–24 hours), flurazepam (40–250 hours), and quazepam (40–250 hours).*

445. Answer: B

Educational objective: Describe the features of expired end-tidal carbon dioxide (PetCO$_2$) monitoring.

Explanation: *Infrared spectrophotometers or respiratory mass spectrometers can be utilized to continuously monitor airway carbon dioxide (PetCO$_2$) levels. The measured level of PetCO$_2$ at the end of a complete expiration is related to PaCO$_2$. PetCO$_2$ may underestimate PaCO$_2$ when the dead space to tidal volume ratio is increased during sleep, and may be less accurate during supplemental oxygen or positive airway pressure therapy.*

446. Answer: C

Educational objective: Describe the clinical features of benign epilepsy of childhood with centrotemporal spikes (benign rolandic epilepsy).

Explanation: *The features of benign epilepsy of childhood with centrotemporal spikes (benign rolandic epilepsy) include perioral numbness and clonic focal twitching of the face and mouth during drowsiness and sleep. Secondarily generalized tonic-clonic seizures may develop. Electroencephalography demonstrates rolandic or centrotemporal spike and sharp waves. Interictal discharges increase during sleep. Onset is during childhood, with spontaneous resolution during the teenage years or adulthood.*

447. Answer: C

Educational objective: Describe the effects of sleep on the levels of the various hormones.

Explanation: *Parathyroid hormone levels increase during sleep. Levels of testosterone in adult men increase at night during sleep. Plasma levels of renin increase during NREM sleep and decrease during REM sleep. Antidiuretic hormone secretion increases during the night but secretion is not related to sleep. Levels of aldosterone increase in the early morning prior to awakening. Among pubescent children, there is a sleep-related increase in levels of luteinizing hormone (LH). LH secretion occurs mainly during NREM sleep. In adult men, the increase in secretion of LH continues to be related to sleep. In contrast, sleep does not appear to have a prominent effect on LH secretion in adult women, in whom LH secretion may even decline during sleep, particularly during the follicular phase of the menstrual cycle.*

448. Answer: A

Educational objective: Define obstructive hypoventilation in children.

Explanation: *Obstructive hypoventilation in children is defined by the presence of prolonged periods of hypoventilation, with hypercapnia and hypoxemia, due to persistent but partial upper airway obstruction. They can occur with or without arousals.*

449. Answer: A

Educational objective: Describe the different methods of measuring respiratory effort during polysomnography.

Explanation: *Respiratory effort can be identified using esophageal pressure monitoring, surface diaphragmatic electromyography, strain gauges, respiratory inductance plethysmography, or thoracic impedance. Measurement of respiratory effort is important in distinguishing central from obstructive apneas. Respiratory effort is accompanied by changes in pleural pressure, which can be accurately measured by esophageal pressure monitoring using either traditional esophageal balloons or newer catheter transducers. This method is particularly useful in distinguishing between obstructive and central apneas. Measurement of esophageal pressures during polysomnography is the reference standard for detecting respiratory effort.*

450. Answer: B

Educational objective: Identify the different types of generalized seizures.

Explanation: *Generalized seizures can occur during awakenings from sleep. They consist of three major seizure disorders. Generalized tonic-clonic seizures are characterized by both tonic (sustained muscle contraction) and clonic (muscle jerks) phases. Absence seizures (petit mal) consist of periods of unconsciousness and blank staring with typical diffuse 3 to 4 Hz spike and wave electroencephalographic discharges. Juvenile myoclonic seizures present with muscle jerks after awakenings from sleep. Complex frontotemporal seizures are considered partial epilepsies.*

451. Answer: C

Educational objective: Describe the relationship between sleep and thyroid-stimulating hormone.

Explanation: *Secretion of thyroid-stimulating hormone (TSH) appears to be linked to both circadian rhythms and sleep. TSH levels are lowest during the daytime; increase progressively during the night, reaching its peak prior to sleep onset; and decline thereafter. Sleep, particularly NREM stages 3 and 4 sleep, inhibits the secretion of TSH. Levels of TSH increase with awakenings and during sleep deprivation. Thyroid hormone levels are high during the daytime and low at night.*

452. Answer: D

Educational objective: *Describe the clinical features of sleep-onset association disorder.*

Explanation: *The patient with sleep-onset association disorder is incapable of falling asleep without the presence of certain desired conditions. This condition is typically seen in a child who is unable to sleep unless a feeding bottle, pacifier, or a favorite toy is available. It is estimated to affect 15% to 20% of children 6 months to 3 years of age. Boys appear to be affected more often than girls. This disorder commonly remits at 3 to 4 years of age but may persist into adulthood (eg, dependence on a television set or radio). Two possible polysomnographic patterns can be expected in patients with sleep-onset association disorder. In the absence of desired circumstances, there is an increase in both sleep latency and frequency of awakenings. Sleep quantity and quality are normal when the required associations are met.*

453. Answer: C

Educational objective: *Describe the mechanisms responsible for the changes in body temperature during sleep.*

Explanation: *A decrease in thermoregulation occurs during sleep with readjustment of the thermal set point to a lower level. The responsiveness to thermal challenges declines during NREM sleep and diminishes further during REM sleep. Sweating and shivering are still present during NREM sleep. Heat production with shivering is absent during REM sleep because of the associated muscle atonia.*

454. Answer: C

Educational objective: *Describe the polysomnographic features of "movement time."*

Explanation: *Epochs in which sleep stage scoring is not possible because more than 50% of the epoch is obscured by movement artifact (if it occurs between two epochs of sleep) is scored as movement time. An epoch is scored as stage wake if it meets criteria for movement time but is between two epochs of wake.*

455. Answer: D

Educational objective: *Identify the best time to provide photic stimulation to entrain the circadian sleep-wake cycle.*

Explanation: *Greatest phase shifting is seen when light exposure occurs closest to the minimum core body temperature(Tmin). A phase delay is produced when light is presented before the Tmin, and a phase advance follows light exposure after the Tmin. Exposure to light during the subjective day generates either no phase shifts (dead zone) or much lesser amounts of phase shifts compared to exposure during the subjective night.*

456. Answer: A

Educational objective: *Identify the risk factors for infant sleep apnea.*

Explanation: *Infant sleep apnea is seen is infants greater than 37 weeks of gestation. Both obstructive and central sleep apneas or hypopneas can occur during infancy. Respiratory events can be associated with hypoxemia, bradytachycardia, and arousals. Factors increasing the risk and severity of infant sleep apnea include low-birth weight, comorbid medical disorders (anemia, lung disease, gastroesophageal reflux, metabolic derangements, or infection), neurologic disorders, and medication use, including anesthesia. Infant sleep apnea is not an independent risk factor for sudden infant death syndrome, and a family history of the latter is not known to predispose to infant sleep apnea.*

457. Answer: C

Educational objective: *Understand which classes of medications can exacerbate or decrease cataplexy in patients with narcolepsy.*

Explanation: *Cataplexy is exacerbated by α_1-receptor antagonists (prazosin) and α_2-receptor agonists; and reduced by α_2-receptor antagonists (yohimbine) and α_1-agonists (methoxamine).*

458. Answer: B

Educational objective: *Distinguish among the different disorders that cause leg movements during the sleep period.*

Explanation: *Hypnagogic foot tremor (HFT) is characterized by rhythmic tremors of the feet or toes that occur during the transition between wakefulness and sleep, or during NREM stages 1 and 2 sleep. HFT appears to be a common and usually incidental finding noted during polysomnography performed for other reasons. The course is generally benign. Polysomnographic findings consist of repetitive leg or foot electromyography (EMG) bursts or movements lasting several seconds to minutes and occurring during drowsy wakefulness or light stages of sleep. With alternating leg muscle activation, brief activity of the anterior tibialis muscle of one leg alternates with activity of the same muscle in the other leg, usually prior to or following an arousal or awakening. It can also occur without any associated arousals from sleep. It diminishes gradually with return to sleep. Polysomnography demonstrates repetitive, brief, and alternating activations of the anterior tibialis EMGs. Each activation has a duration of 0.1 to 0.5 seconds, with at least four muscle activations occurring in sequence lasting from 1 to 30 seconds, and with less than 2 seconds between activations.*

459. Answer: C

Educational objective: *Describe the changes in sleep architecture associated with the use of barbiturates.*

Explanation: *Barbiturates (eg, pentobarbital and phenobarbital) act via the gamma-aminobutyric acid receptors. They can cause excessive sleepiness and may worsen obstructive sleep apnea. Polysomnographic features include a decrease in sleep latency, an increase in total sleep time, a decrease in wake time after sleep onset, an* increase in NREM stage 2 sleep (increase in spindle density), a decrease in NREM stages 3 and 4 sleep, an increase in REM sleep latency, and a decrease in REM sleep. Drug withdrawal can cause rebound insomnia.

460. Answer: D

Educational objective: Describe the features of the retinohypothalamic pathway of the suprachiasmatic nuclei.

Explanation: The main afferent pathway for photic stimuli in the suprachiasmatic nucleus is the retinohypothalamic pathway, which involves the photosensitive retina ganglion cells containing the photopigment, melanopsin. Signals are relayed to the hypothalamus via the retinohypothalamic tract. It uses glutamate and pituitary adenylate cyclase–activating polypeptide as its neurotransmitters. Retinal photoreceptors involved with circadian processes are most sensitive to visible light of shorter wavelengths (from 450 nm [blue] to 500 nm [blue-green]).

461. Answer: B

Educational objective: Describe the pharmacologic properties of the benzodiazepines.

Explanation: Benzodiazepines typically reduce sleep latency, increase total sleep time, and decrease the frequency of awakenings in patients with insomnia. They also increase NREM stage 2 sleep (more sleep spindles), decrease NREM stages 3 and 4 sleep, and decrease REM sleep.

462. Answer: B

Educational objective: Enumerate the clinical features of cluster headaches.

Explanation: Cluster headaches consist of excruciating, unilateral (periorbital or temporal) headaches with a rapid onset and peak within several minutes. They occur more frequently among men. During cluster periods, one to three headache attacks occur daily, often at the same hour each day, over a 1- to 2-month period. Individual attacks typically last a few hours. Associated features include lacrimation, conjunctival injection, rhinorrhea or nasal stuffiness, miosis, ptosis, and increased ipsilateral forehead sweating. Headaches tend to occur during sleep, particularly during REM sleep. Obstructive sleep apnea is a known trigger.

463. Answer: B

Educational objective: Describe the mechanisms responsible for the changes in body temperature during sleep.

Explanation: Core body temperature peaks in the late afternoon and early evening from 6:00 to 8:00 PM, and falls at the onset of sleep. This is due to a number of factors, including greater heat loss mediated by sweating and peripheral vasodilatation, less heat generation secondary to a decrease in both metabolism and wake-related muscle

activity, and decrease in thermoregulation with a readjustment of the thermal set point to a lower level.

464. Answer: A

Educational objective: Describe the use of melatonin in the therapy of delayed sleep phase syndrome.

Explanation: Melatonin given in the evening to patients with delayed sleep phase syndrome is effective in inducing a phase advance of the sleep period with a decrease in sleep latency. Its phase shifting effect is less potent than that of bright light. Melatonin also has a mild hypnotic effect when ingested in supraphysiologic (> 0.5 mg) doses. The U.S. Food and Drug Administration (FDA) does not approve melatonin as a therapy for circadian sleep disorders. Melatonin may worsen asthma symptoms. Its use should be avoided in pregnant or breast-feeding women.

465. Answer: D

Educational objective: Describe the methods for measuring oxygenation and ventilation during sleep.

Explanation: Direct measurements of arterial oxygen tension (PaO_2), arterial carbon dioxide tension ($PaCO_2$), and SaO_2 via arterial blood sampling are more accurate than estimates derived from noninvasive methods. However, they afford only a static measure of oxygenation and ventilation at discrete points of time rather than continuous monitoring. Oxygenation and ventilation changes rapidly during sleep in patients with sleep-related breathing disorders. Thus, to be accurate and reliable, methods to assess blood gases must be capable of rapid and repetitive measurements. However, repetitive sampling of arterial blood during sleep is painful, time-consuming, inconvenient, expensive, and intrusive of the subject's sleep. Noninvasive assessments include pulse oximetry, transcutaneous oxygen tension ($PtcO_2$) measurement, transcutaneous carbon dioxide tension ($PtcCO_2$) measurement, or airway CO_2 ($PetCO_2$) monitoring.

466. Answer: C

Educational objective: Define the phenomenon of blood pressure "dipping."

Explanation: Both heart rate and systolic blood pressure decrease at night. Nighttime systolic blood pressure is often about 10% less than that during the daytime ("dipping" phenomenon). This is believed to be secondary to circadian rhythm–related nocturnal reductions in catecholamine levels.

467. Answer: C

Educational objective: Describe the features of respiratory effort–related arousals.

Explanation: A respiratory effort–related arousal is accompanied by a reduction in airflow and increasing inspiratory effort for at least 10 seconds that does not meet the criteria for either apnea or hypopnea, and is not associated with significant oxygen desaturation. They are identified as a transient flattening of the nasal pressure signal or increasing negative deflections on esophageal pressure monitoring followed by a sudden change in pressure to a less negative level and an arousal.

468. Answer: C

Educational objective: *Describe the changes in the cardiovascular system associated with phasic REM sleep.*

Explanation: *Compared with NREM and tonic REM sleep, phasic REM sleep is associated with an increase in heart rate; minimal change in stroke volume; an increase in peripheral vascular resistance; an increase in cardiac output; an increase in systemic blood pressure; an increase in coronary circulation; and unchanged or slightly increased splanchnic, renal, or skeletal circulation.*

469. Answer: D

Educational objective: *Describe the characteristics of the free-running circadian rhythm.*

Explanation: *Circadian rhythms free-run at their genetically determined frequency in the absence of synchronizing environmental time cues. Most free-running intrinsic human circadian rhythms have been shown to not be exactly 24 hours. This endogenous circadian period is referred to as tau.*

470. Answer: B

Educational objective: *Describe the changes in sleep associated with the neurodegenerative disorders.*

Explanation: *The cerebral degenerative disorders constitute a large group of neurologic conditions having, in common, abnormalities in movement and behavior. Included in this category are Huntington disease, dystonia, ataxia, olivopontocerebellar and spinocerebellar degeneration, spastic torticollis, and musculorum deformans. Muscular contractions and gross body movements are prominent during sleep. REM sleep behavior disorder may develop. Affected individuals may complain of both sleep-onset and sleep-maintenance insomnia. Polysomnographic features include an increase in frequency of awakenings as well as a decrease in NREM stages 3 and 4 sleep and REM sleep. Sleep efficiency is diminished.*

471. Answer: B

Educational objective: *Describe the changes in autonomic nervous system during sleep.*

Explanation: *During REM sleep, compared with NREM sleep, there is an increase in sympathetic tone, especially during phasic REM sleep, resulting in a higher average heart rate and blood pressure. However, an increase in parasympathetic tone during tonic REM sleep can give rise to relative bradycardia and periods of asystole.*

472. Answer: D

Educational objective: *Describe the different artifacts that might be encountered during polysomnography.*

Explanation: *Artifacts can arise from faulty electrode placement or unwanted contamination by physiologic variables and environmental factors. A 60 Hz artifact is due to interference from 60 Hz electrical activity from power lines, high and unequal electrode impedance, or lead failure. It produces a dense, almost square-shaped electroencephalographic tracing. Fixing the electrode placement or changing leads to correct high and unequal electrode impedance can correct 60-Hz interference. A 60-Hz filter can be used as a last resort to correct the artifact.*

473. Answer: C

Educational objective: *Identify the medications that can change REM sleep latency.*

Explanation: *Factors that increase REM latency include an advance in bedtime or first-night effect, acute alcohol ingestion, and medication use (clonidine, REM sleep suppressant agents [monoamine oxidase inhibitors, selective serotonin reuptake inhibitors, tricyclic antidepressants, trazodone, and venlafaxine] and amphetamine). Mirtazapine and nefazodone do not change REM sleep latency. Depression decreases REM sleep latency.*

474. Answer: D

Educational objective: *Describe the effects on melatonin on circadian rhythms.*

Explanation: *Melatonin influences the suprachiasmatic nucleus and alters the phase of circadian rhythms. Appropriately timed administration of melatonin can phase shift the circadian sleep-wake rhythms. It causes a phase delay when taken in the morning, and a phase advance when given in the afternoon or early evening. Melatonin is less effective in phase shifting the circadian rhythm than light exposure. Melatonin also possesses a mild hypnotic effect that helps promote sleep onset.*

475. Answer: B

Educational objective: *Describe the different artifacts that might be encountered during polysomnography.*

Explanation: *Sweat artifact consists of a slow-frequency undulating movement present in most channels that is often synchronous with respiration. It is due to alterations in electrode potentials by salt in sweat. Sweat artifact may resemble delta waves and may result in overscoring of NREM stages 3 and 4 sleep. It can be prevented and minimized by decreasing room temperature.*

476. Answer: A

Educational objective: *Describe the clinical features of hypnic headaches.*

Explanation: *Hypnic headaches are generalized or unilateral headaches that occur during sleep and awaken the patient. Headaches occur more frequently among the elderly and can be accompanied by nausea but not autonomic manifestations. They respond to therapy with lithium. Hypnic headaches are most common during REM sleep.*

477. Answer: C

Educational objective: *Describe the changes in gastrointestinal physiology that occur during sleep.*

Explanation: *Swallowing, salivary production, and esophageal motility decrease during sleep. These changes delay esophageal acid clearance and prolong mucosal acid contact in patients with gastroesophageal reflux. Basal gastric acid secretion displays a circadian rhythmicity with a peak secretion between 10:00 PM and 2 AM (as a result of increased parasympathetic activity) and a nadir in the morning between 5:00 and 11:00 AM. Gastric acid secretion increases during sleep in patients with peptic ulcer disease with no difference in secretion between NREM sleep and REM sleep. Intestinal motility (ie, migrating motor complex) has a lower velocity during sleep.*

478. Answer: B

Educational objective: *Identify the factors that can cause a phase advance or a phase delay of the circadian sleep-wake rhythm.*

Explanation: *A phase shift is a forward or backward displacement of intrinsic circadian rhythms in response to entrainment by a zeitgeber. A phase delay is produced when light is presented near the start of the subjective night (ie, before the core body temperature nadir) whereas a phase advance follows light exposure near the end of the subjective night (ie, after the core body temperature nadir). Physical exercise in the evening can phase delay rhythms, whereas physical exercise in the morning can give rise to phase advancement of rhythms. A phase delay can also result from passive body heating in the evening.*

479. Answer: A

Educational objective: *Describe the features of REM sleep latency.*

Explanation: *REM sleep latency is defined as the period from the first epoch of sleep (sleep onset) to the first epoch of REM sleep. REM sleep latency usually ranges from 60 to 120 minutes. A sleep-onset REM period is generally defined as the occurrence of REM sleep within 10 to 15 minutes of sleep onset.*

480. Answer: A

Educational objective: *Identify the neurotransmitters involved in the regulation of REM sleep.*

Explanation: *The main REM sleep neurotransmitter is acetylcholine. Other neurotransmitters involved with REM sleep regulation include gamma-aminobutyric acid and glycine.*

481. Answer: C

Educational objective: *Describe the features of the neurons of the locus ceruleus, midbrain reticular formation, thalamus, lateral hypothalamus, and basal forebrain.*

Explanation: *Noradrenaline-containing neurons are located in the locus ceruleus in the dorsal pontine tegmentum, which, in turn, project to the cerebral cortex, subcortical areas, brainstem, and spinal cord. Discharge rates increase during waking, decrease during NREM sleep stages 3 and 4, and are absent during REM sleep.*

The substantia nigra and ventral tegmental area contain dopamine and project to the frontal cortex and basal ganglia. Serotonin neurons are located in the dorsal raphe.

482. Answer: A

Educational objective: *Identify the location of the suprachiasmatic nuclei.*

Explanation: *In mammals, the suprachiasmatic nuclei in the anterior hypothalamus, located dorsal to the optic chiasm, serves as the master neural generator of circadian rhythms. Other anatomical sites may also harbor endogenous clocks.*

483. Answer: D

Educational objective: *Describe the indications for split-night polysomnography.*

Explanation: *A split-night polysomnography with an initial diagnostic portion followed by continuous positive airway pressure (CPAP) titration on the same night is an acceptable alternative to a full-night polysomnography with CPAP titration for patients with an apnea hypopnea index (AHI) > 40 during a minimum of 2 hours of sleep time in a diagnostic polysomnography. An AHI of 20 to 40 may also be acceptable based on clinical judgment such as the presence of repetitive prolonged obstructions or marked desaturations. The duration of CPAP titration should be greater than 3 hours. CPAP should eliminate or nearly eliminate respiratory events during sleep, including REM sleep in a supine position. A second full-night polysomnography with CPAP titration is recommended if the duration available for CPAP titration is less than 3 hours, or if CPAP titration fails to successfully eliminate respiratory events during both NREM and REM sleep.*

(From Kushida CA; Littner MR; Morgenthaler T, et al. Practice parameters for the indications for polysomnography and related procedures: an update for 2005. Sleep. 2005;28(4):499–521.)

484. Answer: B

Educational objective: *Know where the hypocretin neurons are located.*

Explanation: Hypocretin neurons are located in the perifornical region of the lateral hypothalamus. The laterodorsal tegmentum/pedunculopontine tegmentum contain acetylcholine, whereas the locus ceruleus and raphe nuclei contain norepinephrine and serotonin, respectively.

485. Answer: B

Educational objective: Describe the role of the various respiratory neuron groups in the control of breathing.

Explanation: The nucleus ambiguus is located parallel to the ventrolateral respiratory group and modulates respiration by its action on laryngeal and pharyngeal muscles.

486. Answer: C

Educational objective: Describe the role of chronotherapy in the treatment of delayed sleep phase syndrome.

Explanation: Chronotherapy for delayed sleep phase syndrome involves either a progressive phase delay or progressive phase advancement of the major sleep episode. With the progressive phase delay approach, bedtime and wake times are delayed usually by about 2 to 3 hours each day on successive days until the desired or conventional bedtime is reached. Napping should be avoided. Physical activities, meal times, and light exposure should be timed to coincide with the progressive delay in wake times. Progressive phase advance, on the other hand, is achieved by gradually advancing bedtimes and the time of awakening (usually by 30 to 60 minutes) over several days until more conventional sleep-wake schedules are attained.

487. Answer: B

Educational objective: Describe the common clinical features of narcolepsy.

Explanation: Automatic behavior (eg, driving or writing) during sleep episodes can occur in about 20% to 40% of persons with narcolepsy. There is no recall of the event. Disruption of nighttime sleep with repetitive awakenings and poor sleep quality can be seen in up to 70% to 80% of persons with narcolepsy. Other common features include a greater prevalence of REM sleep behavior disorder, periodic limb movements of sleep, and sleep apnea. Sleep apnea, both obstructive and central, can occur in about 30% of persons with narcolepsy and can contribute to the severity of excessive sleepiness. REM sleep behavior disorder can be precipitated or aggravated by therapy of cataplexy with tricyclic antidepressants and stimulant agents. Sleep drunkenness, defined by confusion and diminished alertness immediately following an awakening, is observed in approximately 10% of persons with narcolepsy.

488. Answer: C

Educational objective: Define the polysomnographic characteristics of periodic limb movements of sleep.

Explanation: Polysomnography is required for the diagnosis of periodic limb movements of sleep. Limb movements are detected using surface electromyography (EMG) recordings over the anterior tibialis muscles (ie, anterolateral calves). Movements are counted if they occur during sleep and have a duration of 0.5 to 5 seconds, and if they occur in a series of four or more consecutive contractions with intervals between movements of 5 to 90 seconds from the onset of one limb movement to the onset of the next. The amplitude of the EMG is at least 25% greater than that of baseline during biocalibrations.

489. Answer: C

Educational objective: Describe the adverse effects of chronic use of benzodiazepines.

Explanation: Chronic use of benzodiazepines can lead to tolerance and/or dependency. During abrupt drug withdrawal of benzodiazepines, insomnia, sleep fragmentation, and REM sleep rebound (with nightmares) may develop. Rebound insomnia related to sudden discontinuation of chronic benzodiazepine use is characterized by difficulty in both initiating and maintaining sleep that lasts for several days and appears to more severe with drugs with short half-lives than with longer-acting agents.

490. Answer: B

Educational objective: Describe the clinical features of mucopolysaccharidosis.

Explanation: Hurler syndrome is an autosomal recessive disorder characterized by the presence of dwarfism, mental retardation, and increased urinary levels of chondroitin sulfate B and heparin sulfate. On the other hand, Hunter syndrome, a rare X-linked recessive disorder, can have skeletal abnormalities, hepatosplenomegaly, macroglossia, adenotonsillar hypertrophy, tracheomalacia, and high arched palate.

491. Answer: A

Educational objective: Describe the polysomnographic features of obstructive sleep apnea.

Explanation: Polysomnography is required for the diagnosis of obstructive sleep apnea. Features include an increase in frequency of arousals, an increase in NREM stages 1 and 2 sleep, a decrease in NREM stages 3 and 4 sleep, and a decrease in REM sleep.

492. Answer: B

Educational objective: Identify the neurotransmitter associated with the retinohypothalamic pathway of the suprachiasmatic nucleus.

Explanation: The retinohypothalamic pathway is the main photic afferent conduit of the suprachiasmatic nucleus. Its neurotransmitters include glutamate and pituitary adenylate cyclase–activating polypeptide.

493. Answer: C

Educational objective: *Describe the features of arousals from sleep.*

Explanation: *An arousal is defined as a sudden and brief (3 to 14 seconds) change in electroencephalogram (EEG) from sleep to wakefulness or from a "deeper" (stages 3 and 4) to a "lighter " (stages 1 and 2) NREM sleep stage. It may be accompanied by an increase in electromyographic (EMG) activity, body movements, or heart rate. An arousal is usually identified during NREM sleep by an abrupt change in EEG frequency of at least 3 seconds in duration, including alpha, theta, or beta activity (but not spindles or delta waves), following at least 10 seconds of continuous sleep. NREM sleep arousals do not need to be accompanied by changes in chin EMG. During REM sleep arousals, EEG changes are accompanied by changes in chin EMG (increase in amplitude). Isolated increases in chin EMG amplitude without changes in EEG do not constitute an arousal. "Movement arousal" is defined as a body movement associated with an EEG arousal (increase in alpha wave activity, decrease in wave amplitude, or paroxysmal high-voltage waveforms) and increase in EMG activity.*

494. Answer: B

Educational objective: *Describe the two major ascending reticular formation pathways to the forebrain.*

Explanation: *The reticular formation has two major ascending projections into the forebrain. First, a dorsal or thalamocortical pathway projects to the thalamus then to the cerebral cortex. Second, a ventral pathway projects to the subthalamus and posterior hypothalamus, then to the basal forebrain and septum, and finally ends in the cerebral cortex.*

495. Answer: D

Educational objective: *Describe the role of glycine in the regulation of sleep and wakefulness.*

Explanation: *Glycine is the main inhibitory neurotransmitter in the spinal cord. Neurotransmitter release occurs during REM sleep. It causes REM sleep-related paralysis via hyperpolarization of spinal motoneurons.*

496. Answer: C

Educational objective: *Understand the differences between the various treatment modalities for positive airway pressure.*

Explanation: *Treatment modalities for positive airway pressure therapy include continuous positive airway pressure (provides a constant pressure throughout the respiratory cycle), bilevel positive airway pressure (provides two pressure levels during the respiratory cycle: a higher level during inspiration and a lower pressure during expiration), autotitrating positive airway pressure (provides variable pressures using device-specific diagnostic and therapeutic*

algorithms), and nocturnal noninvasive positive pressure ventilation (provides two pressure levels at a set rate to assist ventilation).*

497. Answer: D

Educational objective: *Identify the efferent neurotransmitters of the suprachiasmatic nucleus.*

Explanation: *Transforming growth factor-α and prokineticin 2 are among the efferent suprachiasmatic nuclei neurotransmitters.*

498. Answer: C

Educational objective: *Describe the role of the various respiratory neuron groups in the control of breathing.*

Explanation: *The pontine respiratory group, located in the parabrachial region of the dorsolateral pons, is not essential for the generation of the basic respiratory rhythm. Lesions of this neuron group cause apneustic breathing. The dorsal respiratory group consists primarily of inspiratory neurons and is located in the dorsal medulla (ventrolateral section of the solitary tract nucleus). Neurons of the nucleus ambiguus modulate respiration by its action on laryngeal and pharyngeal muscles. Finally, neurons located in the ventrolateral reticular formation of the dorsal brainstem and upper spinal cord are involved with the maintenance of the respiratory rhythm and the regulation of inspiration and expiration.*

499. Answer: A

Educational objective: *Describe the relationship between sleep and the release of growth hormone.*

Explanation: *Biosynthesis and secretion of growth hormone (GH) by the anterior pituitary gland is stimulated by GH–releasing hormone (GHRH) and inhibited by somatostatin. Release of growth hormone is linked to sleep, occurring among adults during NREM stages 3 and 4 sleep. However, GH secretion can also occur without NREM stages 3 and 4 sleep. In young healthy adults, the daily peak in GH secretion occurs near the onset of sleep, often associated with the first period of NREM stages 3 and 4 sleep. GH secretion is lower during the second half of the sleep period. Unlike in men, in whom there is one peak in secretion of GH at sleep onset, there may be several peaks in GH secretion in women throughout the day and night. GHRH promotes sleep in men (in women GHRH may inhibit sleep), and increases NREM stages 3 and 4 sleep. Somatostatin, by antagonizing GHRH, inhibits sleep.*

500. Answer: B

Educational objective: *Identify the factors that can change REM sleep latency.*

Explanation: *A decrease in REM latency is associated with delays in bedtime, depression, narcolepsy (sleep* onset REM periods), medications (bupropion), obstructive sleep apnea syndrome (secondary to sleep deprivation), REM sleep deprivation, schizophrenia, and sudden withdrawal of REM-suppressing agents.

501. Answer: D

Educational objective: Identify the medications that can alter the percentage of REM sleep.

Explanation: REM sleep is increased by reserpine and following withdrawal of REM suppressants. Bupropion and nefazodone increase REM sleep in depressed patients. Medications that can decrease REM sleep include alcohol, amphetamines, benzodiazepines, clonidine, lithium, monoamine oxidase inhibitors, selective serotonin receptor inhibitors, tricyclic antidepressants, and methylphenidate. Monoamine oxidase inhibitors are the most potent inhibitors of REM sleep. Mirtazapine and trazodone do not change percentage REM sleep.

502. Answer: A

Educational objective: Know the indications for sleep position therapy of obstructive sleep apnea.

Explanation: For many patients with obstructive sleep apnea (OSA), the upper airway is most vulnerable to collapse during supine sleep. Positional sleep apnea has been defined as OSA in which the supine sleep-related apnea hypopnea index (AHI) is at least twice that during sleep in a nonsupine (eg, lateral recumbency) position. Patients with positional sleep apnea are more likely to be less overweight and to have lower apnea hypopneas indices compared to patients whose apnea is present in all sleep positions. In selected patients in whom respiratory events occur exclusively or predominantly during a supine sleep position and if polysomnography demonstrates a normal AHI in the lateral posture, elevation of the head or restricting sleep to lateral recumbency might be tried. Sleep position training alone may be sufficient for patients with OSA whose AHIs are normal during lateral recumbency sleep. However, long-term adherence to and the enduring efficacy of sleep position training are not well established. Patients whose apnea is not position dependent do not generally benefit from this kind of intervention.

503. Answer: C

Educational objective: Describe the American Academy of Sleep Medicine recommendations regarding behavioral treatment of bedtime problems and night wakings in infants and young children.

Explanation: According to the American Academy of Sleep Medicine Practice parameters for behavioral treatment of bedtime problems and nightwakings in infants and young children (Sleep. 2006;29(10):1277–1281), effective interventions recommended for treating bedtime problems and night wakings in young children include unmodified extinction and extinction of undesired behavior with parental presence, parent education and prevention, graduated extinction of undesired behavior, delayed bedtime with removal from bed and positive bedtime routines, and scheduled awakenings. There is insufficient evidence to formulate recommendations on any single therapy over another or on combination interventions over single therapies.

504. Answer: A

Educational objective: Identify which pharmacologic agents used for the therapy of restless legs syndrome are more likely to give rise to augmentation.

Explanation: Dopaminergic medications are considered the first-line therapy for both restless legs syndrome and periodic limb movement disorder. They include dopamine precursors (eg, carbidopa/levodopa) and dopamine agonists (eg, pergolide, pramipexole or ropinirole). Dopamine agonists are less likely to cause augmentation than carbidopa/levodopa. Augmentation resulting from dopamine agonists also tends to be less severe than that due to carbidopa/levodopa.

505. Answer: A

Educational objective: Identify the action of the different receptors of the gamma-aminobutyric acid-A receptor complex.

Explanation: Benzodiazepines act via the gamma-aminobutyric acid-A receptor complex, which consists of several receptors, including BZ1, BZ2, and BZ3. The receptor primarily related to sedation is the BZ1. Eszopiclone, zaleplon and zolpidem also act via the BZ1 receptor.

506. Answer: C

Educational objective: Describe the patterns of prolactin secretion during sleep.

Explanation: Levels of prolactin increase shortly following the onset of sleep, with peak levels occurring during the second half of the evening prior to awakening. Prolactin secretion increases during NREM stages 3 and 4 sleep and it decreases during REM sleep. Secretion of prolactin is suppressed by sleep fragmentation. Administration of benzodiazepines can increase prolactin secretion during sleep.

507. Answer: B

Educational objective: Describe the characteristics of dreaming.

Explanation: Dreaming can occur during both REM (accounting for 80% of dreams) and NREM (20% of dreams) sleep. Compared with REM sleep-related dreams, which tend to be more complex and irrational, NREM dreams are generally simpler and more realistic. Dreams are thought to be associated with processing and consolidation of memory as well as activation and stimulation of central nervous system neural networks. Theories of dreaming include the cognitive hypothesis (dreaming is an extension of awake thought that are governed by different processes) and the activation synthesis hypothesis (dreaming is produced by cortical interpretation of randomly generated intrinsic subcortical activity).

508. Answer: B

Educational objective: Discuss the indications for polysomnography.

Explanation: Polysomnography is indicated for diagnosing sleep-related breathing disorders (SRBDs); titrating continuous positive airway pressure for SRBD; determining therapeutic benefits after upper airway surgery or therapy with dental devices for SRBD; monitoring resolution or recurrence of SRBD following significant weight loss or gain, respectively; diagnosing narcolepsy (followed by multiple sleep latency testing); and evaluation of atypical or injurious parasomnias, seizures, suspected periodic limb movements during sleep or insomnia that persists despite pharmacologic and nonpharmacologic interventions. Polysomnography is not routinely indicated for the diagnosis of chronic lung disease, restless legs syndrome, depression, and circadian rhythm sleep disorders.

(From Kushida CA; Littner MR; Morgenthaler T, et al. Practice parameters for the indications for polysomnography and related procedures: an update for 2005. Sleep. 2005;28(4):499–521.)

509. Answer: D

Educational objective: Describe the results of animal studies of sleep deprivation.

Explanation: In animal models of sleep deprivation, one or more of the following have been described: an increase in homeostatic sleep drive with sleep rebound; changes in metabolism with decrease in anabolic hormones; weight loss despite high amounts of food intake; an increase in metabolic rate; neuroendocrine abnormalities such as increase in plasma norepinephrine levels; impaired response to infectious agents; skin lesions, including hyperkeratosis and ulcerations; an increase in heart rate; a decrease in body temperature and failure of thermoregulation; and death with prolonged sleep deprivation.

510. Answer: C

Educational objective: Describe the features of the Multiple Sleep Latency Test.

Explanation: The study is terminated if no sleep is recorded for 20 minutes. If sleep is recorded, the test is continued for another 15 minutes to allow REM sleep to develop. The test is stopped after the first epoch of unequivocal REM sleep. If no sleep occurs during a nap, its sleep latency is recorded as 20 minutes.

511. Answer: C

Educational objective: Understand the consequences of sleep deprivation in humans.

Explanation: Changes in metabolism associated with sleep deprivation in humans include an increase in sympathetic activation, evening levels of cortisol, and levels of ghrelin; blunting of sleep-dependent secretion of growth hormone and prolactin; decrease in glucose tolerance; decrease in levels of thyroxine and leptin; increase in metabolic rate; and hypothermia.

512. Answer: D

Educational objective: Identify the efferent projections of the suprachiasmatic nucleus.

Explanation: The suprachiasmatic nucleus has efferent projections to several central nervous system areas, including the hypothalamus, locus ceruleus, ventrolateral preoptic nucleus, basal forebrain, hypocretin neurons, pineal gland, and thalamus.

513. Answer: D

Educational objective: Describe the mechanisms responsible for the reduction in urine volume that occurs during sleep.

Explanation: There is a reduction in urine volume accompanied by an increase in urine concentration as a result of an increase in water reabsorption, decrease in glomerular filtration and increase in release of renin. There is generally no significant change, or a slight increase, in renal circulation during sleep.

514. Answer: D

Educational objective: Describe the changes in autonomic nervous system during sleep.

Explanation: There is a reduction in sympathetic tone, an increase in parasympathetic tone, a decrease in heart rate and blood pressure, and vasoconstriction during NREM sleep relative to wakefulness.

515. Answer: C

Educational objective: Describe the American Academy of Sleep Medicine recommendations for the use of light therapy for sleep disorders.

Explanation: American Academy of Sleep Medicine Recommendations for the use of light therapy for sleep disorders include the following:

a) A physician planning to use light therapy should know recommended dosages and intensity limits, as well as the adverse effects of this form of treatment.

b) When used within recommended guidelines regarding intensity and duration of exposure, light therapy used for some circadian rhythm disorders is generally safe.

c)   Light therapy appears to have potential utility for the treatment of the following circadian rhythm disorders:
   d)   Delayed sleep phase syndrome
   e)   Advanced sleep phase syndrome
   f)   Some blind patients with non–24-hour sleep-wake syndrome
g)   Neither the minimum nor optimal duration of light therapy is known for the following circadian rhythm disorders:
   h)   Delayed sleep phase syndrome
   i)   Advanced sleep phase syndrome
   j)   Non–24 sleep-wake syndrome
k)   For jet lag, light therapy at destination appears potentially useful for travelers across multiple time zones.
l)   For shift workers:
   m)   Light exposure before the core body temperature minimum may be helpful for a day to evening to night rotating work schedule.
   n)   Light exposure after the core body temperature minimum may be helpful for a night to evening to day schedule.
o)   No recommendations are provided regarding the use of light therapy for patients with dementia, or other causes of insomnia among the healthy elderly.

(From Chesson, et al. Practice parameters for the use of light therapy in the treatment of sleep disorders. Sleep. 1999;22:5.)

516. Answer: A

Educational objective: *Describe the phenomenon of nocturnal blood pressure "dipping."*

Explanation: *Both heart rate and systolic blood pressure decrease at night. "Dipping" phenomenon refers to the decrease in nighttime systolic blood pressure by about 10% relative to daytime blood pressure.*

517. Answer: D

Educational objective: *Describe the features of paradoxical intention therapy for insomnia.*

Explanation: *Patients with insomnia often display performance anxiety over their inability to fall asleep. Paradoxical intention involves instructing patients with insomnia to go to bed and to try to stay awake as long as they possibly can at night. By persuading the patient with insomnia to remain awake at night rather than trying to sleep, paradoxical intention attempts to decrease the performance anxiety associated with efforts to fall asleep. Paradoxical insomnia might reduce sleep latency. Specific subsets of patients with insomnia that would respond to this therapy have not been defined.*

518. Answer: B

Educational objective: *Describe the differences in respiration between wakefulness and sleep.*

Explanation: *Respiration is controlled by metabolic (ie, pH, PaO_2, and $PaCO_2$) and behavioral systems during wakefulness; in contrast, only the metabolic system operates during NREM sleep. Hypoxic and hypercapnic ventilatory responses decrease during sleep relative to wakefulness, with a greater reduction seen during REM sleep than during NREM sleep. Upper airway muscle tone is diminished during sleep secondary to decreased respiratory neuron excitatory activity to pharyngeal motor neurons. Sleep also blunts the ventilatory response to added inspiratory resistance. There are gender differences in respiratory control. The hypoxic ventilatory response may be similar during both wakefulness and NREM sleep among women (ie, there is a greater fall in hypoxic drive in men than in women from wakefulness to sleep).*

519. Answer: D

Educational objective: *Describe changes in cardiovascular parameters during sleep.*

Explanation: *Compared with wakefulness, NREM sleep is characterized by a decrease in heart rate; minimal change in stroke volume; minimal change or slight decrease in peripheral vascular resistance; a decrease in cardiac output; a decrease in systemic blood pressure; a decrease in coronary circulation; and no significant change in renal, splanchnic, and skeletal circulation.*

520. Answer: C

Educational objective: *Describe the characteristics of melatonin synthesis and secretion.*

Explanation: *Melatonin is synthesized and released by the pineal gland in a rhythmic fashion with greatest secretion at night and suppression of secretion in the daytime. Production and secretion of melatonin is regulated by light stimuli via the suprachiasmatic nuclei. Exposure to light inhibits melatonin secretion. In the pineal gland, the amino acid tryptophan is enzymatically converted into serotonin (5-hydroxytryptamine), which is in turn converted into melatonin (N-acetyl-5-methoxytryptamine). Production of melatonin decreases with aging. The liver metabolizes melatonin.*

521. Answer: A

Educational objective: *Identify the causes of excessive sleepiness in children.*

Explanation: *Insufficient sleep is the most common cause of excessive sleepiness in children. In this syndrome, the child regularly has a sleep duration that is shorter than is expected for age. Sleepiness secondary to insufficient sleep duration generally resolves following a trial of sleep extension. Other causes of sleepiness in children include sleep fragmentation (eg, obstructive sleep apnea or periodic limb movement disorder); alteration in circadian sleep-wake rhythms (eg, delayed sleep phase syndrome); medical, neurologic, and psychiatric disorders (eg, narco-*

lepsy or idiopathic hypersomnia); or use and abuse of substances or medications (eg, alcohol, use of sedative agents or withdrawal from stimulants).

522. Answer: C

Educational objective: Determine the appropriate therapy for patients with advanced sleep phase syndrome.

Explanation: Advanced sleep phase syndrome (ASPS) involves a stable shift in the major sleep period to an earlier time relative to desired or conventional bed times. This results in a marked inability to delay sleep time and a spontaneous morning awakening that is several hours earlier than desired. Patients generally report being most alert in the morning. Sleep typically occurs between 6:00 and 9:00 PM and wake time occurs between 2:00 and 5:00 AM. Sleep, itself, is normal for age and undisturbed. Typical complaints include excessive sleepiness in the late afternoon or early evening and an inability to remain asleep until the desired morning awakening time. Onset is typically during middle age. Prevalence increases with age and the elderly are at greater risk of developing ASPS due to their tendency for mild phase advancement. Diagnosis relies on sleep logs or actigraphy performed over several days. If polysomnography is performed over the usual advanced sleep schedule, sleep latency, duration and quality are normal. In contrast, a short sleep latency and decrease in total sleep time are observed if polysomnography is recorded during conventional sleep-wake times.

Bright light therapy for 30 to 45 minutes or longer during the early evening (7:00 to 9:00 PM) prior to the body temperature nadir, along with restricting light exposure in the early morning, can be tried. Chronotherapy involves gradually shifting usual sleep time until the desired bedtime is achieved. Administration of melatonin during the early morning has been proposed but, given its hypnotic properties, can lead to unwanted daytime sleepiness.

523. Answer: B

Educational objective: Describe the polysomnographic features of stage REM sleep.

Explanation: Electroencephalography (EEG), electromyography (EMG), and electro-oculography do not necessarily change simultaneously at the start or end of REM periods. Any epoch contiguous with stage REM sleep with an EEG showing a relatively low-amplitude, mixed-frequency activity are scored as REM sleep if the EMG shows atonia or hypotonia and if no intervening arousals occur, whether or not rapid eye movements are observed. If an arousal occurs at the transition between NREM and REM sleep, the epochs prior to the arousal with REM-like EEG and EMG are considered stage REM sleep unless the arousal occurred less than 3 minutes after a sleep spindle or K-complex, in which case the epoch is scored as NREM stage 2 sleep.

524. Answer: A

Educational objective: Understand the factors influencing the secretion of melatonin.

Explanation: Melatonin receptors are present in the suprachiasmatic nuclei and hypothalamus. Melatonin is released by the pineal gland during the night. Its secretion is inhibited by light exposure.

525. Answer: B

Educational objective: Describe the neural systems regulating NREM sleep.

Explanation: NREM sleep is regulated by neurons located in the forebrain (anterior hypothalamus-preoptic region, including ventrolateral preoptic area) and basal forebrain), solitary tract nuclei, midbrain raphe, orbitofrontal cortex, amygdala, anterior and dorsomedial thalamic nuclei, and reticular nucleus of the thalamus. The reticular nucleus of the thalamus is responsible for the generation of spindles.

526. Answer: B

Educational objective: Identify the medications used for the treatment of restless legs syndrome and periodic limb movement disorder.

Explanation: Symptoms of restless legs syndrome (RLS) and periodic leg movement disorder (PLMD) often respond to the same medications. Dopaminergic medications are considered the first-line therapy for both RLS and PLMD. These agents decrease the frequency of PLMS, diminish RLS symptoms, and improve sleep quality.

527. Answer: A

Educational objective: Describe the clinical course of narcolepsy.

Explanation: Onset of narcolepsy is generally during adolescence and early adulthood (between 15 and 25 years of age). Excessive sleepiness is often the first symptom to appear, followed one to several years later by cataplexy, sleep paralysis, and sleep hallucinations. Excessive sleepiness is generally persistent and unrelenting, whereas the severity of cataplexy and other manifestation of abnormal REM sleep regulation may wax and wane over time.

528. Answer: D

Educational objective: Describe the polysomnographic features of obsessive-compulsive disorder.

Explanation: Polysomnographic features of obsessive-compulsive disorder include a decrease in sleep efficiency, a decrease in total sleep time, an increase in frequency of awakenings, a decrease in NREM stages 3 and 4 sleep, a decrease in REM sleep latency, and an increase in REM density.

529. Answer: A

Educational objective: *Describe the clinical features of the irregular sleep-wake pattern.*

Explanation: *In the irregular sleep-wake pattern syndrome, stable circadian sleep-wake rhythms are absent. Sleep and wake times are disorganized with three or more short "naps" comprising the fragmentary remnants of the major sleep episode. There is temporal variability in sleep and wake activity from one day to the next with inconsistent and unpredictable sleep onsets and wake times throughout the day. Nonetheless, the aggregate sleep time over a 24-hour period is typically near normal or normal for age. Affected individuals may complain of insomnia, daytime sleepiness and/or cognitive impairment. The disorder is rare in the general population and is most frequently encountered in persons with severe brain dysfunction (eg, mental retardation, dementia, head injury, or recovery from coma). Onset can occur at any age. It appears to affect both genders equally and has no identified familial pattern.*

530. Answer: D

Educational objective: *Describe the changes in the cardiovascular system associated with tonic REM sleep.*

Explanation: *Compared with NREM sleep, tonic REM sleep is associated with a decrease in heart rate; minimal change in stroke volume; a decrease in peripheral vascular resistance; a decrease in cardiac output; a decrease in systemic blood pressure; an increase in coronary circulation; and unchanged or slightly increased splanchnic, renal, and skeletal circulation.*

531. Answer: C

Educational objective: *Describe the changes in hormone levels associated with age-related alterations in sleep.*

Explanation: *Except for prolactin, most hormones have reduced amplitudes with aging. Growth hormone–releasing hormone activity and growth hormone secretion decrease in parallel with the reduction of NREM stages 3 and 4 sleep. Other hormones that are reduced during aging include testosterone (among males) and melatonin.*

532. Answer: C

Educational objective: *Describe the clinical features of childhood narcolepsy.*

Explanation: *Narcolepsy often manifests initially as excessive sleepiness (eg, resumption of daytime napping) during the second decade of life. Cataplexy, sleep paralysis, hypnagogic hallucinations, and sleep-onset REM periods may not be present in young children. In addition, unlike the repetitive short naps that can be seen in adult patients, children with narcolepsy may have prolonged sleep periods. Because of the evolving nature of narcolepsy in this age group, several polysomnographic studies performed over several months to years may be required for diagnosis.*

Multiple sleep latency test parameters have not been standardized in children younger than 8 years of age.

533. Answer: B

Educational objective: *Identify the muscle groups affected by sleep paralysis.*

Explanation: *In sleep paralysis, there is a generalized transient inability to move the head, body and extremities, with sparing of the ocular and respiratory muscles, occurring either at sleep onset (hypnagogic) or on awakening (hypnopompic). Individuals are unable to speak during these episodes. Skeletal muscle atonia is accompanied by areflexia. Fright, profound anxiety, and hallucinations may accompany these attacks, but consciousness and recall are typically unaffected. Paralysis spontaneously resolves after several seconds to several minutes; resolution can be hastened by external stimulation, such as a touch or sound.*

534. Answer: A

Educational objective: *Characterize sleep among older adults.*

Explanation: *Normal aging is associated with changes in sleep, including greater sleep fragmentation, decreased strength of homeostatic sleep drive, greater prevalence of insomnia, obstructive sleep apnea, periodic limb movements in sleep, restless legs syndrome, REM sleep behavior disorder, increase in risk of developing advanced sleep phase syndrome, and decrease in arousal threshold with greater sensitivity to adverse environmental factors.*

535. Answer: B

Educational objective: *Describe the changes in sleep following administration of tricyclic antidepressants.*

Explanation: *Tricyclic antidepressants may precipitate or exacerbate periodic limb movements during sleep or restless legs syndrome. They can cause abnormal dreams and nightmares. Protriptyline may enhance upper airway muscle tone. Sudden tricyclic antidepressant withdrawal can produce REM sleep rebound and insomnia.*

536. Answer: C

Educational objective: *Understand the relationship between the endogenous circadian sleep-wake rhythm and the external 24-hour environment in patients with non–24-hour sleep-wake disorder.*

Explanation: *In free-running or nonentrained type (non–24-hour sleep-wake disorder or hypernyctohemeral syndrome), there is abnormal synchronization between the endogenous sleep-wake circadian rhythm and the 24-hour environmental light-dark cycle. Sleep-wake patterns seem to rely solely on intrinsic biologic rhythms. Freed of exogenous entraining influences such as light and social activities, the free-running internal rhythms behave with a periodicity of slightly over 24 hours.*

Sleep onset and wake times are delayed by about 1 hour or more each day. Less commonly, longer cycles may be observed resulting in greater daily delays. The major sleep period therefore progressively "marches" throughout the day into the afternoon and onto the evening. The relationship between the external 24-hour world and the internal 25-hour clock then tends to vary from one extreme of total asynchrony to the other extreme of complete conformity. The severity of symptoms shares this cyclic variability and ranges from considerable sleep and daytime disturbances to the complete, albeit brief, disappearance of symptoms.

Despite the progressive delay in sleep schedules, sleep duration and daytime performance may be normal if patients are allowed to sleep ab libitum. As sleep onset and offset are progressively delayed, affected individuals complain of periodically recurring problems of insomnia or excessive daytime sleepiness.

This syndrome is rarely encountered in the general population and most reported cases involved totally blind individuals who lack photic entrainment, many of whom also have psychiatric or behavioral disorders. Less commonly, it can affect sighted individuals with severely schizoid or avoidant personality disorders, mental retardation, or dementia. When polysomnography is recorded at a fixed time over several days, sleep latency becomes progressively longer, and total sleep time becomes commensurately shorter. A thorough neurologic evaluation is recommended for sighted persons to exclude any occult central nervous system pathology.

537. Answer: D

Educational objective: *Identify the upper airway dilator muscles.*

Explanation: *Upper airway dilator muscles consists of the Alai nasi (nose); Levator veli palatini, Palatoglossus and Tensor veli palatini (palate); Genioglossus, Geniohyoid, Sternohyoid and Sternothyroid (oropharynx); and Cricothyroid and*

The upper airway dilator muscles include the levator veli palatini palatoglossus, tensor veli palatini, alai nasi, genioglossus, geniohyoid, sternohyoid, sternothyroid, cricothyroid and posterior cricoarytenoid.

538. Answer: B

Educational objective: *Enumerate the changes in respiration that accompany REM sleep.*

Explanation: *REM sleep is associated with a variable and irregular pattern of respiration with variability in respiratory rates and tidal volumes, occurrence of central apneas or periodic breathing during phasic REM sleep, diminished activity of the motor neurons (eg, hypoglossal nerve) innervating the pharyngeal dilator muscle genioglossus, atonia or hypotonia of the intercostal muscles, and decrease in functional residual capacity. The activity of*

the phrenic motor neurons innervating the diaphragm remains intact. Arterial blood gas demonstrates increase in $PaCO_2$ and decrease in PaO_2.

539. Answer: C

Educational objective: *Identify the medications used for the treatment of restless legs syndrome and periodic limb movement disorder.*

Explanation: *Compared with the dopamine agonists, carbidopa/levodopa has a more rapid onset of action. Because of its short duration of action, repeated dosing during the night may be required if symptoms recur later in the night or if morning (end-of-dose) rebound of symptoms occurs. Ropinirole and pramipexole have a longer duration of action than regular formulations of carbidopa/levodopa and are less likely to cause augmentation than carbidopa/levodopa.*

540. Answer: A

Educational objective: *Understand the changes in sleep that occur during the postpartum period.*

Explanation: *The postpartum period is generally defined as the first 6 months following birth of the infant. Changes in sleep architecture include a decrease in sleep efficiency, a decrease in total sleep time, an increase in frequency of awakenings, and an increase in wake time after sleep onset. There is often an increase in NREM stages 3 and 4 sleep, which returns to baseline prepregnancy levels at 1 to 3 months postpartum. Primiparas (first-time mothers) have greater sleep disruption, more interrupted sleep, less total sleep time, and lower sleep efficiency than multiparas. Sleep disruption is also more severe after delivery by cesarean section than after vaginal delivery. Awakenings are frequently related to the infant's intrinsic schedule of sleep-wakefulness and feeding. Finally, there is an increase in the frequency of napping.*

541. Answer: A

Educational objective: *Describe the different circadian rhythm sleep disorders seen in children.*

Explanation: *In delayed sleep phase syndrome (DSPS), the major nocturnal sleep period is chronically delayed in relation to the desired bedtime, with an inability to advance sleep onset to an earlier time. Sleep onset occurs at about the same delayed time each night. Onset of DSPS is often during adolescence. Advanced sleep phase syndrome is characterized by an advance in the major nocturnal sleep period in relation to the desired bedtime and an inability to delay sleep onset at night. The preadolescent child often has a mild degree of phase-advancement in their sleep schedules. Irregular sleep wake schedule is defined by variable periods of sleep and wakefulness throughout the 24-hour day. This sleep-wake variability is common* *among newborn infants and is not considered pathologic until after 6 months of age when consolidation of nighttime sleep develops. The sleep-wake schedule relies on endogenous circadian rhythms and results in incremental delays in the major sleep period. This condition is more commonly observed in blind children, but it may also be encountered in children with mental retardation, severely schizoid or avoidant personality disorder, and, rarely in sighted individuals.*

542. Answer: D

Educational objective: *Describe the clinical features of sleep talking.*

Explanation: *Sleep talking or somniloquy refers to the vocalization or utterance of sounds, words or sentences during sleep. It can occur in all stages of sleep but is most commonly described in NREM stages 1 and 2 sleep and REM sleep. It is common in the general population and is of no apparent clinical or psychologic significance. It affects all age groups with no gender difference. There is a substantial genetic influence in both childhood and adult sleep talking. A number of sleep disorders, including obstructive sleep apnea, REM sleep behavior disorder, sleep terrors, and confusional arousals, can trigger sleep talking.*

543. Answer: C

Educational objective: *Describe the changes in cardiovascular parameters that accompany each episode of obstructive sleep apnea.*

Explanation: *During each episode of obstructive sleep apnea, respiratory efforts against an occluded upper airway can result in a decrease in intrathoracic pressure, which in turn can give rise to reductions in blood pressure and cardiac output. Systemic and pulmonary artery blood pressures then rise as apnea progresses, reaching their peak in the immediate postapneic period. Relative bradycardia may develop during airway obstruction followed by tachycardia during termination of apnea. Respiratory events occurring during REM sleep tend to be longer in duration and associated with greater falls in oxygen saturation.*

544. Answer: D

Educational objective: *Describe the polysomnographic features of shift work sleep disorder.*

Explanation: *Polysomnography is rarely required to diagnose shift work sleep disorder. However, if polysomnography is indicated to exclude other sleep disorders, it is preferable to perform the recording during the usual shift work schedule. Common polysomnographic features include increase in sleep latency, decrease in total sleep time, and decrease in sleep efficiency with frequent arousals and awakenings. Reductions in NREM stage 2 sleep and REM sleep are also seen.*

545. Answer: D

Educational objective: *Understand how the clinical features of Crouzon syndrome contribute to the increased risk of obstructive sleep apnea.*

Explanation: *In Crouzon syndrome, abnormally early fusion of the cranial bones lead to a small head. Additional features include a small jaw, nasal septal deviation, exophthalmos, short upper lip, and, in some cases, a cleft palate. Obstructive sleep apnea can develop secondary to upper airway obstruction occurring as a result of choanal stenosis, maxillary hypoplasia, posterior displacement of the tongue, and lengthened soft palate.*

546. Answer: B

Educational objective: *Describe the factors that increase the likelihood of developing sleep paralysis.*

Explanation: *Predisposing and precipitating factors include sleep deprivation, irregular sleep patterns (eg, shift work), a supine sleep position, use of anxiolytic agents, and, possibly, stress.*

547. Answer: D

Educational objective: *Provide the mechanisms responsible for nocturia among older adults.*

Explanation: *Increased frequency of voiding during the night among older adults may be due to age-related physiologic changes such as decrease in urinary bladder capacity, greater urine production (decrease in urinary concentrating ability), prostatic enlargement (in men), and detrusor overactivity.*

548. Answer: B

Educational objective: *Identify the adverse effects of dopaminergic therapy of restless legs syndrome.*

Explanation: *Development of pleuropulmonary and cardiac valve fibrosis has been described following the use of pergolide. Side effects of ropinirole include nausea, sedation, and postural hypotension. Side effects of pramipexole include nausea, sedation, orthostatic hypotension, leg edema, and headaches. Side effects of bromocriptine include hypotension.*

549. Answer: C

Educational objective: *Describe the clinical features of nightmares.*

Explanation: *Nightmares are unpleasant and frightening dreams, often involving threats to life or security, that occur during REM sleep and that commonly abruptly awaken the sleeper out of sleep. Episodes typically occur in the latter half of the night. Once awakened, the person is fully alert and profoundly fearful and anxious, can recall vividly the preceding dream, and has difficulty returning to sleep. Some minor autonomic* activation, such as tachycardia and tachypnea, is evident. Nightmares may also occur during NREM sleep particularly in persons who have experienced a traumatic event (eg, acute stress disorder or post-traumatic stress disorder).

550. Answer: B

Educational objective: Describe the polysomnographic features of secondary amine tricyclic antidepressants.

Explanation: Secondary amine tricyclic antidepressants include desipramine and protriptyline. Polysomnographic features of secondary amines include an increase in sleep latency, a decrease in sleep efficiency, an increase in wake time after sleep onset, an increase in REM sleep latency, a decrease in REM sleep, and an increase in REM density.

551. Answer: C

Educational objective: Describe the countermeasures for sleepiness among shift workers.

Explanation: Intermittent exposure to bright lights in the workplace, administration of psychostimulants (eg, caffeine or modafinil) during evening work hours, and scheduled napping can enhance alertness and reduce sleepiness among shift workers.

552. Answer: D

Educational objective: Describe the pharmacologic properties of benzodiazepine receptor agonists.

Explanation: Effects of benzodiazepine receptor agonists (benzodiazepine and nonbenzodiazepine benzodiazepines receptor agonists) on sleep architecture include a decrease in sleep latency, a decrease in frequency of awakenings, an increase in total sleep time, an increase in NREM stages 3 and 4 sleep (benzodiazepines), and a decrease in REM sleep (benzodiazepines).

553. Answer: D

Educational objective: Describe the changes in autonomic nervous system that accompanies NREM and REM sleep.

Explanation: The sympathetic nervous system originates in the thoracolumbar portion of the spinal cord, whereas the parasympathetic nervous system originates in the brain stem and sacral portion of the spinal cord. There is an overall reduction in sympathetic activity and increase in parasympathetic activity during the transition from wakefulness to NREM sleep. There is a further increase in parasympathetic activity and reduction in sympathetic activity during REM sleep (except for the transient increases in sympathetic tone during phasic REM sleep).

554. Answer: D

Educational objective: Understand the consequences of sleep deprivation in humans.

Explanation: Sleep deprivation in humans is associated with the following:

a) Sleepiness and an increase in homeostatic sleep drive, a decrease in sleep latency during polysomnography, Multiple Sleep Latency Test (MSLT), and Maintenance of Wakefulness Test (MWT)

b) Increase in polysomnographic slow wave activity and NREM stages 3 and 4 sleep

c) Increase in morbidity and mortality

d) Negative impact on mood

e) Irritability, nervousness and impulsiveness; paradoxic hyperactivity in children;

f) Diminished attention, alertness, vigilance, vigor, cognition, concentration, learning, memory, psychomotor performance, executive function, reaction time and motivation

g) Increase in fatigue and errors of both omission and commission

h) Fall in cerebral glucose metabolism

i) Ptosis, nystagmus, slurring of speech, hyperactive gag reflexes, and tremors

j) Hyperactive deep tendon reflexes

k) Increase in pain sensitivity

l) Increase in cardiovascular morbidity

m) Decrease in febrile response to endotoxin

n) Decrease in antibody titers to influenza vaccination

o) Increase in risk of motor vehicle accidents

555. Answer: B

Educational objective: Describe the pathophysiology of upper airway closure in patients with obstructive sleep apnea.

Explanation: Severity of daytime sleepiness appears to correlate better with the extent of sleep fragmentation than with the apnea hypopnea index, whereas the degree of arterial oxygen desaturation may be related to the subsequent development of pulmonary artery hypertension. The upper airway, from the nares to the larynx, is a flexible collapsible tube that performs various functions in respiration, swallowing, and phonation. An obstructive apnea or hypopnea occurs when the forces that maintain upper airway patency such as activation of dilator muscles (genioglossus, tensor palatini, geniohyoid, and sternohyoid) are insufficient to counteract the factors that promote upper airway closure during sleep (eg, negative intraluminal pressure). The upper airways of patients with obstructive sleep apnea (OSA) tend to be narrower (due to altered anatomical structures, fat accumulation in soft tissues, mucosal swelling, or muscle hypertrophy) and are more vulnerable to collapse compared to that among persons without this disorder. The critical closing pressure is the pressure at which collapse the upper airway occurs and is less negative among patients with OSA compared to normal persons. The most common sites of upper airway obstruction are the airspaces behind the palate (retropalatal) and behind the tongue (retrolingual).

556. Answer: B

Educational objective: *Describe the clinical features of sleep-related dissociative disorders.*

Explanation: *Dissociative disorder can occur during the daytime, during sleep, or both. Nighttime episodes of violent or sexualized behavior, self-mutilation, screaming, running, eating, or driving a car may last several minutes or hours, and they can recur several times nightly. There is generally amnesia for the event. Women are affected more commonly then men. Many patients have a history of psychiatric disorders (mood, anxiety, or post-traumatic stress disorders; suicide attempts; or self-mutilation) or abuse (ie, sexual, physical or emotional), and demonstrate daytime dissociative behaviors. Sustained electroencephalographic wakefulness is present during these episodes. Abnormal behaviors tend to begin several seconds after an arousal, unlike disorders of arousal, wherein activity starts immediately with the arousal from sleep.*

557. Answer: C

Educational objective: *Enumerate the different neuronal systems that are responsible for the development of narcolepsy.*

Explanation: *Hypocretins are neuropeptides that appear to have multiple functions, including regulation of sleep-wake cycle, appetite, body temperature, and blood pressure. Loss of hypocretin (also known as orexin) neurons in the lateral hypothalamus appears to be the major underlying mechanism responsible for narcolepsy. The hypocretin neurotransmitter system is located in the perifornical area of the hypothalamus, with wide projections to several wake-promoting areas of the central nervous system (locus ceruleus, medullary reticular formation, raphe nuclei, and thalamus). A majority of patients with narcolepsy have decreased levels of hypocretin-1. Low cerebrospinal levels of hypocretin in patients with narcolepsy with cataplexy have been described.*

558. Answer: B

Educational objective: *Describe the characteristic features of sleep during infancy and childhood.*

Explanation: *Sleep spindles first appear after 4 weeks to 3 months of age.*

559. Answer: B

Educational objective: *Describe the effects of therapy using benzodiazepines in patients with restless legs syndrome and periodic limb movement disorder.*

Explanation: *Benzodiazepines can decrease periodic limb movement disorder-related complaints of insomnia and arousals but does not reduce the frequency of leg movements. It can improve sleep quality in restless legs syndrome.*

560. Answer: C

Educational objective: *Describe the features of the regions of the suprachiasmatic nucleus.*

Explanation: *The core region is located in the ventrolateral portion of the suprachiasmatic nucleus, utilizes vasoactive intestinal peptide as its neurotransmitter, has smaller neurons (30 μm²), and functions to reset the endogenous circadian rhythms. The shell region is located in the dorsomedial portion of the suprachiasmatic nucleus, utilizes arginine vasopressin as its neurotransmitter, has larger neurons (45 μm²), and controls the endogenous circadian rhythms.*

561. Answer: B

Educational objective: *Identify the factors that determine susceptibility to developing jet lag.*

Explanation: *Rapid eastward or westward air travel across multiple time zones can precipitate both transient insomnia and hypersomnolence. In time zone change syndrome or jet lag, the person's intrinsic circadian rhythm remains temporarily aligned to the home time zone and has not synchronized to the external cues in the new local time zone. Individuals traveling westward are phase-advanced relative to the new clock time and those traveling eastward are phase-delayed. A westward flight is associated with an early evening sleepiness as well as increased wakefulness during the early morning hours. Conversely, eastward flights result in both difficulty falling asleep and difficulty awakening the next day. There are individual differences in susceptibility, and not every traveler develops jet lag. Symptoms tend to increase in severity with greater amounts and rates of time zone transitions, and with increasing age. The direction of travel (symptoms may be more pronounced with eastward travel that entails a phase advance) and factors associated with travel itself, such as prior sleep deprivation, psychologic stress, and prolonged inactivity during flights, may influence symptom severity as well. North-south travel does not lead to jet lag symptoms.*

562. Answer: A

Educational objective: *Describe the relationship between sleep and cortisol.*

Explanation: *Release of corticotropin-releasing hormone (CRH) from the hypothalamus stimulates the secretion of adrenocorticotropic-hormone (ACTH) by the anterior pituitary, which, in turn increases cortisol release in a pulsatile fashion from the adrenal cortex. Secretion of cortisol appears to be linked to the circadian rhythm rather than to sleep. Levels increase in the early morning, peak at midmorning (ie, 8:00 AM), and declines to its nadir in the evening. Sleep is associated with a modest decline in cortisol secretion. The nadir of cortisol levels occurs following the onset of sleep. Cortisol is then released in pulses* starting in the early morning (ie, between 2:00 and 4:00 AM) until final awakening. Sleep fragmentation and awakenings give rise to increased secretion of cortisol. CRH increases vigilance and inhibits sleep. Administration of CRH, ACTH, or cortisol decreases REM sleep. CRH decreases NREM stages 3 and 4 sleep, whereas cortisol enhances NREM stages 3 and 4 sleep.

563. Answer: B

Educational objective: Describe the changes in respiration that occur during NREM sleep.

Explanation: During NREM sleep, breathing becomes regular in amplitude and frequency due to the loss of the wake-related stimulus for breathing and the absence of nonrespiratory factors affecting respiration. Respiration is controlled solely by centrally driven processes. Periodic breathing, with hypopneas and hyperpneas, can occur at sleep onset and may persist until NREM stage 2 sleep. NREM stages 3 and 4 sleep is associated with a stable and regular pattern of respiration, a decrease or no change in respiratory rate, a decrease in tidal volume and functional residual capacity, a reduction in minute ventilation (relative hypoventilation), an increase in $PaCO_2$, a decrease in PaO_2, a decrease in inspiratory airflow, and an increase in upper airway resistance. In addition, diminished activity of the accessory muscles of respiration (intercostal muscles) and dilator muscles of the nose, pharynx, and larynx occurs.

564. Answer: C

Educational objective: Describe the clinical features of delayed sleep phase syndrome.

Explanation: Delayed sleep phase syndrome (DSPS) is characterized by a chronic or recurrent inability to sleep during desired hours, with a delayed habitual bedtime coupled with an equally delayed arising time (ie, the major nocturnal sleep period occurs later than the conventional or socially acceptable bedtime). Individuals complain of being unable to fall asleep until the early morning hours (eg, 1:00 to 6:00 AM) as well as difficulty arising until late morning or early afternoon (e.g., 10:00 AM to 2:00 PM). Patients often report feeling most alert late in the evening and most sleepy in the morning. If they attempt to sleep and arise at times closer to socially accepted norms, both sleep-onset insomnia and morning sleepiness occur. They typically have no difficulty in remaining asleep following the onset of sleep, with normal (or prolonged) sleep duration and quality for age during their preferred sleep schedules, if sleep is allowed to continue ad libitum until spontaneous awakening. Prevalence appears to be highest among adolescents and young adults. Polysomnography is not routinely indicated for the diagnosis of DSPS.

565. Answer: C

Educational objective: Describe the pharmacologic properties of zaleplon.

Explanation: Zaleplon has a rapid onset of action and an ultra-short duration of action with a half-life of only about 1 hour. Except for a shortened sleep latency, it is associated with minimal effects on sleep architecture. There is no tolerance to its sleep-promoting effects and no rebound insomnia on its discontinuation. Zaleplon is administered at a dose of 5 to 10 mg at bedtime. It may also be given during prolonged middle-of-the-night awakenings as long as there is at least 4 hours remaining prior to rising time.

566. Answer: C

Educational objective: Describe the features of continuous positive airway pressure therapy.

Explanation: Continuous positive airway pressure (CPAP) is effective in symptomatic patients with moderate to severe OSA. CPAP treatment is generally recommended for all patients with an apnea hypopnea index (AHI) > 15/hour, and symptomatic patients (eg, excessive daytime sleepiness, insomnia, impaired cognition, mood disorder, insomnia, hypertension, ischemic heart disease, or stroke) with an AHI between 5/hour and 30/hour. Less than optimal CPAP utilization is a significant problem in clinical practice. Patterns of nightly use are often discernible by the first few days or weeks of initiating treatment. Intermittent use of CPAP should be avoided, because virtually all of the sleep and daytime alertness gains derived from sleeping with CPAP are rapidly reversed with CPAP discontinuation.

567. Answer: A

Educational objective: Identify the different factors that are capable of entraining the circadian sleep-wake rhythm.

Explanation: Entrainment is the process by which external time cues adjust the phase of the endogenous circadian rhythms. Zeitgebers (from the German word "time-giver") are environmental cues that are capable of entraining endogenous circadian rhythms. Environmental light is the dominant synchronizer for the circadian sleep-wake pacemaker. Several nonphotic synchronizers are also capable of entraining circadian sleep-wake rhythms, such as meals, activities, social cues, and ambient temperature. These nonphotic stimuli have a weaker influence on the sleep-wake cycle than environmental light.

568. Answer: B

Educational objective: Identify the risk factors for sudden infant death syndrome.

Explanation: Sudden infant death syndrome (SIDS) is defined by an abrupt unexpected death in an apparently healthy infant, the cause of which is not determined by history, postmortem examination, and death scene investigation. A majority of victims are believed to have died during their sleep. It is more prevalent in males and occurs predominantly before 6 months of age. Risk of SIDS is elevated with prematurity, prone (and to a lesser extent, side) sleeping position, pre- and postnatal exposure to tobacco smoke, maternal substance abuse, preterm births, multiple births, teenage pregnancies, siblings with SIDS, lower socioeconomic status, and the occurrence of apnea of infancy. Having infants sleep on their backs reduces the incidence of SIDS.

569. Answer: D

Educational objective: Describe the clinical features of disorders of arousal.

Explanation: The disorders of arousal are believed to result from abnormal arousal processes (during which motor activity is restored without an accompanying full consciousness) and consist of confusional arousals, sleepwalking, and sleep terrors. They occur out of NREM sleep, particularly stages 3 and 4 sleep, during the first third of the night. These disorders are most commonly encountered during childhood and their frequency diminishes with increasing age as NREM stages 3 and 4 sleep decline. There is often a strong familial pattern.

570. Answer: A

Educational objective: Enumerate the factors contributing to the genesis of primary sleep enuresis.

Explanation: Primary enuresis commonly results from an impaired arousal response secondary to very deep sleep and high nighttime urine volume due to impaired release of vasopressin during sleep. Other contributory factors include inappropriate or inadequate toilet training and residence in disorganized families.

571. Answer: D

Educational objective: Describe the polysomnographic features of tertiary amine tricyclic antidepressants.

Explanation: Tertiary amine tricyclic antidepressants include amitriptyline, clomipramine, doxepin, and imipramine. Polysomnographic features of tertiary amines include a decrease in sleep latency, an increase in sleep efficiency, an increase in total sleep time, a decrease in frequency of arousals, an increase in NREM stage 1 and 2 sleep, a decrease in NREM stages 3 and 4 sleep, an increase in REM sleep latency, a decrease in REM sleep, and an increase in REM density.

572. Answer: C

Educational objective: Describe the features of the suprachiasmatic nuclei.

Explanation: The suprachiasmatic nuclei oscillate independently of the environment, firing more frequently during the daytime relative to nighttime and during wake and REM sleep relative to NREM sleep. They promote wakefulness during the day and enhance sleep consolidation during the night.

573. Answer: A

Educational objective: Describe the pharmacologic properties of eszopiclone.

Explanation: Eszopiclone is a cyclopyrrolone, nonbenzodiazepine agent that has received U. S. Food and Drug Administration (FDA) approval without a restriction to short-term usage. Long-term pharmacologic treatment of chronic primary insomnia using eszopiclone does not appear to be associated with drug tolerance.

574. Answer: B

Educational objective: Describe the duration of ultradian sleep cycles in various age groups.

Explanation: NREM-REM cycle length increases progressively during childhood. It is about 50 minutes during infancy, 60 to 70 minutes during childhood, and 90 to 120 minutes during adulthood.

575. Answer: C

Educational objective: Explain the changes in circadian rhythms associated with aging.

Explanation: Changes in circadian rhythms associated with aging include a decrease in melatonin levels, a change in relationship between sleep-wake rhythms and timing of melatonin output with sleep onset and offset occurring earlier relative to melatonin secretion, a dampening of circadian sleep-wake rhythms, and an advancement in phase of circadian rhythms. Compared with younger adults, the zone of increased alertness may occur earlier after the nadir of core body temperature.

576. Answer: C

Educational objective: Describe the clinical features of childhood obstructive sleep apnea.

Explanation: Although many children with obstructive sleep apnea (OSA) may present with excessive sleepiness, others may not. It has been estimated that only about 30% of children with OSA complain of excessive sleepiness. Childhood OSA may manifest as behavioral problems and academic difficulties.

577. Answer: A

Educational objective: Describe the polysomnographic features of obstructive sleep apnea in children.

Explanation: An obstructive apnea or hypopnea in children is defined by the presence of pauses in breathing or reduction in airflow (> 30% to 50% relative to baseline) lasting two normal respiratory cycles or longer. One or more scorable respiratory event per hour of sleep is considered significant. These events may be accompanied by paradoxical rib cage–abdominal wall excursions and increasingly negative esophageal pressure swings. Electroencephalographic arousals may or may not occur following respiratory events.

578. Answer: D

Educational objective: Describe the role of iron supplementation in the therapy of patients with restless legs syndrome.

Explanation: Restless legs syndrome (RLS) related to iron deficiency may improve with iron supplementation in some patients. Ferritin levels greater than 50 μg/1 are associated with fewer RLS symptoms.

579. Answer: A

Educational objective: Identify which of the psychiatric disorders can give rise to excessive sleepiness or insomnia.

Explanation: Psychiatric disorders associated with insomnia include bipolar disorder, depression, generalized anxiety disorder, obsessive-compulsive disorder, panic disorder, personality disorders, post-traumatic stress disorder, and schizophrenia.

On the other hand, atypical depression and seasonal affective disorders can give rise to excessive daytime sleepiness.

580. Answer: B

Educational objective: Describe the changes in sleep architecture following the administration of nefazodone.

Explanation: Nefazodone is a serotonin reuptake inhibitor and serotonin-2 antagonist. Polysomnographic features include an increase in sleep efficiency, increase in total sleep time, decrease in wake time after sleep onset, and increase in NREM stages 3 and 4 sleep. It does not increase REM sleep latency or decrease REM sleep; it may increase REM sleep and REM density.

581. Answer: D

Educational objective: Identify the physiologic variables that peak during the circadian periods of sleep or wakefulness.

Explanation: Peak activity of adrenocorticotropic hormone, cortisol, follicle-stimulating hormone, luteinizing hormone, melatonin, growth hormone and prolactin occurs during the sleep phase. In contrast, body temperature, forced expiratory volume, and insulin levels peak during the active phase.

582. Answer: A

Educational objective: Describe the effect of obstructive sleep apnea on the course of chronic obstructive pulmonary disease.

Explanation: Patients with the "overlap syndrome" have both chronic obstructive pulmonary disease and obstructive sleep apnea (OSA). Compared with those with OSA alone, patients with overlap syndrome have lower nighttime PaO_2 levels, higher $PaCO_2$ and higher pulmonary artery mean pressures.

583. Answer: A

Educational objective: Identify the medications that increase REM sleep.

Explanation: REM sleep is enhanced by cholinergic medications and suppressed by monoaminergic medications. Both selective serotonin reuptake inhibitors and lithium reduce REM sleep.

584. Answer: B

Educational objective: Describe the adverse effects associated with pemoline administration.

Explanation: Pemoline is a dopamine agonist that increases alertness. It has been withdrawn from the market due to concerns regarding liver failure.

585. Answer: A

Educational objective: Describe the features of dim light melatonin onset.

Explanation: Two biological markers have been utilized to estimate the timing of circadian rhythms, namely dim light melatonin onset (DLMO), and minimum of the core body temperature rhythm(Tmin). DLMO, defined as the time when melatonin levels stars to rise (> 3 and 10 pg/ml for salivary and plasma melatonin, respectively), generally occurs 2 to 3 hours before bedtime in normally entrained persons.

586. Answer: D

Educational objective: Describe the pharmacologic features of ecstasy.

Explanation: Ecstasy is chemically related to methamphetamine and its use has been associated with both an increase in wakefulness and a decrease in REM sleep.

587. Answer: B

Educational objective: Describe the pharmacologic features of chloral hydrate.

Explanation: Chloral hydrate acts via the gamma-aminobutyric receptor complex and causes a decrease in sleep latency and increase in total sleep time. It has a relatively short half-life. Chronic ingestion of chloral hydrate can be complicated by rapid development of tolerance as well as the occurrence of rashes, gastric discomfort, and hepatic toxicity.

588. Answer: C

Educational objective: Define the terms used to describe rhythms.

Explanation: Period length is the time interval between two consecutive events (eg, between two peaks) in a cycle. Phase is the temporal position of a cycle (eg, circadian rhythm) in relation to an external cue (eg, light-dark cycle). Amplitude is defined as the maximal excursion from peak to trough of a cycle. Acrophase is the peak of an amplitude.

589. Answer: D

Educational objective: *Describe the pharmacologic features of haloperidol.*

Explanation: *Haloperidol is a typical antipsychotic. Changes in sleep architecture associated with the use of haloperidol include a decrease in sleep latency, an increase in sleep efficiency, an increase in total sleep time, and an increase in REM sleep latency. There are no consistent changes in NREM stages 3 and 4 sleep.*

590. Answer: A

Educational objective: *Determine what levels of oxygen desaturation and hypercapnia related to respiratory events in children are considered significant.*

Explanation: *The following levels of oxygen desaturation and hypercapnia related to respiratory events are significant in children: oxygen desaturation nadir < 92% or change in oxygen desaturation nadir from baseline > 4%; maximal end-tidal CO_2 > 53 to 55 mm Hg, increase in end-tidal CO_2 > 45 mm Hg for greater than 60% of total sleep time, or increase in end-tidal CO_2 > 50 mm Hg for greater than 10% of total sleep time.*

591. Answer: B

Educational objective: *Define the terms that characterize circadian rhythms.*

Explanation: *Amplitude is defined as the maximal excursion from peak to trough of a cycle. It can be subdivided into an acrophase (peak), mesor (mean), and nadir (trough).*

592. Answer: B

Educational objective: *Describe the changes in sleep following administration of mirtazapine.*

Explanation: *Mirtazapine, a serotonin and alpha 2-receptor, histamine, and norepinephrine blocker, can cause excessive sleepiness, abnormal dreams, and nightmares. Polysomnographic features include a decrease in sleep latency, an increase in total sleep time, an increase in sleep efficiency, a decrease in wake time after sleep onset, a decrease in NREM stage 1 sleep, an increase in NREM stages 3 and 4 sleep, and an increase in REM sleep latency.*

593. Answer: C

Educational objective: *Describe the clinical features of a long sleeper.*

Explanation: *The sleep of a long sleeper is substantially lengthier than is typical for his or her age group, often consistently greater than 10 hours during a 24-hour period for a young adult. Patients may present with complaints of daytime sleepiness if they habitually obtain less than this*

amount of sleep. Onset is generally during childhood. It has an unrelenting, chronic course. Polysomnography documents a normal sleep efficiency, an increase in total sleep time (ie, 10 hours or longer), normal amounts of NREM stages 3 and 4 sleep, and increases in NREM stage 2 and REM sleep. Mean sleep latency on the Multiple Sleep Latency Test (MSLT) is normal if the patient has obtained the usual amount of nighttime sleep prior to the test.

594. Answer: C

Educational objective: *Identify the genetic features of animal models of narcolepsy.*

Explanation: *Animal models of narcolepsy have included canine mutations of hypocretin receptor-2 gene (Hcrt2) in lateral hypothalamic neurons, and hypocretin knockout rodents with null mutation of the prepohypocretin gene. In canine narcolepsy, the mode of inheritance of narcolepsy appears to be recessive. Finally, increase in pontine cholinergic M_2 muscarinic receptors, and basal ganglia and amygdala M_1 receptors have been reported in narcoleptic dogs.*

595. Answer: C

Educational objective: *Identify the annual spontaneous cure rate of primary sleep enuresis.*

Explanation: *Spontaneous cure rate in children with primary sleep enuresis is estimated at 15% annually.*

596. Answer: B

Educational objective: *Identify the parasomnias classified as disorders of arousal.*

Explanation: *Disorders of arousal from NREM sleep include confusional arousals, sleepwalking, and sleep terrors.*

597. Answer: D

Educational objective: *Describe sleep during pregnancy, labor, and the postpartum period.*

Explanation: *There is an increase in progesterone, estrogen, and prolactin levels during pregnancy. The increase in levels of progesterone during pregnancy can give rise to excessive sleepiness (sedative effect) and urinary frequency (smooth muscle inhibitory effect). Estrogen decreases REM sleep. The cephalad displacement of the diaphragm by the enlarging uterus and changing hormonal milieu can significantly affect respiratory patterns. Pregnant women often complain of dyspnea. However, oxygen saturation remains relatively stable during sleep in most women without significant sleep-related breathing disorders. Shorter nighttime sleep duration in the period before labor and delivery is associated with longer labor and increased likelihood of cesarean delivery.*

598. Answer: A

Educational objective: Describe the essential features of parasomnias.

Explanation: Parasomnias are undesirable physical phenomena or behavior that develop predominantly or exclusively during the sleep period. These abnormal events or experiences are not principally abnormalities of the states of sleep and wakefulness, and are not generally associated with major complaints of excessive sleepiness or insomnia. Parasomnias can manifest as activation of skeletal muscles or of the autonomic nervous system during sleep. They usually occur intermittently or episodically either within sleep or during its transition to and from wakefulness.

599. Answer: A

Educational objective: Identify when infants achieve nocturnal sleep consolidation.

Explanation: Sleep is distributed equally across the day and night in newborns. Nocturnal sleep consolidation and the ability to sleep through the night develops by 6 to 9 months of age.

600. Answer: A

Educational objective: Describe the demographics of narcolepsy.

Explanation: Narcolepsy affects an estimated 0.05% of the general population in the United States. The prevalence in other population groups includes:

Israel—1/50,000 (0.002%)

Japan—1/600 (0.17% to 0.18%)

North America and Europe—1/4,000 (0.025%)

Finland—26/100,000 (0.026%)

Onset is often during adolescence or early adulthood (in the second decade of life). Narcolepsy with cataplexy appears to affect males slightly more frequently than females. Excessive sleepiness is usually being the presenting symptom, followed months to years later by cataplexy, sleep paralysis, and hypnagogic hallucinations.

Index

abnormal dreams, 466t, 468t, 485b

abnormal movements, 372, 373t

abnormal swallowing syndrome, sleep-related, 37, 82t, 96, 97t, 397

absence seizures, 139, 366

absolute extinction. *See* extinction techniques

acetazolamide, 91, 191t, 221, 224

acetylcholine, 11t, 13t, 251t

achondroplasia, 176t, 409t, 410t, 428t

acquired immunodeficiency syndrome (AIDS), 341–342

acrocephalosyndactyly, types I/V, 178t, 179t

acromegaly, 23t, 122, 176–177t, 191t, 193t, 339–341

actigraphy, 65–67, 110, 162t, 193t

activation synthesis hypothesis, 26

acute insomnia, 75, 77–78, 80, 347

acute pain, 344

acute stress disorder, 279, 385–386t

adaptive servoventilation (ASV), 196, 222

Addison disease, 158t, 341

adenoidectomy, 207t

adenosine, 13t, 112, 471, 472t

adenotonsillar enlargement, 410–413

adenotonsillectomy, 412–414

adjustment sleep disorder, 79–80. *See also* insomnia

    characteristics of, 156t

    in children, 418, 431t

    clinical course, 79

    consequences of, 80

    definition of, 79

    demographics, 79

    differential diagnosis of, 80

    evaluation of, 80

adolescents, 408t

    and circadian rhythm sleep disorders, 60t

    delayed sleep-phase syndrome in, 255, 425

    excessive sleepiness in, 134

    and sleep deprivation, 29t

    sleep stages in, 8t

adrenergic agonists, 316

adrenocorticotropic hormone (ACTH), 21, 23t, 24t

advanced sleep-phase syndrome (ASPS), 258–260. *See also* circadian rhythm disorders; delayed sleep-phase syndrome (DSPS)

    characteristics of, 87t, 156t

    in children, 425–426

    clinical features, 259

    demographics, 259

    evaluation of, 259

    genetics of, 259

    pathophysiology of, 259

    therapies for, 259–260

age, 402–405

    and advanced sleep-phase syndrome, 259

    and central sleep apnea, 215

    and delayed sleep-phase syndrome, 255

    duration of sleep, 4, 402

    number of sleep phases, 402

    and obstructive sleep apnea, 176t

    percentage of REM sleep time, 404t

    proportion of NREM-REM sleep, 404t

    sleep distribution, 402

    sleep electrophysiology, 402–403

    sleep patterns, 407–408t

    sleep stages, 403–404t

    ultradian sleep cycles, 404t

aggressive behavior, 38

aging, 438–442

    change in sleep architecture with, 438

    and circadian rhythms, 439–440

    and endocrine system, 23–24

    and primary sleep disorders, 440–441

        insomnia, 440

        obstructive sleep apnea, 440–441

        periodic limb movement disorder, 441

        rapid eye movement sleep behavior disorder, 441

    sleep disturbance with, 438–439

    sleep in, 438

agoraphobia, 387

agrypnia excitata, 284

airflow measurement, 43

akathisia, 307, 380

albuterol, 480t

alcohol, 38, 112, 177t, 464–465

alcohol-dependent sleep disorder, 105t, 160t, 465

alcoholism, 103t, 159t, 388

aldosterone, 22

allergies. *See* food allergy insomnia

almitrine, 191t

alpha-2 adrenergic agonists, 316

alpha-2 antagonist hypertensives, 479t

alpha-dihydroergocryptine, 314b

alpha-NREM sleep anomaly, 345, 346b, 347, 350t

alprazolam, 315

alternating leg muscle activation (ALMA), 395, 507t

demographics, 75
differential diagnosis of, 111
evaluation of, 106
factors, 78t
fatal familial insomnia, 82t,
99–101, 275
food allergy insomnia, 81t, 90,
409t, 418
idiopathic insomnia, 85–86
medical interview, 107–108
in older adults, 440
paradoxical insomnia, 85, 110, 116
pathophysiology of, 76–77
primary, 83–86
psychophysiologic, 78, 83–84, 263
rebound insomnia, 108, 119, 120,
467, 469
and sleep-endocrine activity, 24t
therapies for, 111–125
general measures, 111–125
nonpharmacologic therapy,
111–117
pharmacologic therapy, 117–125
transient insomnia, 79, 263–264
in women, 454
inspiratory positive airway pressure,
202–203
institutionalized older adults, 441–442
sleep disturbance in, 442
sleep in, 441
therapy for, 442
insufficient sleep syndrome, 153–154
in children, 421
clinical features, 153
consequences of, 153
definition of, 153
demographics, 153
evaluation of, 153
multiple sleep latency features
of, 153t
polysomnographic features of, 153t
therapy for, 154
insulin/insulin resistance, 22, 29t,
183t, 334
intensive care unit (ICU) sleep
disturbance, 347–350
diagnostic/therapeutic factors,
348–349
environmental noise, 349
improving sleep in, 349
patient factors, 348
polysomnographic features of, 349

interleukins, 12t, 14t, 24, 334, 489b
intermediate sleep, 49, 404t
International Classification of Sleep
Disorders (ICSD), 281, 395
interstitial lung disease, 328t
intestinal motility, 19
iron therapy, 316
irregular sleep-awake pattern
syndrome (ISWP), 260.
See also circadian rhythm
disorders
characteristics of, 87t, 156t
in children, 426
demographics, 260
evaluation of, 260
sleep disturbance in, 87t
therapies for, 260
irritable bowel syndrome, 158t, 214,
338, 409t, 427t

Jacksonian march, 367t
jet lag, 80. See also circadian rhythm
disorders; time zone change
syndrome; transient insomnia
characteristics of, 157t
clinical features, 262–263
sleep-endocrine activity in, 24t
therapies for, 263
juvenile myoclonic epilepsy, 366, 367t
juvenile rheumatoid arthritis, 428t

kava, 125, 481t, 484t
K complexes, 6, 7b, 42t, 101, 105t,
158t, 344b, 405t
Kleine-Levin syndrome, 154, 280, 429t
Klüver-Bucy syndrome, 280
kyphoscoliosis, 328t

labetalol, 478t, 479t, 484t
lai tai, 398
lamotrigine, 104b, 476t, 481t, 483t
laryngomalacia, 178t, 418t
laryngospasm, sleep-related, 397
laser-assisted uvulopalatoplasty,
208t, 210t
lateral hypothalamus, 11t
leg cramps. See nocturnal leg cramps
leptin, 23, 24t, 29t, 176
levodopa, 111, 281, 313b, 314,
314b, 315
Lewy bodies, 282, 363
Lewy body dementia, 290, 294t

light therapy, 113, 258t
limit-setting sleep disorder, 88–89
characteristics of, 156t
in children, 416
clinical features, 88–89
definition of, 88–89
demographics, 88–89
differential diagnosis of, 88–89
evaluation of, 88–89
lingualplasty, 207t
lithium, 52t, 154, 280, 293, 306, 365t,
384, 465, 466t
locus ceruleus, 11t, 13t, 252
long sleepers, 152, 159, 395.396b
losartan, 479t
lovastatin, 479t
lower airway obstruction, 227t
L-tryptophan, 192t, 194t, 253, 490b.
See also melatonin
luteinizing hormone, 22, 100,
249t, 448
Lyme disease, 27t, 343

macroglossia, 41t, 94–95t, 176t,
180, 410t
magnesium, 281, 316
Maintenance of Wakefulness Test
(MWT), 64–65, 145, 162t, 474t
major depressive disorder, 382, 430t
major depressive episode, 381t,
383t, 384
mammalian sleep, 5
mandibular advancement, 180t,
207–208t, 441
mandibular hypoplasia, 176t,
179–180, 410t, 411
mandibular repositioners, 204
manic episode, 382–383t
maprotiline, 466t, 483t, 489t, 490t
maxillary hypoplasia, 178–179
maxillomandibular osteotomy,
206, 208t
mazindol, 146t, 471
medical disorders, 92–99
cardiovascular disorders, 92, 96t
in children, 426–429
effects on sleep, 82t, 158t
and excessive sleepiness, 155
gastrointestinal disorders, 96–97
respiratory disorders, 92, 94–96t
medical interview, 107–108
consequences of insomnia, 107

Sleep Medicine: Essentials and Review is a valuable new book that can be used both as a highly practical, concise text for managing sleep disorders and as a "high yield" review for preparing for the Sleep Medicine Certification Examination and the Board of Registered Polysomnographic Technologists Examination. Noted authority Dr Teofilo Lee-Chiong also includes over 600 board-type multiple choice questions with answers and explanations. The book offers these important and useful features:

- Presents comprehensive, yet concise coverage of both basic science and all clinical areas of sleep medicine

- Based on the current American Academy of Sleep Medicine International Classification of Sleep Disorders

- Discusses all the latest Practice Parameters related to Sleep Medicine that often form the basis of the questions on the Sleep Medicine Certification Examination

- Features easy-to-use approaches for the management of sleep disorders

- Summarizes the new American Academy of Sleep Medicine scoring rules for sleep stages, respiratory movements, and cardiovascular events

- Contains in-depth discussions of behavioral medicine, a topic increasingly covered on board examinations

- Includes 600 board-type multiple choice questions with answers and complete explanations

- Features a unique chapter format to enhance readability

There is no book in the field that is so practical and clinically useful, and none better to help you prepare for board examinations. It will be valuable to sleep specialists, pulmonologists, neurologists, psychiatrists, internists, family practice physicians, otolaryngologists, respiratory therapists, nurses, sleep technologists, and other health providers interested in learning more about sleep neurophysiology and sleep disorders.

Teofilo Lee-Chiong, MD, is Head of the Section of Sleep Medicine at National Jewish Medical and Research Center in Denver, Colorado, and Associate Professor of Medicine at the University of Colorado Health Sciences Center. He is editor of the popular major texts, Sleep Medicine (Elsevier), Sleep: A Comprehensive Handbook (Wiley-Liss), and Fundamentals of Sleep Technology (Lippincott Williams & Wilkins). He also serves as Consulting Editor for the Sleep Medicine Clinics (Saunders).

Cover Design: Kathryn Houghtaling

ISBN 978-0-19-530659-0

9 780195 306590

90000

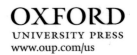

OXFORD
UNIVERSITY PRESS
www.oup.com/us